GAMSAT-Prep.com

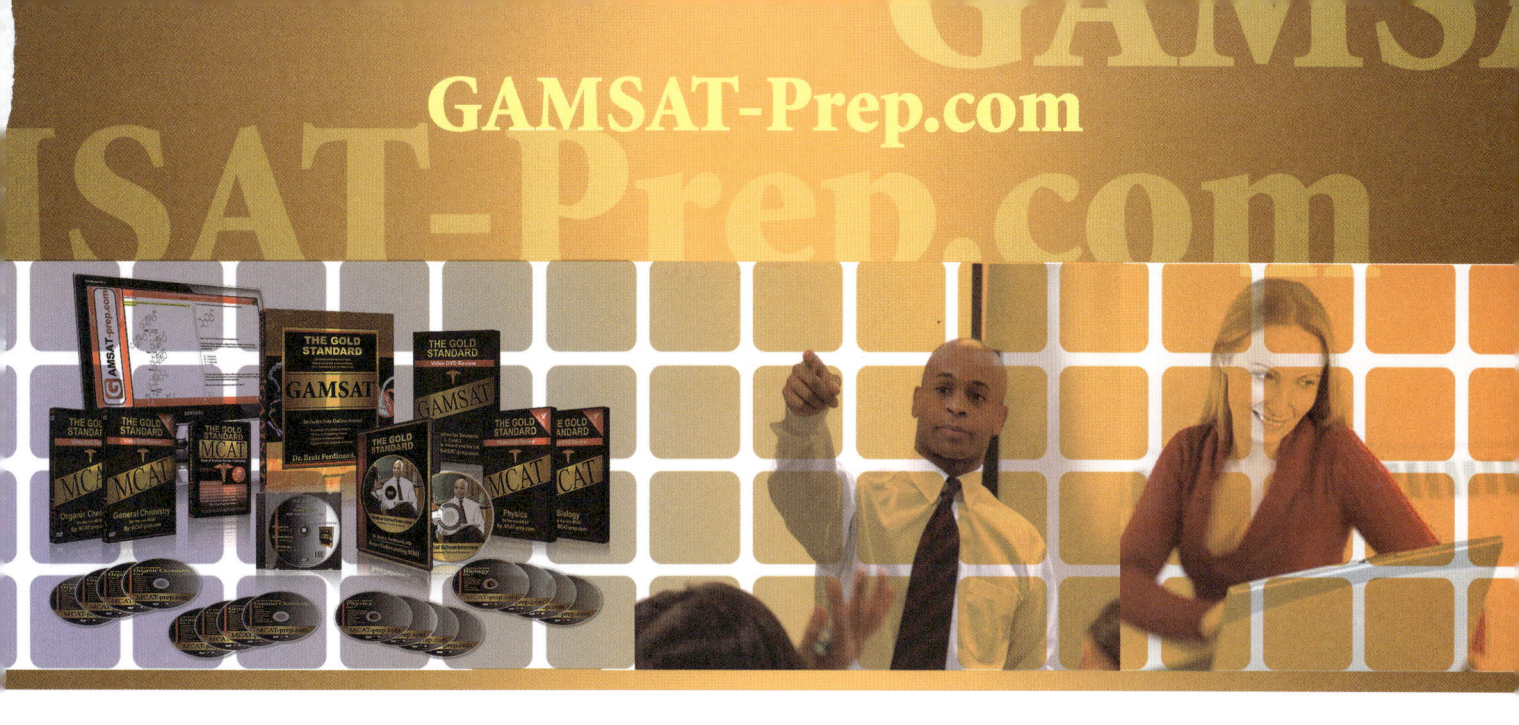

The Gold Standard textbook is a critical component of a multimedia experience including MP3s, DVDs, online interactive programs, practice GAMSATs and a lot more.

GAMSAT-Prep.com

The only prep you need.™

SAVE MONEY!

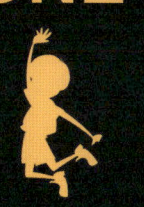

This coupon can be used to save $50 AUD or 30 £ or 36 € off the Live Gold Standard Complete GAMSAT Course OR $50 AUD or 30 £ or 36 € off our online teaching course: The Platinum Program.

To learn more about these programs, go to GAMSAT-prep.com, click on GAMSAT Courses in the top Menu and then scroll down to see "Complete GAMSAT Course".

Expiry Date: August 30, 2016   **Coupon Code: 839XVC9835**

Not redeemable for cash. Not valid in conjunction with another discount offer, non-refundable and not for re-sale. This coupon is governed by the Terms of Use found at GAMSAT-prep.com.

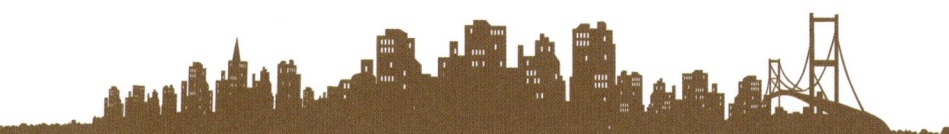

Gold Standard Live GAMSAT Courses are held in the following cities:
Sydney • Melbourne • Dublin • London • Brisbane • Perth • Adelaide • Cork

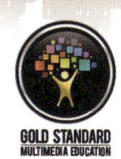

GOLD STANDARD MULTIMEDIA EDUCATION

* GAMSAT is administered by ACER which does not endorse this study guide.

THE GOLD STANDARD

GAMSAT

Editor and Author

Brett Ferdinand BSc MD-CM

Contributors

Lisa Ferdinand BA MA
Sean Pierre BSc MD
Kristin Finkenzeller BSc MD
Ibrahima Diouf BSc MSc PhD
Brigitte Bigras BSc MSc PhD
Naomi Epstein BEng
Charles Haccoun BSc MD-CM
Timothy Ruger BA MA

Illustrators

Daphne McCormack
Nanjing Design
 • Ren Yi, Huang Bin
 • Sun Chan, Li Xin

RuveneCo inc

Free Online Access Features
(For the original owner of this textbook)

10 Hours of Teaching Videos
Chapter Review Questions
Explanations to GS-1 Exam
Physics Equation List
Organic Chemistry Summary

Be sure to register at www.GAMSAT-prep.com by clicking on Register in the top right corner of the website. Once you login, click on GAMSAT Textbook Owners in the right column and follow directions. Please Note: benefits are for 1 year from the date of online registration, for the original book owner only and are not transferable; unauthorized access and use outside the Terms of Use posted on GAMSAT-prep.com may result in account deletion; if you are not the original owner, you can purchase your virtual access card separately at GAMSAT-prep.com.

Visit The Gold Standard's Education Center at www.gold-standard.com.

Copyright (c) 2012 RuveneCo (Worldwide), 3rd Edition

ISBN 978-1-927338-05-6

Portions of this book are copyright © 1994, 1995, 1996, 1997, 1998, 1999, 2000, 2001, 2002, 2003, 2004, 2005, 2006, 2007, 2008, 2009, 2010, 2011, 2012 by RuveneCo Inc.
All rights reserved. No part of this book may be reproduced, stored in a retrieval system, or transmitted in any form or by any means, electronic or mechanical, including photocopying, recording, or otherwise, without permission in writing from the publisher.

Material protected under copyright in Section I and Section III of The Gold Standard GAMSAT Exams were reproduced with permission; credits follow each passage.

Address all inquiries, comments, or suggestions to the publisher. For Terms of Use go to: www.GAMSAT-prep.com

RuveneCo Publishing
559-334 Cornelia St
Plattsburgh, NY, USA 12901
E-mail: learn@ruveneco.com
Online at www.ruveneco.com

The reviews on the back cover represent the opinions of individuals and do not necessarily reflect the opinions of the institutions they represent.

RuveneCo Inc. is neither associated nor affiliated with the Australian Council for Educational Research (ACER) who has developed and administers the Graduate Australian Medical School Admissions Test (GAMSAT) nor The University of Sydney. Printed in China.

GAMSAT-Prep.com
THE GOLD STANDARD

PREFACE

No science background in university? Great in the sciences but little experience reading from the humanities or writing essays? Had a bad experience with a high school physics teacher? Full-time arts student? Full-time mom? Part-time job? It's OK. The Gold Standard has you covered. This is not just a textbook, it is a learning experience.

The Gold Standard has integrated textbook reading with many free features including online problem solving with explanations, essays for you to review in the book and online, 10 hours of online teaching videos with ideas presented in clear terms, online equation lists and organic reaction summary, hundreds of additional practice questions, a full-length paper practice test with online detailed explanations and a forum thread to discuss every individual question - for free - and much more. We also offer - separately or in packages - the Gold Standard GAMSAT DVD with helpful strategies for all test sections; 16 science review DVDs prepared for the MCAT which, thankfully, contain all the major GAMSAT science topics clearly explained; and to increase study efficiency: flashcards, MP3s and an iPhone application.

The flashcards and iPhone App point to which section in the book you can find more details. The book points to which DVD you can use as a lecture. The videos and the explanations to the practice tests also point to specific sections of the book should you require clarification. We have also added options like an essay correction service and live courses in classrooms in Australia, Ireland and the UK. Thus we created a multimedia integrated approach so you can choose the tools that help you study best.

Now let's discuss medical school admissions. Your GPA and GAMSAT score can write the ticket for a medical school interview where success opens the door for admissions. Our aim is to be of help every step of the way. Herein lies a comprehensive section by section review for the GAMSAT, a concise examination as to how you can improve your grades at school, and a 'to the point' approach on the non-academic aspects of the admissions process: in particular, medical school interviews and, for those that require them, autobiographical materials and letters of reference. The medical interview section can stand alone or can be used in conjunction with The Gold Standard Medical School Interview DVD where I conduct a live interview in front of a class on campus and then analyze each response - question by question.

Truly, The Gold Standard has evolved into a complete reference textbook for the premedical student and other students who may need to sit the GAMSAT. Learn well and it will be reflected in your performance.

Good luck!

– B.F., MD

GAMSAT-Prep.com

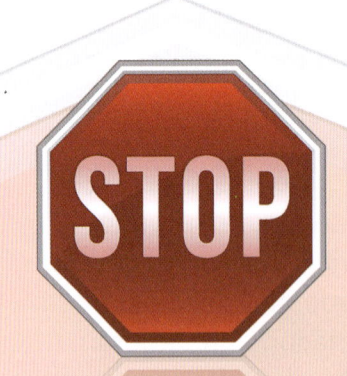

GAMSAT SCORE!

Good, we have your attention! We just want to be sure that you understand that not every student needs the same Section 3 (science) score in order to be admitted to medical school. Some science students must ace Section 3 to be admitted while some non-science students can gain admittance with an average Section 3 score because of an exceptional performance in the non-science sections. This book is for all students. This means that there may be some science chapters that might not be "worth it" for the non-science student. So we have colour-coded the importance of chapters in providing pertinent background information based on our experience.

    HIGH   MEDIUM   LOW

Now you can use your own judgement based on how much time you have to study and our assessment of the <u>importance</u> of that chapter. You will find this coding system particularly helpful when studying Biology. Also, if you have no science background in any of the subjects then we highly recommend taking advantage of the 10 hours of online video time that comes with this textbook. In addition, we suggest that all students complete the non-science problem sets in this textbook as well as the science chapter review questions with worked solutions that are online. Reviewing content only provides the background needed for science reasoning. In order to move to the next level, you must do problem sets followed by timed full-length practice beginning with the GS-1 test which is at the back of this textbook. Review, practice and full-length testing can help you obtain an exceptional GAMSAT score.

As of the publication date of this textbook, calculators are no longer permitted.

To further discuss any of the issues above: gamsat-prep.com/forum.

GAMSAT-Prep.com

Table of Contents

Preface v
Introduction I

Part I: MEDICAL SCHOOL ADMISSIONS

1. Improving Academic Standing 5
2. The Medical School Interview 11
3. Autobiographical Materials and References 19

Part II: UNDERSTANDING THE GAMSAT

1. The Structure of the GAMSAT 25
2. The Recipe for GAMSAT Success 33
3. Review for Section I 39
    How to Improve Your Score 40
    Types of Questions 44
    Warm-up Exercises 55
4. Review for Section II 71
    The 5 Minute, 5 Step Plan 75
    Warm-up Exercises 79
    Corrected Essays 88
    Common Grammatical Errors 95

Part III: THE PHYSICAL SCIENCES

A. General Chemistry CHM-01

1. Stoichiometry CHM-03
2. Electronic Structure and the Periodic Table CHM-13
3. Bonding CHM-25
4. Phases and Phase Equilibria CHM-35
5. Solution Chemistry CHM-47
6. Acids and Bases CHM-57
7. Thermodynamics CHM-71
8. Enthalpy and Thermochemistry CHM-79
9. Rate Processes in Chemical Reactions CHM-89
10. Electrochemistry CHM-101

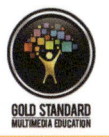

B. Physics PHY-01

1. Translational Motion PHY-03
2. Force, Motion, and Gravitation PHY-11
3. Particle Dynamics PHY-19
4. Equilibrium PHY-25
5. Work and Energy PHY-33
6. Fluids and Solids PHY-39
7. Wave Characteristics and Periodic Motion PHY-49
8. Sound PHY-61
9. Electrostatics and Electromagnetism PHY-67
10. Electric Circuits PHY-77
11. Light and Geometrical Optics PHY-89
12. Atomic and Nuclear Structure PHY-99

Part IV: THE BIOLOGICAL SCIENCES

A. Biology BIO-01

1. Generalized Eukaryotic Cell BIO-03
2. Microbiology BIO-21
3. Protein Synthesis BIO-29
4. Enzymes and Cellular Metabolism BIO-35
5. Specialized Eukaryotic Cells and Tissues BIO-47
6. Nervous and Endocrine Systems BIO-61
7. The Circulatory System BIO-81
8. The Immune System BIO-91
9. The Digestive System BIO-97
10. The Excretory System BIO-105
11. The Musculoskeletal System BIO-113
12. The Respiratory System BIO-121
13. The Skin as an Organ System BIO-127
14. Reproduction and Development BIO-133
15. Genetics BIO-145
16. Evolution BIO-155

B. Organic Chemistry ORG-01

1. Molecular Structure of Organic Compounds ORG-03
2. Stereochemistry ORG-13

—viii—

3. Alkanes ORG-21
4. Alkenes ORG-29
5. Aromatics ORG-37
6. Alcohols ORG-45
7. Aldehydes and Ketones ORG-53
8. Carboxylic Acids ORG-61
9. Carboxylic Acid Derivatives ORG-67
10. Ethers and Phenols ORG-75
11. Amines ORG-81
12. Biological Molecules ORG-87
13. Separations and Purifications ORG-101
14. Spectroscopy ORG-107

APPENDICES TO THE GOLD STANDARD TEXT

Appendix A: GAMSAT Math Review 601
Appendix B: The SI, Metric and Imperial Systems 606
Appendix C: The Experiment 607
Appendix D: Study Aids for the GAMSAT 608

Part V: GOLD STANDARD GAMSAT* EXAM

1. The Gold Standard GAMSAT 611
2. Practice Test GS-1 .... GS1-1

Part VI: ANSWER KEYS & ANSWER DOCUMENTS

1. Cross-referenced Answer Keys AK-3
2. Answer Documents AK-5

GAMSAT-Prep.com
THE GOLD STANDARD

INTRODUCTION

The GAMSAT (Graduate Australian Medical School Admissions Test), developed by the Australian Council for Educational Research (ACER), helps determine whether a student with at least a bachelor's degree can advance their studies in medicine, dentistry, pharmacy and veterinary science. In many ways, modeled after the MCAT which has a 70 year history, the GAMSAT was developed for the universities in Australia in the mid-1990s and, more recently, has been used as a component of the admissions procedure at a growing number of institutions in the UK and Ireland.

The GAMSAT is divided into 3 sections: (i) Section I: Reasoning in the Humanities and Social Sciences; (ii) Section II: Written Communication (two essays); and (iii) Section III: Reasoning in the Biological Sciences (biology and organic chemistry) and the Physical Sciences (physics and general chemistry).

The Gold Standard will expose the GAMSAT section by section - both within the pages to come and with the help of the Gold Standard Online Access Card, which can be found on the inside back cover of this textbook. Exam-taking tips for the GAMSAT, the Recipe for GAMSAT Success, and a review with strategies for Section I and Section II will all be explored. After which, a comprehensive and fully illustrated science review will follow. The science review contains physics, general chemistry, biology, and organic chemistry - all in the necessary detail but with colour-coded chapters in the Index to improve study efficiency. Hundreds of chapter review questions are online and you will also be able to use the pull-out full-length simulated GAMSAT test at the back of this textbook. Thus the information you learned will be put into practice. You will also have online access to 10 hours of teaching videos which most students find very helpful. This book, in combination with the free online videos or the more comprehensive Gold Standard science review DVDs, will be able to teach the student without a science background from the bottom up or serve as a fresh basic review for the advanced student in science. You will not be required to consult any textbooks and, if you are doing so, you are likely chasing salient details that are not required for the GAMSAT.

The GAMSAT is a reasoning test. You must master some basic scientific principles but memorization alone will not get you far. You are to do a "science survey" to get a foundation NOT a marathon of memorization. We understand this tenet and we have designed this book to emphasize this reality by describing in front of each chapter: what to memorize, what to understand and what is simply not required.

Your formula for success comes in 3 parts: content review, practice problems and full-length testing. We will guide you through the process.

Let's begin...

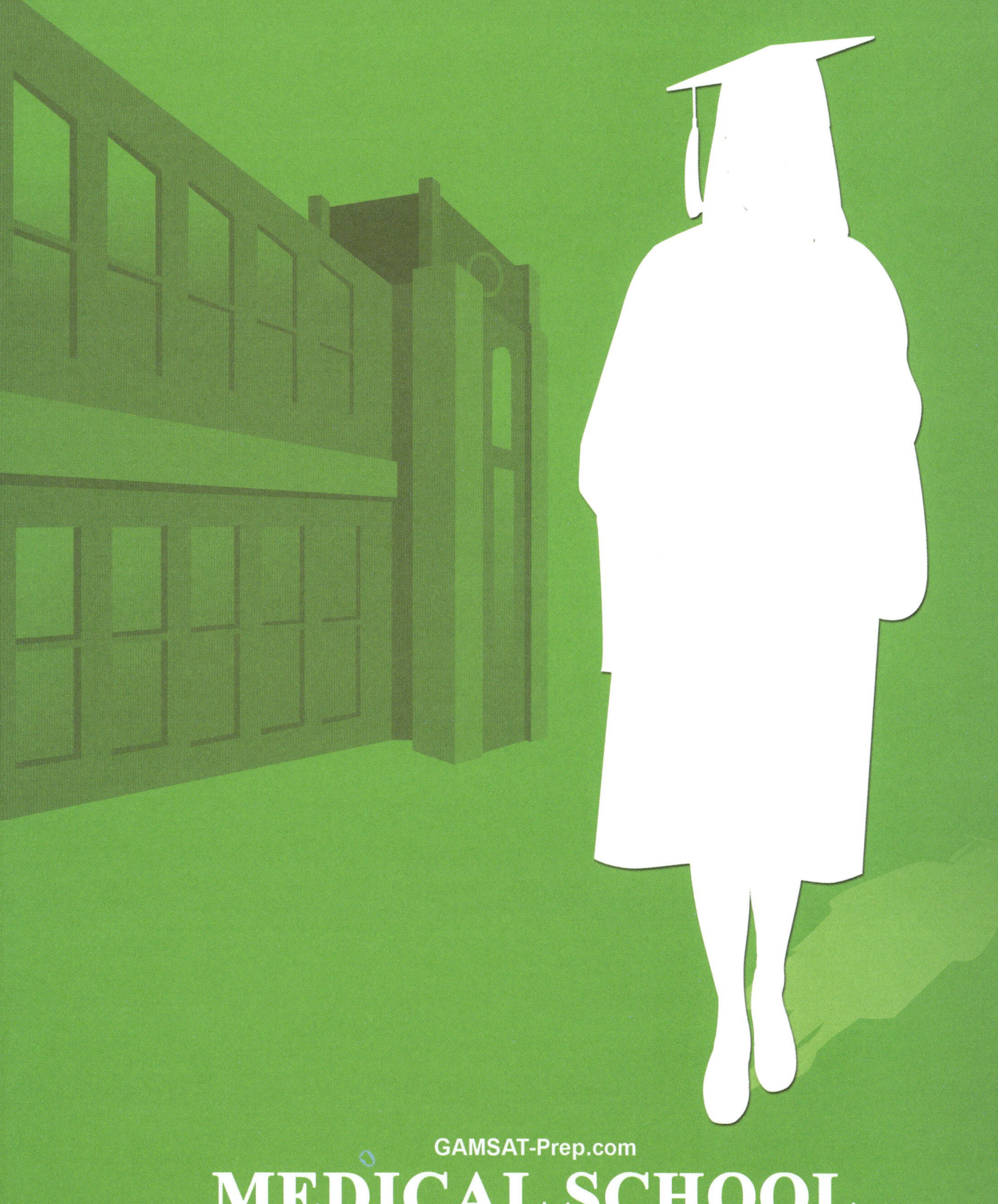

GAMSAT-Prep.com
MEDICAL SCHOOL ADMISSIONS
PART I

IMPROVING ACADEMIC STANDING

1.1 Lectures

Before you set foot in a classroom you should consider the value of being there. Even if you were taking a course like 'Basket-weaving 101', one way to help you do well in the course is to consider the <u>value</u> of the course to **you**. The course should have an *intrinsic* value (i.e. 'I enjoy weaving baskets'). The course will also have an *extrinsic* value (i.e. 'If I do not get good grades, I will not be accepted...'). <u>Motivation</u>, a <u>positive attitude</u>, and an <u>interest in learning</u> give you an edge before the class even begins.

Unless there is a student 'note-taking club' for your courses, your <u>attendance record</u> and the <u>quality of your notes</u> should both be as excellent as possible. Be sure to choose seating in the classroom which ensures that you will be able to hear the professor adequately and see whatever she may write. Whenever possible, do not sit close to friends!

Instead of chattering before the lecture begins, spend the idle moments quickly reviewing the previous lecture in that subject so you would have an idea of what to expect. Try to <u>take good notes</u> and <u>pay close attention</u>. The preceding may sound like a difficult combination (esp. with professors who speak and write quickly); however, with practice you can learn to do it well.

And finally, do not let the quality of teaching affect your interest in the subject nor your grades! Do not waste your time during or before lectures complaining about how the professor speaks too quickly, does not explain concepts adequately, etc... When the time comes, you can mention such issues on the appropriate evaluation forms! In the meantime, consider this: despite the good or poor quality of teaching, there is always a certain number of students who **still** perform well. You must strive to count yourself among those students.

1.2 Taking Notes

Unless your professor says otherwise, if you take excellent notes and learn them inside out, you will *ace* his course. Your notes should always be <u>up-to-date</u>, <u>complete</u>, and <u>separate</u> from other subjects.

GAMSAT-Prep.com
THE GOLD STANDARD

To be safe, you should try to write everything! You can fill in any gaps by comparing your notes with those of your friends. You can create your own shorthand symbols or use standard ones. The following represents some useful symbols:

|·|	between
=	the same as
≠	not the same as
∴	therefore
Δ	difference, change in
cf.	compare
c̄ or w	with
c̄out or w/o	without
esp.	especially
∵	because
i.e.	that is
e.g.	for example

Many students rewrite their notes at home. Should you decide to rewrite your notes, your time will be used efficiently if you are paying close attention to the information you are rewriting. In fact, a more useful technique is the following: during class, write your notes only on the right side of your binder. Later, rewrite the information from class in a <u>complete</u> but <u>condensed</u> form on the left side of the binder (*this condensed form should include mnemonics which we will discuss later*).

Some students find it valuable to use different color pens. Juggling pens in class may distract you from the content of the lecture. Different color pens would be more useful in the context of rewriting one's notes.

1.3 The Principles of Studying Efficiently

If you study efficiently, you will have enough time for extracurricular activities, movies, etc. The bottom line is that your time must be used efficiently and effectively.

During the average school day, time can be found during breaks, between classes, and after school to quickly review notes in a library or any other quiet place you can find on campus. Simply by using the available time in your school day, you can keep up to date with recent information.

You should design an individual study schedule to meet your particular needs. However, as a rule, a certain amount of time every evening should be set aside for more in depth studying. Weekends can be set aside for special projects and reviewing notes from the beginning.

On the surface, the idea of regularly reviewing notes from the beginning may sound like an insurmountable task which would take forever! The reality is just the opposite. After all, if you continually study the information, by the time mid-terms approach you would have seen the first lecture so many times that it would take only moments to review it again. On the other hand, had you not been reviewing regularly, it would be like reading that lecture for the first time!

You should study wherever you are comfortable and effective studying (i.e. library, at home, etc.). Should you prefer studying at home, be sure to create an environment which is conducive to studying.

Studying should be an active process to memorize and understand a given set of material. Memorization and comprehension are best achieved by the **elaboration** of course material, **attention, repetition,** and practising **retrieval** of the information. All these principles are borne out in the following techniques.

1.4 Studying from Notes and Texts

Successful studying from either class notes or textbooks can be accomplished in three simple steps:

- **Preview the material**: read all the relevant headings, titles, and sub-titles to give you a general idea of what you are about to learn. You should never embark on a trip without knowing where you are going!

- **Read while questioning**: **passive studying** is when you sit in front of a book and just read. This can lead to boredom, lack of concentration, or even worse - difficulty remembering what you just read! **Active studying** involves reading while actively questioning yourself. For example: how does this fit in with the 'big picture'? How does this relate to what we learned last week? What cues about these words or lists will make it easy for me to memorize them? What type of question would my professor ask me? If I was asked a question on this material, how would I answer? Etc...

- **Recite and consider**: put the notes or text away while you attempt to recall the main facts. Once you are able to recite the important information, consider how it relates to the entire subject.

N.B. if you ever sit down to study and you are not quite sure with which subject to begin, always start with either the most difficult subject or the subject you like least (usually they are one in the same!).

GAMSAT-Prep.com
THE GOLD STANDARD

1.5 Study Aids

The most effective study aids include practice exams, mnemonics and audio MP3s.

Practice exams (*exams from previous semesters*) are often available from the library, upper level students, online or directly from the professor. They can be used like maps which guide you through your semester. They give you a good indication as to what information you should emphasize when you study; what question types and exam format you can expect; and what your level of progress is.

One practice exam should be set aside to do one week before 'the real thing.' You should time yourself and do the exam in an environment free from distractions. This provides an ideal way to uncover unexpected weak points.

Mnemonics are an effective way of memorizing lists of information. Usually a word, phrase, or sentence is constructed to symbolize a greater amount of information (i.e. LEO is A GERC = Lose Electrons is Oxidation is Anode, Gain Electrons is Reduction at Cathode). An effective study aid to active studying is the creation of your own mnemonics.

Audio MP3s can be used as effective tools to repeat information and to use your time efficiently. Information from the left side of your notes (*see 1.2 Taking Notes*) including mnemonics, can be dictated and recorded. Often, an entire semester of work can be summarized into one 90 minute recording.

Now you can listen to the recording on an iPod while waiting in line at the bank, or in a bus or with a car stereo on the way to school, work, etc. You can also listen to recorded information when you go to sleep and listen to another one first thing in the morning. You are probably familiar with the situation of having heard a song early in the morning and then having difficulty, for the rest of the day, getting it out of your mind! Well, imagine if the first thing you heard in the morning was: "Hair is a modified keratinized structure produced by the cylindrical down growth of epithelium..."! Thus MP3s become an effective study aid since they are an extra source of repetition.

Some students like to **record lectures**. Though it may be helpful to fill in missing notes, it is not an efficient way to repeat information.

Some students like to use **study cards** (flashcards) on which they may write either a summary of information they must memorize or relevant questions to consider. Then the cards are used throughout the day to quickly flash information to promote thought on course material.

IMPROVING ACADEMIC STANDING

1.5.1 Falling Behind

Imagine yourself as a marathon runner who has run 25.5 km of a 26 km race. The finishing line is now in view. However, you have fallen behind some of the other runners. The most difficult aspect of the race is still ahead.

In such a scenario some interesting questions can be asked: Is now the time to drop out of the race because 0.5 km suddenly seems like a long distance? Is now the time to reevaluate whether or not you should have competed? Or is now the time to remain faithful to your goals and give 100%?

Imagine one morning in mid-semester you wake up realizing you have fallen behind in your studies. What do you do? Where do you start? Is it too late?

Like a doctor being presented with an urgent matter, you should see the situation as one of life's challenges. Now is the worst time for doubts, rather, it is the time for action. A clear line of action should be formulated such that it could be followed.

For example, one might begin by gathering all pertinent study materials like a complete set of study notes, relevant text(s), sample exams, etc. As a rule, to get back into the thick of things, notes and sample exams take precedence. Studying at this point should take a three pronged approach: i) a regular, consistent review of the information from your notes from the beginning of the section for which you are responsible (i.e. *starting with the first class*); ii) a regular, consistent review of course material as you are learning it from the lectures (*this is the most efficient way to study*); iii) regular testing using questions given in class or those contained in sample exams. Using such questions will clarify the extent of your progress.

It is also of value, as time allows, to engage in extracurricular activities which you find helpful in reducing stress (i.e. sports, piano, creative writing, etc.).

MEDICAL SCHOOL ADMISSIONS

THE MEDICAL SCHOOL INTERVIEW

2.1 Introduction

The application process to most medical schools includes interviews. Only a select number of students from the applicant pool will be given an offer to be interviewed. The medical school interview is, as a rule, something that you *achieve*. In other words, after your school grades and GAMSAT scores (and/or references and autobiographical materials for international schools) have been reviewed, you are offered the ultimate opportunity to put your foot forward: a personalized interview.

Depending on the medical school, you may be interviewed by one, two or several interviewers. You may be the only interviewee or there may be others (i.e., *a group interview*). There may be one or more interviews lasting from 20 minutes to two hours. And, of course, there is the increasingly popular multiple mini-interview (MMI) which includes many short assessments in a timed circuit.

Despite the variations among the technical aspects of the interview, in terms of substance, most medical schools have similar objectives. These objectives can be arbitrarily categorized into three general assessments: (i) your personality traits, (ii) social skills, and (iii) knowledge of medicine.

Personality traits such as maturity, integrity, compassion, sincerity, honesty, originality, curiosity, self-directed learning, intellectual capacity, confidence (*not arrogance!*), and motivation are all components of the ideal applicant. These traits will be exposed by the process of the interview, your mannerisms, and the substance of what you choose to discuss when given an ambiguous question. For instance, bringing up *specific* examples of academic achievement related to school and related to self-directed learning would score well in the categories of intellectual capacity and curiosity, respectively.

Motivation is a personality trait which may make the difference between a high and a low or moderate score in an interview. A student must clearly demonstrate that they have the enthusiasm, desire, energy, and interest to survive (typically) four long years of medical school and beyond! If you are naturally shy or soft-spoken, you will have to give special attention to this category.

Social skills such as leadership, ease of communication, ability to relate to others and work effectively in groups, volunteer work, cultural and social interests, all constitute skills which are often viewed as critical for future physicians. It is not sufficient to say

GAMSAT-Prep.com
THE GOLD STANDARD

in an interview: "I have good social skills"! You must display such skills via your interaction with the interviewer(s) and by discussing specific examples of situations which clearly demonstrate your social skills.

Knowledge of medicine includes <u>at least</u> a general understanding of what the field of medicine involves, the curriculum you are applying to, and a knowledge of popular medical issues like abortion, euthanasia, AIDS, the health care system, etc. It is striking to see the number of students who apply to medical school each year whose knowledge of medicine is limited to headlines and popular TV shows! It is not logical for someone to dedicate their lives to a profession they know little about.

Doing volunteer work in a hospital is a good start. Alternatively, getting a part-time job in a hospital or having a relative who is a physician can help expose you to the daily goings-on in a hospital setting. An even better strategy to be informed is the following: (i) keep up-to-date with the details of medically related controversies in the news. You should also be able to develop and support opinions of your own; (ii) skim through a medical journal at least once; (iii) read the medical section of a popular science magazine (i.e. Scientific American, Discover, etc.); (iv) keep abreast of changes in medical school curricula in general and specific to the programs to which you have applied. You can access such information at most university libraries and by writing individual medical schools for information on their programs; (v) do a First-Aid course.

2.2 Preparing for the Interview

If you devote an adequate amount of time for interview preparation, the actual interview will be less tense for you and <u>you will be able to control most of the content of the interview.</u>

Reading from the various sources mentioned in the preceding sections would be helpful. Also, read over your curriculum vitae and/or any autobiographical materials you may have prepared. Note highlights in your life or specific examples that demonstrate the aforementioned personality traits, social skills or your knowledge of medicine. Zero in on qualities or stories which are either important, memorable, interesting, amusing, informative or "all of the above"! Once in the interview room, you will be given the opportunity to elaborate on the qualities you believe are important about yourself.

Email or call the medical school and ask them about the structure of the interview (i.e., one-on-one, group, MMI, etc.) and ask them if they can tell you who will interview you. Many schools have no qualms volunteering such information. Now you can determine the person's expertise by either asking or looking through staff members of the different faculties or medical specialties

THE MEDICAL SCHOOL INTERVIEW

MEDICAL SCHOOL ADMISSIONS

at that university or college. A cardiac surgeon, a volunteer from the community, and a medical ethicist all have different areas of expertise and will likely orient their interviews differently. Thus you may want to read from a source which will give you a general understanding of their specialty.

Choose appropriate clothes for the interview. Every year some students dress for a medical school interview as if they were going out to dance! Medicine is still considered a conservative profession, you should dress and groom yourself likewise. First impressions are very important. Your objective is to make it as easy as possible for your interviewer(s) to imagine you as a physician.

Do practice interviews with people you respect but who can also maintain their objectivity. Let them read this entire chapter on medical school interviews. They must understand that you are to be evaluated *only* on the basis of the interview. On that basis alone, one should be able to imagine the ideal candidate as a future physician.

2.3 Strategies for Answering Questions

Always remember that the interviewer controls the *direction* of the interview by his questions; you control the *content* of the interview through your answers. In other words, once given the opportunity, you should speak about the topics that are important to you; conversely, you should avoid volunteering information which renders you uncomfortable. You can enhance the atmosphere in which the answers are delivered by being polite, sincere, tactful, well-organized, outwardly oriented and maintaining eye contact. Motivation, enthusiasm, and a positive attitude must all be evident.

As a rule, there are no right or wrong answers. However, the way in which you justify your opinions, the topics you choose to discuss, your mannerisms and your composure all play important roles. It is normal to be nervous. It would be to your advantage to channel your nervous energy into a positive quality, like enthusiasm.

Do not spew forth answers! Take your time - it is not a contest to see how fast you can answer. Answering with haste can lead to disastrous consequences as happened to a student I interviewed:

Q: *Have you ever doubted your interest in medicine as a career?*
A: *No!*
Well,...ah...I guess so. Ah ... I guess everyone doubts something at some point or the other...

Retractions like that are a bad signal but it illustrates an important point: there are usually no right or wrong answers in an interview; however, there are right or wrong ways of answering. Through the example we can conclude the following: <u>listen carefully to the question</u>, <u>try to relax</u>, and <u>think before you answer</u>!

Do not sit on the fence! If you avoid giving your opinions on controversial topics, it will be interpreted as indecision which is a negative trait for a prospective physician. You have a right to your opinions. However, you must be prepared to defend your point of view in an objective, rational, and informative fashion. It is also important to show that, despite your opinion, you understand both sides of the argument. If you have an extreme or unconventional perspective and if you believe your perspective will not interfere with your practice of medicine, <u>you must let your interviewer know that</u>.

For example, imagine a student who was against abortion under *any* circumstance. If asked about her opinion on abortion, she should clearly state her opinion objectively, show she understands the opposing viewpoint, and then use data to reinforce her position. If she felt that her opinion would not interfere with her objectivity when practising medicine, she might volunteer: "If I were in a position where my perspective might interfere with an objective management of a patient, I would refer that patient to another physician."

Carefully note the reactions of the interviewer in response to your answers. Whether the interviewer is sitting on the edge of her seat wide-eyed or slumping in her chair while yawning, you should take such cues to help you determine when to continue, change the subject, or when to stop talking. Also, note the more subtle cues. For example, gauge which topic makes the interviewer frown, give eye contact, take notes, etc.

Lighten up the interview with a well-timed story. A conservative joke, a good analogy, or anecdote may help you relax and make the interviewer sustain his interest. If it is done correctly, it can turn a routine interview into a memorable and friendly interaction.

It should be noted that because the system is not standardized, a small number of interviewers may ask overly personal questions (i.e., about relationships, religion, etc.) or even questions which carry sexist tones (i.e., *What would you do if you got pregnant while attending medical school?*). Some questions may be frankly illegal. If you do not want to answer a question, simply maintain your composure, express your position diplomatically, and address the interviewers <u>real</u> concern (i.e. *Does this person have the potential to be a good doctor?*). For example, you might say in a non-confrontational tone of voice: "I would rather not answer such a question. However, I can assure you that whatever my answer may have been, it would in no way affect either my prospective studies in medicine nor any prerequisite objectivity I should have to be a good physician."

MEDICAL SCHOOL ADMISSIONS

2.4 Sample Questions

There are an infinite number of questions and many different categories of questions. Different medical schools will emphasize different categories of questions. Arbitrarily, ten categories of questions can be defined: ambiguous, medically related, academic, social, stress-type, problem situations, personality oriented, based on autobiographical material, miscellaneous, and ending questions. We will examine each category in terms of sample questions and general comments.

Ambiguous Questions:

- *Tell me about yourself.*
  How do you want me to remember you?
  What are your goals?
  There are hundreds if not thousands of applicants, why should we choose you?
  Convince me that you would make a good doctor.
  Why do you want to study medicine?

COMMENTS: These questions present nightmares for the unprepared student who walks into the interview room and is immediately asked: "Tell me about yourself." Where do you start? If you are prepared as previously discussed, you will be able to take control of the interview by highlighting your qualities or objectives in an informative and interesting manner.

Medically Related Questions:

What are the pros and cons to our health care system?
If you had the power, what changes would you make to our health care system?
Do doctors make too much money?
Is it ethical for doctors to strike?
What is the Hippocratic Oath?
Should fetal tissue be used to treat disease (i.e. Parkinson's)?
If you were a doctor and an under age girl asked you for the Pill (or an abortion) and she did not want to tell her parents, what would you do?
Should doctors be allowed to 'pull the plug' on terminally ill patients?
If a patient is dying from a bleed, would you transfuse blood if you knew they would not approve (i.e. Jehovah Witness)?

COMMENTS: The health care system, euthanasia, cloning, abortion, and other ethical issues are very popular topics in this era of technological advances, skyrocketing health care costs, and ethical uncertainty. A well-informed opinion can set you apart from most of the other interviewees.

Questions Related to Academics:

Why did you choose your present course of studies?
What is your favorite subject in your present course of studies? Why?
Would you consider a career in your present course of studies?
Can you convince me that you can cope with the workload in medical school?
How do you study/prepare for exams?
Do you engage in self-directed learning?

COMMENTS: Medical schools like to see applicants who are well-disciplined, committed to medicine as a career, and who exhibit self-directed learning (i.e. such a level of desire for knowledge that the student may seek to study information independent of any organized infrastructure). Beware of any glitches in your academic record. You may be asked to give reasons for any grades they may deem substandard. On the other hand, you should volunteer any information regarding academic achievement (i.e. prizes, awards, scholarships, particularly high grades in one subject or the other, etc.).

Questions Related to Social Skills or Interests:

Give evidence that you relate well with others.
Give an example of a leadership role you have assumed.
Have you done any volunteer work?
What would you do as Prime Minister with respect to the trade imbalance with China?
Is the monarchy a legitimate institution?
What are the prospects for a lasting peace in Afghanistan? Iraq? the Sudan? the Middle-East?
What do you think of the regional free-trade agreements?

COMMENTS: Questions concerning social skills should be simple for the prepared student. If you are asked a question that you cannot answer, say so. If you pretend to know something about a topic in which you are completely uninformed, you will make a bad situation worse.

Stress-Type Questions:

How do you handle stress?
What was the most stressful event in your life? How did you handle it?
The night before your final exam, your father has a heart-attack and is admitted to a hospital, what do you do?

COMMENTS: The ideal physician has positive coping methods to deal with the inevitable stressors of a medical practice. Stress-type questions are a legitimate means of determining if you possess the raw material necessary to cope with medical school and medicine as a career. Some interviewers go one step further. They may decide to introduce stress <u>into</u> the interview and see how you handle it. For example, they may decide to ask you a confrontational question or try to back you into a corner (i.e. *You do not know anything about medicine, do you?*). Alternatively, the interviewer might use silence to introduce stress into the interview. If you have completely and confidently answered a question and silence falls in the room, <u>do not</u> retract previous statements, mutter, or fidget. Simply wait for the next question. If the silence becomes unbearable, you may consider asking an intelligent question (i.e. a specific question regarding their curriculum).

MMI-Type Problem Situations:

A 68 year-old married woman has a newly discovered cancer. Her life expectancy is 6 months. How would you inform her?

A 34 year-old man presents with AIDS and tells you, as his physician, that he does not want to tell his wife. What would you do?

You are playing tennis with your best friend and the ball hits your friend in the eye. What do you do?

A 52 year-old female diabetic comes to your ER in a coma but dies almost immediately. You are the physician who must now inform her husband and daughter. Enter the room and talk to them.

Your best friend in med-school has a part-time job to support herself. She has been unable to make it to some compulsory seminars because of her job and has asked you to mark her name present on the roll. What do you do and why?

COMMENTS: Some programmes have a few MMI stations with an actor in the room or other students. As for the other questions, listen carefully (or in the case of MMI, read the question posted on the door carefully) and take your time to consider the best possible response. Keep in mind that the ideal physician is not only knowledgeable, but is also <u>compassionate</u>, <u>empathetic</u>, <u>honest</u> and is objective enough to understand <u>both sides</u> of a dilemma. Be sure such qualities are clearly demonstrated.

Personality-Oriented Questions:

If you could change one thing about yourself, what would it be?
How would your friends describe you?
What do you do with your spare time?
What is the most important event that has occurred to you in the last five years?
If you had three magical wishes, what would they be?
What are your best attributes?

COMMENTS: Of course, most questions will assess your personality to one degree or the other. However, these questions are quite direct in their approach. Forewarned is forearmed!

Question Based on Autobiographical Materials:

COMMENTS: Any autobiographical materials you may have provided to the medical schools is fair game for questioning. You may be asked to discuss or elaborate on any point the interviewer may feel is interesting or questionable.

Miscellaneous Questions:

Should the federal government reinstate the death penalty? Explain.
What do you expect to be doing 10 years from now?
How would you attract physicians to rural areas?
Why do you want to attend our medical school?
What other medical schools have you applied to?
Have you been to other interviews?

COMMENTS: You will do fine in this grab-bag category as long as you stick to the strategies previously iterated.

Ending Questions:

What would you do if you were not accepted to a medical school?
How do you think you did in this interview?
Do you have any questions?

COMMENTS: The only thing more important than a good first impression is a good finish in order to leave a positive lasting impression. They are looking for students who are so committed to medicine that they will not only re-apply to medical school if not accepted, but they would also strive to improve on those aspects of their application which prevented them from being accepted in the first attempt. All these questions should be answered with a quiet confidence. If you are given an opportunity to ask questions, though you should not flaunt your knowledge, you should establish that you are well-informed. For example: "I have read that you have changed your curriculum to a more patient-oriented and self-directed learning approach. I was wondering how the medical students are getting along with these new changes." Be sure, however, not to ask a question unless you are genuinely interested in the answer.

2.5 The Interview: Questions, Answers and Feedback

Specific interview questions can be found online for free at futuredoctor.net. Dr. Ferdinand reproduced and captured the intense experience of a medical school interview on video to be used as a learning tool. "The Gold Standard Medical School Interview: Questions, Tips and Answers" DVD was filmed live in HD on campus in front of a group of premedical students - most of whom were invited for medical school interviews. A volunteer is interviewed in front of the class and the entire interview is conducted as if it were the real thing. After the interview, an analysis of each question and the mindset behind it is discussed in an open forum format. If you are not sure that you have the interviewing skills to be accepted to medical school, then it is a must-see video.

Whenever Dr. Ferdinand is conducting his live Medical School Interview seminar in Sydney, London or Dublin, the dates will be posted at GAMSAT-prep.com.

Autobiographical Materials and References

3.1 Autobiographical Materials

Autobiographical materials include resumes, CVs, personal statements, questionnaires and other written materials that may be required when applying to medical school or a graduate program. In general, these materials and letters of reference are required by almost all institutions in the US and Canada but relatively few institutions in Australia, Ireland and the UK. Consult individual institutions regarding their requirements. Just in case the information can serve you well, we have included it. Autobiographical materials are a sort of *written interview*. Thus the same objectives, preparation, and strategies apply as previously mentioned for interviews. However, there are some unique factors.

For example, you can begin writing long in advance of the deadline. The ideal way to prepare is to use your computer or to have a few sheets of paper at home where you continually write any accomplishments or interesting experiences you have had anytime in your life! By starting this process early, months later you should, hopefully(!), have a long list from which to choose information appropriate for the autobiographical materials. Your resume or curriculum vitae may also be of value.

Be sure to write rough drafts and have qualified individuals proofread it for you. Spelling and grammatical errors should not exist.

The document should be written on the appropriate paper and/or in the format as stated in the directions. Do not surpass your word and/or space limit. Usually the submission is online but if they require it on paper, ideally, it would be laser printed on business paper. The document should be so pretty that your parents should want to frame it and hang it in the living room! Handwritten or typed material with 'liquid paper' or 'white-out' is simply not impressive.

Your document must be clearly organized. If you are given directive questions then organization should not be a problem. However, if you are given open-ended questions or if you are told, for example, to write a 1000 word essay about yourself, adequate organization is key. There are two general ways you can organize such a response: *chronological* or *thematic*. However, they are not mutually exclusive.

In a **chronological** response, you are organized by doing a systematic review of important events through time. In writing an essay or letter, one could start with an interesting or amusing story from childhood and then highlight important events chronologically and in concordance with the instructions.

In the **thematic** approach a general theme is presented from the outset and then verified through examples at any time in your life. For example, imagine the following statement somewhere in the introduction of an autobiographical letter/essay:

My concept of the good physician is one who has a solid intellectual capacity, extensive social skills, and a creative ability. I have strived to attain and demonstrate such skills.

Following such an introduction to a thematic response, the essayist can link events from anytime to the general theme of the essay. Each theme would thus be examined in turn.

And finally, keep in mind the advice given for interviews since much of it applies here as well. For example, the appropriate use of an amusing story, anecdote, or an interesting analogy can make your document an interesting one to read. And, as for interviews, specific examples are more memorable than overly generalized statements.

3.2 Letters of Reference

Letters of reference (a.k.a. *assessments* which are written by *referees*) are required by most medical schools in North America. It provides an opportunity for an admissions committee to see what other people think of you. Consequently, it is often viewed as an important aspect of your application package.

Choose the people who will submit your letter of reference in accordance with instructions from the medical schools to which you are applying. If no such instructions are given, then construct a list of possible referees. Choose from this list individuals who: (i) you can trust; (ii) are reliable; (iii) can write, at least, reasonably well; (iv) understand the importance of your application; and (v) can present with some confidence attributes you have which are consistent with those of a good physician. A good balance would be to have one referee who is a professor, another a physician and a third who has experience with your social skills or achievements.

Often students either want or are told to have someone as a referee who they do not know well (i.e. a professor). In such a case choose your referee prudently. If they agree to give you a recommendation, give them your resume, curriculum vitae, or any other autobiographical materials you may have. Alternatively, you may ask to arrange a mini-interview. Either way, you would have armed your referee with information which can be used in a specific and personal manner in the letter of reference.

People are not paid to write you a letter of reference! Therefore, make it as easy as possible for them. Give them an ample amount of time before the deadline for submission. Also, supply them with a stamped envelope with the appropriate address inscribed. Besides being the polite thing to do, they may also be impressed by your organization. And finally, once the letter of reference has been sent, do not forget to send a "Thank-you" card to your referee.

$$\mathcal{A} + \mathcal{B} = ?$$

UNDERSTANDING THE GAMSAT

THE STRUCTURE OF THE GAMSAT

1.1 Introduction

The Graduate Australian Medical School Admissions Test (GAMSAT) is a prerequisite for admission to participating medical and dental schools in Australia, Ireland and the UK. Each year thousands of applicants submit GAMSAT test results to medical, dental and graduate schools as well as other programmes (i.e. pharmacy, optometry, veterinary science, etc.). While the actual weight given to GAMSAT scores in the admissions process varies from school to school, often they are regarded in a similar manner to your university GPA (i.e. your academic standing).

The GAMSAT is available to any student who has already completed a bachelor's degree, or who will be enrolled in their penultimate (second to last) or final year of study for a bachelor's degree, at the time of sitting the test. The test is administered as follows: test dates in Australia and Ireland are conventionally in March; the test date in the UK is usually in September. Students can sit the GAMSAT twice in one year. As examples, in Australia: GAMSAT Australia (March) then GAMSAT UK in Melbourne (September); in the UK: GAMSAT UK (September) and then GAMSAT Ireland (March).

GAMSAT results are generally valid for 2 years. There is no restriction on the number of times you may sit the GAMSAT. Currently, results from sitting the GAMSAT in any one country can be used in applying to any other country that requires the GAMSAT.

To access the most up to date information and to register for the GAMSAT, consider visiting one of the following websites:

> **Australia:** www.gamsat.acer.edu.au
> **Ireland:** www.gamsat-ie.org
> **UK:** www.gamsatuk.org

1.1.1 The *new* MCAT for International Applicants or for US/Canada

The new Medical College Admission Test (MCAT) is a prerequisite for admission to nearly all the medical schools in North America. Each year, over 50,000 applicants to American and English Canadian medical schools submit MCAT test results.

The MCAT is a computer based test (CBT) administered on a Saturday or a weekday, more than 20 times per year. To register for the MCAT, you should consult your undergraduate adviser and register online: www.aamc.org.

GAMSAT-Prep.com
THE GOLD STANDARD

The MCAT can be used by international students applying to medical schools that accept GAMSAT scores. Only international students have the option of sitting the MCAT instead of the GAMSAT. Consult individual programmes for confirmation.

1.2 The Format of the GAMSAT

The GAMSAT aims to test your skills in problem solving, critical thinking, writing as well as mastery and application of concepts in the basic sciences. The exam is divided into three sections. All questions, save for Section II, are multiple choice with 4 options per question. Ten minutes reading time is given for Sections I and III, and five minutes for Section II. The following is your schedule for the test day:

Section I	
Reasoning in the Humanities and Social Sciences	
Questions	75
Time	100 minutes

Section II	
Written Communication	
Questions	2
Time	60 minutes
Lunch	60 minutes

Section III	
Reasoning in Biological and Physical Sciences	
Questions	110
Time	170 minutes

Biological and Physical Sciences collectively include biology, general and organic chemistry at the introductory university level, and physics at essentially the Grade 12 level. Overall, the subject material is weighted as follows:

Biology	40%
Chemistry	40%
Physics	20%

The layout of Section I and Section III are similar with separate "Units" containing stimulus material followed by multiple choice questions. Section I may use excerpts from poems, novels, articles, a cartoon, etc. However, for Section III, the stimulus material can also include a passage, graph, equation(s), text, data, etc.

THE STRUCTURE OF THE GAMSAT

UNDERSTANDING THE GAMSAT

1.2.1 GAMSAT vs MCAT

The MCAT used to be longer (more questions, more time) compared with the GAMSAT but that has changed since 2007. Like the GAMSAT, the MCAT also used to be a pencil, pen and paper test but also since 2007, it has changed and has become a Computer Based Test (CBT). The value of understanding the differences and similarities between the two exams is as follows: (1) some students who are citizens of Australia, Ireland or the UK may choose to also sit the MCAT in order to apply to one of the majority of medical schools in the US and Canada that require the MCAT; (2) currently, international students

Table 1: Comparing the two standardized tests for medical school admissions.

	GAMSAT	MCAT (before 2007)	MCAT (2007-2014)
Testing method	Paper	Paper	Computer
Total test time	5½ hours	8 hours	5½ hours
Name of Verbal Section	Section 1	Verbal Reasoning	Verbal Reasoning
# Questions; Time	75 questions; 100 min.	65 questions; 85 min.	40 questions; 60 min.
Writing Section	Section 2	Writing Sample	Writing Sample
# Questions; Time	2 questions; 60 min.	2 questions; 60 min.	2 questions; 60 min.
Physical and Biological Sciences*	Section 3	1) Physical Sciences 2) Biological Sciences	1) Physical Sciences 2) Biological Sciences
# Questions; Time	110 questions; 170 min.	154 questions (total); 200 min. (total)	104 questions (total); 140 min. (total)
Breaks	• None between Section I and II • 1 hour for lunch	• 5 min. between sections • 1 hour for lunch	• 5 min. between sections • Lunch optional (max. 1 hour)
Countries	Australia, Ireland, UK	US, Canada	US, Canada
Test Frequency	Once or twice annually per country	Twice annually per country	More than 20 test dates annually
Official Practice Materials	4 booklets (e-books)	10 booklets	1 manual, 8 CBTs (practice tests #3 to #11)

* Physical Sciences includes physics and general or inorganic chemistry. Biological Sciences includes biology and organic chemistry. The AAMC is expected to announce major changes to the MCAT which would not come into effect before 2015. This table was used with permission from GAMSATtestpreparation.com.

have the option to sit either the GAMSAT or MCAT in order to submit applications to Australia, Ireland or the UK, some choose to sit the MCAT (or both tests) in order to also apply to North American medical programmes.

The 2 tests have both significant similarities and significant differences. The GAMSAT makes it possible for a student with little science background to learn independently and, with strong reasoning skills, succeed. Whereas, the MCAT requires formal training in the sciences because of the number of equations and facts that must be memorized.

Thus the GAMSAT leans on reasoning while the MCAT contains more memorization (though nowhere near as much memorization as required for an average introductory level university science course). It is the issue of memorization that makes some students say that the MCAT is more difficult but clearly that depends on your pre-exam reading history and learning experiences.

1.2.2 English as a Second Language (ESL)

Many ESL students will need to pay extra attention to Section I and Section II of the GAMSAT. Specific advice for all students will be presented in the chapters that follow. This advice should be taken very seriously for ESL students.

Having said that, GAMSAT scores are subjected to a statistical analysis to check that each question is fair, valid and reliable. Test questions in development are scrutinized in order to minimize gender, ethnic or religious bias, in order to affirm that the test is culturally fair.

Candidates whose native language is not English are permitted to bring a printed bilingual dictionary on test day for use in Section I and Section II only. The pages must be unmarked and all paper notes removed. Any candidate using this option must submit the dictionary to the Supervisor for inspection before the test begins.

Depending on your English skills, you may or may not benefit from an English reading or writing summer course. Of course, you would have the option of deciding whether or not you would want to take such a course for credit. GAMSAT-prep.com also offers an online speed reading/comprehension program with extra practice questions.

1.3 How the GAMSAT is Scored

The GAMSAT is scored for each of the three sections individually. The sections consisting of multiple choice questions are first scored right or wrong resulting in a raw

UNDERSTANDING THE GAMSAT

score. Note that wrong answers are worth the same as unanswered questions so ALWAYS ANSWER ALL THE QUESTIONS even if you are not sure of certain answers. The raw score is then converted to a scaled score ranging from 0 (lowest) to 100 (highest). Essentially, the scores are scaled to ensure that the same proportion of individual marks within each section are given from year to year (using Item Response Theory). The scaled score is neither a percentage nor a percentile. It is not possible to accurately replicate this scoring system at home.

Section II is marked by three independent markers from each zone. A scale of 10 points is used. Should there be a difference of 5 or more in two scores then an additional marker will be used. Ultimately, the three closest scores are totaled for the Section II raw score which is then converted to a scaled score.

You will receive a score for each of the three sections, together with an Overall GAMSAT Score. The Overall Score is a weighted average of the three component scores.

The Overall GAMSAT Score is determined using the following formula:

Overall Score = (1 × Section I + 1 × Section II + 2 × Section III) ÷ 4

Standards for interviews or admissions may vary for both Sectional Scores and the Overall GAMSAT Score. For example, one particular medical school may establish a cutoff (minimum) of 50 for any given section and 60 for the Overall GAMSAT Score. Contact individual programmes for specific score requirements.

The GAMSAT may include a small number of questions which will not be scored. These questions are either used to calibrate the exam or were found to be either too ambiguous or too difficult to be counted or are trial questions which may be used in the future. So if you see a question that you think is off the wall, unanswerable or inappropriate for your level of knowledge, it could well be one of these questions so never panic! And of course, answer every question because guessing provides a 25% chance of being correct while not answering provides a 0% chance of being correct!

1.3.1 GAMSAT Scores in Different Countries

GAMSAT scores are interchangeable and can be used to apply to any university that requires the GAMSAT. You may sit GAMSAT UK, Australia or Ireland to apply to universities in any of these countries.

You must ensure that your scores have not expired if you are using a score from a previous sitting of the GAMSAT (i.e. GAMSAT scores cannot be more than two years old). Otherwise, you choose the GAMSAT score

GAMSAT-Prep.com
THE GOLD STANDARD

that you wish to submit for consideration for admissions.

Since there is no limit to the number of times you can sit the GAMSAT, you may even choose to sit the exam twice in one year: for example, GAMSAT Australia or Ireland in March and then GAMSAT UK in September.

Any two tests on different examination dates will have, essentially, the same format; however, the questions are different for each exam.

How many times did you sit the GAMSAT?	
Once	67%
Twice	27%
3 Times	6%

2010 Gold Standard GAMSAT survey at the University of Sydney (Usyd Medical Science Society), n>100, average reported GAMSAT score (most recent): 62.2.

1.3.2 Average, Good and High GAMSAT Scores

Please keep in mind that the percentile rank indicates your test performance relative to all the students who sat the same test on the same day. It records the percentage of students whose scores were lower than yours.

Score	Percentile	Score
56-58	50th	average
61-63	75th	usually good*
73 or higher	98th	very high

*Please note, a "good" score may be good enough for admittance to one particular medical school but below the cutoff of another. Consult the websites of the medical institutions to which you intend to apply. Click on your national icon at the following webpage to get a summary of scores required at institutions near you: www.gamsat-prep.com/GAMSAT-scores.

THE STRUCTURE OF THE GAMSAT

UNDERSTANDING THE GAMSAT

An average GAMSAT score is often around 56-58 and a high GAMSAT score is over 63. Please keep in mind when evaluating the statistics provided and the graphic: this data is meant to give you a general idea of the process. The numbers can vary somewhat from one exam sitting to another. And as mentioned previously, you cannot replicate the scoring system at home since there is no formula provided to convert raw scores into official GAMSAT scores.

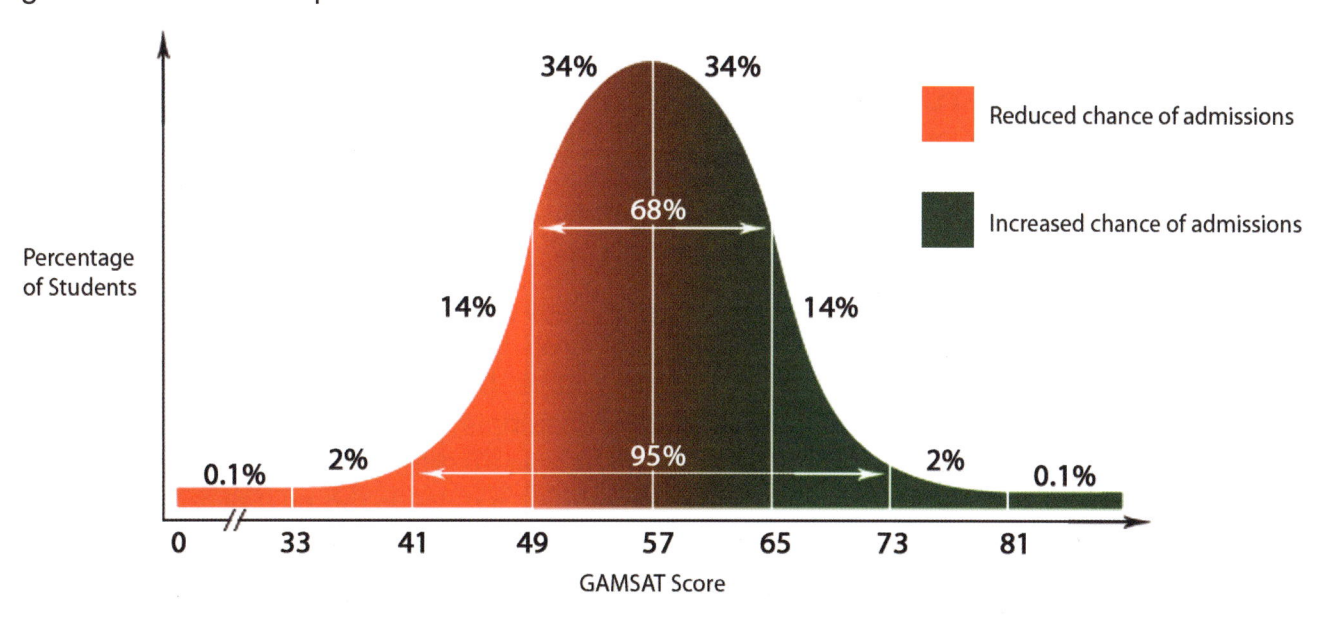

Figure 1: Typical Overall GAMSAT Score Distribution (Approx.)

1.3.3 When are the scores released?

The test date in Australia and Ireland is traditionally in March while it is usually in September for the UK. GAMSAT results are released within 2 months of sitting the exam. Candidates are emailed login information to access their personal results report. Should there be any changes to the exam dates or any other modifications, get the up to date information online at one of the ACER websites listed in Section 1.4.

1.4 ACER

The GAMSAT has been developed by the Australian Council for Educational Research (ACER) with the Consortium of Graduate Medical Schools to help in the selection of students to graduate-entry programmes. ACER administers the GAMSAT and publishes several important sets of materials which are available on their website: i) GAMSAT Practice Questions; ii) GAMSAT Sample Questions; and iii) GAMSAT Practice Test and GAMSAT Practice Test 2 which are released operational full-length tests. GAMSAT Practice Test 2 was released in 2010 for the very first time.

These materials can be obtained online:

Australia: www.gamsat.acer.edu.au
Ireland: www.gamsat-ie.org
UK: www.gamsatuk.org

Some students purchase commercially available simulated GAMSAT exams without ever having seen the materials from ACER. This is often a serious mistake. If you are looking to sit an actual GAMSAT, you go to the source. The source of the GAMSAT is ACER. Once you have been exposed to their style of questions and stimulus material, you will be in a better position to accurately assess other simulated practice material should you require it.

There are some students who feel that their experience with the real GAMSAT was not well represented by ACER's practice materials. Usually, this is not a problem with the materials; rather, it is a problem with the technique used in preparation. We will discuss this in detail in the next chapter.

Did you feel the ACER practice tests accurately represented the real exam?	
YES	63%
NO	37%
2010 Gold Standard GAMSAT survey at the University of Sydney (Usyd Medical Science Society), n>100, average reported GAMSAT score (most recent): 62.2.	

UNDERSTANDING THE GAMSAT

THE RECIPE FOR GAMSAT SUCCESS

2.1 The Important Ingredients

- Time, Motivation
- Read from varied sources
- The Gold Standard GAMSAT DVD
- A review of the 4 basic GAMSAT sciences

GAMSAT-Specific Information
- The Gold Standard GAMSAT textbook
- *optional:* The Gold Standard DVDs, MP3s or online programs (GAMSAT-prep.com)
- *optional:* GS Essay Correction Service or GAMSAT University online.

- *AVOID:* textbooks (too much detail), upper level courses for the purpose of improving GAMSAT scores

GAMSAT-Specific Problems
- Free chapter review problems
- The Gold Standard GAMSAT test (GS-1)
- Official ACER practice materials and full-length tests
- *optional:* more full-length GAMSAT practice tests (GAMSAT-prep.com)

If you could prepare all over again, what would you do differently?	
Top 5 Responses	
1	Study more
2	More practice essays
3	Newspapers, current events
4	More multiple choice questions
5	More science review
2010 Gold Standard GAMSAT survey at the University of Sydney (Usyd Medical Science Society), n>100, average reported GAMSAT score (most recent): 62.2.	

2.2 The Proper Mix

1) Study regularly and start early. There is a lot of material to cover and you will need sufficient time to review it all adequately. Creating a study schedule is often effective. Starting early will reduce your stress level in the weeks leading up to the exam and may make your studying easier. Depending on your English skills and the quality of your science background, a good rule of thumb is: 3-6 hours/day of study for 3-6 months.

2) Keep focused and enjoy the material you are learning. Forget all past negative learning experiences so you can open your mind to the information with a positive attitude. Given an open mind and some time to consider what you are learning, you will find most of the information tremendously interesting. Motivation can be derived from a sincere interest in learning and by keeping in mind your long term goals.

3) Section I and II preparation: Begin by reading the advice given in Chapters 3 and 4 in this textbook as well as The Gold Standard GAMSAT DVD. Time yourself and practice, practice, practice with various resources for Section I as needed at GAMSAT-prep.com and of course the ACER materials. You can also review free corrected Writing Sample essays at GAMSAT-prep.com/forum.

For Section I, you should be sure to understand each and every mistake you make as to ensure there will be improvement. For Section II, you should have someone who has good writing skills read, correct, and comment on your essays. Have the person read Chapter 4 for guidance on what they should be evaluating. And finally, you also have the option of having your essays corrected, scored and returned to you with personal advice (GAMSAT-prep.com).

4) Section III preparation: The Gold Standard is not associated with ACER in any way; however, contained herein is each and every topic that you are responsible for in the Biological and Physical Sciences, as evidenced by past testing patterns. Thus the most directed and efficient study plan is to begin by reviewing - not memorizing - the science sections in this textbook. While doing your science survey, you should take notes specifically on topics that are marked Memorize or Understand on the first page of each chapter. Your notes, we call them Gold Notes (!!), should be very concise (no longer than one page per chapter). Every week, you should study from your Gold Notes at least a few times.

As you are incorporating the information from the science review, do the Biological and Physical Sciences problems included in the free chapter review questions online at GAMSAT-prep.com. This is the best way to more clearly define the depth of your understanding and to get you accustomed to the most challenging of the questions you can expect on the GAMSAT.

UNDERSTANDING THE GAMSAT

5) Do practice exams. Ideally, you would finish your science review in The Gold Standard text and/or the science review DVDs at least a couple of months prior to the exam date. Then each week you can do a practice exam under simulated test conditions and thoroughly review each exam after completion. Scores in practice exams should improve over time. Success depends on what you do between the first and the last exam. You can start with ACER's "GAMSAT Practice Questions" then continue with The Gold Standard (GS) practice exams and then complete the practice materials from ACER.

==You should do practice exams as you would the actual test: in one sitting within the expected time limits.== Doing practice exams will increase your confidence and allow you to see what is expected of you. It will make you realize the constraints imposed by time limits in completing the entire test. It will also allow you to identify the areas in which you may be lacking.

Some students can answer all GAMSAT questions quite well if they only had more time. Thus you must time yourself during practice and monitor your time during the test. On average, you will have 1.3 minutes per question in Section I and 1.5 minutes per question for Section III. In other words, ==every 30 minutes, you should check to be sure that you have completed approximately 23 questions (Section I) or 20 questions (Section III).== If not, then you always guess on "time consuming questions" in order to catch up and, if you have time at the end, you return to properly evaluate the questions you skipped.

Set aside at least the equivalent of a full day to review the explanations for EVERY test question. Do NOT dismiss any wrong answer as a "stupid mistake." You made that error for a reason so you must work that out in your mind to reduce the risk that it occurs again. You can reduce your risk by testproofing answers (a technique first described in the GAMSAT DVD: spending 5-10 seconds being critical of your response) and by considering the questions in the table below.

6) Big on concepts, small on memorization: Remember that the GAMSAT will

1. Why did you get the question wrong (or correct)?
2. What question-type or passage-type gives you repeated difficulty?
3. What is your mindset when facing a particular passage?
4. Did you monitor your time during the test?
5. Are most of your errors at the beginning or the end of the test?
6. Did you eliminate answer choices when you could and actually cross them out?
7. For Section I, what was the author's mindset and main idea for each passage?
8. Was your main problem a lack of content review or a lack of practice?
9. In which specific science content areas do you need improvement?
10. Have you designed a study schedule to address your weaknesses?

GAMSAT-Prep.com
THE GOLD STANDARD

primarily test your understanding of concepts. The GAMSAT is not designed to measure your ability to memorize tons of scientific facts and trivia, but both your knowledge and understanding of concepts are critical.

Evidently, some material in this textbook must be memorized; for example, some very basic science equations (i.e. weight W = mg, Ohm's Law, Newton's Second Law, etc.), rules of logarithms, trigonometric functions, the phases in mitosis and meiosis, naming organic compounds and other basic science facts. Based on past testing patterns, we will guide you. Nonetheless, ==for the most part,== ==your objective should be to try to understand, rather than memorize== the biology, physics and chemistry material you review. This may appear vague now, but as you immerse yourself in the science review chapters and practice material, you will more clearly understand what is expected of you.

7) Relax once in a while! While the GAMSAT requires a lot of preparation, you should not forsake all your other activities to study. Try to keep exercising, maintain a social life and do things you enjoy. If you balance work with things which relax you, you will study more effectively overall.

2.3 It's GAMSAT Time!

1) On the night before the exam, try to get a good night sleep. The GAMSAT is physically draining and it is in your best interest to be well rested when you sit the exam.

2) Avoid last minute cramming. On the morning of the exam, do not begin studying ad hoc. You will not learn anything effectively, and noticing something you do not know or will not remember might reduce your confidence and lower your score unnecessarily. Just get up, eat a good breakfast, consult your Gold Notes (the top level information that you personally compiled) and go do the exam.

3) Eat breakfast! It will make it possible for you to have the food energy needed to go through the first two parts of the exam.

4) Pack a light lunch. Avoid greasy food that will make you drowsy. You do not want to feel sleepy for the afternoon section. Avoid sugar-packed snacks as they will cause a 'sugar low' eventually and will also make you drowsy. A chocolate bar or other sweet highly caloric food could, however, be very useful during the last section when you may be tired. The 'sugar low' will hit you only after you have completed the exam when you do not have to be awake!

5) Make sure you answer all the questions! You do not get penalized for incorrect answers, so always choose something even if you have to guess. If you run out of time, pick a letter and use it to answer all the remaining questions. ACER performs statistical analyses on every test so no one letter will give you an unfair advantage so just choose your "lucky" letter and move on!

6) Pace yourself. Do not get bogged down trying to answer a difficult question. If the question is very difficult, make a mark beside it, guess, move on to the next question and return later if time is remaining.

7) Remember that some of the questions may be thrown out as inappropriate, used solely to calibrate the test or trial questions. If you find that you cannot answer some of the questions, do not despair. It is possible they could be questions used for these purposes.

8) Do not let others psyche you out! Some people will be saying between exam sections, 'It went great. What a joke!' Ignore them. Often these types may just be trying to boost their own confidence or to make themselves look good in front of their friends. Just focus on what you have to do and tune out the other examinees.

9) Do not study at lunch. You need the time to recuperate and rest. Eat, avoid the people discussing the test sections and relax! At most, you can review your Gold Notes.

10) Before reading the "stimulus material" of the problem (the passage, article, etc.), some students find it more efficient to quickly read the questions first. In this way, as soon as you read something in the stimulus material which brings to mind a question you have read, you can answer immediately (this is especially helpful for Section I). Otherwise, if you read the text first and then the questions, you may end up wasting time searching through the text for answers.

11) Read the text and questions carefully! Often students leave out a word or two while reading, which can completely change the sense of the problem. Pay special attention to words in italics, CAPS, bolded, or underlined. Underline or circle anything you believe might be important in the passage.

12) You must be both diligent and careful with the way you fill out your answer document because you will not be given extra time to either check it or fill it in later.

13) If you run out of time, just do the questions. In other words, only read the part of the passage which your question specifically requires in order for you to get the correct answer.

14) Expel any relevant equation onto your exam booklet! Even if the question is of a theoretical nature, sometimes equations contain the answers and they are much more objective than the reasoning of a nervous pre-medical student! In physics, it is often helpful to draw a picture or diagram. Arrows are valuable in representing vectors.

15) Consider having the following on test day: a watch (mobile phones are not permitted in the exam room) and layers of clothes so that you are ready for too much heat or an overzealous air conditioning unit.

16) Solving the problem may involve algebraic manipulation of equations and/or numerical calculations. Be sure that you know what all the variables in the equation stand for and that you are using the equation in the appropriate circumstance.

In chemistry and physics, the use of **dimensional analysis** will help you keep track of units <u>and</u> solve some problems where you might have forgotten the relevant equations. Dimensional analysis relies on the manipulation of units and is the source of many easy GAMSAT marks every year. For example, if you are asked for the energy involved in maintaining a 60 watt bulb lit for two minutes you can pull out the appropriate equations <u>or</u>: i) recognize that your objective (unknown = energy) is in joules; ii) recall that a watt is a joule per second; iii) convert minutes into seconds. {note that minutes and seconds cancel leaving joules as an answer}

$$60 \frac{\text{joules}}{\text{second}} \times 2 \text{ minutes} \times 60 \frac{\text{seconds}}{\text{minutes}}$$

$$= 7200 \text{ joules} \quad \text{or} \quad 7.2 \text{ kilojoules}$$

17) The final step in problem solving is to ask yourself: *is my answer reasonable*? For example, if you would have done the preceding problem and your answer was 7200 kilojoules, intuitively this should strike you as an exorbitant amount of energy for an everyday light bulb to remain lit for two minutes! It would then be of value to recheck your calculations. {*'intuition' in science is often learned through the experience of doing many problems*}

18) Whenever doing calculations, the following will increase your speed: (i) manipulate variables but plug in values only when necessary; (ii) avoid decimals, use fractions wherever possible; (iii) square roots or cube roots can be converted to the power (*exponent*) of 1/2 or 1/3, respectively; (iv) before calculating, check to see if the possible answers are sufficiently far apart such that your values can be approximated (i.e. 19.2 ≈ 20, 185 ≈ 200). Since 2012, calculators ceased being permitted for the GAMSAT. We will show you throughout the book how to be quick and efficient with your calculations.

19) Are you great in biology and organic chemistry but weak in the physical sciences? Since biology and organic chemistry represent more than 1/2 your science score, you should attack those problems from the outset to ensure that you have fully benefitted from your strengths. Now you can go back and complete the physics and general chemistry. This is just an example of 'examsmanship': managing the test to maximize your performance.

20) Learn to relax or at least you must learn to manage your anxiety. Channel that extra energy into acute awareness of the information being presented to you. If you have a history of anxiety during exams to the extent that you feel that it affected your score, then you should start learning relaxation techniques now. You can search online regarding various methods such as visualization, deep breathing and other techniques that can even be used during the exam if needed.

UNDERSTANDING THE GAMSAT

REVIEW FOR SECTION I

3.1 Overview

Section I of the GAMSAT is, for many applicants, the most difficult section to do well. This can be explained by the absence of an overall set of facts to study in order to prepare. Some applicants, due to the lack of review material, neglect to prepare for this section.

While the best preparation is regular reading from a variety of sources throughout your high school and undergraduate studies, it is also possible to improve your ability to do well in this section as you approach the test date. You should not neglect to prepare for this section as it accounts for one of your final GAMSAT numerical scores!

Section I is called "Reasoning in Humanities and Social Sciences." You are provided 100 minutes to complete 75 questions. This section consists of a number of "Units" where each Unit presents stimulus material and a number of multiple choice questions (4 options per question).

The stimulus material in Section I can be anything from a poem, a cartoon, a picture, an extract from a play, novel, song, instructional manual or magazine. Essentially anything that involves words or symbols and thinking is fair game. There is no specific presumed knowledge required to answer any of the questions. ==Reasoning, analysis, timing and pacing are all key components to success.==

Which GAMSAT section was the easiest?	
Section I	5%
Section II	54%
Section III	41%
2010 Gold Standard GAMSAT survey at the University of Sydney, n>100, <5% with a non-science background; average reported GAMSAT score (most recent): 62.2.	

3.2 How to Improve your Section I Score

3.2.1 One Year or More Before the GAMSAT

Read! Be known as a "voracious reader"! Read any novel that interests you. Read editorials from national, international and local newspapers (among your options: the reference section of the library or online).

For those of you with a short attention span: Ted.com. With Ted.com you will have short, powerful lectures on a great range of topics - many of which will stick to you and create new tools in your use of language: analogies, examples, stories which span the globe as well as time. Ted.com is a free website. We will always update further suggestions on GAMSAT-prep.com which you can find by clicking on FREE GAMSAT in the top menu.

At least once per week, for 1-3 hours, you should read among the following (all of which are available in a university library or online):

- **Novels**
- **Philosophy** (i.e. The Meaning of Things by AC Grayling)
- **Local Newspapers** Most popular conservative and liberal national newspapers: editorials (because they tend to be argumentative) and newspaper cartoons since they use a style of humour and presentation that is fair game for the GAMSAT.

- **The Economist**
- **The New York Times**

Your exposure to knowledge outside of the sciences, creativity, culture, poetry, current affairs, political cartoons and more will have a significant impact on your performance in Section I and Section II. The added benefit - which you may only appreciate later - will be your improved performance in the medical school interviews and possibly even less obvious at the moment - an increased well-roundedness.

Be sure that when you are reading, especially opinion pieces, you are reading actively. Continually ask questions ...

1) How would you summarize or simplify what is being presented?
2) Identify the main points.
3) How would you describe the author's attitude to the topic?

UNDERSTANDING THE GAMSAT

3.2.2 One Year or Less Before the GAMSAT

Read section 3.2.1 one more time! Even at this point in your preparation, being a voracious reader - with all that it entails - should be your goal. Besides reading, you need to practice. The best strategy is to take ACER's GAMSAT Practice Questions (it is not a full-length test) and do Section I as a timed exam and then review your mistakes. If you performed well and understood the source of your errors then you will only require ACER and the Gold Standard (GS) GAMSATs in order to complete your preparation for Section I. If, on the other hand, you struggled in the test or struggled to understand your mistakes then you may need additional work on strategies, practice or, as mentioned previously, a formal course for or without credit. An optional Section I GAMSAT program can be found at GAMSAT-prep.com.

Practice Problems
• ACER materials
• GS book and online

Practice Exams
• ACER materials
• GS book and online

Additional Practice Options
• GAMSAT-prep.com

3.2.3 Exam Strategies

1) Read carefully and annotate. The test is yours. You paid for it so do not be afraid to strike-out, circle or more rarely, to make notes. Doing so helps you to read actively and then later, to find keywords or points without having to search aimlessly.

2) Always try to identify the main points of each paragraph, the idea behind the text and the structure of the passage as you read. Doing this will make it easier for you to answer the questions. Some students find it helpful to do the following: just before you read from each Unit, imagine someone young that you know - for example, a younger brother, sister, cousin, etc. Imagine that once you finish reading the stimulus material, you will have to explain it to them in words that they understand. Keep that imagery during your evaluation of the material so you have a heightened sense of awareness and responsibility for what you are reading.

3) The "Questions First, Passage Once Technique": some applicants like to quickly scan the questions prior to reading the text. Then they read the passage and answer questions as they read the information (usu. the questions are placed in the same order as you would find the answers in the passage). You may find it more efficient to work in that way. Try one of the practice exams this way and, if you find it easier to answer the questions correctly, you should use this method on the actual GAMSAT.

4) Pace yourself. A major problem in this section is that test takers run out of time. Read at a reasonable speed. You want to read carefully but quickly. You will have about 1.3 minutes per question in Section I. Every 30 minutes, you should check your watch to be sure that you have completed approximately 23 questions. Of course you can judge time in any way you want (20, 25, 30 minute intervals, etc.). But decide on a system when you are practicing then stick to that system on exam day. Of course, if you have not completed the desired number of questions in the interval that you have set for yourself, then you consistently guess on time consuming questions in order to catch up and, if you have time at the end, you return to properly evaluate the questions you skipped or marked.

5) Do not skim through the stimulus material. Ideally, you only want to read through once in order to answer the questions correctly. This way you will be able to finish in the allotted time. Of course, referring back to material that you annotated is not the same as having to re-read a passage because you read too quickly the first time.

6) We have already established that reading diverse material in the period leading up to the exam will be useful since the stimulus material will be from a variety of sources. Use this reality to help you create a mindset that, in the exam, you are prepared for "edutainment." You are ready to learn interesting, vibrant material which sometimes borders on a form of entertainment (novels, poems, cartoons, some articles, etc.). After completing a Unit, look forward to what you can learn and discover in the next Unit. Having properly prepared and then to sit the exam with the right attitude will give you an edge.

3.2.4 Question and Answer Techniques

1) Process of Elimination (PoE): cross out any answers that are obviously wrong.

2) Beware of the Extreme: words such as *always, never, perfect, totally*, and *completely* are often (but not always) clues that the answer choice is incorrect.

3) Comfortable Words: moderate words such as *normally, often, at times,* and *ordinarily* are often included in answer choices that are correct.

4) Mean Statements: mean or politically incorrect statements are highly unlikely to be

included in a correct answer choice. For example, if you see any of the following statements in an answer choice, you can pretty much guarantee that it is not the correct answer:

    Parents should abuse their children.
    Poor people are lazy.
    Religion is socially destructive.
    Torture is usually necessary.

5) Never lose sight of the question. By the time students read answer choices **C**. and **D**., some have forgotten the question and are simply looking for "true" sounding statements; you can then fall into the next trap:

True but False and False but True: for example,

Answer Choice D.: Most people are of average height. ⟶ This is a true statement.

However, the question was: What is the weight of most people?

Therefore, the true statement becomes the incorrect answer!

Continually check the question and check or cross out right and wrong answers.

3.3 Style of Questions

i) Comprehension: Identify key concepts and/or facts in a passage either directly taken from the text or inferred from it.

ii) Evaluation: Consider the validity, accuracy, value, etc. of ideas and facts presented.

iii) Application: Use the information presented in the passage to solve new problems described in the questions.

iv) Incorporation of new information: Reevaluate the passage based on new facts associated with the questions.

3.4 Online Help

You can get Section 1 help online including speed reading/comprehension and over 15 mini-tests through GAMSAT University at GAMSAT-prep.com. You can find general advice for written verbal skills at About.com.

To access our latest suggestions for all GAMSAT sections including Section 1, go to GAMSAT-prep.com and click FREE GAMSAT in the top menu.

3.5 Types of Questions

Main Idea Questions

These test your comprehension of the theme of the article. Questions may ask you for the main idea, central idea, purpose, a possible title for the passage, and so on. You may be asked to determine which statement best expresses the author's arguments or conclusions.

Inference Questions

These require you to understand the logic of the author's argument and then to decide what can be reasonably inferred from the article and what cannot be reasonably inferred.

Analysis of Evidence Questions

These ask you to identify the evidence the author uses to support his/her argument. You may be required to analyze relationships between given and implied information. You may be asked not only to understand the way the author uses different pieces of information but also to evaluate whether the author has built sound arguments.

Implication Questions

You may be asked to make judgments about what would follow if the author is correct in his/her argument or what a particular discovery might lead to. You may be given new information and then asked how this affects the author's original argument.

Tone Questions

You may be asked to judge the attitude of the author towards the subject.

Hybrid Questions

Often more than one question type is used in the same instance. An "implication" question can be answered through the "tone" or "evidence" which is presented within the material. In addition, an assessment of material such as a "main idea" often includes "an analysis of evidence." There may be a number of "hybrid" type questions, which include one or more of all the question types discussed. In logically deducing and ruling out answers, two central ideas are very helpful: the most "encompassing" of the answers, and which of the answers has the most "explanatory power" in relation to the others. This will become more clear as we do some exercises.

UNDERSTANDING THE GAMSAT

3.5.1 Main Idea Questions

Since this is very common, we will do some exercises to ensure that you can successfully deal with these question types. Please take a piece of paper (i.e. Post-it note) to cover the answers while you are responding to the questions. To find the main idea, ask the following three questions.

> 1. What is this passage about (the topic)?
> 2. What is the most important thing the author says about the topic (the main idea)?
> 3. Do all of the other ideas in the passage support this main idea?

Read the following passage and find the main idea.

For most immigrants, the journey to America was long and often full of hardships and suffering. The immigrants often walked the entire distance from their villages to the nearest seaport. There the ships might be delayed and precious time and money lost. Sometimes ticket agents or ship captains fleeced the immigrants of all they owned.

The most important idea in this paragraph is:
A. immigrants had to walk long distances to get to seaports.
B. ship schedules were very irregular.
C. ship captains often stole all the possessions of immigrants.
D. the journey of immigrants to America was very difficult and often painful.

1. *What is this passage about?*
   _____
   _____

2. *What is the most important thing the author says about the topic (the main idea)?*
   _____
   _____

3. *Do all of the other ideas in the passage support this main idea?*
   _____
   _____

1. This paragraph is about the immigrants' journey to America. This is the topic of the paragraph.
2. The author says that the immigrants' journey "was long and often full of hardships and suffering." This is the main idea of the paragraph.
3. To be absolutely sure that this is the main idea, ask yourself: Do all of the other ideas in the passage support this main idea? There are other ideas in the paragraph, but each one is an example of some kind of hardship suffered by the immigrants. Thus, the correct choice is D.

The Main Idea at the Beginning of a Passage

Did you notice that the main idea was contained in the first sentence? Often the main idea is in the first sentence.

Read the following passage and find the main idea.

Working conditions in the factories were frequently unpleasant and dangerous. A workday of 14 or 16 hours was not uncommon.

GAMSAT-Prep.com
THE GOLD STANDARD

The work was uncertain. When the factory completed its orders, the men were laid off. Often the pay was inadequate to feed a man's family. This meant that often an entire family had to work in factories in order to survive.

This paragraph is most concerned with:
A. dangerous and difficult working conditions in factories.
B. the passage of child-labor laws.
C. the lack of job security in early factories.
D. the low pay scale of early factories.

1. *What is this passage about?*
   _____
   _____

2. *What is the most important thing the author says about the topic (the main idea)?*
   _____
   _____

3. *Do all of the other ideas in the passage support this main idea?*
   _____
   _____

> 1. The topic of the passage is working conditions in the factories.
> 2. Working conditions in the factories were frequently dangerous and unpleasant.
> 3. All of the other sentences give examples of dangerous or unpleasant working conditions. The correct choice is A.

The Main Idea in the Middle of a Passage

Sometimes the main idea is stated somewhere in the middle of a paragraph. That is why the three questions about the main idea are so helpful.

What is this passage about? → will help you focus on the main idea.

What is the most important thing the author says about the topic? → will point out the main idea.

Do all of the other ideas in the passage support this main idea? → will help you to be sure you have chosen the most important idea rather than one of the less important ideas.

If you can answer these three questions, you will find the main idea no matter where it is placed in the paragraph.

Read the following passage carefully and ask yourself the three key questions. Then answer the question following the passage.

Many who had left the Catholic Church during the Protestant upheaval eventually returned to their original faith. However, the religious struggle of the sixteenth century destroyed the unity of Western Christendom. No longer was there one Church, nor one people, or one empire.

The main point the author makes in this paragraph is that:
A. the Protestant Reformation destroyed the Catholic Church.
B. the Protestant Reformation did not affect the Catholic Church.
C. some Protestants rejoined the Catholic Church.
D. Western Christendom was never again unified after the Protestant Reformation.

UNDERSTANDING THE GAMSAT

1. *What is this passage about?*
   _____
   _____

2. *What is the most important thing the author says about the topic (the main idea)?*
   _____
   _____

3. *Do all of the other ideas in the passage support this main idea?*
   _____
   _____

> The topic is the Protestant upheaval. The most important thing the author says about the Protestant upheaval is that it destroyed the unity of Western Christendom. The first sentence gives an example of unity. The second sentence points out that this example of unity was of very minor importance compared to the disunity. The third sentence expands this idea of disunity and tells how extensive the disunity was. The main idea is contained in the second sentence. All of the other ideas support that sentence. Thus, the correct choice is D.

The Main Idea in Several Sentences

The main idea is not always contained in a single sentence. Sometimes it takes more than one sentence to express a complex idea. Then you must piece together ideas from two or more sentences to find the main idea. The three questions are particularly helpful with paragraphs like this one:

Locke, of course, was no lone voice. The climate was right for him. He was a member of the Royal Society, and was thus intimately concerned with the work of the great seventeenth-century scientists. He argued that property, the possession of land and the making of money was a rational consequence of human freedom. This promise linked him to other great developments of the period: the formation of the powerful banks, the agricultural revolution, the new science, and the Industrial Revolution.

The main idea of this paragraph is:
A. John Locke believed that property was a product of human freedom.
B. John Locke was linked to the agricultural and industrial revolutions as well as to the new science and the formation of banks.
C. Property is the possession of land and the making of money.
D. John Locke's views on property linked him to all the other great developments of the seventeenth century.

1. *What is this passage about?*
   _____
   _____

2. *What is the most important thing the author says about the topic (the main idea)?*
   _____
   _____

3. *Do all of the other ideas in the passage support this main idea?*
   _____
   _____

UNDERSTANDING THE GAMSAT 47

GAMSAT-Prep.com
THE GOLD STANDARD

You probably took a little more time to piece together the main idea. Notice that all of the choices are true statements. All of them are found in the passage. But now you are asked to judge which is the most important.

1. The topic is John Locke. More precisely, the passage is about how John Locke was linked to the great events of the seventeenth century.

2. What is the most important thing the author says about John Locke and the events of his time? Locke's idea that property was a natural result of human freedom linked him to the great developments of his period.

3. The first sentence says that Locke was not "a lone voice"; the second sentence says that the "climate was right for him." These sentences support the idea that Locke was linked to the developments of his period. The third sentence states explicitly that Locke was "intimately concerned with the work of seventeenth-century scientists." The fourth sentence states Locke's ideas on property (part of the main idea). The last sentence links Locke with the great developments of his period (part of the main idea) and it lists those developments. Since all of the sentences in the paragraph support your statement of the main idea, you may be confident that you have the complete main idea. All of the other statements support the main idea, but they do not state it completely. Choice D is therefore correct.

The Main Idea in Several Paragraphs

So far, you have learned to find the main idea of paragraphs. To find the main idea of passages consisting of several paragraphs, first find the main idea of each paragraph. In the passage below, the main idea of each paragraph has been underlined.

Americans have long believed that George Washington died of injuries he received from a fall from a horse. <u>We now know that his doctors killed him.</u> Oh, it was no political assassination. They killed him by being what they were; physicians practicing good eighteenth-century medicine (which prescribed bleeding for every disease and injury). Washington, was bled of two quarts of blood in two days.

It is commonly thought that the practice of blood-letting died with the eighteenth century, but even today leeches are sold in every major city in the United States. <u>These blood-sucking little worms are still used by ignorant people to draw off "bad blood,"</u> the old-world treatment for every disease of body and spirit.

The cities of America are infested with an even worse kind of bloodsucker than the leech. Like the leech, he is not a cure-all, but a cure-nothing. Like the leech, he transmits diseases more dangerous than those he is supposed to cure. And like his brother, the primordial worm, he kills more often than he cures. His name is "pusher". <u>His treatment is not blood-letting, but addiction.</u>

The purpose of the passage is to:
A. explain how George Washington died.
B. describe the eighteenth-century practice of using leeches to treat diseases.
C. denounce the practice of blood-letting.
D. make a comparison between leeches and drug pushers.

UNDERSTANDING THE GAMSAT

Re-read only the underlined portions of the passage. These sentences can be used to form a summary of the passage:

George Washington died of bleeding. Leeches are still used by ignorant people for treating diseases.

The cities of America are infested with an even worse kind of bloodsucker than the leech. His name is "pusher."

Now ask yourself the same questions you used to find the main idea of a single paragraph.

1. *What is this passage about?*
   _____
   _____

2. *What is the most important thing the author says about the topic (the main idea)?*
   _____
   _____

3. *Do all of the other ideas in the passage support this main idea?*
   _____
   _____

> 1. The topic is leeches, blood-letting, and drug pushers.
> 2. Drug pushers are worse than leeches and do more harm than blood-letting.
> 3. The first paragraph explains that leeches were used in the eighteenth century and could kill people. The second paragraph explains that ignorant people still use leeches. The third paragraph compares leeches and drug pushers and stresses that drugs are the more harmful.
> The answer is D.

In addition to asking the three questions, you could also ask whether each of the answer choices is too narrow or too broad. For example, in the previous question choices A, B, and C are all too narrow to be the main idea.

3.5.2 Inference Questions

Some questions ask you to make inferences. An inference is a conclusion not directly stated in the text, but implied by it. Read the following passage. The topic is not directly stated, but you can infer what the paragraph is about.

Dark clouds moved swiftly across the sky blotting out the sun. With no further warning, great cracks of thunder and flashes of lightning disturbed the morning's calm. Fortunately, the deckhands had already tied everything securely in place and closed all portholes and hatches or we would have lost our gear to the fury of wind and water.

GAMSAT-Prep.com
THE GOLD STANDARD

1. This passage most likely describes:
   A. a storm during an African safari.
   B. a storm at sea.
   C. an Antarctic expedition.
   D. a flash flood.

2. Which of the following statements is false?
   A. The storm was unexpected.
   B. The storm came suddenly.
   C. It was windy.
   D. It was cloudy.

Nowhere in the paragraph are the words "sudden storm at sea" but, obviously, that is what the paragraph is about. The words dark clouds, thunder, lightning, wind, and water all suggest a storm. The word deckhands suggests a ship at sea. Several other words give you the feeling of the suddenness of the storm. You are justified in inferring that the writer was caught in a sudden and terrible storm at sea. The answer to question 1 is B.

Are you justified in concluding that the storm was unexpected? You know that things that happen suddenly are often unexpected. Was that the case with this storm? The last sentence tells you that the deckhands had already tied everything down and closed all portholes and hatches. That sentence indicates the storm was expected. The answer to question 2 is A.

Read the following paragraph. You will be asked to examine the cause-effect relationships implied by it later.

Bo went to the playoff game with several of his friends. At the stadium Bo ate four frankfurters with mustard and relish, two hamburgers with chili, drank several bottles of soda, and ate an assortment of candy, potato chips, pretzels, and ice cream. Suddenly Bo felt dizzy, feverish, and sick. When he got home, he took something to calm his stomach and went to bed.

3. Bo got sick because:
   A. he took something to calm his stomach.
   B. he went to the playoff game.
   C. he felt dizzy and feverish.
   D. he ate too much.

It is easy to see that Bo got sick because he ate too much → choice D. What is wrong with the other answers?

Choice A is wrong because the cause and effect are mixed up. Bo took something to calm his stomach because he was sick. He was not sick because he took something to calm his stomach.

Choice B is wrong because going to the playoff game really had nothing to do with his nausea later. If he had eaten the same food at home, he probably would have been just as sick. There is no real causal connection between the game and the sickness.

Choice C is incorrect because the feverishness and dizziness probably had the same cause as Bo's sickness. They were signs or symptoms of his illness, but not its cause.

UNDERSTANDING THE GAMSAT

Read the following paragraph. The question following it is concerned with the relationships between the main idea and supporting details.

Do we live in a revolutionary age? Our television and newspapers seem to tell us that we do. The late twentieth century has seen the governments of China and Cuba, among others, overthrown. The campuses of our universities erupted into violence; above the confusion of voices could be heard slogans of social revolution. We are constantly reminded that we live in a time of scientific and technological revolution. Members of militant racial groups cry for the necessity and inevitability of violent revolution. Even a new laundry detergent is described as "revolutionary!" Many causes, many voices, all use the same word.

4. Revolutionary ages are generally marked by:
   A. violence, slogans, science.
   B. violence, television coverage, governments overthrown.
   C. peace, science, technology.
   D. violence, confusion, governments overthrown.

Notice that the author does not answer his own question in the first sentence (the main idea). All of the other sentences give illustrations or examples of "revolution." The question asks you to make a generalization about the nature of revolution from these examples. Choices A and B include examples from a particular revolution (if one does exist). They are not true generalizations. Choice C is patently contrary to the ideas of the passage. Choice D is correct.

3.5.3 Analysis of Evidence Questions

Some questions ask you to check back in the text to see if the passage confirms or refutes a particular detail. This is the easiest kind of question to answer. In fact, the answer may be so obvious, you may be tempted to feel that some kind of trick is involved. Relax! If you can find the answer in the passage, you are almost certainly right.

The Fertile Crescent has been called the cradle of civilization. The Fertile Crescent is that sickle-shaped area of land between the Tigris and Euphrates rivers. The waters of these rivers changed the Asian desert into rich land with abundant crops. Many people believe that this is the land where man first settled down to farming after ages as a wandering hunter and later as a herder. Some even believe that the fabulous Garden of Eden was located somewhere in the Fertile Crescent.

5. The Fertile Crescent is located in:
   A. Africa.
   B. Europe.
   C. Asia.
   D. the West.

6. A crescent is:
   A. shaped like a sickle.
   B. always fertile.
   C. round.
   D. deserted.

7. The land between the Tigris and Euphrates rivers:
   A. has good soil and abundant water for irrigation.
   B. is populated by hunters.
   C. was extremely overpopulated.
   D. is shaped like a full moon.

> 5. C is correct → 3rd sentence.
> 6. A → 2nd sentence.
> 7. A → 3rd sentence.

3.5.4 Implication Questions

Sometimes you will have to apply one of the ideas in a passage to another situation. Sometimes this type of question takes a broad generalization from the passage and asks you to apply it to a specific situation. Attempt the passage below.

In December 1946, full-scale war broke out between French soldiers and Viet Minh forces. The people tended to support the Viet Minh. Communist countries aided the rebels, especially after 1949 communist regime came to power in China. The United States became involved in the struggle in 1950, when the United States declared support of Vietnamese independence, under Bao Dai.

Finally, in 1954, at the battle of Dien Bien Phu, the French suffered a shattering defeat and decided to withdraw. The 1954 Geneva Conference, which arranged for a cease-fire, provisionally divided Vietnam into northern and southern sectors at the 17th parallel. The unification of Vietnam was to be achieved by general elections to be held in July 1956 in both sectors under international supervision. In the north, the Democratic Republic of Vietnam was led by its president, Ho Chi Minh, and was dominated by the Communist party.

In the south, Ngo Dinh Diem took over the government when Bao Dai left the country in 1954. As the result of a referendum held in 1955, a republic was established in South Vietnam, with Diem as President.

8. A good title for this passage would be (main idea question):
   A. "The United States and Vietnam"
   B. "The Geneva Conference"
   C. "The Vietnamese Fight for Independence"
   D. "The Career of Bao Dai"

UNDERSTANDING THE GAMSAT

9. In the second paragraph the word "provisionally" means (implication question):
   A. temporarily.
   B. permanently.
   C. with a large, outfitted army.
   D. helplessly.

10. Bao Dai was in 1950 (implication question):
    A. a possible Vietnamese independence leader.
    B. the leader of the French.
    C. the brother of Dien Bien Phu.
    D. the President of South Vietnam.

11. The tone of this passage is (tone question):
    A. objective.
    B. partial to the French.
    C. partial to the North Vietnamese.
    D. cynical.

12. From the passage we might assume that in 1946 the Viet Minh were (implication question):
    A. South Vietnamese.
    B. Vietnamese rebels.
    C. North Vietnamese.
    D. French-supporting Vietnamese.

12. B
11. A
10. D
9. A
8. C

3.5.5 Tone Questions

An author may express his feelings or attitudes toward a subject. This expression of emotion imparts a tone to the writing. To determine the tone of a passage, think of the emotions or attitudes that are expressed throughout the passage. Below are some terms used to describe tone.

Term	Meaning
Admiring	respectful, approving
Belittling	making small, depreciating
Cynical	unbelieving, sneering

Term	Meaning
Denigrating	blackening, defamatory
Didactic	instructive, authoritarian
Ebullient	exuberant, praising
Lampooning	satirical, making fun of
Laudatory	praising
Mendacious	untruthful, lying
Objective	factual
Optimistic	hopeful

Term	Meaning
Praising	commending, laudatory
Reverential	exalted, regarding as sacred
Ridiculing	deriding, mocking, scornful
Saddened	sorrowful, mournful
Sanguine	confident, hopeful
Sarcastic	bitter, ironic
Sardonic	mocking, bitter, cynical
Satiric	ridiculing, mocking
Tragic	sad

A tragic tone reflects misfortune and unfulfilled hopes. A satiric tone mocks and ridicules its subject. An author may use an ironic tone to develop a contrast between (1) what is said and what is meant, (2) what actually happens and what appears to be happening, or (3) what happens and what was expected to happen. These are just a few of the emotions or attitudes that influence the tone.

Attempt the questions below.

A certain baseball team took the pennant for the first time in many years. Different people reacted differently.

13. "Wow! I can't believe it! This is the best thing that could have happened in this city!" The tone of this remark is:
    A. serious.
    B. excited.
    C. sarcastic.
    D. amazed.

14. "Ah! This is like it was when I was a boy. It makes my chest swell with pride again and brings tears to my eyes."
    The tone of this remark is:
    A. sentimental.
    B. excited.
    C. sarcastic.
    D. amazed.

15. "The team's manager and coach have had a lot of influence throughout the season. They deserve a lot of credit for this victory."
    The tone of this remark is:
    A. serious.
    B. excited.
    C. sarcastic.
    D. amazed.

16. "What!? They won!? And they started off so poorly this season. I just can't believe it!"
    The tone of this remark is:
    A. serious.
    B. excited.
    C. sarcastic.
    D. amazed.

17. "It couldn't have been skill since they don't have that. It couldn't have been bribery, since they don't have any money. The other team must all have been sick. It's the only way they could have won."
    The tone of this remark is:
    A. serious.
    B. excited.
    C. sarcastic.
    D. amazed.

UNDERSTANDING THE GAMSAT

13. B
14. A
15. A
16. D
17. C

3.6 Warm-up Exercises

These short, relatively easy passages will help consolidate the principles and techniques explained in Section 3.5.

Passage 12

As the mid-century approached, the women of America were far from being acclimated to their assigned dependent role. In fact, leaders of the growing suffrage movement were seeking equality under the law. Incredible as it seems now, in early nineteenth-century America a wife, like a black slave, could not lawfully retain title to property after marriage. She could not vote, and she could legally be beaten by her master.

18. One of the goals of the suffrage movement was:
    A. dependence on a master.
    B. equality with men.
    C. recognition of divorce.
    D. abolition of slavery.

19. Which sentence describes American women of the early 19th century?
    A. They were against marriage.
    B. They were satisfied with their role in society.
    C. They were victims of a male-dominated society.
    D. They had many slaves to do their work.

18. B
19. C

Passage 13

No dwelling in all the world stirs the imagination like the tipi of the Plains Indian. It is without doubt one of the most picturesque of all shelters and one of the most practical movable dwellings ever invented. Comfortable, roomy, and well ventilated, it was ideal for the roving life these people led in following the buffalo herds up and down the country. It also proved to be just as ideal in a more permanent camp during the long winters on the prairies.

20. What is a tipi?
    A. A buffalo
    B. An Indian
    C. A prairie
    D. A residence

UNDERSTANDING THE GAMSAT 55

21. What kind of life did the Plains Indians lead?
    A. They wandered with the buffaloes.
    B. They led comfortable and ideal lives.
    C. They spent their lives in one place.
    D. They lived in large, airy caves.

24. What delighted the narrator's wife?
    A. The invitation to the White House
    B. Wilder's compliment
    C. A double old-fashioned
    D. Attending the dinner with Wilder

20. D
21. A

22. C
23. A
24. B

Passage 14

A dozen years ago, Thornton Wilder and I made the happy discovery that we were both invited to a White House dinner for the French Minister of Culture, Andre Malraux. We decided at once to go together. He was to pick up my wife and me at our hotel, and specified that I should have a double old-fashioned ready for him. Thornton did justice to the drink. He also delighted my wife. She was nervous about the dress she was wearing, and he told her it reminded him of the black swan of Tasmania and was so graceful that it danced almost by itself. He illustrated in long, slow undulations, his arms waving. My wife was ham all evening.

22. Who is the narrator of the passage?
    A. Andre Malraux
    B. Thornton Wilder
    C. The passage does not say.
    D. Tasmania

23. What does "happy" mean in the expression "happy discovery"?
    A. Fortunate
    B. Contented
    C. Optimistic
    D. Clever

Passage 15

Nobody knows with certainty how big a proportion of the world's population is suffering from the basic problem of chronic undernourishment. But the commonly quoted United Nations estimate of 460 million sufferers is, if anything, on the low side. This represents 15 percent of the global population. Many more suffer from other deficiencies, making global totals even more difficult to calculate.

25. The paragraph indicates that:
    A. malnutrition is the number one problem in modern society.
    B. relatively few people suffer from malnutrition.
    C. the United Nations is supplying food to those suffering from malnutrition.
    D. it is not easy to count the number of people in the world who are undernourished.

25. D

Passage 16

Another way to fight insomnia is to exercise every day. Muscular relaxation is an important part of sleep. Daily exercise leaves your muscles pleasantly relaxed and ready for sleep.

26. What is insomnia?
    A. Muscular relaxation
    B. Inability to sleep
    C. Exercise
    D. Sleep

27. According to the passage, daily exercise:
    A. helps a person fall asleep more readily.
    B. is harmful for the muscles.
    C. prepares a person for fighting.
    D. is unnecessary.

26. B
27. A

Passage 17

The decade was erected upon the smoldering wreckage of the 60's. Now and then, someone's shovel blade would strike an unexploded bomb; mostly the air in the 70's was thick with a sense of aftermath, of public passions spent and consciences bewildered. The American gaze turned inward. It distracted itself with diversions trivial or squalid. The U.S. lost a President and a war, and not only endured those unique humiliations with grace, but showed enough resilience to bring a Roman-candle burst of spirit to its Bicentennial celebration.

28. What image is used to describe the 70's?
    A. A celebration
    B. A race
    C. A postwar period
    D. A long movie full of passion

29. What is the author's attitude regarding the events of the 70's?
    A. He is pessimistic.
    B. He is bewildered.
    C. He is optimistic.
    D. He is afraid.

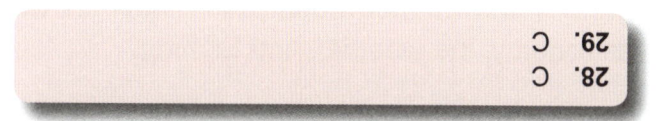

28. C
29. C

Passage 18

One bright spot in the U.S. economy in 1979 was the surprising decline in gasoline use. Rising fuel costs are finally prodding Americans to cut back on consumption, and the need for this becomes more acute all the time.

30. How does the author view the decline in gas consumption?
    A. He is indifferent.
    B. He thinks it is a good sign.
    C. He doesn't see the need for it.
    D. He is unhappy about it.

31. Why are Americans using less gasoline?
    A. The economy is good.
    B. They do not need as much.
    C. They want to spend more time at home.
    D. Gasoline is becoming very expensive.

Passage 19

During the early part of the colonial period, living conditions were hard, and people had little leisure time for reading or studying. Books imported from abroad were expensive and were bought mainly by ministers, lawyers, and wealthy merchants. The only books to be found in most homes were the Bible and an almanac, a book giving general information about such subjects as astronomy, the weather, and farming.

32. The early colonists did not do much reading because:
    A. they did not know how to read.
    B. the Bible told them that reading was sinful.
    C. they did not have time.
    D. they were not interested in reading.

33. Books were bought primarily by:
    A. the nobility.
    B. professional and wealthy people.
    C. the lower class.
    D. sellers of almanacs.

Passage 20

Never before in history have people been so aware of what is going on in the world. Television, newspapers, radio keep us continually informed and stimulate our interest. The sociologist's interest in the world around him is intense, for society is his field of study. As an analyst, he must be well acquainted with a broad range of happenings and must understand basic social processes. He wants to know what makes the social world what it is, how it is organized, why it changes in the way that it does. Such knowledge is valuable not only for those who make great decisions, but also for you, since this is the world in which you live and make your way.

34. The passage chiefly concerns:
    A. the work of a sociologist.
    B. the news media.
    C. modern society.
    D. decision-makers.

35. It can be inferred that a good sociologist must be:
    A. persistent.
    B. sensitive.
    C. objective.
    D. curious.

36. According to the passage, modern society is more aware of world events than were previous societies because:
    A. the news media keep us better informed.
    B. travel is easier and faster.
    C. there are more analysts.
    D. today's population is more sociable.

Passage 21

Whatever answer the future holds, this much I believe we must accept: there can be no putting the genie back into the bottle. To try to bury or to suppress new knowledge because we do not know how to prevent its use for destructive or evil purposes is a pathetically futile gesture. It is, indeed, a symbolic return to the methods of the Middle Ages. It seeks to deny the innermost urge of the mind of men; the desire for knowledge.

37. The author believes that:
    A. new ideas should not be encouraged.
    B. we should return to the methods of the Middle Ages.
    C. new knowledge is always used for evil purposes.
    D. to suppress knowledge is a useless act.

38. What is the meaning of "no putting the genie back into the bottle"?
    A. Once new discoveries have been made, it is impossible to deny their existence and to control the consequences which might result from them.
    B. We cannot be sure that knowledge will be used for humanitarian purposes.
    C. The desire for knowledge was not strong during the Middle Ages.
    D. We cannot answer tomorrow's questions today.

39. According to the author, man's most basic desire is:
    A. to know the future.
    B. to prevent destruction and evil.
    C. to become less ignorant.
    D. to avoid useless activity.

40. The passage was written:
    A. to convince us that the Middle Ages contributed little to modern society.
    B. to inspire us to meet challenges wisely.
    C. to persuade us to mistrust new ideas.
    D. to show us what we can expect in the future.

37. D
38. A
39. C
40. B This answer remains after eliminating the others.

Passage 22

It is important to distinguish among communication, language, and speech. These terms may, of course, be used synonymously, but strictly speaking, communication refers to the transmission or reception of a message, while language, which is usually used interchangeably with speech, is here taken to mean the speech of a population viewed as an objective entity, whether reduced to writing or in any other form.

41. According to the author, which word could be best used to replace "speech"?
   A. Communication
   B. Transmission
   C. Language
   D. Reception

42. The author understands "language" to mean:
   A. the totality of the way a given people expresses itself.
   B. the giving or receiving of a message.
   C. the exchange of words between two people.
   D. the written works of a population.

Answers (inverted): 41. C 42. A

Passage 23

The long, momentous day of John Glenn began at 2:20 a.m. when he was awakened in his simple quarters at Cape Canaveral's hangars by the astronauts' physician, Dr. William K. Douglas. Glenn had slept a little over seven hours. He shaved, showered, and breakfasted. Outside, the moon was obscured by fleecy clouds; the weather, responsible for four of the nine previous postponements, looked rather ominous.

43. At approximately what time did Glenn go to sleep?
   A. 5 p.m.
   B. 7 p.m.
   C. 9 a.m.
   D. 7 a.m.

44. Which statement about the weather is true?
   A. It was perfect for the occasion.
   B. It was cloudy and rainy.
   C. It had caused delays in the past.
   D. The passage does not say.

45. Who is John Glenn?
   A. A doctor
   B. A weatherman
   C. A spaceman
   D. A sailor

Answers (inverted): 43. B 44. C 45. C

3.7 Short Test and Analysis

The multiple choice Section I of the GAMSAT, as described before, is organized into Units. Now that you have worked through all the warm up exercises, you can proceed to test yourself with GAMSAT-style Units with appropriate stimulus material. We will work through the answers when you are finished.

There are 7 Units with 15 questions: choose the best answer for each question. You have 20 minutes. Please time yourself.

UNDERSTANDING THE GAMSAT

BEGIN ONLY WHEN TIMER IS READY

Unit 1

Questions 1–2

The Global Economy

Marked by a rise of technology, the global economy can be thought of as a complex international system, interlinked through the flow of goods, services, and information. Geographically, there are spatial changes, in labor and production, and the global economy is marked by a lifting of trade barriers and restrictions. Globalization has to some extent leveled out the competitive labor between major industrial countries and emerging countries. While prior to globalization, the United States dominated the global economy to a great extent, with the advent of information technologies, such as computers, the internet and the Web, the relocation of jobs from high wage to low wage countries, the emergence of economic blocs, such as NAFTA, and the nascent beginning of industrialization in Southeast Asia, the U.S. is purportedly dwindled to roughly one quarter of the global economy's flow of goods, services and information.

1. The best metaphor listed below used in describing the global economy would be?
   A. Medium
   B. River
   C. Network
   D. Hypertext

2. In Sentence 2, one can make the inference that the spatial changes in labor and production, are not only due to the lifting of trade barriers and restrictions, but also because of:
   A. the production of goods and services in the US only.
   B. the advent of information technologies, such as the internet.
   C. the rise of the minimum wage in the United States.
   D. terrorism and wars.

Unit 2

Question 3

Oxymorons are literary devices, which bring two contradictory terms together, to establish a nuance of meaning, or use, for effect. "Cheerful pessimist," "Wise fool," and "Sad Joy," are all examples of oxymorons. This device is used in literary classics, but also in everyday speech.

3. Which of the following phrases, used in everyday speech, would not be considered an oxymoron?
    A. Working Holiday
    B. Silent scream
    C. Limitless extension
    D. Virtual Reality

Unit 3

Questions 4–5

Morning at the Window (T.S. Eliot)   1
    They are rattling breakfast plates in basement kitchens,
    And along the trampled edges of the street
    I am aware of the damp souls of housemaids
    Sprouting despondently at area gates.   5

    The brown waves of fog toss up to me
    Twisted faces from the bottom of the street,
    And tear from a passer-by with muddy skirts
    An aimless smile that hovers in the air
    And vanishes along the level of the roofs.   10

4. After reading this poem, one could make a general comparison based on which of the following elements or attributes?
    A. Vapor
    B. Liquid
    C. Shadow
    D. Light

5. After studying the verbs, adverbs, and adjectives in this poem, one could make the general assessment that the tonality of the poem indicates a sense of:
    A. a detached observation of randomness.
    B. involved despair but superior attitude.
    C. quiet desperation, yet engaged.
    D. distanced and disconnected reception.

UNDERSTANDING THE GAMSAT

Unit 4

Questions 6–10

Cyberterrorism

Cyberterrorism, simply defined, is a convergence of computers, the internet, and terrorism. A specialist in cyberterrorism, Dorothy Denning, defines cyberterrorism as, "unlawful attacks and threats of attack against computers, networks, and the information stored therein when done to intimidate or coerce a government or its people in furtherance of political or social objectives." Further, to qualify as cyberterrorism, an attack should result in violence against persons or property, or at least cause enough harm to generate fear.

To some extent, differentiation is made between cyber crimes, such as phishing and cyber sapping from cyberterrorism, but the line of demarcation becomes less accurate when major corporations are being hacked into.

The line between the two usually focuses on the "level of danger" or "threat" which is usually not an individual hacker, but a "premeditated use of disruptive activities, or the threat thereof, against computers and/or networks, with the intention to cause harm or further social, ideological, religious, political or similar objectives, or to intimidate any person in furtherance of such objectives." This definition is a merger of cyber and definitions of terrorism by the United States Department of Defense. The line between cyber crime and cyberterrorism becomes quite arbitrary when considering that such a "cyber crime" as "identity theft" could be used by a terrorist to establish another identity, or multiple identities. The use of bots, malware, spy ware, viruses, and worms, provides another example, in which one must distinguish whether the purported use on computer networks is by an alienated teenager, or a terrorist.

Many countries (U.S., U.K., and India) will admit to "hacking" or internet intrusions from the same suspects: China and/or Russia, and admit that the internet must be thought of as a utility, in the same manner, as water, power, and possibly vulnerable to cyber-attack. There have been other "intrusions" in the past few years. The U.S. Power grid was invaded by software (by China or Russia), Estonia, Chechnya and Kyrgyzstan have all come under cyber attack, an estranged employee dumped massive amounts of sewage in Australia through a rigged computer program, air control traffic in Alaska was hacked, causing a partial shutdown of the airport. These are notable examples that are quite real to those who would proclaim that cyberterrorism is a myth. "Hackers" theorize an attack on vulnerable businesses and corporations within the infrastructure of countries, instead of government "intrusions." One has to admit that the private sector and government sector are intertwined, interdependent, and possibly vulnerable to cyberterrorism.

6. According to the passage, the difference between "cyber crime" and "cyberterrorism" seems to be:
   A. categorical and convincing.
   B. academic and undefined.
   C. unsubstantial and congruent.
   D. tenuous, yet well-defined.

7. From your reading of the passage, we can surmise that the author is:
   A. strongly opposed to hacking and cyber crime.
   B. just sticking to the facts.
   C. very opinionated.
   D. striving to be impartial and objective.

8. From your reading of the passage, why do you surmise the internet must be thought of as a public utility, much the same as water or power?
   A. Because it is run by both public and private companies
   B. Because governments and the internet are connected
   C. Because it could be a likely target by terrorists
   D. Because everyone has access to the internet globally

9. What would be the best argument listed below to formulate the opinion that cyberterrorism is a myth?
   A. There is no real war being fought on the internet.
   B. Terrorism is marked by violence and fear.
   C. Real terrorism blows up buildings and kills people.
   D. There is a difference between cyber crime and cyberterrorism.

10. What does the author mean by "infrastructure" in line 28, paragraph 3?
    A. The vulnerable aspects of valuable commodities
    B. A network of private businesses and corporations
    C. The interior aspects of governmental departments
    D. Governmental operations of internet sites

Unit 5

Question 11

Two very short stories by Franz Kafka

The Wish to be a Red Indian
If one were only an Indian, instantly alert, and on a racing horse, leaning against the wind, kept on quivering jerkily over the quivering ground, until one shed one's spurs, for there needed no spurs, threw away the reins, for there needed no reins, and hardly saw that the land before one was smoothly shorn heath when horse's neck and head would be already gone.

The Trees
For we are like tree trunks in the snow. In appearance they lie sleekly and a little push should be enough to set them rolling. No, it can't be done, for they are firmly wedded to the ground. But see, even that is only appearance.

11. A wise literary critic remarked that the whole point of reading Kafka was to re-read. Indeed, he presents us with an abstract world of images which almost seem to operate on their own volition. After re-reading these two very short stories, which of the following abstract terms, by way of ratio, would best describe the stories respectively?
    A. Initiation – Naturalization
    B. Transformation – Simulation
    C. Alienation – Perception
    D. Being - Becoming

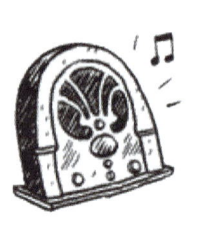

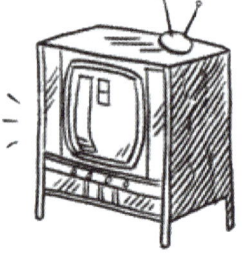

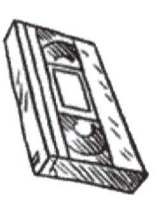

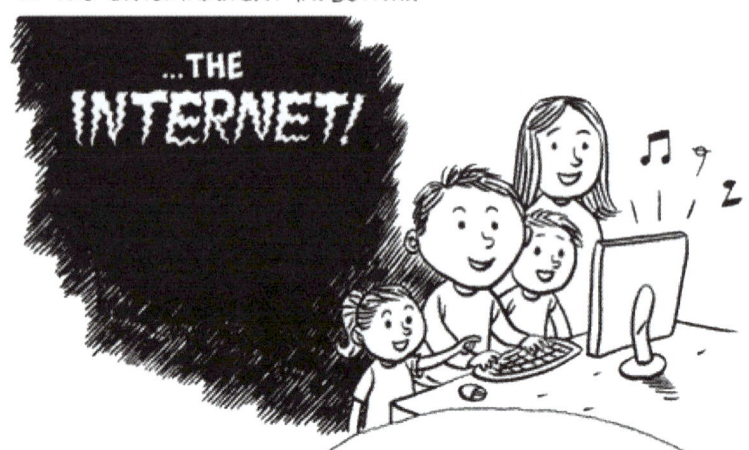

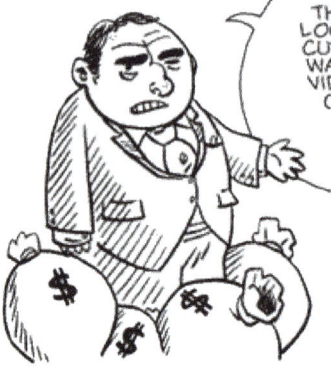

Unit 6

Questions 12–14

12. Undoubtedly biased for the free exchange of copyrighted material, which of the following groups of subjects would most adequately represent the contentious ideas presented within the cartoon?
    A. Popular Media, Hypertextuality, File-Sharing
    B. Intellectual Property, The Internet, Piracy
    C. Corporate Greed, Data Transfer, Representation
    D. Human Rights, Copyrights, Media

13. There is a logical fallacy, in the over-exaggeration, stated by the corporate character with the bags of money: "That's why we need to ban you from the internet . . ." This over-exaggeration is a figure of speech, or trope, stylistically known as:
    A. alliteration.
    B. rhetoric.
    C. hyperbole.
    D. simile.

14. Comparing the use of the Internet to other forms of media historically, is an argument by:
    A. definition.
    B. synthesis.
    C. deduction.
    D. analogy.

Unit 7

Question 15

Nietzsche quote: "Without chaos, how could one create a dancing star?"

After reading the above aphorism from the philosopher Nietzsche, one immediately notices the existence of two seemingly asymmetrical terms; namely chaos and the ability to create, or the functioning of the act of creation. Given this odd pairing, one can make certain assumptions and inferences about Nietzsche's beliefs. Which of the following would not be a highly likely inference to be drawn?

   A. Chaos precedes an act of Creation.
   B. Chaos and Creativity are interlinked.
   C. Chaos is necessary for Creation.
   D. Chaos precludes Creativity.

If time remains, you may review your work. If your allotted time (20 minutes) is complete, please proceed to the Answer Key.

GAMSAT-Prep.com
THE GOLD STANDARD

3.7.1 Units 1–7 Answer Key and Explanations

1.	C	4.	A	7.	D	10.	B	13.	C
2.	B	5.	D	8.	C	11.	B	14.	D
3.	C	6.	B	9.	D	12.	B	15.	D

1. A controlling metaphor can be thought of as a "Main Idea" type of question, in relation to section 3.5. In addition, this metaphor must be "inferred" based on the logic presented within the paragraph. (C) A metaphor can be inferred through the main idea within the first sentence. In describing the global economy, it can "be thought of as a complex international system, interlinked through the flow of goods, services, and information." The two terms "interlinked" and "flow" particularly stand out, indicating the metaphor of a "network." While (A) "Medium" and (D) "Hypertext" are certainly related, they do not encompass the complexity of the global economy. The metaphor of (B) "River" indicates the general notion of a flow and the possibilities of interlinkage, but is limited by one direction – that is a river is linear, while a complex network would have a flow, in many different directions.

2. This is most certainly an "analysis of evidence" type of question in relation to section 3.5. We are asked to make logical connections in relation to the evidence, as an example is being presented and extended. The correct choice (B) "The evolution of digital technologies," would effect the spatial redistribution of labor and production – communication and the flow of information could be accomplished with relative ease on a global level. This line of thought follows logically from the first sentence, in terms of a "flow of . . . information," i.e., not only the "outsourcing" of labor and production to different companies. Since information is also a commodity, in many instances, this would be the correct choice. (A) can be ruled out as a non-sequiter. Although (C) "the rise of the minimum wage" and (D) "terrorism" may have consequential effects on the rise of the global economy geographically, the more encompassing influence adhering to the idea of "global" would most certainly be advances in technology and digital communications.

3. All of the word pairings are oxymorons, and stand in juxtaposition as opposites, except for (C) "limitless extension" which implies a freeing of reservations, qualifications, or limits. An oxymoron could be fashioned in this pairing as a "limitless closure" or a "closed extension." This is also an "analysis of evidence" type of question (section 3.5) based on logically deducing which terms stand in opposition dialectically to each other.

4. (A) Vapor is the correct choice, as indicated by "the brown waves of fog" which enters and controls the imagery of the poem, in the second stanza, which also "toss," "tear," "hover," and finally "vanish" as a vapor. (C) "Shadow" and (D) "Light" are certainly implied by the title, but are not referred to within the internal composition of the poem. (B) "Liquid" is evidently in line with "the damp souls" which are "sprouting" but a vapor would be a more encompassing idea which is also inclusive of a sense of liquidity. This question is a "tone" type of question, in which assessments must be made logically on the basis of how and what images are presented. Usually when doing analysis of poetry, imagery is paramount to interpretation. Keep this in mind, when reviewing and analyzing poetry since poems are a regular feature of GAMSAT Section I. The images not only control the tonality of the poetry, but contribute to the overall main idea as well.

5. As evidenced in the above analysis, this question concerns "tone" and on the basis of these verbs, adverbs and adjectives, we can infer the correct choice of (D). There is a remote, "distanced and disconnected reception" as evidenced by the words, "rattled," "trampled," "despondently," and "aimless." Within the poem, there is nothing to suggest (A) "detached observation" (which would be more in line with "the scientific method") because the speaker is "aware," and subjectively involved and perceptive, nor is there anything suggesting (B) "despair" or superiority, or (C) desperation which can be ruled out.

6. (B) "Academic and undefined" is the correct answer. Much of the discussion is of a theoretical nature and focuses on "definitions." The discussion is certainly not (A), (C), or (D), but the answers require a certain level of understanding in terms of vocabulary and the terminology used. This question is certainly an "analysis of evidence" question. Defining the terms is a tactful way of presenting evidence and used often to provide clarity in an exposition, as well as necessary qualifications, reservations concerning the topic, and limits and controls the discussion.

7. (D) The author is striving to be impartial and objective, not sticking to just the facts (B) for certain value judgments are inferred and assumed within the assessment. The author is not (C) very opinionated, for generalizations concerning the subject is supported with evidence in the use of examples and testimony. Though the author (A) may be strongly against hacking and cyberterrorism, as activities which he or she may find reprehensible, there are no calls to action for countermeasures, nor is the language used emotionally-charged. For these reasons, this is a hybrid question which corresponds to both "analysis of evidence" and the general "tone" of the argument in relation to section 3.5.

8. Even though (A), (B),& (D) are all true to some extent, the concepts do not necessarily relate to both of the ideas advanced in the question: the internet as a public utility within the context of terrorism; so by way of deduction, we find that (C) is the correct answer in that the internet shared by many, such as a public utility, is a likely, easily accessible, and vulnerable target to terrorist attacks. This is an "analysis of evidence" type of question as presented in section 3.5. One makes assessments in a logical and deductive manner, by ruling out certain choices based on the evidence presented and its logical extension.

9. (D) "There is a difference between cyber crime and cyberterrorism" is the correct choice. Many have argued that the inflated cyber crimes have been unnecessarily associated with terrorism, and have lacked many of the defining characteristics of a terrorist attack. Following this line of reasoning, (A) could be inferred, and very close to being the correct answer, but only as inclusive of answer (D). The two other choices can be easily ruled out, as too general (B) to be applicable or (C) much too specific. This question also corresponds to "an analysis of evidence," most notably in how both are "defined" as mentioned above in relation to question 6. On another level, it hints of an "implication question" because it questions the reader not only to assess the evidence, but implies that the author may or may not be correct in his evaluation of the subject.

10. (B) This can be surmised very quickly after a brief re-read. All the other answers may or may not be part and/or parcel of the notion of "infrastructure" and so lack the explanatory power in relation to the question. Again this is an "analysis of evidence" type of question, most notably by using "definitional" terms to delimit the notion of "infrastructure." When abstract ideas such as the notion of "infrastructure" are used, one can usually make a choice based on "explanatory power." Which choice is inclusive of the logic which is presented? How do the other choices inadequately assess or represent the evidence which is presented?

11. This is probably one of the most difficult questions presented in this section - due to Kafka's writings, the issues of interpretation, and the abstract

ratios given as answers. (B) "Transformation-Simulation" is the correct answer. Undoubtedly, a transformation is occurring in the first passage, and an association of a tree's appearance with a representation, or in more general terms, simulation, simulacra, and simulacrum. It does help to know Latin and Greek etymological roots in this instance. Answer (D) would be a close answer if the ratio was reversed to Becoming-Being, but not as it is respective to the order of the passages. Though there may or may not be an (A) Initiation, within the passage, and the term Naturalization, though having connections to Nature – the tree - is vague and lacks specificity, so this is not correct. (C) Alienation-Perception is also very close, but the term "Alienation" carries negative connotations, when in fact the first passage, is a "wish" that results in a sense of liberated freedom and movement. Perception would be quite correct, in assessing Kafka's 2nd passage, since perception is so interlinked with appearance. But given the ratio, (C) can be ruled out as not as qualified or encompassing as (B). This is also a hybrid type of question, which presents abstract terms to define a main idea based on tone. So not only is the reader asked to relate an abstract term to a "main idea" type of question, but also review the "tone" of the passage by examining the dominant images.

12. All of the answer choices are at least partially correct. The most encompassing and specific in relation to the cartoon's contentions is (B). Through "an analysis of evidence" in assessing the "main ideas" presented within the material, this answer can be deduced. Again, we must determine what the most encompassing answer choice is while possessing the most explanatory power.

13. (C) Hyperbole is the correct answer. As a figure of speech or stylistic device it represents over-exaggeration. Alliteration (A) is a repetition of consonants, usually in the beginning of words. Rhetoric (B) has a number of definitions, the art of persuasion, the use of stylistic devices, and a pejorative connotation as empty words or bombast. Simile (D) is a sub-species of metaphor; a comparison using "like" or "as" –within this question, a certain degree of familiarity with poetry and public speaking is assumed. In order to assess the correct answer of a logical fallacy, we need to base our deductions on "an analysis of evidence" presented.

14. These comparisons are certainly an argument by "analogy" (D) by contrasting different forms of media throughout the years with the internet. (A) "definition" is not correct, because the internet is not being defined or interpreted as a specific media or medium. (C) an argument from "synthesis" would be a clash of ideas, in proper terms, dialectic and the result of this clash. This can be ruled out as well in relation to the cartoon. (C) "deduction" is finding the correct answer, by ruling out others –a logical process of subtraction, of which, this cartoon does not. As such, this question is "an analysis of evidence" type of question as referred to in section 3.5.

15. All of the answers in relation to the Nietzsche quote can be inferred to some extent except (D), the correct choice. A certain degree of familiarity with vocabulary, particularly the term "precludes" is assumed and necessary to make the correct choice in (D). This phrase essentially would be antipodal – in opposition to the other assessments, meaning Chaos limits or rules out Creativity. This is an "inference" type of question, as presented in section 3.5. We infer that all of the choices are correct, in relation, to the quote except for (D), which negates, instead of affirms a relation between the two: chaos and creativity.

UNDERSTANDING THE GAMSAT

REVIEW FOR SECTION II

4.1 Overview

GAMSAT Section II, or "Written Communication," is comprised of 2 essays.

Why write an essay?

The GAMSAT included an essay section likely in part because the MCAT introduced essays in 1992 due to complaints from deans of US med-schools concerning communication skills of med-students. Ironically, 2015 is the end of MCAT essays but Section II is a well-established part of the GAMSAT.

Section II will measure your ability to:
1) develop a central idea
2) synthesize ideas and concepts
3) express ideas in a logical and cohesive way
4) write clearly, using standard English and appropriate grammar, spelling and punctuation.

You are not expected to write a short polished essay of final draft quality. The people grading your exam are aware that you only had 30 minutes to write the essay. Nevertheless, you will be expected to write a 'good' essay. Please refer to Section 4.4 for a scoring key. You may also consult Section 4.5 and GAMSAT-prep.com for examples of what a 'good' essay is in the eyes of the markers.

Section II, being the only non-multiple choice section of the GAMSAT, includes two separately timed hand-written thirty minute essays. You are provided 5 minutes reading time. Each essay is on a theme which is conveyed through a group of five quotes. Your essay must address the theme and may include 1 or more of the given quotations. The first essay "Task A" and the second essay "Task B" have different themes.

	Writing Task A	Writing Task B
Writing style	• expository • argumentative	• reflective • discursive
Theme	• philosophical • political	• interpersonal • social
Topics (examples)	• censorship • human nature • education • progress • wealth	• hatred • youth • self-discovery • conformity • humour

GAMSAT-Prep.com
THE GOLD STANDARD

4.1.1 The Statement

Both Task A and Task B offer a number of ideas relating to a common, general theme. Task A deals with socio-cultural issues while Task B deals with more personal and social issues. In selecting topics, ACER makes an effort to minimise factors which might disadvantage candidates from non-English speaking backgrounds.

The statements will not be about your reasons for entering medical school, the application process, emotionally-charged religious or ethical issues (i.e. abortion).

While you do not need any specific knowledge to do well in this section, you should read from varied sources (see Section 3.2.1) to familiarize yourself with current political and social concerns.

4.1.2 General Pointers for Section II

You are expected to write a first draft quality essay. A few grammatical, punctuation or spelling errors will not affect your mark greatly. However, a large number of such errors to the extent that your ideas become difficult to follow, will harm you. You are allowed to cross out words, sentences or passages. Do not try to recopy your essay. You are not expected to and you will not have the time to do this. However, please be sure that your writing is legible.

A title is not mandated but it could be helpful especially if it were catchy or intriguing. Both Tasks must have at least 3 paragraphs: an introduction, the body and the conclusion.

The use of creativity can be great. For example, some students choose to write the essay (especially Task A) as though it is a conversation between two people. Other students use metaphors. For example, using a video camera as a metaphor of an objective observer that switches from scene to scene. In the final scene (the conclusion or resolution), one could begin by saying: "And now, the camera is truly in focus" as one describes how the conflict is resolved.

Though such creative expressions can be quite powerful, they cannot make up for the following basic fact: you must address the needs of the essay. You must clearly deal with the concerns of ACER which includes: (1) addressing the central theme clearly; (2) applying at least one of the quotations to your essay; (3) control of thought, ideas and expression; and to a lesser extent, (4) organization and technical issues. Of course, being "overly" creative could have its own risks (i.e. inappropriate distraction).

If you can, since this is formal writing, minimize your use of contractions as well as first-person and second-person pronouns ("I," "me," "you") in Task A though you can and should be more personal in Task B.

Typically, the most interesting ideas will get the most marks.

Specific examples can be powerful from history or from current affairs. Both will be greatly bolstered with the advice in Sections 3.2.1 and 3.2.2 of the previous chapter - irrespective of your academic background.

4.1.3 Focussing on Task A

Let "A" be Argumentative!

An argumentative essay has three tasks. These tasks can be summarized as follows:

> **1. Thesis:** the first paragraph should provide an explanation or an interpretation of the quotation or quotations that you have chosen.

> **2. Antithesis:** the second paragraph (and sometimes a 3rd and/or 4th) provides an example, real or hypothetical, that demonstrates a point of view opposite to the one presented in the Thesis.

> **3. Synthesis:** the final paragraph concludes with a way for the conflict between the viewpoint expressed in the Thesis and the one presented in the Antithesis to be reconciled.

These three tasks should keep you quite busy for the 30 minutes you have to write the essay. The tasks, however, once you are familiar with them, will help you by structuring your essay automatically for you.

All MCAT Writing Samples (see Section 1.2.1 for details) follow the same rules as GAMSAT Section II, Task A. You will get access to at least a dozen officially corrected real Writing Samples at GAMSAT-prep.com to provide you with examples of both poor and great argumentative essays written in 30 minutes.

GAMSAT-Prep.com
THE GOLD STANDARD

4.1.4 Focussing on Task B

Let "B" be Bersonal? OK, it does not exactly spell "personal" but it's close enough! The important point is to understand that they are expecting a different approach from Task A.

Why so different?

Consider some of the criticisms aimed at young doctors: impressive "book knowledge" and technical ability but lacking skills in listening, communication and empathy. Is it a fact that younger people are less empathetic because of a lack of experience? Can interpersonal skills - including empathy - be the focus of a section of a standardized exam? How does one evaluate empathy?

Ideas and imagination.

They need to know whether you can imagine someone else's perspective. This does not mean that you need to write a creative story using the imagination of Isaac Asimov! It simply means that you have to be able to visualise and explain how other people may be feeling and experiencing life; thus the interpersonal and social theme.

The organization of the Task B essay can be summarized as follows:

1 Introduction: the first paragraph should acquaint the reader with the topic. In addition, it should give the markers a glimpse of what to expect from the body of your text, which you can do by clearly stating your specific assertion and point of view. Make sure your introduction is written in an active tone, with strong verbs and powerful statements.

2 The body: the second paragraph (and sometimes a 3rd and/or 4th) should focus on one main idea that supports your assertions in the Introduction. Dissect that main idea into three distinct parts: the main assertion, a specific supporting example or examples, and a summary (each could be one paragraph depending on how much you can write effectively in the limited time).

3 Conclusion: the last paragraph summarizes the main point(s), reasserts your view and ends the essay with impact. This will be the last thing markers will get from your essay, so make sure it ties everything together succinctly as well as creates a lasting impression in their mind.

Remember that Task B should be written with feeling.

UNDERSTANDING THE GAMSAT

4.1.5 Practice Materials

It is great to know the structure, as previously described, for Task A and Task B. However, you must practice generating ideas and expressing yourself.

Practice Problems
• Brainstorm using famous quotes (Section 4.3)
• ACER
• GS

Full-length practice tests
• GS
• ACER

If you are very concerned about your performance and feel that you need personalized comments from an expert, you can find an essay correcting service available at GAMSAT-prep.com.

4.2 The Five Minute, Five Step Plan

Normally, an essay would be written over a considerable period of time. You would think about your essay, plan what you would write, write, correct and polish your essay, and perhaps rewrite sections. However, a timed essay is not normal. It is a situation where your thoughts have to be ordered, structured and organized straight out of your head! You have to plan what you will write quickly and efficiently. You have 30 minutes to write an essay, but if you spend a few minutes planning first, your essay should greatly improve. It is possible to write a structured complete essay in 30 minutes, but for most students, it requires practice.

The objective of the Five Minute, Five Step Plan is to take 5 minutes to prepare and 5 steps to complete the essay.

Step 1: Read the instructions and the stimulus material.

This may seem obvious, but you would be surprised by the number of students who misread or misinterpret what is expected of them. Carefully read the quotations. Underline or circle keywords.

Consider the following quotations and create an essay in response to one or more of them.

Example of a quotation that could be chosen from stimulus material in Writing Task A:

The government is best that governs least.
Henry David Thoreau

Now, in your mind, you should be thinking of writing a comprehensive essay in which you accomplish the following objectives. Explain what you think the statement means. Describe a specific example in which the government's powers should be increased. Discuss the basis for increasing or decreasing the government's powers.

Step 2: Prewrite your Thesis (Task 1), Antithesis (Task 2) and Synthesis (Task 3).

You should jot down notes in the margin of your test booklet or below the quotation (you will not be permitted "scrap" or "scratch" paper). Generating ideas at this early stage will have the greatest impact on your final score.

Task 1: Usually, you will have to explain a statement which will not be simply factual or self-evident. For example, the statement, "The government is best which governs least," has to be explained and terms have to be defined. Make notes as the information comes to mind:

Ex.: Government: -federal, state, provincial, municipal
-authority, power
-a ruling body

Governs: -rules, delegates, guides
-creates laws
-exerts control, authority

When it comes time to <u>write</u> (Step 4), you will formulate a statement which clearly addresses Task 1: *"Explain what you think the statement means."* You should choose one clear definition from amongst the possibilities. You may also want to use an example to further illustrate the point of view you are presenting:

The ideal ruling body would strive to maintain, at a minimum, its exertion of authority over the population. Clearly, a government representing the people should not have the right to indiscriminately curb the freedom of an individual. The consequence would be a contradiction of democratic principles. Thus a government should avoid extending its powers; rather, government should use its authority prudently.

There are many different interpretations and examples which can be used to explain what the statement means. One possibility is to suggest that 'big' government produces excessive 'red tape' or bureaucracy which eventually may lead to higher taxes and a greater deficit. Also consider using a quotation about government (e.g. from John F. Kennedy).

Another possibility would be to mention that 'big' government leads to too much power, and "absolute power corrupts absolutely." There are an endless number of possibilities. The key is to choose one line of thinking and present it in a clear manner.{*Note how the structure and length of the sentences vary in the example*}

Task 2: Follow a similar approach for tasks two and three. Write down any points you may want to include in your essay which contradict the statement even if you completely agree with it. You should be able to see the other side. If you cannot think of something to challenge the statement, try to think what someone who actively disagrees with the statement would say.

Ex.: i> *Rights of one person begins where another person's rights end: government ensures that happens.*
ii> *National crisis*
iii> *War/draft*

Choose one specific example and elaborate. Take (iii) as a case in point. The writer may use World War II as a specific example. The fact that the U.S. government increased its powers by legislating that certain members of the population must go to war (= *draft*) could be explored. The war prevented the Nazi government from becoming an even greater destructive force and its reign of terror ended. Thus the U.S. government expanded its powers for the greater good.

Task 3: For the third task, look back at the ideas you wrote down to address the first two tasks. You should then be able to reconcile the two opposing views. Write down what you think is the key component of your answer to the third task. Remember that you are not expected to solve all the problems in the world. Simply try to find the best way you know to solve the dilemma outlined by the first two tasks. There are no right or wrong answers for this assignment. What is being graded is your reasoning and your ability to express your thoughts.

Ex.: i> *When the survival of the community is endangered*
ii> *Government should govern for the benefit of its citizens*

Prewriting the tasks is not like writing a formal outline. It is simply a way to structure your ideas in order to enable you to write a well-organized essay in 30 minutes. While prewriting might seem like a waste of time, it is the key to helping you complete all three tasks in the time allowed.

Step 3: Organize your notes

Once you have completed the three tasks, you will want to organize and clarify your ideas. This will allow you to review your ideas before you write and to see how they fit together. You may want to remove some ideas and reformulate others. At this stage, you will decide in which order you will address the three tasks (normally, however, you will keep the order as Tasks 1, 2, 3, respectively). Once you have done this, you will be ready to write the essay. At this point, you will have spent five or six minutes prewriting the tasks. In doing so, you will have created a structure for your essay which will make writing it much easier.

Step 4: Write

When you write, pace yourself. This will be much easier as your notes will provide a framework to work with in writing. You will want to ensure you have a few (about five) minutes to review your masterpiece! Make sure that your essay flows. Use transition words and phrases between your paragraphs. Pay attention to your spelling, punctuation and grammar. Be sure to vary the *structure* and *length* of the sentences in your text.

Do not assume that the reader can read your mind! Be explicit in your presentation. Providing a specific, well-illustrated example can impress the marker. And finally, be sure to not digress from the theme of your essay.

Step 5: Proofread

Reread your text. You want to spend your last five minutes proofreading your essay. Look for and correct mistakes and ensure you followed the plan you established as you prewrote the tasks. At this point you want to simply polish your essay.

By following these five steps, you should be able to write an essay which successfully addresses all three tasks in the time allowed. In combination with relevant ideas, this approach ensures a good score.

4.3 The Power of Quotations

"I quote others only in order to better express myself," DeMontaigne once said. A properly placed quotation can have a powerful effect on your Writing Sample. If used improperly, you will have inadvertently confirmed that you misunderstood the statement provided.

You can choose to use a quotation to support your position or to provide the opposite point of view. But remember: a quote is *word for word*. They will not be impressed if you misquote John F. Kennedy or The Constitution. If you only forgot the name of someone who is not well known, you can get away with saying something like: "It has been said that . . ."

We have placed 50 quotations for you to work through. Half for Writing Task A and the other half for Writing Task B. Please consider re-reading Sections 4.1.3 and 4.1.4. Your aim is to quickly key in on the theme being presented and generate ideas in point form in less than 5 minutes. Frankly, your efficiency should increase in the last 10 essays in each section. Do not try to complete all the exercises in one sitting.

Please keep in mind: Section 2 is not a spectator sport. You can't improve significantly just by reading this book or glancing at some quotations. To improve, you must practice. The following exercises have been carefully chosen to help you express your key ideas briefly - as if to plan your essay. Also, you can discuss the way you structured your essay with other students at gamsat-prep.com/forum.

UNDERSTANDING THE GAMSAT

4.3.1 Writing Task A: Structure 25 Essays

1. Let us never negotiate out of fear. But let us never fear to negotiate.
   John F. Kennedy
   Thesis _____
   Antithesis _____
   Synthesis _____

2. We live in a moment in history where change is so speeded up that we begin to see the present only when it is already disappearing.
   R.D. Laing
   Thesis _____
   Antithesis _____
   Synthesis _____

3. All diplomacy is a continuation of war by other means.
   Chou En-Lai
   Thesis _____
   Antithesis _____
   Synthesis _____

4. It is better that ten guilty persons escape than one innocent suffer.
   William Blackstone
   Thesis _____
   Antithesis _____
   Synthesis _____

5. Money is like the sixth sense without which you cannot make a complete use of the other five.
   W. Somerset Maugham
   Thesis _____
   Antithesis _____
   Synthesis _____

6. That man is richest whose pleasures are the cheapest.
   Henry David Thoreau
   Thesis _____
   Antithesis _____
   Synthesis _____

7. The technologies which have had the most profound effects on human life are usually simple.
   Freeman Dyson
   Thesis _____
   Antithesis _____
   Synthesis _____

8. The great growling engine of change - technology.

Alvin Toffler

Thesis _____
Antithesis _____
Synthesis _____

9. Ability is a poor man's wealth.

John Wooden

Thesis _____
Antithesis _____
Synthesis _____

10. The mother of revolution and crime is poverty.

Aristotle quotes

Thesis _____
Antithesis _____
Synthesis _____

11. It is better to be defeated on principle than to win on lies.

Arthur Calwell

Thesis _____
Antithesis _____
Synthesis _____

12. Those who make peaceful revolution impossible will make violent revolution inevitable.

John F. Kennedy

Thesis _____
Antithesis _____
Synthesis _____

13. Injustice anywhere is a threat to justice everywhere.

Martin Luther King, Jr.

Thesis _____
Antithesis _____
Synthesis _____

14. ...government of the people, by the people, for the people, shall not perish from the earth.

Abraham Lincoln

Thesis _____
Antithesis _____
Synthesis _____

15. In the long-run every Government is the exact symbol of its People, with their wisdom and unwisdom.

Thomas Carlyle

Thesis _____
Antithesis _____
Synthesis _____

16. The cost of liberty is less than the price of repression.

 W. E. B. Du Bois

 Thesis _____
 Antithesis _____
 Synthesis _____

17. I have to follow them, I am their leader.

 Alexandre-Auguste Ledru-Rollin

 Thesis _____
 Antithesis _____
 Synthesis _____

18. I would rather be exposed to the inconveniences attending too much liberty than those attending too small a degree of it.

 Thomas Jefferson

 Thesis _____
 Antithesis _____
 Synthesis _____

19. Those who expect to reap the blessings of freedom, must, like men, undergo the fatigues of supporting it.

 Thomas Jefferson

 Thesis _____
 Antithesis _____
 Synthesis _____

20. The only way to make sure people you agree with can speak is to support the rights of people you don't agree with.

 Eleanor Holmes Norton

 Thesis _____
 Antithesis _____
 Synthesis _____

21. I disapprove of what you say, but I will defend to the death your right to say it.

 Voltaire

 Thesis _____
 Antithesis _____
 Synthesis _____

22. He that would make his own liberty secure must guard even his enemy from oppression.

 Thomas Paine

 Thesis _____
 Antithesis _____
 Synthesis _____

23. War settles nothing.

Dwight D. Eisenhower

Thesis _____
Antithesis _____
Synthesis _____

24. You can't hold a man down without staying down with him.

Booker T. Washington

Thesis _____
Antithesis _____
Synthesis _____

25. Men prize the thing ungained, more than it is.

Shakespeare

Thesis _____
Antithesis _____
Synthesis _____

4.3.2 Writing Task B: Structure 25 Essays

1. It is amazing how complete the delusion that beauty is goodness.

Leo Tolstoy

Introduction _____
Body _____
Conclusion _____

2. Whether you think you can or think you can't - you are right.

Henry Ford

Introduction _____
Body _____
Conclusion _____

3. From the deepest desires often come the deadliest hate.

Socrates

Introduction _____
Body _____
Conclusion _____

4. The error of youth is to believe that intelligence is a substitute for experience, while the error of age is to believe that experience is a substitute for intelligence.

Lyman Bryson

Introduction _____
Body _____
Conclusion _____

5. Conform and be dull.

   James Frank Dobie

   Introduction _____
   Body _____
   Conclusion _____

6. You can stay young as long as you can learn, acquire new habits and suffer contradictions.

   Marie von Ebner-Eschenbach

   Introduction _____
   Body _____
   Conclusion _____

7. Hatred is the coward's revenge for being intimidated.

   George Bernard Shaw

   Introduction _____
   Body _____
   Conclusion _____

8. The young always have the same problem – how to rebel and conform at the same time. They have now solved this by defying their parents and copying one another.

   Quentin Crisp

   Introduction _____
   Body _____
   Conclusion _____

9. Youth is the best time to be rich, and the best time to be poor.

   Euripides

   Introduction _____
   Body _____
   Conclusion _____

10. Some people say they haven't yet found themselves. But the self is not something one finds; it is something one creates.

    Thomas Szasz

    Introduction _____
    Body _____
    Conclusion _____

11. My youth is escaping without giving me anything it owes me.

    Ivy Compton-Burnett

    Introduction _____
    Body _____
    Conclusion _____

12. You can't get rid of poverty by giving people money.

P.J. O'Rourke

Introduction _____
Body _____
Conclusion _____

13. Nobody can make you feel inferior without your consent.

Eleanor Roosevelt

Introduction _____
Body _____
Conclusion _____

14. Youth is something very new: twenty years ago no one mentioned it.

Coco Chanel

Introduction _____
Body _____
Conclusion _____

15. There are three things extremely hard: steel, a diamond, and to know one's self.

Benjamin Franklin

Introduction _____
Body _____
Conclusion _____

16. Comedy is the last refuge of the nonconformist mind.

Edward Albee

Introduction _____
Body _____
Conclusion _____

17. When she stopped conforming to the conventional picture of femininity she finally began to enjoy being a woman.

Betty Naomi Friedan

Introduction _____
Body _____
Conclusion _____

18. When you can't remember why you're hurt, that's when you're healed.

Jane Fonda

Introduction _____
Body _____
Conclusion _____

UNDERSTANDING THE GAMSAT

19. Laughter is the shortest distance between two people.

   Victor Borge

   Introduction _____
   Body _____
   Conclusion _____

20. In prison, those things withheld from and denied to the prisoner become precisely what he wants most of all.

   Eldridge Cleaver

   Introduction _____
   Body _____
   Conclusion _____

21. People travel to wonder at the height of mountains, at the huge waves of the sea, at the long courses of rivers, at the vast compass of the ocean, at the circular motion of the stars, and they pass themselves by without wondering.

   St. Augustine

   Introduction _____
   Body _____
   Conclusion _____

22. Ask the young. They know everything.

   Joseph Joubert

   Introduction _____
   Body _____
   Conclusion _____

23. A sense of humor is a major defense against minor troubles.

   Mignon McLaughlin

   Introduction _____
   Body _____
   Conclusion _____

24. If the misery of the poor be caused not by the laws of nature, but by our institutions, great is our sin.

   Charles Darwin

   Introduction _____
   Body _____
   Conclusion _____

25. They can't hurt you unless you let them.

   Multiple attributions

   Introduction _____
   Body _____
   Conclusion _____

4.4 The Scoring Key

Your score in the Written Communication section will mostly be based on how you present your ideas. Although technical issues - like occasional grammar and spelling errors - essentially influence the quality of your writing, these are only assessed relative to the effectiveness of your general response. Your personal stand and attitude towards the subject matter will not be part of the assessment. The following are two primary criteria on which Section II is assessed: thought and content, and organisation and expression.

Thought and content refers to the substance of your ideas in response to a text. The GAMSAT gives emphasis on *generative thinking,* which is basically about generating values and innovative ideas in your writing within the thirty minutes per essay time limit. The way you effectively carry out your thoughts and feelings as responses to the task give weight to this criterion.

Organisation and expression is how you develop those fresh ideas in a logical and coherent manner. Control of language, i.e. grammar and fluency, is an inherent consideration in the assessment. However, your skills in this area will only be secondary to the overall content of your response.

Most papers are evaluated on common scoring descriptions. It is advisable that you ask someone to correct your essay to get a general idea. Have this person go through the following guide. Please be reminded that this is not endorsed by ACER and should only be considered as a guide to provide you with a general idea of the process.

Typical Essay Grade	Characteristics of a Paper	Estimated Conversion to a GAMSAT Score
6/6	Thought and content shows clear and coherent transitions of ideas. The writer stays focused on the subject or issue. There is evidence of a logical build-up of arguments (i.e. normally just Task A but possibly Task B) or reflective discussion (i.e. Task B). Command of the language is excellent.	≥ 72
5/6	Writing shows clarity of ideas with a certain extent of complexity. The argument stays focused on the issue while main ideas are well-developed. Control of the language is strong.	65–71

UNDERSTANDING THE GAMSAT

Typical Essay Grade	Characteristics of a Paper	Estimated Conversion to a GAMSAT Score
4/6	The essay observes clarity of thought and some depth in ideas. There is also a development of major points and some focus. Control of the language is adequate.	58–64
3/6	There is evidence of some problems with integration and transition of ideas. Major ideas need to be organized and discussed clearly. Errors in grammar and mechanics are evident.	51–57
2/6	Thought and content are disorganized and unclear. There is a lack of logical organization of main ideas. There are numerous errors in grammar, usage and structure.	44–50
1/6	The essay shows a lack of comprehension about the writing task. There is no development and organization of ideas. Poor handling of the language prevents the reader from following the points of the writer.	≤ 43

GAMSAT-Prep.com
THE GOLD STANDARD

4.5 Corrected Essays

In this section, you will find two response essays with corresponding comments. More corrected essays can be accessed at GAMSAT-prep.com/forum. If you wish, use this as yet another exercise. Get a pen and some lined paper. Time yourself (30 minutes) and create an essay in response to the instructions below. Subsequently, compare your response to the graded essays that follow.

WRITING TASK A

Consider the following comments and develop a piece of writing in response to one or more of them.

Your writing will be judged on the quality of your response to the theme; how well you organise and present your point of view, and how effectively you express yourself. You will not be judged on the views or attitudes you express.

* * * * * *

"Laws made by common consent must not be trampled on by individuals."

George Washington

"The final test of civilization of a people is the respect they have for law."

Lewis F. Korns

"In matters of conscience, the law of the majority has no place."

Mahatma Gandhi

"In Republics, the great danger is that the majority may not sufficiently respect the rights of the minority."

James Madison

"All, too, will bear in mind this sacred principle, that though the will of the majority is in all cases to prevail, that will to be rightful must be reasonable; that the minority possess their equal rights, which equal law must protect, and to violate would be oppression."

Thomas Jefferson

A A A A A

The law of the majority Unimportant?

"In matters of concience the law of the majority has no place". For instance, a h.s. student, greatly feels peer pressure would choose not to smoke eventhough the majority of his peers feel that it is a desirable thing to do. According to the statement this student should make his choice based on what he believes not to be right, regardless of the general consesnus of his peers.

There are some situations in which the law of majority is important in matters of conscience. For instance, a politician that believes in firearms can not make a law to force his constituents to carry guns, if they are horrible opposed to such weapons in the first place. Therefore the politician, in doing what he feels is right wouldn't be able to ignore the general consensus of the people of his province about firearms because his decision about such a law would affect them as well as him.

Certain circumstances would govern whether the law of majority is important or not in matters of conscience. If a person acts in such a way that he can live with, and it doesn't have adverse effects on other people who may

SAMPLE ESSAY #1

A A A A A

feel quite differently, then the law of majority is unimportant. If a person's conscience tells them to act in ways that hurt others, then the conscience of the majority must be taken into account. For instance, a Christian school teacher can't force her class that is majority Jewish to sing christmas songs because she believes it's the proper thing to do during the christmas holidays. That would antagonize the class, which would have been taken into consideration when she wanted to do what's right.

IF YOU NEED MORE SPACE, CONTINUE ON THE BACK OF THIS PAGE.

UNDERSTANDING THE GAMSAT

Analysis of Sample Essay #1

Score
2/6   44–50

Task 1 – not really achieved. Although the statement was used in the first sentence, it was never really defined as a thesis nor otherwise defined. Encountering the typographical error "concience" instead of "conscience" or the mistake in spelling the quote in the beginning, seriously hurts the credibility of the writer. Peer evaluation or pressure is somewhat analogous to the making of laws by the majority, but quite loose as an association. For these reasons, clarity of thought and concrete examples to support a given thesis seem cloudy and unfocused.

Task 2 – an antithesis is never really developed to the extent needed. While the politician example whom is juxtaposed in relation to a general consensus, could be developed, the idea of "forcing" people to carry weapons, seems an example, a bit absurd and reaching. The credibility of the writer is also questioned, when the use of "horrible" instead of the correct "horribly" (Para. 2, Line 2) is used adding to a general tone of inconsistency in care of grammar, and overall approach to the subject.

Task 3 – Because neither of the above tasks were completed with the necessary organizational and supportive devices and materials, providing a synthesis of arguments presented is impossible. A touchy feely context-based qualification in the surmounting to a "well, it all depends on the circumstance," is an intellectual and academic cop-out. The example of the Christian school teacher with Jewish students not forcing them to sing Christian songs, could be developed in more detail, if such an example is chosen.

Overall – some good ideas, but unfocused, not organized to the extent needed. There seems to be some misunderstanding of the quote. The writer needs to reveal the Gandhi meaning that non-violent resistance to certain political repressions was not only necessary, but morally correct and in opposition to the laws of the majority. Hypothetical examples could be explored also: suppose that there was a law passed that said you could not protest or peaceably assemble to protest, or a law prohibiting you from enjoying "life, liberty, and the pursuit of happiness.' In many ways, the subject of the essay concerns "personal liberty" vs. "collective responsibility" or "subjective reactions" to "legislative mandates or laws." This juxtaposition, or fulcrum needs to be explored and balanced to a larger degree.

Technical errors, spelling, and typographical errors deflated the essay – as previously noted. A stronger organizational pattern is needed, which follows a sequential and logical progression.

Evaluation (*see* Section 4.5): 2/6. This essay completely fails to address adequately one or more of the tasks. There may be recurring mechanical errors (i.e. spelling and grammar). Problems with analysis and organization are typical (though organization was fine in this instance).

2	These essays may show some problems with clarity or complexity of thought. The treatment of the writing assignment may show problems with integration or coherence. Major ideas may be underdeveloped. There may be numerous errors in mechanics, usage, or sentence structure.

SAMPLE ESSAY #2

A A A A A

My Rights Begin Where Yours End

In our democratic society, we have created many laws or rules gained through legislation. These rules are discussed, developed and enacted by elected officials who represent the majority of their constituents. However, the laws produced in this manner may be in conflict with a particular individual's beliefs or values. Thus the statement suggests that when such a conflict is evident, the individuals beliefs superceed the law, rendering the rules of the majority irrelevant. "In matters of conscience, the law of the majority has no place," spoken by a man of peace regarding a non violent struggle. However, there are those who have used such ideas for darker purposes...

For example, in 1996 many churches frequented by the African-American community were set ablaze by individuals — some of whom were members of racist movements. Both arson and such race-based acts are illegal in America. As in this case, the individuals who acted in defiance of the law of majority claimed they were abiding by their own beliefs and values. Thus they acted with a clear conscience destroying the lives and communities of innocent victims. Such a crime is immoral, unacceptable and — according to the rules of

IF YOU NEED MORE SPACE, CONTINUE ON THE NEXT PAGE.

A A A A A

the majority — illegal. Clearly, the law of majority must supercede the conscience of the perpetrators of such a crime.

The dividing line becomes clear. Life, liberty and the pursuit of happiness are the foundations of Constitution. The concept is both logical and moral. Our conscience should be our guide as we excercise our our freedom. However, since our neighbors and fellow Americans share the same rights, someone's conscience should never be used as a reason why someone's Constitutionally protected rights are stripped away. In conclusion, one's conscience should be one's guide but when it interferes with the rights of others, the law of majority becomes more important.

GAMSAT-Prep.com
THE GOLD STANDARD

Analysis of Sample Essay #2

Score
5/6   65–71

Task 1 – A quick example could help buttress Task 1 in outlining the thesis matter, where subjective liberties are at odds with social, legislative, or governmental mandates. As noted in Essay #1, hypothetical examples could be used in supporting the thesis outline. Identifying the source of the quote as Gandhi, as a man of peace, helps further establish the credibility as a writer.

Task 2 – effective transition into an antithetical notion of when a sinister turn is taken between the dialectic of individual rights-beliefs and governmental mandates. Very good *specific* example and portrayal of the paradoxes of such a balance.

Task 3 – follows a logical progression, sequential with good analysis and reasoning. Good use of quotes in relation to a most relevant document concerning this juxtaposition: The Constitution (naturally, there are many effective international, national or regional examples depending on where you live or where you attend school).

Overall – good logical sequence, completion of tasks to an above average extent, clarity of focus, good development of ideas, clear and simple style of language.

The title did not necessarily - nor correctly - represent the outline of the ideas presented to the adequacy needed. The title is somewhat ambiguous and polysemantic, having several ways to interpret. Another minor observation – rules and laws are conflated to some extent, they could be differentiated more effectively, or simply omit the use of the word "rules".

Examples of some minor technical and typographical errors – "gained" in Paragraph (P) 1, Line (L) 2 is redundant, omit; P1, L9 – "supercede" not "superceed"; P3, L2 – insert "the" before "Constitution"; P3, L3 should be "These concepts are . . ."; P3, L4 doubled "our our"; P3, L9 – "constitutionally" – use lower case.

Evaluation (*see* Section 4.5): 5/6: All tasks are addressed by this essay. The treatment of the subject is substantial but not as thorough as for a 6 point essay. While some depth, structure and good vocabulary and sentence control is exhibited, this is at a lower level than for a 6 point essay.

> **5** These essays show clarity of thought, with some depth or complexity. The treatment of the rhetorical assignment is generally focused and coherent. Major ideas are well developed. A strong control of language is evident.

UNDERSTANDING THE GAMSAT

4.6 Common Grammatical Errors

Please do not read the following section unless either it is more than 6 weeks before the real exam or you have done some practice essays and you find that generating ideas and producing a well-structured essay is no longer challenging. At this point, improving details such as grammar and flexibility in the use of language can now become more interesting to explore as you aim to go from a very good score to an excellent score.

Some Basic Concepts

By definition, a sentence has the following properties:
- it contains a *subject*
- it contains a *verb*
- it expresses a *complete thought*

E.g., the sentence *"China prospers."* has a subject: "China"; a verb: "prospers"; and it conveys a complete thought or idea that makes sense.

Most sentences also have an *object* (receiver of the action); e.g., in the sentence "Mary baked a cake," the object is "a cake."

Run-on Sentences (fused sentences)

Incorrect usage	Correct usage	Explanation
He watched the movie ten times he really loved it.	He watched the movie ten times. He really loved it. He watched the movie ten times; he really loved it. He watched the movie ten times, for he really loved it. Since he really loved the movie, he watched it ten times.	Run-on sentences occur when two main clauses have no punctuation between them. Separate the two main ideas into separate complete sentences and punctuate each properly. Use a conjunction preceded by a comma to combine two ideas. Subordinate one of the main ideas into a clause.

Comma Faults (comma splices)

Incorrect usage	Correct usage	Explanations
He watched the movie ten times, he really loved it.	He watched the movie ten times, for he really loved it. He watched the movie ten times; he really loved it.	Comma faults occur when two main clauses are joined by only a comma. Use comma before a conjunction (*and, but, for, nor, or, so,* or *yet*) to join two complete thoughts (sentences). Use a semicolon to join two sentences. Omit the use of a conjunction, and start the second sentence in lowercase. Form two complete thoughts as separate sentences with the proper end marks. (See preceding example.) Join two thoughts by subordinating one of them. (See preceding example.)

Sentence Fragments

Incorrect usage	Correct usage	Explanation
Luke can read a book. And memorize it right after.	Luke can read a book and memorize it right after.	A sentence must have a subject and a verb.

Faulty Subordination

Incorrect usage	Correct usage	Explanation
I gazed out of the bus window, noticing a person getting mugged.	Gazing out of the bus window, I noticed a person getting mugged.	Place what you want to emphasize in the main clause, not the subordinate clause. Here the mugging should be emphasized and so should be in the main clause.

Errors in Subject-Verb Agreement

Rule: The verb should agree with the subject in terms of number (singular or plural) and person (first, second, or third).

Incorrect usage	Correct usage	Explanation
There is no glasses.	There are no glasses.	In this sentence, the subject is *glasses*, not there. *glasses* is plural; therefore, the verb should be plural (i.e. *are*).
She like diamonds.	She likes diamonds.	The subject *she* is in the second person, and is singular; therefore, the verb should also be in the second person, and be singular (i.e. *likes*).
Neither Emma nor Harry were there.	Neither Emma nor Harry was there.	In sentences where subjects are joined by *or* or *nor*, the verb agrees with the subject closer to it. In this example, "Harry" is the nearer subject. It is singular, so the verb should be also.
Neither Mary nor the others was there.	Neither Mary nor the others were there.	"Others" is the subject that is nearer to the verb. It is plural, so the verb should be also.
All of the team were there.	All of the team was there.	"Team" is singular, so the verb should be also.
All the players was present.	All the players were present.	"Players" is plural, so the verb should be also.
There are a variety of fruits.	There is a variety of fruits.	"Variety" is singular.
	There is a lot of birds here *or* there are a lot of birds here.	Both are correct. The first is correct since "lot" is singular. The second is correct because it is gaining acceptance through popular use.
Here is your shoes and tie.	Here are shoes and tie.	This sentence is in the inverted order, i.e., the subject/s come/s after the verb. When re-stated in the normal order, this sentence will be: *Your shoes and tie are here.* Subjects joined by *and* always take the plural form. Therefore, "shoes and tie" is plural, so the verb should be also.

Incorrect usage	Correct usage	Explanation
Fiona is one of the worst singers who has performed in this bar.	Fiona is one of the worst singers who have performed in this bar.	When relative pronouns *who*, *which*, or *that* are used as subjects of dependent adjective clauses, the verb of the adjective clause must agree in number with the antecedent of the pronoun. In this sentence, the antecedent of *who* is *singers*. "Singers" is plural, so the verb should be also (i.e. "have").
"I forget" or "I forgot".	I've forgotten.	Note that "I often forget" and "I forgot my umbrella yesterday" are correct.
Everybody are happy with the results.	Everybody is happy with the results.	Words like *everybody, everyone, everything, somebody, someone, each, either, nothing* and *anything* are examples of indefinite pronouns in singular form. Always remember that only the following are indefinite pronouns that are plural in form: *both, few, many, others,* and *several*. *All, any, more, most, none, some* may take singular or plural forms depending on the context of the sentence.
The queen, together with invited guests, face the media.	The queen, together with together with invited guests, faces the media.	The subject in this sentence is "queen". "Invited guests" is a noun of the intervening phrase that merely adds information about the subject. "Queen" is singular, so the verb should be also Expressions of amount:.
Two-thirds of the project were assigned to me.	Two-thirds of the project was assigned to me.	When the subject is a fraction, the verb agrees with the noun in the of-phrase (i.e. "project").
The number of applicants remain unaccounted.	The number of applicants remains unaccounted.	*The number of* is always singular. *A number of* is always plural.

Errors in Noun-Pronoun Agreement

Rule: Pronouns should agree with their nouns in terms of number (singular or plural), person (first, second, or third), and gender (masculine or feminine).

Incorrect usage	Correct usage	Explanation
Did everyone remember their assignment?	Did everyone remember his assignment?	*Everyone* is singular, so the pronoun should be as well.
It was them who apologized.	It was they who apologized.	The nominative case (I, you, he, she, it, we, you, they, who) is used following some form of the verb *to be*.
If I were him, I would go.	If I were he, I would go.	As above.
It is me.	It is I.	As above.
Whom will succeed?	Who will succeed?	A simple rule-of-thumb is to use "who" when "he" would also make sense; and use "whom" when "him" would also make sense (e.g. "Him will succeed" does not sound right, while "he will succeed" does).
Who did you give it to?	Whom did you give it to?	As above. "You gave it to he" does not sound right, while "you gave it to him" does. Thus, use "whom".
It belongs to he and I.	It belongs to him and me.	The *objective* case of pronoun (i.e. me, you, him, her, it, us, you, them, whom) is used as the object of a preposition, such as "to".
Hugh fired he.	Hugh hired him.	The *objective* case of pronoun (i.e. me, you, him, her, it, us, you, them, whom) is used as the *object* of a verb.
He is as proficient as me.	He is as proficient as I.	Try stretching the sentence out: "He is as proficient as *I am proficient*, not "he is as proficient as *me am proficient*."
He was in the same class as us.	He was in the same class as we.	Try stretching the sentence out: "He was in the same class as *we were in*."
I trust Bob more than he.	I trust Bob more than him.	Try stretching the sentence out: "I trust Bob more than *I trust him*."
Now sing without me coaching you.	Now sing without my coaching you.	Use the *possessive* case of the pronoun (i.e. my, your, his, her, its, our, your, their, whose) in sentences like this.

Special Problems in Pronoun Agreement

Incorrect usage	Correct usage	Explanation
The movie was disappointing because *they* never made the plot seem realistic.	The *movie* was disappointing because *it* never made the plot seem realistic. The movie was disappointing because *the writers* never made the plot seem realistic.	Pronoun must agree with antecedents that are either clearly stated or understood. Otherwise, use a specific noun.
In 17th century England, *you* had to choose between following the Church or the King.	In 17th century England, *Puritans* had to choose between following the Church or the King.	Use *YOU* only when the reference is truly addressed to the reader.
Charles asked *William* about the state of his marriage. William tried to evade the topic, but confused about the situation, *he* tried to carry on a pleasant conversation.	*Charles* asked *William* about the state of his marriage. *William* tried to evade the topic, but confused about the situation, *Charles* tried to carry on a pleasant conversation.	Always use a pronoun close enough to its antecedent to avoid confusion.
I placed my passport in my bag, but I can't find *it*.	I placed my passport in my bag, but I can't find *my bag*.	Use pronouns to refer to an obvious antecedent.

Dangling Modifiers

Rule: Avoid dangling modifiers (i.e. adjectives or adverbs that do not refer to the noun or pronoun they are intended to refer to).

Incorrect usage	Correct usage	Explanation
While dialling the phone, the lights went out.	While *I was* dialling the phone, the lights went out.	The modifying phrase "while walking in the garden" does not refer to a particular noun or pronoun (i.e. it dangles).
After attending the mass, pizza was eaten.	After attending the mass, we ate pizza.	As above.

Misplaced Modifiers

Incorrect usage	Correct usage	Explanation
Nina won almost 1 million euros.	Nina almost won 1 million euros.	The first sentence does not mean what it is intended to mean. The modifier "nearly" is misplaced.
I only want you.	I want only you.	Same as above.

"Were" to be used in the Subjunctive Mood

Rule: Use *"were"* in the subjunctive mood, i.e. when expressing a wish, regret, or a condition that does not exist.

Incorrect usage	Correct usage	Explanation
If I was prettier, I would be famous.	If I were prettier, I would be famous.	This sentence is in the subjunctive mood.
Mum treats him as if he is a slave.	Mum treats him as if he were a slave.	As above.

That, Which, and Who

Incorrect usage	Correct usage	Explanation
This is the novel which he loved.	This is the novel that he loved.	When commas are not used, use "that".
This gown, that is designed by Monique, is expensive and elegant.	This gown, which is designed by Monique, is expensive and elegant.	When commas are used, use "which".
She is the person that designed the gown.	She is the person who designed the gown.	For persons, use "who". Do not use "who" for animals.
The President, which is an avid golfer, was on the course.	The President, who is an avid golfer, was on the course.	For persons, use "who", even when commas are used.

Note: Often the above pronouns can be omitted making a sentence more concise. Thus:

This is the novel he loved. ("That" is implied.) This gown, designed by Monique, is expensive and elegant. She designed the gown. The President, an avid golfer, was on the course.

Faulty Parallelism

Incorrect usage	Correct usage	Explanation
She likes to read, swim and shopping a lot.	She likes to read, swim and shop a lot. She likes to read, to swim and to shop a lot.	Similar ideas should be expressed in grammatically similar forms. (E.g., nouns with nouns, adjectives with adjectives, words with words, phrases with phrases)
The professor was asked to submit his report quick and accurately.	The professor was asked to submit his report quickly and accurately.	Similar ideas should be expressed in grammatically similar structures (i.e. same word order, consistent verb tenses).

Mixed Constructions

Incorrect usage	Correct usage	Explanation
Will asked Lizzie to marry him?	Will asked Lizzie to marry him?	Don't mix a statement with a question.
The reason is because I don't have a nanny.	The reason is that I don't have a nanny.	Don't mix two different sentence constructions.

Split Infinitives

Incorrect usage	Correct usage	Explanation
I need to mentally prepare.	I need to prepare mentally.	"To prepare" is an infinitive. Splitting infinitives with other words tends to be awkward.

Commas

Incorrect usage	Correct usage	Explanation
Uncle has money, wealth and power.	Uncle has money, wealth, and power.	Use a comma before the last item in a series to avoid any confusion.
The food was served late cold and smelly.	The food was served late, cold, and smelly.	Use commas to separate adjectives that could be joined with "and." You could say that "the food was served late and cold and smelly."
Jonas is a popular, varsity player.	Jonas is a popular varsity player.	Don't use commas to separate adjectives that could not be joined with "and." It would be ridiculous to say that " Jonas is a popular and varsity player."

UNDERSTANDING THE GAMSAT

Incorrect usage	Correct usage	Explanation
You wait here, and I'll get your coat.	You wait here and I'll get your coat.	Don't use a comma to set off clauses that are short or have the same subject. However, always use a comma before "for", "so," and "yet" to avoid confusion.
The doctor gave detailed precise instructions to the nurse.	The doctor gave detailed, precise instructions to the nurse.	Use commas to separate adjectives of same or equal rank.
India has a rigid, social caste system.	India has a rigid social caste system.	Do not use commas to separate adjectives that must stay in a specific order.

Semicolons

Incorrect usage	Correct usage	Explanation
The car is old, however, it is in good condition.	The car is old; however, it is in good condition. The car is old; it is, however, in good condition.	Use a semicolon with a conjunctive adverb (e.g. nevertheless, however, otherwise, consequently, thus, therefore, meanwhile, moreover, furthermore).

Apostrophes

Correct usage	Explanation
Maggie Holmes' dog is lost. Maggie Holmes 's dog is lost.	Since there is disagreement on which is correct, both are acceptable.
The girl's doll fell in the mud. The girls' doll fell in the mud.	Common errors arise when apostrophes are misplaced in singular and plural nouns. In the first sentence, placing the apostrophe in between the noun and an *s* indicates a singular noun. In the second sentence, an apostrophe placed after a plural noun hints that the "doll" is commonly owned by at least two girls.

Troublesome Verbs

TRANSITIVE (followed by an object)	INTRANSITIVE (not followed by an object)
raise, raising, raised: The farmer is raising chickens.	**rise, rising, rose**: The moon is rising.
lay, laying, laid: I am laying the dress on the bed.	**lie, lying, lain**: I am lying on the bed.

GAMSAT-Prep.com
THE GOLD STANDARD

"A" or "The"

Correct usage	Explanation
I dated **the** cheerleader back in college.	The definite article **the** is used when referring to a specific subject or member of a group. The speaker in the sentence could have been acquainted with many cheerleaders; but he was able to date only one particular cheerleader.
I dated **a** cheerleader back in college.	Use the indefinite article **a** to refer to a non-specific subject. The sentence implies that the speaker dated someone who could have been any member of a cheerleading group.

Proper Usage of *"The"*

• The Thames flow through Oxford and London. • The Gibson Desert is home to indigenous Australians. • Myths say that Santa Claus lives in the North Pole. • The equator is approximately 3,500 miles from the southernmost part of the United Kingdom. • The Chinese are hardworking people.	USE **the** when referring to • the proper names of rivers, oceans and seas; • deserts, forests, gulfs, and peninsulas • geographical areas • points on the globe • some countries like *the* Netherlands, *the* Dominican Republic, *the* Philippines, *the* United States • the people of a nation
Anna shops in Bond Street. Blue Lake attracts many tourists in Australia. St. Patrick's Island is a sanctuary for seabirds. Galtymore ranks 14th among Ireland's highest mountain peak. English is the main language used in the United Kingdom.	DO NOT USE **the** when referring to • street names • names of lakes except with a group of lakes • bays • most countries/territories but NOT cities, states or towns • names of mountains in general • names of continents • names of islands except with island chains • names of languages and nationalities

Verb or Participle

Not all verbs demonstrate an action. There are those that merely express a condition or an existence. These are called linking verbs. Words that describe (adjectives) or identify (another noun) should follow the linking verb.

Examples:

Incorrect Usage	Correct Usage
Nicole Kidman **sounds** sarcastically in the interview.	Nicole Kidman **sounds** sarcastic in the interview. 　The verb "sounds" expresses the state of emotions (sarcastic) of the subject (Nicole Kidman) at the time of the interview.
	Sir Edward Hallstrom **is** a philanthropist. 　The verb "is" connects the noun "philanthropist" to the subject "Sir Edward Hallstrom".

Participles are words that look like verbs but function in the sentence as nouns.

Example: **Exploring** Lake Argyle is one of the most wonderful outdoor adventures in Australia.
"Exploring" is a participle that functions as the noun-subject in the sentence and should not be confused with the main verb "is".

Common errors involving confusion between verbs and participles lead to **Sentence Fragments.**

Incorrect Usage	Correct Usage	Explanation
Dancing on her toes. The ballerina **was** superb.	**Dancing** on her toes, the ballerina **was** superb.	The main thought of the sentence is a description of the level of performance of the subject (ballerina) - "superb". The action word "dancing" merely adds information about what the subject (ballerina) does.

GAMSAT-Prep.com

GENERAL CHEMISTRY
PART III.A: PHYSICAL SCIENCES

IMPORTANT: Before doing your science survey for the GAMSAT, be sure you have read the Preface, Introduction and Part II, Chapter 2. The beginning of each science chapter provides guidelines as to what you should Memorize, Understand and what is Not Required. These are guides to get you a top score without getting lost in the details. Our guides have been determined from an analysis of all ACER materials plus student surveys. Additionally, the original owner of this book gets a full year access to many online features described in the Preface and Introduction including an online Forum where each chapter can be discussed.

STOICHIOMETRY

Chapter 1

Memorize	Understand	Not Required*
Define: molecular weight Define: empirical/molecular formula Rules for oxidation numbers	* Composition by % mass * Mole concept, limiting reactants * Avogadro's number * Calculate theoretical yield * Basic types of reactions * Calculation of ox. numbers	* Advanced level college info * Balancing complex equations * Stoichiometric coefficients in competing reactions

GAMSAT-Prep.com

Introduction

Stoichiometry is simply the math behind the chemistry involving products and reactants. The math is quite simple, in part, because of the law of conservation of mass that states that the mass of a closed system will remain constant throughout a chemical reaction.

Additional Resources

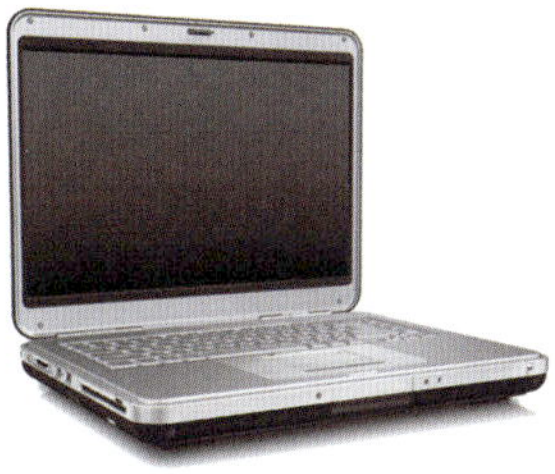

Free Online Q&A + Forum

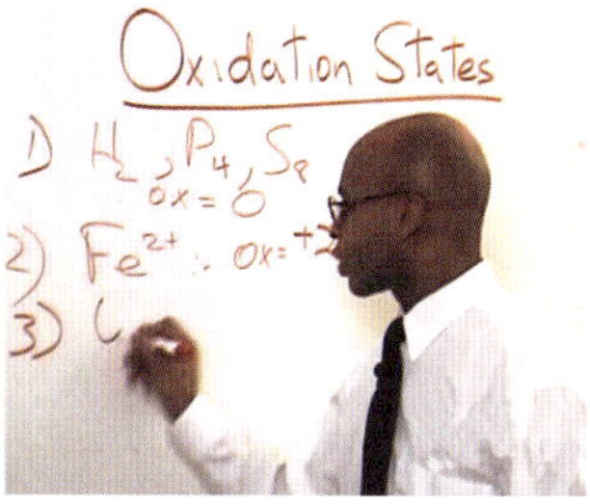

Video: Online or DVD 1, 4

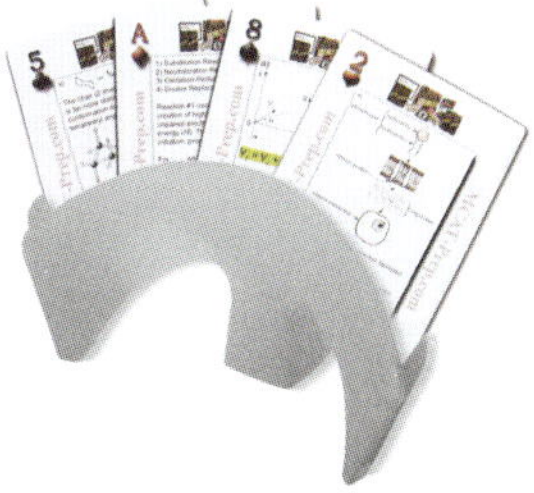

Flashcards

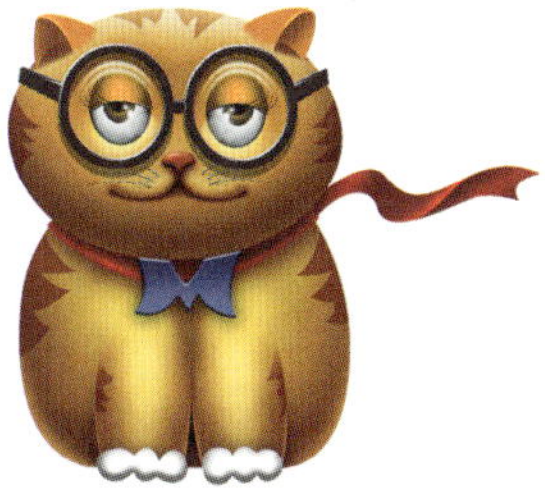

Special Guest

THE PHYSICAL SCIENCES   CHM-03

* The real GAMSAT may have advanced level information presented (ie. in a passage) but previous knowledge of said information is not required to answer the questions that would follow. Practice ACER and GS practice GAMSATs can help you clarify this point.

GAMSAT-Prep.com
THE GOLD STANDARD

1.1 Generalities

Most substances known to us are mixtures of pure compounds. Air, for instance, contains the pure compounds nitrogen (~78%), oxygen (~21%), water vapor and many other gases (~1%). The compositional ratio of air or any other mixture may vary from one location to another. Each pure compound is made up of molecules which are composed of smaller units: the *atoms*.

Atoms combine in very specific ratios to form molecules. During a chemical reaction molecules break down into individual or fragments of atoms which then recombine to form new compounds. Stoichiometry establishes relationships between the above-mentioned specific ratios for individual molecules or for molecules involved in a given chemical reaction.

1.2 Empirical Formula vs. Molecular Formula

The molecules of oxygen (O_2) are made up of two atoms of the same element. Water molecules on the other hand are composed of two different elements: hydrogen and oxygen in the specific ratio 2:1. Note that water is not a mixture of hydrogen and oxygen since this ratio is specific and does not vary with the location or the experimental conditions. The *empirical formula* of a pure compound is the simplest whole number ratio between the numbers of atoms of the different elements making up the compound. For instance, the empirical formula of water is H_2O (2:1 ratio) while the empirical formula of hydrogen peroxide is HO (1:1 ratio). The *molecular formula* of a given molecule states the exact number of the different atoms that make up this molecule. The empirical formula of water is identical to its molecular formula, i.e. H_2O; however, the molecular formula of hydrogen peroxide, H_2O_2, is different from its empirical formula (both correspond to a 1:1 ratio).

1.3 Mole - Atomic and Molecular Weights

Because of the small size of atoms and molecules chemists have to consider collections of a large number of these particles to bring chemical problems to our macroscopic scale. Collections of tens or dozens of atoms are still too small to achieve this practical purpose. For various reasons the number 6.02×10^{23} (Avogadro's number: N_A) was chosen. It is the number of atoms in 12 grams of the most abundant *isotope* of carbon (isotopes are elements which are identical chemically since the number of protons are the same; their masses differ slightly since the number of neutrons differ). A mole of atoms or molecules (or in fact any particles in general) contains an Avogadro number of these particles. The weight in grams of a mole of atoms of a given element is the gram-atomic weight,

GENERAL CHEMISTRY

GAW, of that element (sometimes weight is measured in atomic mass units - see Physics section 12.2, 12.3). Along the same lines, the weight in grams of a mole of molecules of a given compound is its gram-molecular weight, GMW. Here are some equations relating these concepts in a way that will help you solve some of the stoichiometry problems:

For an element:

$$\text{\# moles} = \frac{\text{(weight of sample in grams)}}{\text{GAW}}$$

For a compound:

$$\text{\# moles} = \frac{\text{(weight of sample in grams)}}{\text{GMW}}$$

The GAW of a given element is not to be confused with the mass of a single atom of this element. For instance the mass of a single atom of carbon-12 (GAW = 12 g) is $12/N_A = 1.66051 \times 10^{-24}$ grams. Atomic weights are dimensionless numbers defined as follows:

$$\frac{\text{mass of an atom of X}}{\text{mass of an atom of Y}} = \frac{\text{atomic weight of element X}}{\text{atomic weight of element Y}}$$

Clearly if the reference element Y is chosen to be carbon-12 (which is the case in standard periodic tables) the GAW of any element X is numerically equal to its atomic weight. The molecular weight of a given molecule is equal to the sum of the atomic weights of the atoms that make up the molecule.

1.4 Composition of a Compound by Percent Mass

The percentage composition of a compound is the percent of the total mass of a given element in that compound. For instance, the chemical analysis of a 100 g sample of pure vitamin C demontrates that there are 40.9 g of carbon, 4.58 g of hydrogen and 54.5 g of oxygen. The composition of pure vitamin C is:

%C = 40.9; %H = 4.58; %O = 54.5

The composition of a compound by percent mass is closely related to its empirical formula. For instance, in the case of vitamin C, the determination of the number of moles of atoms of C, H or O in a 100 g of vitamin C is rather straightforward:

\# moles of atoms of C in a 100 g of vitamin C = 40.9/12.0 = 3.41

\# moles of atoms of H in a 100 g of vitamin C = 4.58/1.01 = 4.53

\# moles of atoms of O in a 100 g of vitamin C = 54.5/16.0 = 3.41

[GAW can be determined from the periodic table in Chapter 2]

To deduce the smallest ratio between the numbers above, one follows the simple procedure:

(i) divide each one of the previously obtained numbers of moles by the smallest one of them (3.41 in our case):

for C: 3.41/3.41 = 1.00

for H: 4.53/3.41 = 1.33

for O: 3.41/3.41 = 1.00

(ii) multiply the numbers obtained in the previous step by a small number to obtain a whole number ratio. In our case we need to multiply by 3 (in most cases this factor is between 1 and 5) so that :

for C: 1.00 × 3 = 3;

for H: 1.33 × 3 = 4 and

for O: 1.00 × 3 = 3

Therefore, in this example, the simplest whole number ratio is 3C:4H:3O and we conclude that the empirical formula for vitamin C is: $C_3H_4O_3$.

In the previous example, instead of giving the composition of vitamin C by percent weight we could have provided the raw chemical analysis data and asked for the determination of that composition. For instance, this data would be that the burning of a 4.00 mg sample of pure vitamin C yields 6.00 mg of CO_2 and 1.632 mg of H_2O. Since there are 12.0 g of carbon in 44.0 g of CO_2 the number of milligrams of carbon in 6.00 mg of CO_2 (which corresponds to the number of mg of carbon in 4.00 mg of vitamin C) is simply:

6.00 × (12.0/44.0) = 1.636 mg of C in 6.00 mg of CO_2 or 4.00 mg of vitamin C

To convert this number into a percent mass is then trivial. Similarly, the percent mass of hydrogen is obtained from the previous data and bearing in mind that there are 2.02 g of hydrogen (and not 1.01 g) in 18.0 g of water. {"Burning" means *combustion* which takes place in the presence of excess oxygen as described in ORG 3.2.1}

How many moles are in guacamole? Avocado's number.

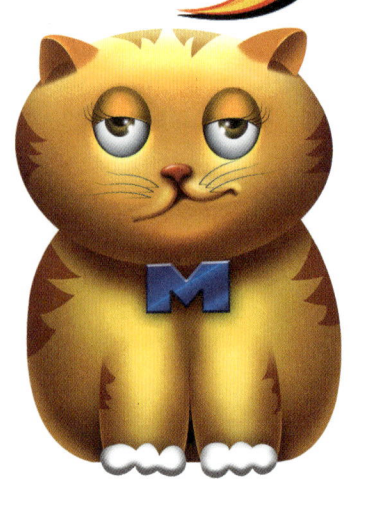

GENERAL CHEMISTRY

1.5 Description of Reactions by Chemical Equations

The convention for writing chemical equations is as follows: compounds which initially combine or <u>react</u> in a chemical reaction are called *reactants*; they are always written on the left-hand side of the chemical equation. The compounds which are <u>produced</u> during the same process are referred to as the *products* of the chemical reaction; they always appear on the right-hand side of the chemical equation. In the chemical equation:

$$2\ BiCl_3 + 3\ H_2O \rightarrow Bi_2O_3 + 6\ HCl$$

the coefficients represent the relative number of moles of reactants that combine to form the corresponding relative number of moles of products: they are the <u>stoichiometric coefficients</u> of the balanced chemical equation. The law of conservation of mass requires that the number of atoms of a given element remains constant during the process of a chemical reaction. Balancing a chemical equation is putting this general principle into practice. It is always easier to balance elements that appear only in one compound on each side of the equation; therefore, as a general rule, always balance those elements first and then deal with those which appear in more than one compound last.

Given the preceding chemical reaction, if H_2O is present in excessive quantity, then $BiCl_3$ would be considered the **limiting reactant.** In other words, since the amount of $BiCl_3$ is relatively small, it is the $BiCl_3$ which determines how much product will be formed. Thus if you were given 316 grams of $BiCl_3$ in excess H_2O and you needed to determine the quantity of HCl produced (theoretical yield), you would proceed as follows:

▸ Determine the number of moles of $BiCl_3$ (*see* CHM 1.3) given Bi = 209 g/mol and Cl = 35.5 g/mol, thus $BiCl_3$ = (1 × 209) + (3 × 35.5) = 315.5 or approximately 316 g/mol:

moles $BiCl_3$ = (316 g)/(316 g/mol)
  = 1.0 mole of $BiCl_3$.

▸ From the stoichiometric coefficients of the balanced equation:

2 moles of $BiCl_3$: 6 moles of HCl; therefore, 1 mole of $BiCl_3$: 3 moles of HCl

▸ Given H = 1 g/mol, thus HCl = 36.5 g/mol, we get:

3 moles × 36.5 g/mol = 110 g of HCl (approx.).

The real GAMSAT does not usually provide a periodic table so the atomic weights (a.m.u.) will be given when required. Also, since calculators are not permitted, you should practice performing all calculations that you see in this textbook.

GAMSAT-Prep.com
THE GOLD STANDARD

1.5.1 Categories of Chemical Reactions

Throughout the chapters in General Chemistry we will explore many different types of chemicals and some of their reactions. The following represents some balanced chemical equations as examples:

Substitution Reaction (CHM 9.4)
$CH_4 + Cl_2 \rightarrow CH_3Cl + HCl$

Neutralization Reaction (CHM 6.9.1)
$2HCl + Ba(OH)_2 \rightarrow Ba^{2+} + 2Cl^- + H_2O$

Redox Reaction (CHM 1.6, 10.1)
$H_2SO_4 + Fe \rightarrow FeSO_4 + H_2$

Disproportionation Reaction (CHM 1.6)
$2CO \rightarrow C + CO_2$

Double Replacement Reaction
$CaCl_2 + Na_2CO_3 \rightarrow CaCO_3 + 2NaCl$

In a disproportionation reaction, the chemical (CO in our example) is simultaneously reduced and oxidized (cf. NaCl in CHM 1.6) forming 2 differerent products. A double replacement reaction involves ions (CHM 5.2) which change partners.

1.6 Oxidation Numbers, Redox Reactions, Oxidizing vs. Reducing Agents

A special class of reactions known as *redox* reactions are better balanced using the concept of <u>oxidation state</u>. This section deals with these reactions in which electrons are transferred from one atom (or a group of atoms) to another.

First of all, it is very important to understand the difference between the ionic charge and the oxidation state of an element. For this let us consider the two compounds sodium chloride (NaCl) and water (H_2O). NaCl is made up of the charged species or ions: Na^+ and Cl^-. During the formation of this molecule, one electron is transferred from the Na atom to the Cl atom. It is possible to verify this fact experimentally and determine that the charge of sodium in NaCl is indeed +1 and that the one for chlorine is −1. The elements in the periodic table tend to lose or gain electrons to different extents. Therefore, even in non-ionic compounds electrons are always transferred, to different degrees, from one atom to another during the formation of a molecule of the compound. The actual partial charges that result from these partial transfers of electrons can also be determined experimentally. The oxidation state is not equal to such partial charges. It is rather an artificial concept that is used to perform some kind of "electron bookkeeping."

In a molecule like H_2O, since oxygen tends to attract electrons more than hydrogen, one can predict that the electrons that

GENERAL CHEMISTRY

allow bonding to occur between hydrogen and oxygen will be displaced towards the oxygen atom. For the sake of "electron bookkeeping" we assign these electrons to the oxygen atom. The charge that the oxygen atom would have in this artificial process would be –2: this defines the oxidation state of oxygen in the H_2O molecule. In the same line of reasoning one defines the oxidation state of hydrogen in the water molecule as +1. The actual partial charges of hydrogen and oxygen are in fact smaller; but, as we will see later, the concept of oxidation state is very useful in stoichiometry.

Here are the general rules one needs to follow to assign oxidation numbers to different elements in different compounds:

1. In elementary substances, the oxidation number of an element is zero. This is, for instance, the case for N in N_2 or Na in sodium element, O in O_2, or S in S_8.

2. In monoatomic ions the oxidation number of the element that make up this ion is equal to the charge of the ion. This is the case for Na in Na^+ (+1) or Cl in Cl^- (–1) or Fe in Fe^{3+} (+3). Clearly, monoatomic ions are the only species for which atomic charges and oxidation numbers coincide.

3. In a neutral molecule the sum of the oxidation numbers of all the elements that make up the molecule is zero. In a polyatomic ion (e.g. SO_4^{2-}) the sum of the oxidation numbers of the elements that make up this ion is equal to the charge of the ion.

4. Some useful oxidation numbers to memorize:

    For H: +1, except in metal hydrides (general formula XH where X is from the first two columns of the periodic table) where it is equal to –1.

    For O: –2 in most compounds. In peroxides (e.g. in H_2O_2) the oxidation number for O is –1, it is +2 in OF_2 and –1/2 in superoxides (e.g. potassium superoxide: KO_2 which contains the O_2^- ion as opposed to the O^{2-} ion).

    For alkali metals (first column in the periodic table): +1.

    For alkaline earth metals (second column): +2.

    Aluminium always has an oxidation number of +3 in all its compounds.
    (i.e. clorides $AlCl_3$, nitrites $Al(NO_2)_3$, etc.)

An element is said to have been *reduced* during a reaction if its oxidation number decreased during this reaction, it is said to have been oxidized if its *oxidation* number increased. A simple example is:

$$Zn(s) + CuSO_4(aq)$$
Oxid.#:   0   +2
$$ZnSO_4(aq) + Cu(s)$$
Oxid.#:   +2   0

During this reaction Cu is reduced (oxidation number decreases from +2 to 0) while

Zn is oxidized (oxidation number increases from 0 to +2). Since, in a sense, Cu is reduced by Zn, Zn can be referred to as the <u>reducing agent</u>. Similarly, Cu is the <u>oxidizing agent</u>.

The redox titrations will be dealt with in the section on titrations (CHM 6.10). Many of the redox agents in the table below will be explored in the chapters on Organic Chemistry.

Common Redox Agents	
Reducing Agents	**Oxidizing Agents**
* Lithium aluminium hydride (LiAlH$_4$) * Sodium borohydride (NaBH$_4$) * Metals * Ferrous ion (Fe^{2+})	* Iodine (I$_2$) and other halogens * Permanganate (MnO$_4$) salts * Peroxide compounds (i.e. H$_2$O$_2$) * Ozone (O$_3$); osmium tetroxide (OsO$_4$) * Nitric acid (HNO$_3$); nitrous oxide (N$_2$O)

GOLD NOTES

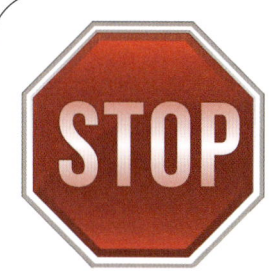

Reminder: Chapter review questions are available online for the original owner of this textbook. Doing practice questions will help clarify concepts and ensure that you study in a targeted way. First, register at gamsat-prep.com, then login and click on GAMSAT Textbook Owners in the right column so you can use your Online Access Card to have access to the Lessons section.

No science background? Consider watching the relevant videos at gamsat-prep.com and you have support at gamsat-prep.com/forum. Don't forget to check the Index at the beginning of this book to see which chapters are HIGH, MEDIUM and LOW relative importance for the GAMSAT.

Your online access continues for one full year from your online registration.

GOLD NOTES

ELECTRONIC STRUCTURE AND THE PERIODIC TABLE
Chapter 2

Memorize	Understand	Not Required*
* Definitions of quantum numbers * Shapes of s, p orbitals * Order for filling atomic orbitals	* Conventional notation, Pauli, Hund's * Box diagrams, IP, electronegativity * Valence, EA * Variation in shells, atomic size *Trends in the periodic table	* Advanced level college info * Memorizing Schroedinger's equation * Memorizing data from the periodic table * IUPAC's systematic element names (gen. chem.)

GAMSAT-Prep.com

Introduction

The periodic table of the elements provides data and abbreviations for the names of elements in a tabular layout. The purpose of the table is to illustrate recurring (periodic) trends and to classify and compare the different types of chemical behavior. To do so, we must first better understand the atom. The periodic table is not usually provided in the real GAMSAT but you are still responsible for knowing the trends and relative locations of the most common atoms.

Additional Resources

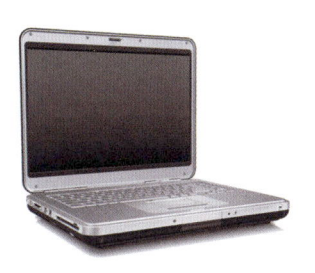

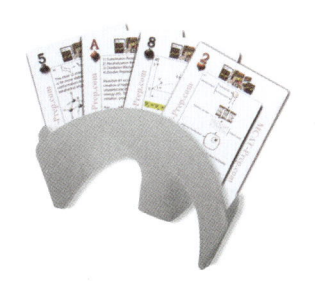

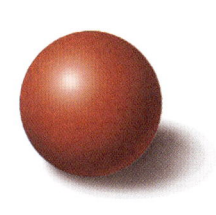

Free Online Q&A + Forum | Video: Online or DVD 1 | Flashcards | Special Guest

THE PHYSICAL SCIENCES CHM-13

* The real GAMSAT may have advanced level information presented (ie. in a passage) but previous knowledge of said information is not required to answer the questions that would follow. Practice ACER and GS practice GAMSATs can help you clarify this point.

2.1 Electronic Structure of an Atom

The modern view of the structure of atoms is based on a series of discoveries and complicated theories that were put forth at the turn of this century. We will only present the main ideas behind these findings that shaped our understanding of atomic structure.

The first important idea is that electrons (as well as any microscopic particles) are in fact waves as well as particles; this concept is often referred to in textbooks as the dual nature of matter.

Contrary to classical mechanics, in this modern view of matter information on particles is not derived from the knowledge of their position and momentum at a given time but by the knowledge of the wave function (mathematical expression of the above-mentioned wave) and their energy. Mathematically, such information can be derived, in principle, by solving the master equation of quantum mechanics known as the Schroedinger equation. In the case of the hydrogen atom, this equation can be solved exactly. It yields the possible states of energy in which the electron can be found within the hydrogen atom and the wave functions associated with these states. The square of the wave function associated with a given state of energy gives the probability to find the electron, which is in that same state of energy, at any given point in space at any given time. These wave functions as well as their geometrical representations are referred to as the *atomic orbitals*. We shall explain further below the significance of these geometrical representations.

Even for a hydrogen atom there is a large number of possible states in which its single electron can be found (when it is subjected to different external perturbations). A labelling of these states is therefore necessary. This is done using the *quantum numbers*. These are:

(i) n: *the principal quantum number*. This number takes the integer values 1, 2, 3, 4, 5… The higher the value of n the higher the energy of the state labelled by this n. This number defines the atomic shells K (n = 1), L (n = 2), M (n = 3) etc…

(ii) *l*: *the angular momentum quantum number*. It defines the shape of the atomic orbital in a way which we will discuss further below. For a given electronic state of energy defined by n, *l* takes all possible integer values between 0 and n − 1. For instance for a state with n = 0 there is only one possible shape of orbital, it is defined by *l* = 0. For a state defined by n = 3 there are 3 possible orbital shapes with *l* = 0, 1 and 2.

All orbitals with *l*=0 are called "s", all with *l* =1 are "p", those with *l* =2 or 3 are "d" or "f" respectively. The important shapes to remember are: i) s = spherical, ii) p = 2 lobes or "dumbbell" (*see the following diagrams*). For values of *l* larger than 3, which occur with an n greater or equal to 4, the corresponding series of atomic orbitals follows the alphabetical order h, i, j,…

GENERAL CHEMISTRY

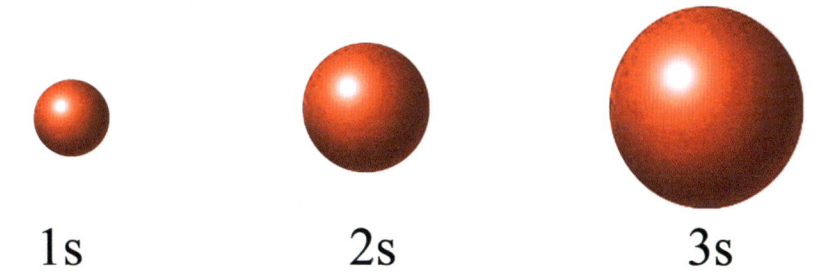

Figure III.A.2.1: Atomic orbitals where $l = 0$. Notice that the orbitals do not reveal the precise location (position) or momentum of the fast moving electron at any point in time (Heisenberg's Uncertainty Principle). Instead, we are left with a 90% chance of finding the electron somewhere within the shapes described as orbitals.

(iii) m_l: *the magnetic quantum number.* It defines the orientation of the orbital of a given shape. For a given value of l (given shape), m_l can take any of the $2l + 1$ integer values between $-l$ and $+l$. For instance for a state with $n = 3$ and $l = 1$ (3p orbital in notation explained in the previous paragraph) there are three possible values for m_l: -1, 0 and 1. These 3 orbitals are oriented along x, y or the z axis of a coordinate system with its origin on the nucleus of the atom: they are denoted as $3p_x$, $3p_y$ and $3p_z$. The diagrams show the representation of an orbital corresponding to an electron in a state ns, np_x, np_y, and np_z. These are the 3D volumes where there is 90% chance to find an electron which is in a state ns, np_x, np_y, or np_z, respectively. This type of diagram constitutes the most common geometrical representation of the atomic orbitals.

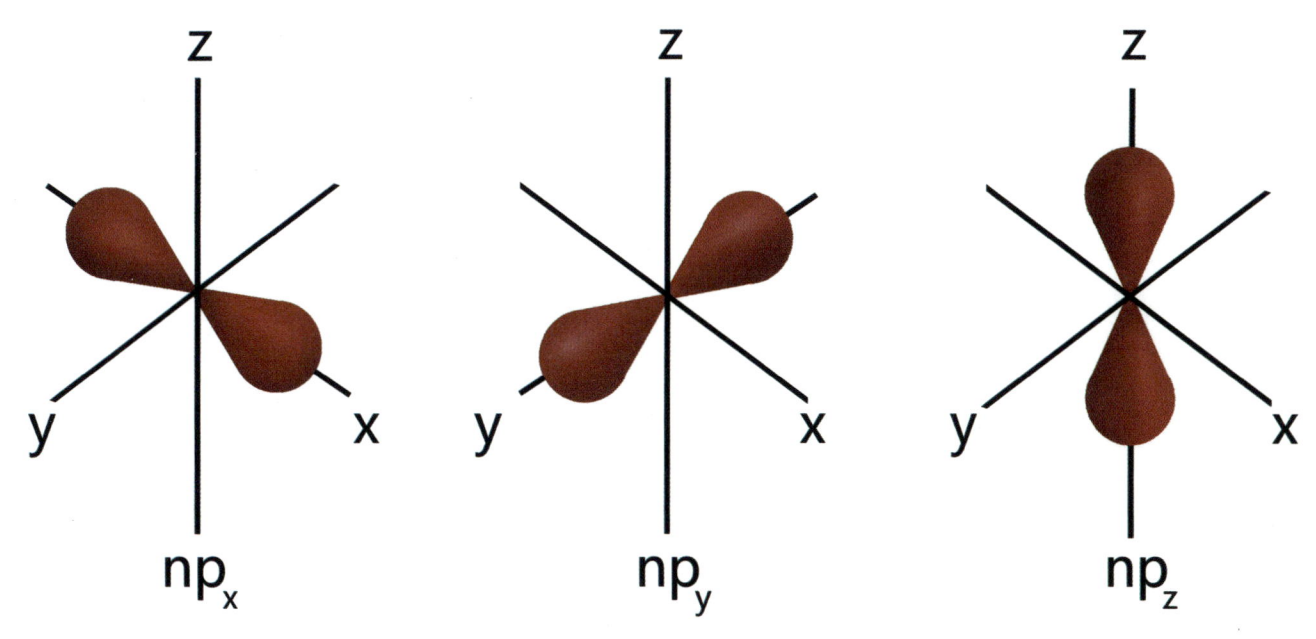

Figure III.A.2.2: Atomic orbitals where $l = 1$.

(iv) m_s: *the spin quantum number*. This number takes the values +1/2 or −1/2 for the electron. Some textbooks present the intuitive, albeit wrong, explanation that the spin angular momentum arises from the spinning of the electron around itself, the opposite signs for the spin quantum number would correspond to the two opposite rotational directions. We do have to resort to such an intuitive presentation because the spin angular moment has, in fact, no classical equivalent and, as a result, the physics behind the correct approach is too complex to be dealt with in introductory courses.

2.2 Conventional Notation for Electronic Structure

The state of an electron in an atom is completely defined by a set of quantum numbers (n, *l*, m_l, m_s). If two electrons in an atom share the same n, *l* and m_l numbers their m_s have to be of opposite signs: this is known as Pauli's exclusion principle. This principle along with a rule known as Hund's rule constitutes the basis for the procedure that one needs to follow to assign the possible (n, *l*, m_l, m_s) states to the electrons of a polyelectronic atom. Orbitals are "filled" in sequence, according to an example below. When filling a set of orbitals with the same n and *l* (e.g. the three 2p orbitals: $2p_x$, $2p_y$ and $2p_z$ which differ by their m_l's) electrons are assigned to orbitals with different m_l's first with parallel spins (same sign for their m_s), until each orbital of the given group is filled with one electron, then, electrons are paired in the same orbital with antiparallel spins (opposite signs for m_s). This procedure is illustrated in an example which follows. The electronic configuration which results from orbitals filled in accordance with the previous set of rules corresponds to the atom being in its lowest overall state of energy. This state of lowest energy is referred to as the ground state of the atom.

The restrictions related to the previous set of rules lead to the fact that only a certain number of electrons is allowed for each quantum number:

for a given n (given shell): the maximum number of electrons allowed is $2n^2$.

for a given *l* (s, p, d, f…): this number is $4l + 2$.

for a given m_l (given orbital orientation): a maximum of 2 electrons is allowed.

There is a **conventional notation** for the electronic structure of an atom:

(i) orbitals are listed in the order they are filled

(ii) generally, in this conventional notation, no distinction is made between electrons in states defined by the same n and l but which do not share the same m_l.

For instance the ground state electronic configuration of oxygen is written as:

$$1s^2 \, 2s^2 \, 2p^4$$

GENERAL CHEMISTRY

When writing the electronic configuration of a polyelectronic atom orbitals are filled (with two electrons) in order of increasing energy: 1s 2s 2p 3s 3p 4s 3d ... according to the following figure:

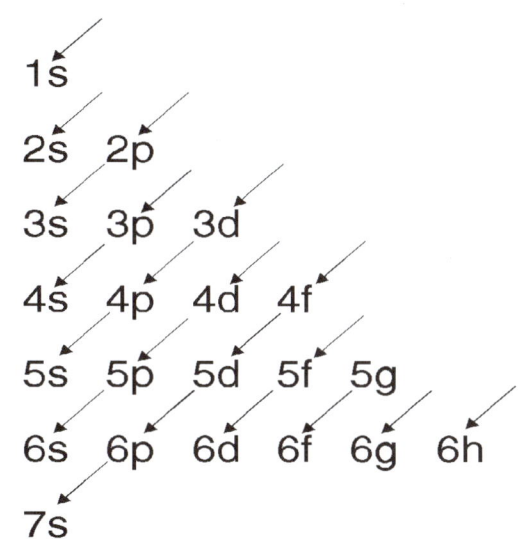

1s
2s 2p
3s 3p 3d
4s 4p 4d 4f
5s 5p 5d 5f 5g
6s 6p 6d 6f 6g 6h
7s

follow the direction of successive arrows moving from top to bottom

Figure III.A.2.3: The order for filling atomic orbitals.

Another illustrative notation is also often used. In this alternate notation orbitals are represented by boxes (hence the referring to this representation as "box diagrams"). Orbitals with the same l are grouped together and electrons are represented by vertical ascending or descending arrows (for the two opposite signs of m_s).

For instance for the series H, He, Li, Be, B, C we have the following electronic configurations:

H: $1s^1$ box diagram: [↑]

He: $1s^2$ box diagram: [↑↓] and not [↑↑]
     (rejected by Pauli's exclusion principle)

Li: $1s^2$ $2s^1$
     [↑↓]   [↑]

Be: $1s^2$ $2s^2$
     [↑↓]   [↑↓]

B: $1s^2$ $2s^2$ $2p^1$
     [↑↓]   [↑↓]   [↑][ ][ ]

C: $1s^2$ $2s^2$ $2p^2$
     [↑↓]   [↑↓]   [↑][↑][ ]

(to satisfy Hund's rule of maximum spin)

To satisfy Hund's rule the next electron is put into a separate 2p "box". The 4th 2p electron (for oxygen) is put in the first box with an opposite spin.

Finally, we should point out that electrons can be promoted to higher unoccupied (or partially occupied) orbitals when the atom is subjected to some external perturbation which inputs energy into the atom. The resulting electronic configuration is called an excited state configuration.

2.3 Elements, Chemical Properties and The Periodic Table

Since most chemical properties of the atom are related to their outermost electrons (valence electrons), it is the orbital occupation of these electrons which is most relevant in the complete electronic configuration. The periodic table (there is one at the end of this chapter with a summary of trends) can be used to derive such information in the following way:

(i) the row or period number gives the "n" of the valence electrons of any given element of the period.

(ii) the first two columns or groups and helium (He) are referred to as the "s" block. The valence electrons of elements in these groups are "s" electrons.

(iii) groups 3A to 8A (13th to 18th columns) are the "p" group. Elements belonging to these groups have their ground state electronic configurations ending with "p" electrons.

(iv) Elements in groups 3B to 2B (columns 3 to 12) are called transition elements. Their electronic configurations end with $ns^2(n-1)d^x$ where n is the period number and x = 1 for column 3, 2 for column 4, 3 for column 5, etc... Note that these elements sometimes have unexpected or unusual valence shell electronic configurations.

This set of rules should make the writing of the ground-state valence shell electronic configuration very easy. For instance: Sc being an element of the "d" group on the 4th period should have a ground-state valence shell electronic configuration of the form: $4s^23d^x$. Since it belongs to group 3B (column 3) x = 1; therefore, the actual configuration is simply: $4s^23d^1$. However, half-filled (i.e. Cr) and filled (i.e. Cu, Ag, Au) d orbitals have remarkable stability. This stability makes for unusual configurations (i.e. by the rules Cr = $4s^23d^4$, but in reality Cr = $4s^13d^5$ creating a half-filled d orbital). Some metal ions form colored solutions due to the transition energies of the d-electrons.

A number of physical and chemical properties of the elements are periodic, i.e. they vary in a regular fashion with atomic numbers. We will define some of these properties and explain their trends:

(i) First ionization energy or potential (1st IE or IP): the energy required to remove one of the outermost electrons from an atom in its gaseous state. The ionization potential increases from left to right in a period and decreases from the top to the bottom of a group or column in the periodic chart. The 1st IP drops sharply when we move from the last element of a period (inert gas) to the first element of the next period. These are general trends, elements located after an element with a half-filled shell, for instance, have a lower 1st IP than expected by these trends.

(ii) Second ionization energy or potential (2nd IE or IP): the previous trends can be used if one remembers the relationship between 1st and 2nd ionization processes of an atom of element X:

$$X + \text{energy} \rightarrow X^+ + 1e^-$$
1st ionization of X

$$X^+ + \text{energy} \rightarrow X^{2+} + 1e^-$$
$$2^{nd} \text{ ionization of X}$$

The second ionization process of X can be viewed as the 1st ionization of X^+. With this in mind it is very easy to predict trends of 2nd IP's. For instance, let us compare the 2nd IP's of the elements Na and Al. This is equivalent to comparing the 1st IP's of Na^+ and Al^+. These, in turn, have the same valence shell electronic configurations as Ne and Mg, respectively. Applying the previous general principles on Ne and Mg we arrive at the following conclusions:

- the 1st IP of Ne is greater than the 1st IP of Mg
- the 1st IP of Na^+ is therefore expected to be greater than the 1st IP of Al^+
- the latter statement is equivalent to the final conclusion that the 2nd IP of Na is greater than the 2nd IP of Al.

(iii) Electron affinity (EA) is the energy change that accompanies the following process for an atom of element X:

$$X(gas) + 1e^- \rightarrow X^-(gas)$$

This property measures the ability of an atom to accept an electron. Halogen atoms (F, Cl, Br…) have a very negative EA because they have a great tendency to form negative ions. On the other hand, alkaline earth metals which tend to form positive rather than negative ions have very large positive EA's. The overall tendency is that EA's become more negative as we move from left to right across a period, they are more negative (less positive) for non-metals than for metals and they do not change considerably within a group or column.

(iv) Atomic radius generally decreases from left to right across a period and increases when we move down a group.

(v) Electronegativity is a parameter that measures the ability of an atom, when engaged in a molecular bond, to pull or repel the bond electrons. This parameter is determined from the 1st IE and the EA of a given atom. Electronegativity follows the same general trends as the 1st IE.

2.3.1 Bond Strength

When there is a big difference in electronegativity between two atoms sharing a covalent bond then the bond is generally weaker as compared to two atoms with little electronegativity difference. This is because in the latter case, the bond is shared more equally and is thus more stable.

Bond strength is inversely proportional to bond length. Thus, all things being equal, a stronger bond would be shorter. Bonds and bond strength is further discussed in ORG 1.3-1.5.1.

GAMSAT-Prep.com
THE GOLD STANDARD

PERIODIC TABLE OF THE ELEMENTS

INCREASING IONIZATION ENERGY OR IONIZATION POTENTIAL
INCREASING NEGATIVITY OF ELECTRON AFFINITY

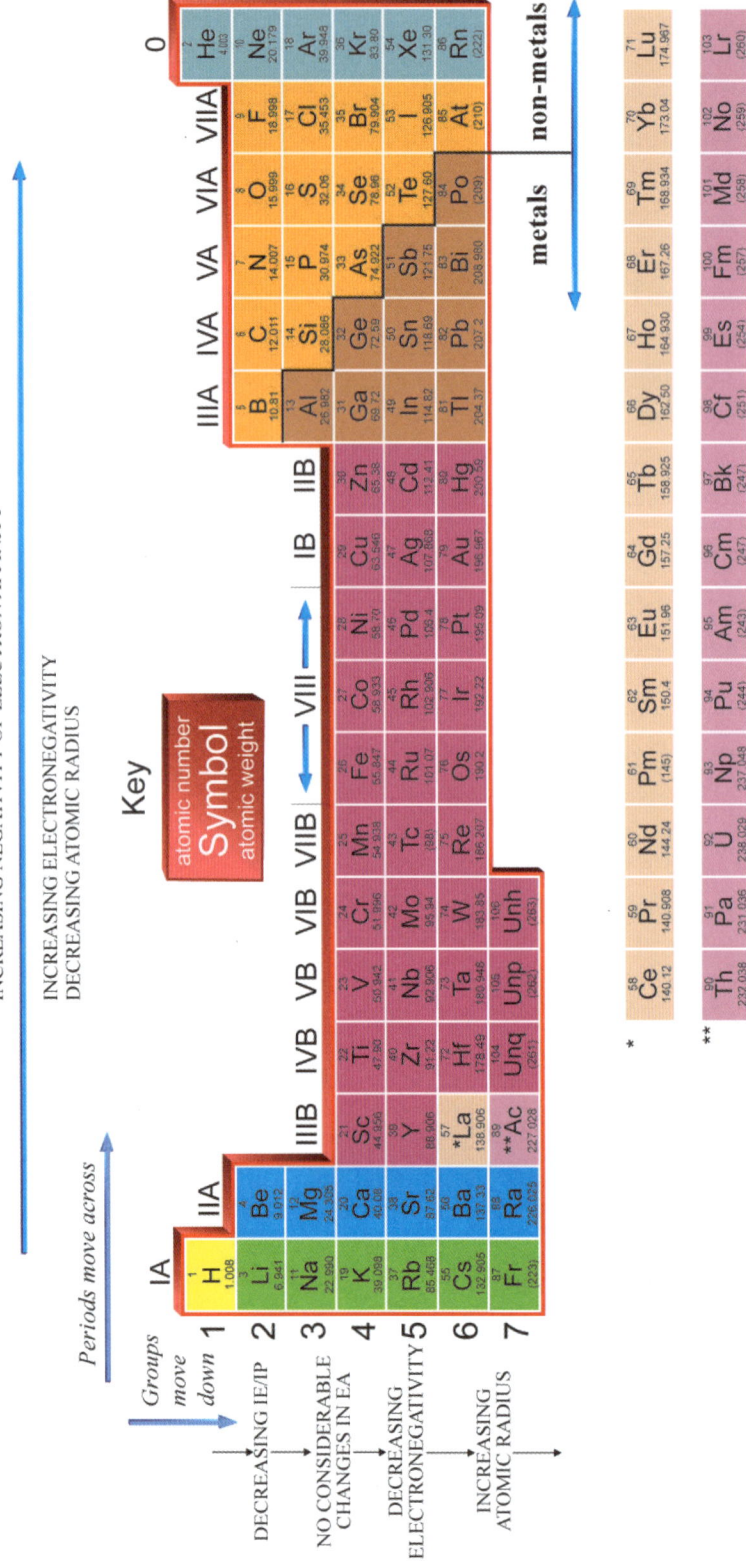

INCREASING ELECTRONEGATIVITY
DECREASING ATOMIC RADIUS

Periods move across
Groups move down

Key: atomic number / Symbol / atomic weight

metals ← → non-metals

	IA	IIA	IIIB	IVB	VB	VIB	VIIB	VIII			IB	IIB	IIIA	IVA	VA	VIA	VIIA	0
1	1 H 1.008																	2 He 4.003
2	3 Li 6.941	4 Be 9.012											5 B 10.81	6 C 12.011	7 N 14.007	8 O 15.999	9 F 18.998	10 Ne 20.179
3	11 Na 22.990	12 Mg 24.305											13 Al 26.982	14 Si 28.086	15 P 30.974	16 S 32.06	17 Cl 35.453	18 Ar 39.948
4	19 K 39.098	20 Ca 40.08	21 Sc 44.956	22 Ti 47.90	23 V 50.942	24 Cr 51.996	25 Mn 54.938	26 Fe 55.847	27 Co 58.933	28 Ni 58.70	29 Cu 63.546	30 Zn 65.38	31 Ga 69.72	32 Ge 72.59	33 As 74.922	34 Se 78.96	35 Br 79.904	36 Kr 83.80
5	37 Rb 85.468	38 Sr 87.62	39 Y 88.906	40 Zr 91.22	41 Nb 92.906	42 Mo 95.94	43 Tc (98)	44 Ru 101.07	45 Rh 102.905	46 Pd 106.4	47 Ag 107.868	48 Cd 112.41	49 In 114.82	50 Sn 118.69	51 Sb 121.75	52 Te 127.60	53 I 126.905	54 Xe 131.30
6	55 Cs 132.905	56 Ba 137.33	57 *La 138.906	72 Hf 178.49	73 Ta 180.948	74 W 183.85	75 Re 186.207	76 Os 190.2	77 Ir 192.22	78 Pt 195.09	79 Au 196.967	80 Hg 200.59	81 Tl 204.37	82 Pb 207.2	83 Bi 208.980	84 Po (209)	85 At (210)	86 Rn (222)
7	87 Fr (223)	88 Ra 226.025	89 **Ac 227.028	104 Unq (261)	105 Unp (262)	106 Unh (263)												

* 58 Ce 140.12 | 59 Pr 140.908 | 60 Nd 144.24 | 61 Pm (145) | 62 Sm 150.4 | 63 Eu 151.96 | 64 Gd 157.25 | 65 Tb 158.925 | 66 Dy 162.50 | 67 Ho 164.930 | 68 Er 167.26 | 69 Tm 168.934 | 70 Yb 173.04 | 71 Lu 174.967

** 90 Th 232.038 | 91 Pa 231.036 | 92 U 238.029 | 93 Np 237.048 | 94 Pu (244) | 95 Am (243) | 96 Cm (247) | 97 Bk (247) | 98 Cf (251) | 99 Es (254) | 100 Fm (257) | 101 Md (258) | 102 No (259) | 103 Lr (260)

DECREASING IE/IP
NO CONSIDERABLE CHANGES IN EA
DECREASING ELECTRONEGATIVITY
INCREASING ATOMIC RADIUS

CHM-20   ELECTRONIC STRUCTURE AND THE PERIODIC TABLE

GENERAL CHEMISTRY

Element	Symbol	Atomic Number
Actinium	Ac	89
Aluminum	Al	13
Americium	Am	95
Antimony	Sb	51
Argon	Ar	18
Arsenic	As	33
Astatine	At	85
Barium	Ba	56
Berkelium	Bk	97
Beryllium	Be	4
Bismuth	Bi	83
Boron	B	5
Bromine	Br	35
Cadmium	Cd	48
Calcium	Ca	20
Californium	Cf	98
Carbon	C	6
Cerium	Ce	58
Cesium	Cs	55
Chlorine	Cl	17
Chromium	Cr	24
Cobalt	Co	27
Copper	Cu	29
Curium	Cm	96
Dysprosium	Dy	66
Einsteinium	Es	99
Erbium	Er	68

Element	Symbol	Atomic Number
Europium	Eu	63
Fermium	Fm	100
Fluorine	F	9
Francium	Fr	87
Gadolinium	Gd	64
Gallium	Ga	31
Germanium	Ge	32
Gold	Au	79
Hafnium	Hf	72
Helium	He	2
Holmium	Ho	67
Hydrogen	H	1
Indium	In	49
Iodine	I	53
Iridium	Ir	77
Iron	Fe	26
Krypton	Kr	36
Lanthanum	La	57
Lawrencium	Lr	103
Lead	Pb	82
Lithium	Li	3
Lutetium	Lu	71
Magnesium	Mg	12
Manganese	Mn	25
Mendelevium	Md	101
Mercury	Hg	80
Molybdenum	Mo	42

Element	Symbol	Atomic Number
Neodymium	Nd	60
Neon	Ne	10
Neptunium	Np	93
Nickel	Ni	28
Niobium	Nb	41
Nitrogen	N	7
Nobelium	No	102
Osmium	Os	76
Oxygen	O	8
Palladium	Pd	46
Phosphorous	P	15
Platinum	Pt	78
Plutonium	Pu	94
Polonium	Po	84
Potassium	K	19
Praseodymium	Pr	59
Promethium	Pm	61
Protactinium	Pa	91
Radium	Ra	88
Radon	Rn	86
Rhenium	Re	75
Rhodium	Rh	45
Rubidium	Rb	37
Ruthenium	Ru	44
Samarium	Sm	62
Scandium	Sc	21

Element	Symbol	Atomic Number
Selenium	Se	34
Silicon	Si	14
Silver	Ag	47
Sodium	Na	11
Strontium	Sr	38
Sulfur	S	16
Tantalum	Ta	73
Technetium	Tc	43
Tellurium	Te	52
Terbium	Tb	65
Thallium	Tl	81
Thorium	Th	90
Thulium	Tm	69
Tin	Sn	50
Titanium	Ti	22
Tungsten	W	74
(Unnilhexium)	(Unh)	106
(Unnilpentium)	(Unp)	105
(Unnilquadium)	(Unq)	104
Uranium	U	92
Vanadium	V	23
Xenon	Xe	54
Ytterbium	Yb	70
Yttrium	Y	39
Zinc	Zn	30
Zirconium	vZr	40

GOLD NOTES

GOLD NOTES

BONDING

Chapter 3

Memorize	Understand	Not Required*
* Hybrid orbitals, shapes * Define Lewis: structure, acid, base * Define: octet rule, formal charge	* Ionic, covalent bonds * VSEPR, Resonance * Dipole, covalent polar bonds * Trends in the periodic table	* Advanced level college info * Details of VSEPR * Memorizing hybrids with d, f * Memorizing dipole moment equation

GAMSAT-Prep.com

Introduction

Attractive interactions between atoms and molecules involve a physical process called chemical bonding. In general, strong chemical bonding is associated with the sharing or transfer of electrons between atoms. Molecules, crystals and diatomic gases are held together by chemical bonds which makes up most of the matter around us.

Additional Resources

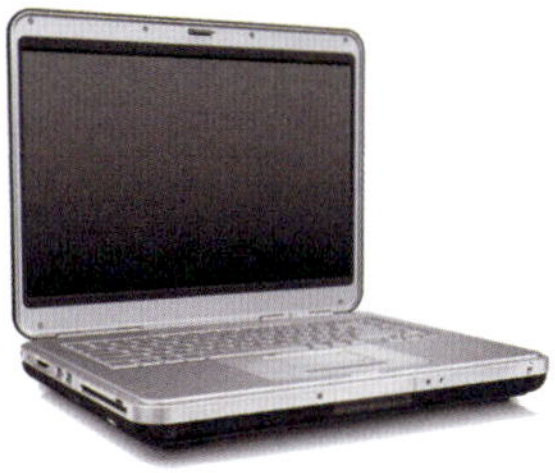

Free Online Q&A + Forum 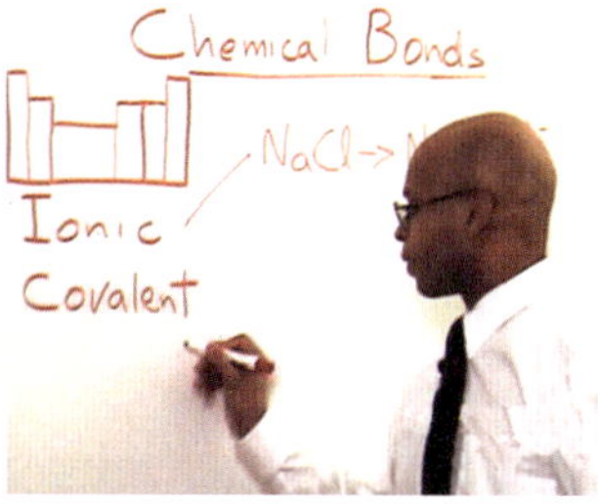   Video: Online or DVD 1, 2 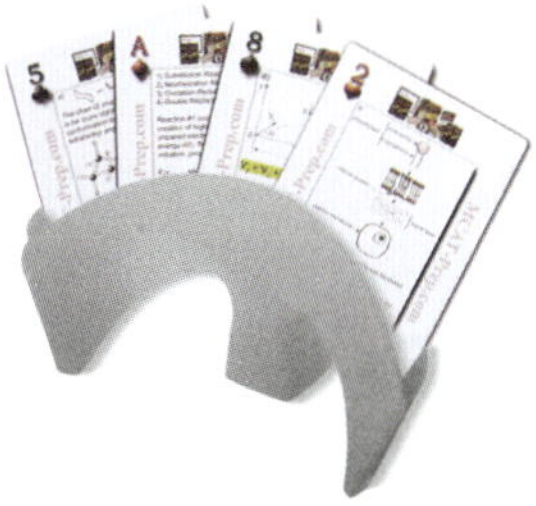   Flashcards 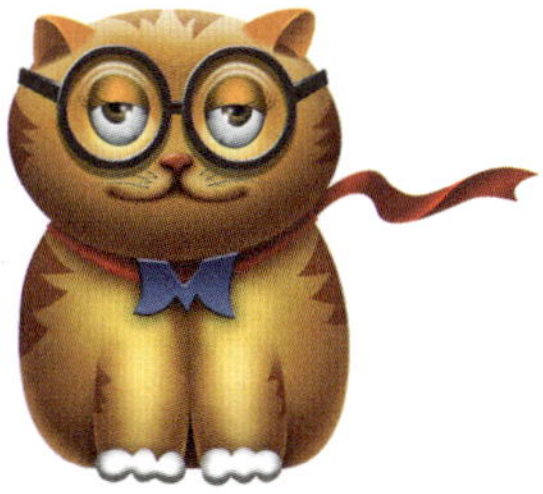   Special Guest

THE PHYSICAL SCIENCES

* The real GAMSAT may have advanced level information presented (ie. in a passage) but previous knowledge of said information is not required to answer the questions that would follow. Practice ACER and GS practice GAMSATs can help you clarify this point.

3.1 The Ionic Bond

When an element X with a low ionization potential is combined with an element Y with a large negative electron affinity one or more electrons are transferred from the atoms of X to the atoms of Y. This leads to the formation of cations X^{n+} and anions Y^{m-}. These ions of opposite charges are then attracted to each other through electrostatic forces. The bonds that hold these ions together are called <u>ionic bonds</u>. Ionic bonding favors the formation of large stable spatial arrangements of ions: <u>crystalline solids</u>. In our general example, note that to maintain electrical neutrality the empirical formula of this ionic compound has to be of the general form: X_mY_n (the total positive charge: $n \times m$ is equal to the total negative charge: $m \times n$ in a unit formula). For instance, since aluminium tends to form the cation Al^{3+} and oxygen the anion O^{2-} the empirical formula for aluminium oxide is Al_2O_3.

3.2 The Covalent Bond

Atoms are held together in non-ionic molecules by <u>covalent bonds</u>. In this type of bonding two valence electrons are shared by two atoms. A <u>Lewis structure</u> is a representation of covalent bonding in which shared electrons are shown either as lines or as pairs of dots between two atoms. For instance, let us consider the H_2O molecule. The valence shell electronic configurations of the atoms that constitute this molecule are:

O: $2s^2 2p^4$

H: $1s^1$

Since hydrogen has only one electron to share with oxygen there is only one possible covalent bond that can be formed between the oxygen atom and each of the hydrogen atoms. 4 of the valence electrons of the oxygen atom do not participate in this covalent bonding, these are called <u>non-bonding electrons or lone pairs</u>. The Lewis structure of the water molecule is:

H:Ö:H or H-Ö-H

Lewis formulated the following general rule known as the <u>octet rule</u> concerning these representations: atoms tend to form covalent bonds until they are surrounded by 8 electrons (except for hydrogen which can be surrounded by a maximum of only 2 electrons). To satisfy this rule (and if there is a sufficient number of valence electrons), two atoms may share more than one pair of electrons thus forming more than one covalent bond at a time. In such instances the bond between these atoms is referred to as a double or a triple bond depending on whether there are two or three pairs of shared electrons, respectively.

Some molecules cannot fully be described by a single Lewis structure. For instance, for the carbonate ion: CO_3^{2-}, the octet rule is satisfied for the central carbon atom if one of the C...O bonds is double (*see* ORG

1.5). While this leads us to thinking that the three C...O bonds are not equivalent, every experimental evidence concerning this molecule show that the three bonds are the same (same length, same polarity, etc...). This suggests that in such instances a molecule cannot be described fully by a single Lewis structure. Indeed, since there is no particular reason to choose one oxygen atom over another we can write three equivalent Lewis structures for the previous ion. These three structures are called <u>resonance structures</u>. It is the full set of resonance structures that describe such a molecule. In this picture, the C...O bonds are neither double nor single, they have both a single and a double bond character. It is often interesting to compare the number of valence electrons that an atom possesses when it is isolated and when it is engaged in a covalent bond within a given molecule. This is often quantitatively described by the concept of <u>formal charge</u>. This concept is defined as follows:

total # of valence e⁻'s in the free atom
− total # of non-bonding e⁻'s in the molecule
− 1/2 (total # bonding e⁻'s) in the molecule
───────────────────────────────────────
= formal charge

Let us apply this definition to the two previous examples: H_2O and CO_3^{2-}. This process is fairly straightforward in the case of the water molecule:

total # of valence e⁻'s in free O: 6
− total # of non-bonding e⁻'s on O in H_2O: 4
− 1/2 (total # of bonding e⁻'s) on O in H_2O: 2
───────────────────────────────────────
Formal charge of O in H_2O = 0

The case of CO_3^{2-} ion is not as obvious. If we consider one of the equivalent resonance forms, for the oxygen with a double bond we have:

total # of valence e⁻'s in free O: 6
− total # of non-bonding e⁻'s on O in the ion: 4
− 1/2 (total # of bonding e⁻) on O in the ion: 2
───────────────────────────────────────
Formal charge of O of C=O in the ion = 0

Similarly, the calculation of the formal charge for O of C−O in the same ion leads to the following: $6 - 6 - 1/2(2) = -1$. Considering that CO_3^{2-} is represented by three resonance forms, the actual formal charge of the oxygen atom is $1/3 (-1 -1 + 0) = -2/3$. This number formally reflects the idea that the oxygen atoms are equivalent and that any one of them has a −1 charge in 2 out of three of the resonance forms of this ion. Here are some simple rules to remember about formal charges:

(i) For neutral molecules, the formal charges of all the atoms should add up to zero.

(ii) For an ion, the sum of the formal charges must equal the ion's charge.

The following rules should help you select a plausible Lewis structure:

(i) If you can write more than one Lewis structure for a given neutral molecule; the most plausible one is the one in which the formal charges of the individual atoms are zero.

(ii) Lewis stuctures with the smallest formal charges on each individual atom are more plausible than the ones that involve large formal charges.

(iii) Out of a range of possible Lewis structures for a given molecule, the most plausible ones are the ones in which negative formal charges are found on the most electronegative atoms and positive charges on the most electropositive ones.

In addition to these rules, remember that some elements have a tendency to form molecules that do not satisfy the octet rule:

(i) When sulfur is the central atom in a molecule or a polyatomic ion it almost invariably does not fulfill the octet rule. The number of electrons around S in these compounds is usually 12 (e.g. SF_6, SO_4^{2-}). This situation (expanded octets) also occurs in other elements in and beyond the third period.

(ii) Molecules that have an element from the 3A group (B, Al..) as their central atom do not generally obey the octet rule. In these molecules there are less than 8 electrons around the central atom (e.g. AlI_3 and BF_3).

(iii) Some molecules with an odd number of electrons can clearly not obey the octet rule (e.g. NO and NO_2).

3.3 Partial Ionic Character

Except for homonuclear molecules (molecules made of atoms of the same element, e.g. H_2, O_3, etc...), bonding electrons are not equally shared by the bonded atoms. Thus a diatomic (= *two atoms*) compound like Cl_2 shares its bonding electrons equally; whereas, a binary (= *two different elements*) compound like CaO (calcium oxide) or NaCl (sodium chloride) does not. Indeed, for the great majority of molecules, one of the two atoms between which the covalent bond occurs is necessarily more electronegative than the other. This atom will attract the bonding electrons to a larger extent. Although this phenomenon does not lead to the formation of two separate ionic species, it does result in a molecule in which there are partial charges on these particular atoms: the corresponding covalent bond is said to possess partial ionic character. This polar bond will also have a dipole moment given by:

$$D = q \cdot d$$

where q is the absolute value of the partial charge on the most electronegative or the most electropositive bonded atom and d is the distance between these two atoms. To obtain the total dipole moment of a molecule one must add the individual dipole moment vectors present on each one of its bonds. Since this is a vector addition, the overall result may

GENERAL CHEMISTRY

be zero even if the individual dipole moment vectors are very large.

Non-polar bonds are generally stronger than polar covalent and ionic bonds, with ionic bonds being the weakest. However, in compounds with ionic bonding, there is generally a large number of bonds between molecules and this makes the compound as a whole very strong. For instance, although the ionic bonds in one compound are weaker than the non-polar covalent bonds in another compound, the ionic compound's melting point will be higher than the melting point of the covalent compound. Polar covalent bonds have a partially ionic character, and thus the bond strength is usually intermediate between that of ionic and that of non-polar covalent bonds. The strength of bonds generally decreases with increasing ionic character.

3.4 Lewis Acids and Lewis Bases

In the previous section we pointed out some exceptions to Lewis' octet rule. Among these were molecules that had a deficiency of electrons around the central atom (e.g. BF_3). When such a molecule is put in contact with a molecule with lone pairs (e.g. NH_3) a reaction occurs. Such a reaction can be interpreted as a donation of a pair of electrons from the second type of molecule to the first, or alternately by an acceptance of a pair of electrons by the first type of molecule. Molecules such as BF_3 are referred to as Lewis acids while molecules such as NH_3 are Lewis bases. {LEwis Acids: Electron Acceptors}

What is the name of 007's northern cousin? Polar Bond.

3.5 Valence Shell Electronic Pair Repulsions (VSEPR Models)

One of the shortcommings of Lewis structures is that they cannot be used to predict molecular geometries. In this context a model known as the <u>valence-shell electronic pair repulsion or VSEPR model</u> is very useful. In this model, the geometrical arrangement of atoms or groups of atoms bound to a central atom A is determined by the number of pairs of valence electrons around A. VSEPR procedure is based on the principle that these electronic pairs around the central atom are arranged in such a way that the repulsions between them are minimized. The general VSEPR procedure starts with the determination of the number of electronic pairs around A:

$$
\begin{array}{l}
\text{\# of valence electrons in a free atom of A} \\
+\ \text{\# of sigma bonds involving A} \\
-\ \text{\# of pi bonds involving A} \\
\hline
=\ (\text{total \# of electrons around A})
\end{array}
$$

The division of this total number by 2 yields the total number of electron pairs around A. Note the following important points:

(i) A single bond counts for 1 sigma bond, a double bond for 1 sigma bond and 1 pi bond and a triple bond for 1 sigma and two pi bonds.

(ii) The general calculation presented above is performed for the purposes of VSEPR modelling; its result can be quite different from the one obtained in the corresponding Lewis structure.

(iii) For all practical purposes, one always assigns a double bond (i.e. 1 sigma bond and one pi bond) to a terminal oxygen (an oxygen which is not a central atom and is not attached to any other atom besides the central atom).

(iv) A terminal halogen is always assigned a single bond.

Once the number of pairs around the central atom is determined, the next step is to use Figure III.A.3.1 to predict the arrangement of these pairs around the central atom.

The next step is to consider the previous arrangement of the electronic pairs and place the atoms or groups of atoms that are attached to the central atom in accordance with such an arrangement. The pairs which are not involved in the bonding between these atoms and the central atom are lone pairs. If we substract the number of lone pairs from the total number of pairs we readily obtain the number of bonding pairs. It is the number of bonding pairs which ultimately determines the molecular geometry in the VSEPR model according to Table III.A.3.1. Let us consider three examples: CH_4, H_2O and CO_2.

1 – CH_4:

$$
\begin{array}{lr}
\text{\# of valence electrons on C:} & 4 \\
+\ \text{\# of sigma bonds:} & +4 \\
-\ \text{\# of pi bonds:} & -0 \\
\hline
 & = 8/2 = 4 \text{ pairs}
\end{array}
$$

According to Figure III.A.3.1 this corresponds to a tetrahedral arrangement. All of these pairs correspond to an H atom attached to the central atom of carbon. Therefore, the 4 pairs are bonding pairs and the molecular geometry is also tetrahedral.

2 – H_2O:

# of valence electrons on O:	6
+ # of sigma bonds on the central O:	+ 2
- # of pi bonds on the central O:	− 0
	= 8/2 = 4 pairs

3 – CO_2:

# of valence electrons on C:	4
+ # of sigma bonds for terminal O's:	+ 2
- # of pi bonds for terminal O's:	− 2
	= 4/2 = 2 pairs

This total number of pairs corresponds to a linear arrangement. Since both of these pairs are used to connect the central C atom to the terminal O's there are no lone pairs left on C. Therefore, the number of bonding pairs is also 2 and the molecular geometry is also linear.

Here are some additional rules when applying the VSEPR model:

(i) When dealing with a cation (<u>positive</u> ion) <u>subtract</u> the charge of the ion from the total number of electrons.

(ii) When dealing with an anion (<u>negative</u> ion) <u>add</u> the charge of the ion to the total number of electrons.

(iii) A lone pair repels another lone pair or a bonding pair very strongly. This causes some deformation in bond angles. For instance, the H–O–H angle is smaller than 109.5°.

(iv) The previous rule also holds for a double bond. Note that in one of our previous examples (CO_2), the angle is still 180° since there are two double bonds and no lone pairs. Indeed, in this geometry, the strong repulsions between the two double bonds are symmetrical.

(v) The VSEPR model can be applied to polyatomic molecules. The procedure is the same as above except that one can only determine the arrangements of groups of atoms around one given central atom at a time. For instance, you could apply the VSEPR model to determine the geometrical arrangements of atoms around C or around O in methanol (CH_3OH). In the first case the molecule is treated as CH_3 – X (where –X is –OH) and in the second it is treated as HO–Y (where –Y is –CH_3). The geometrical arrangement is tetrahedral in the first case which gives HCX or HCH angles close to 109°. The second case corresponds to a bent arrangement (with two lone pairs on the oxygen) and gives an HOY angle close to 109° as well.

Table III.A.3.1: Geometry of simple molecule in which the central atom A has one or more lone pairs of electrons (= e⁻).

Total number of e⁻ pairs	Number of lone pairs	Number of bonding pairs	Arrangement of e⁻ pairs	Geometry	Examples
3	1	2	Trigonal planar	Bent (sp^2)	SO_2
4	1	3	Tetrahedral	Trigonal pyramidal (sp^3)	NH_3
4	2	2	Tetrahedral	Bent (sp^3)	H_2O
5	1	4	Trigonal bipyramidal	Distorted tetrahedron (dsp^3)	SF_4
5	2	3	Trigonal bipyramidal	T-shaped (dsp^3)	ClF_3

Note: dotted lines only represent the overall molecular shape and not molecular bonds. In brackets under "Geometry" is the hybridization, to be discussed in ORG 1.2.

This also corresponds to a tetrahedral arrangement, however only two of these pairs are bonding pairs (connecting the H atoms to the central oxygen atom); therefore, the actual geometry according to Table III.A.3.1 is bent or V-shape geometry.

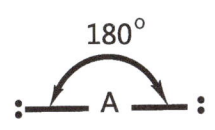

linear arrangement of 2 electron pairs around central atom A

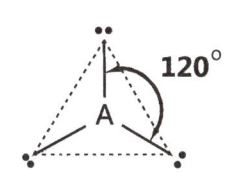

trigonal planar arrangement of 3 electron pairs around central atom A

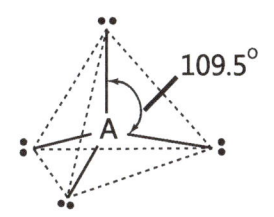

tetrahedral arrangement of 4 electron pairs around central atom A

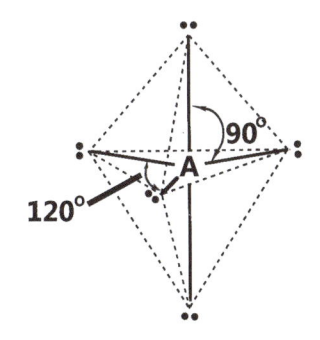

trigonal bipyramidal arrangement of 5 electron pairs around central atom A

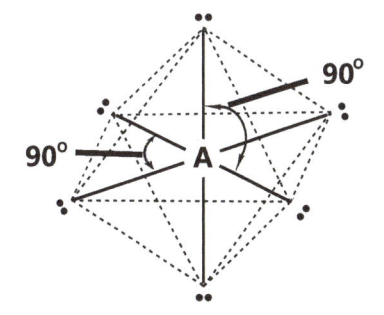

octahedral arrangement of 6 electron pairs around central atom A

Figure III.A.3.1: Molecular arrangement of electron pairs around a central atom A. Dotted lines only represent the overall molecular shape and not molecular bonds.

GOLD NOTES

PHASES AND PHASE EQUILIBRIA
Chapter 4

Memorize
Define: temp. (C, K), gas P and weight
Define: STP, ideal gas, deviation
Define: H bonds, dipole forces

Understand
* Kinetic molecular theory of gases
* Maxwell distribution plot, H bonds, dipole F.
* Deviation from ideal gas behavior
* Equations: ideal gas/Charles'/Boyle's
* Partial Press., mole fraction, Dalton's
* Intermolecular forces, phase change/diagrams

Not Required*
* Advanced level college info
* Memorizing Van der Waals' equation
* Memorizing the gas constant R
* Memorizing values: triple point of H_2O

GAMSAT-Prep.com

Introduction

A phase, or state of matter, is a uniform, distinct and usually separable region of material. For example, for a glass of water: the ice cubes are one phase (solid), the water is a second phase (liquid), and the humid air over the water is the third phase (gas = vapor). The temperature and pressure at which all 3 phases of a substance can coexist is called the triple point.

Additional Resources

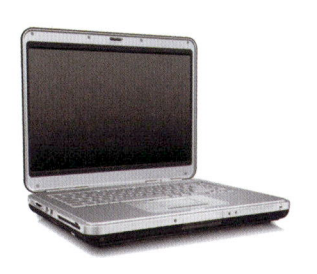

Free Online Q&A + Forum

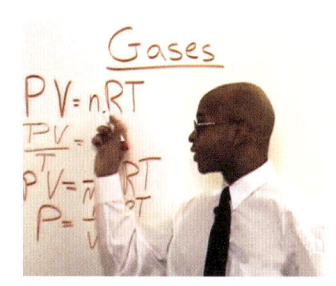

Video: Online or DVD 2

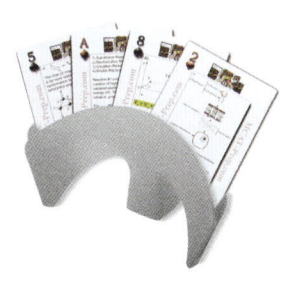

Flashcards

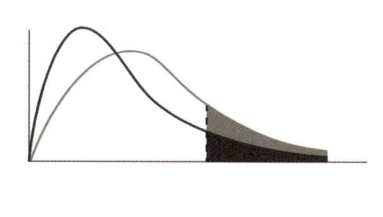

Special Guest

THE PHYSICAL SCIENCES CHM-35

* The real GAMSAT may have advanced level information presented (ie. in a passage) but previous knowledge of said information is not required to answer the questions that would follow. Practice ACER and GS practice GAMSATs can help you clarify this point.

GAMSAT-Prep.com
THE GOLD STANDARD

Elements and compounds exist in one of three states: <u>the gaseous state, the liquid state or the solid state</u>.

4.1 The Gas Phase

A substance in the gaseous state has neither fixed volume nor fixed shape: it spreads itself <u>uniformly</u> throughout any container in which it is placed.

4.1.1 Standard Temperature and Pressure, Standard Molar Volume

Any given gas can be described in terms of four fundamental properties: mass, volume, temperature and pressure. To simplify comparisons, the volume of a gas is normally reported at 0°C (273.15 K) and 1 atm (101.33 kPa = 760 mmHg = 760 torr); these conditions are known as the <u>standard temperature and pressure (STP)</u>.

> The volume occupied by one mole of any gas at STP is referred to as the <u>standard molar volume</u> and is equal to 22.4 l.

4.1.2 Kinetic Molecular Theory of Gases

The <u>kinetic molecular theory of gases</u> describes the behavior of matter in the gaseous state. A gas that fits this theory exactly is called an <u>ideal gas</u>. The essential points of the theory are as follows:

1. Gases are composed of <u>extremely small</u> molecules separated by distances that are relatively large in comparison with the diameters of the molecules.

2. Molecules of gas are in <u>constant motion</u>, except when they collide with one another.

3. Molecules of an <u>ideal gas</u> exert no attractive or repulsive force on one another.

4. The collisions experienced by gas molecules do not, on the average, slow them down; rather, they cause a <u>change</u> in the direction in which the molecules are moving. If one molecule loses energy as a result of a collision, the energy is gained by the molecule with which it collides. <u>Collisions</u> of the molecules of an ideal gas with the walls of the container <u>result in no loss of energy</u>.

5. The average kinetic energy of the molecules (KE = 1/2 mv²) increases in direct proportion to the temperature of the gas (KE = 3/2 kT) when the temperature is measured on an absolute scale (i.e. the Kelvin scale) and k is a constant (the Boltzmann constant).

The plot of the distribution of collision energies of gases is similar to that of liquids. However, molecules in liquids require a minimum escape kinetic energy in order to enter the vapor phase.

The properties of gases can be explained in terms of the kinetic molecular theory of ideal gases.

Experimentally, we can measure four properties of a gas:

1. The weight of the gas, from which we can calculate the number (N) of molecules of the gas present;

2. The pressure (P), exerted by the gas on the walls of the container in which this gas is placed (N.B.: a vacuum is completely devoid of particles and thus has *no* pressure);

3. The volume (V), occupied by the gas;

4. The temperature (T) of the gas.

In fact, if we know any three of these properties, we can calculate the fourth. So the minimum number of these properties required to fully describe the state of an ideal gas is three.

$T_2 > T_1$

Total fraction (shaded area) is larger at the higher temperature

Minimum escape K.E.

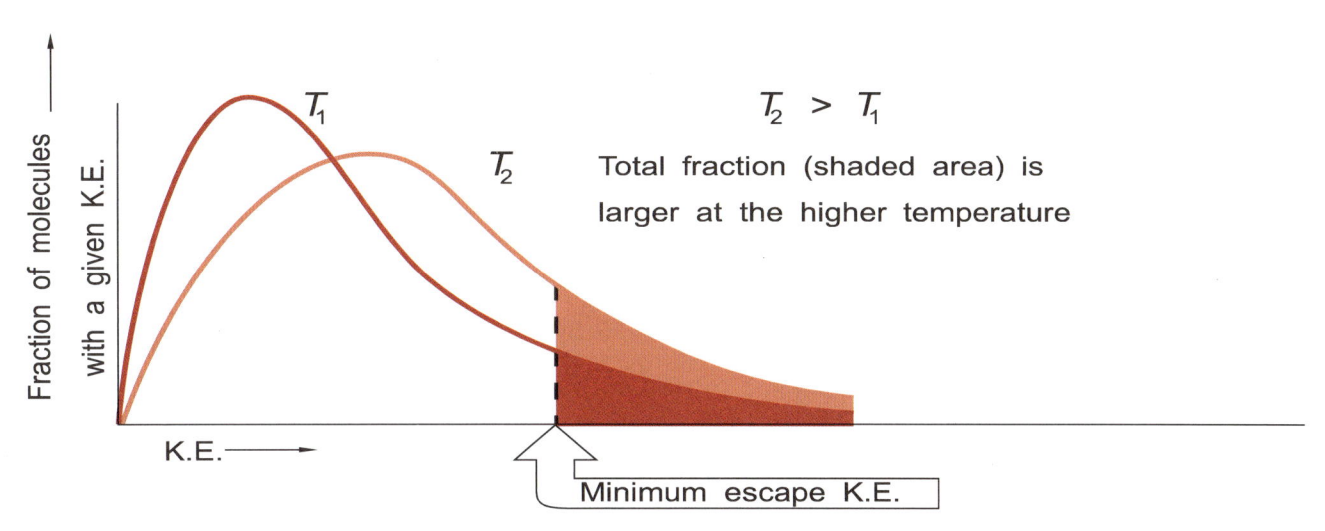

Figure III.A.4.1: The Maxwell Distribution Plot.

THE PHYSICAL SCIENCES   CHM-37

GAMSAT-Prep.com
THE GOLD STANDARD

4.1.3 Charles' Law

The volume (V) of a gas is directly proportional to the absolute temperature (expressed in Kelvins) when P and N are kept constant.

$$V = \text{Constant} \times T \quad \text{or} \quad V_1/V_2 = T_1/T_2$$

4.1.4 Boyle's Law

The volume (V) of a fixed weight of gas held at constant temperature (T) varies inversely with the pressure (P).

$$V = \text{Constant} \times 1/P \quad \text{or} \quad P_1V_1 = P_2V_2$$

4.1.5 Combined Gas Law

For a given mass of gas the product of its pressure and volume divided by its Kelvin temperature is a constant.

$$\frac{P_1V_1}{T_1} = \frac{P_2V_2}{T_2}$$

(at constant mass)

4.1.6 Ideal Gas Law

The combination of Boyle's law and Charles' law yields the ideal gas law:

$$PV = nRT$$

where R is the <u>universal gas constant</u> and n is the number moles of gas molecules.

R = 0.0821 L-atm/K-mole
 = 8.31 kPa-dm³/K-mole

A typical ideal gas problem is: an ideal gas at 27 °C and 380 torr occupies a volume of 492 cm³. What is the number of moles of gas?

<u>Ideal Gas Law problems often amount to mere exercises of unit conversions. The easiest way to do them is to convert the units of the values given to the units of the R gas constant.</u>

CHM-38   PHASES AND PHASE EQUILIBRIA

$$P = 380 \text{ torr} = \frac{380 \text{ torr}}{(760 \text{ torr/atm})}$$

$$= 0.500 \text{ atm}$$

$$T = 27\,°C = 273 + 27\,°C = 300 \text{ K}$$

$$V = 492 \text{ cm}^3 = 492 \text{ cm}^3 \times (1 \text{ liter}/1000 \text{cm}^3)$$

$$= 0.492 \text{ liter}$$

$$PV = nRT$$

$$n = PV/RT$$

$$n = \frac{(0.500 \text{ atm} \times 0.492 \text{ L})}{(0.0821 \text{ L-atm/K-mole} \times 300 \text{ K})}$$

$$n = 0.0100 \text{ mole}$$

Also note that the ideal gas law could be used in the following alternate ways (Mwt = molecular weight):

(i) since n = (mass m of gas sample)/(Mwt M of the gas)

$$PV = (m/M)RT$$

(ii) since m/V is the density d of the gas:

$$P = \frac{dRT}{M}$$

4.1.7 Partial Pressure and Dalton's Law

In a mixture of unreactive gases, each gas distributes evenly throughout the container. All molecules exert the same pressure on the walls of the container with equal force. If we consider a mixture of gases occupying a total volume (V) at a temperature (T) the term <u>partial</u> pressure is used to refer to the pressure exerted by one component of the gas mixture if it were occupying the entire volume (V) at the temperature (T).

<u>Dalton's law</u> states that the total pressure observed for a mixture of gases is equal to the sum of the pressures that each individual component would exert were it alone in the container.

$$P_T = P_1 + P_2 + \ldots + P_i$$

where P_T is the total pressure and P_i is the partial pressure of any component (i).

The mole fraction (X_i) of any one gas present in a mixture is defined as follows:

$$X_i = n_i/n_{(total)}$$

where n_i = moles of that gas present in the mixture and $n_{(total)}$ = sum of the moles of all gases present in the mixture.

Of course, the sum of all mole fractions in a mixture must equal one:

$$\Sigma X_i = 1$$

The partial pressure (Pi) of a component of a gas mixture is equal to:

$$P_i = X_i PT$$

The ideal gas law applies to any component of the mixture:

$$P_i V = n_i RT$$

4.1.8 Deviation of Real Gas Behavior from the Ideal Gas Law

The molecules of an ideal gas have zero volume and no inter-molecular forces. It obeys the ideal gas law. Its molecules behave as though they were moving points exerting no attraction on one another and occupying no space. Real gases deviate from ideal gas behavior as follows:

1. They do not obey $PV = nRT$. We can calculate n, P, V and T for a real gas on the assumption that it behaves like an ideal gas but the calculated values will not agree with the observed values.

2. Their molecules are subject to van der Waal attraction forces which are themselves independent of temperature. But the deviations they cause are more pronounced at low temperatures because they are less effectively opposed by the slower motion of molecules at lower temperatures. Similarly, an increase in pressure at constant temperature will crowd the molecules closer together and reduce the average distance between them. This will increase the attractive force between the molecules and the stronger these forces, the more the behavior of the real gas will deviate from that of an ideal gas. Thus, a real gas will act less like an ideal gas at higher pressures than at lower pressures. {Mnemonic: an ideal Plow and Thigh = an ideal gas exists when Pressure is low and Temperature is high}

3. The particles (i.e. molecules or atoms) occupy space. When a real gas is subjected to high pressures at ordinary temperatures, the fraction of the total volume occupied by the molecules increases. Under these conditions, the real gas deviates appreciably from ideal gas behavior.

4. Their size and mass also affect the speed at which they move. At constant temperature, the kinetic energy ($KE = 1/2\ mv^2$) of all molecules – light or heavy – is nearly the same. This means that the heavier molecules must be moving more slowly than the lighter ones and that the attractive forces between the heavier molecules must be exercising a greater influence on

their behavior. The greater speed of light molecules, however, tends to counteract the attractive forces between them, thus producing a slighter deviation from ideal gas behavior. Thus, a heavier molecule will deviate more widely from ideal gas behavior than a lighter molecule. {The preceding is given by Graham's law, where the rate of movement of a gas (*diffusion* or streaming through a fine hole - *effusion*) is inversely proportional to the square root of the molecular weight of the gas.}

4.2 Liquid Phase (Intra- and Intermolecular Forces)

The most striking properties of a liquid are its viscosity and surface tension (*see Physics section 6.1*). Liquids also distinguish themselves from gases in that they are relatively incompressible. The molecules of a liquid are also subject to forces strong enough to hold them together. These forces are intermolecular and they are weak attractive forces, that is they are effective over short distances only. They are also called Van der Waal forces. The most important ones are:

1. Dipole-dipole forces which depend on the orientation as well as on the distance between the molecules; they are inversely proportional to the fourth power of the distance. In addition to the forces between permanent dipoles, a dipolar molecule induces in a neighboring molecule an electron distribution that results in another attractive force, the dipole-induced dipole force, which is inversely proportional to the seventh power of the distance and which is relatively independent of orientation.

2. London forces are attractive forces acting between nonpolar molecules. They are due to the unsymmetrical instantaneous electron distribution which induces a dipole in neighboring molecules with a resultant attractive force.

3. Hydrogen bonds occur whenever hydrogen is covalently bonded to an atom such as O, N or F that attract electrons strongly. Because of the differences in electronegativity between H and O or N or F, the electrons that constitute the covalent bond are closer to the O, N or F nucleus than to the H nucleus leaving the latter relatively unshielded. The unshielded proton is strongly attracted to the O, N or F atoms of neighboring molecules since these form the negative end of a strong dipole. Hydrogen bonding is a special case of dipole-dipole interaction.

GAMSAT-Prep.com
THE GOLD STANDARD

4.3 Phase Equilibria (Solids, Liquids and Gases)

4.3.1 Phase Changes

Elements and compounds can undergo transitions between the solid, liquid and gaseous states. They can exist in different <u>phases</u> and undergo <u>phase changes</u> which need not involve chemical reactions. A phase is a homogeneous, physically distinct and mechanically separable part of a system. Each phase is separated from other phases by a physical boundary.

A few examples:

1. Ice/liquid water/water vapor (3 phases)

2. Any number of gases mix in all proportions and therefore constitute just one phase.

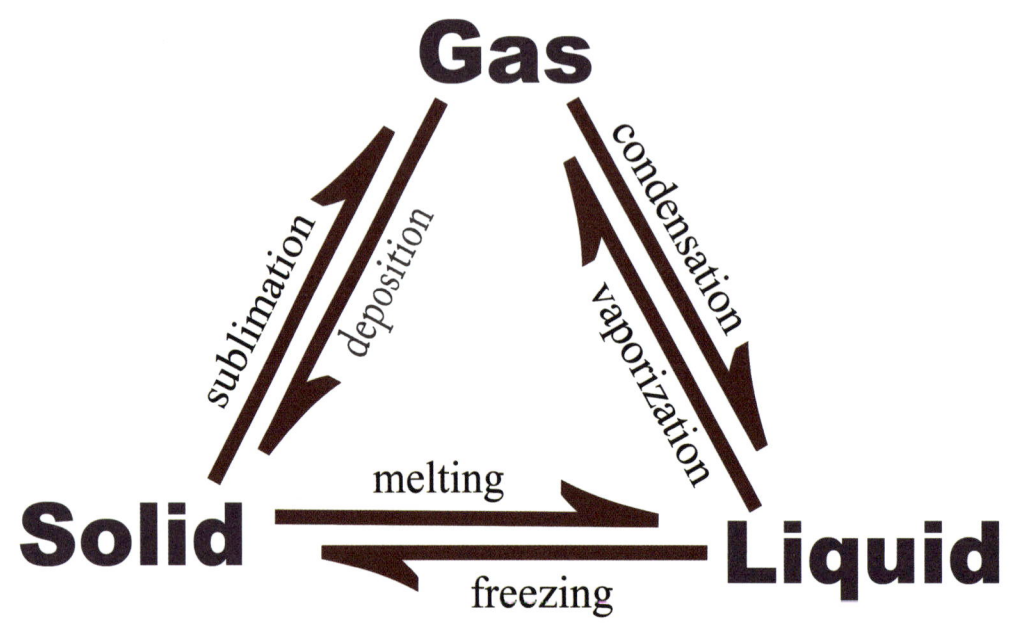

Figure III.A.4.2: Phase Changes

GENERAL CHEMISTRY

3. The system CaCO$_3$ → CaO + CO$_2$ (2 phases, i.e. 2 solids: CaCO$_3$ and CaO and a gas: CO$_2$)

4. A saturated salt solution (3 phases: solution, undissolved salt, vapor)

An example of phase change is the vaporization of water into its vapor state. A system is considered <u>homogeneous</u> when it is uniform throughout its volume so that its properties are the same in all parts. This does not imply a single molecular species: a solution of sodium chloride is homogeneous provided its concentration is the same throughout.

4.3.2 Freezing Point, Melting Point, Boiling Point

The conversion of a liquid to a gas is called <u>vaporization</u>. We can increase the rate of vaporization of a liquid by i) increasing the temperature ii) reducing the pressure, or iii) both. Molecules escape from a liquid because, even though their average kinetic energy is constant, not all of them move at the same speed (*see Figure III.A.4.1*). A fast-moving molecule can break away from the attraction of the others and pass into the vapor state. When a tight lid is placed on a vessel containing a liquid, the vapor molecules can not escape and some revert back to the liquid state. The number of molecules leaving the liquid at any given time equals the number of molecules returning. Equilibrium is reached and the number of molecules in the fixed volume above the liquid remains constant. These molecules exert a constant pressure at a fixed temperature which is called the <u>vapor pressure</u> of the liquid.

Boiling and evaporation are similar processes but they differ as follows: the vapor from a boiling liquid escapes with sufficient pressure to push back any other gas present, rather than diffusing through it. The <u>boiling point</u> of a liquid is the temperature at which the vapor pressure of the liquid equals the opposing pressure (atmospheric, thus it is usually air). Under a lower pressure, the boiling point is reached at a lower temperature. Increased intermolecular interactions (i.e. H$_2$O *see* CHM 4.2, alcohol *see* ORG 6.1, etc.) will decrease the vapor pressure thus raising the boiling point. Other factors being equal, as a molecule becomes heavier (increasing molecular weight), it becomes more difficult to push the molecule into the atmosphere thus the boiling point increases (i.e. alkanes *see* ORG 3.1.1). The <u>freezing point</u> of a liquid is the temperature at which the vapor pressure of the solid equals the vapor pressure of the liquid. Increases in the prevailing atmospheric pressure decreases the melting point and increases the boiling point.

When a solid is heated, the kinetic energy of the components increases steadily. Finally, the kinetic energy becomes great enough to overcome the forces holding the components together and the solid changes to a liquid. For pure crystalline solids, there is a fixed temperature at which this transition from solid to liquid occurs. This temperature is called the melting point. Pure solids melt completely at one temperature. Impure solids begin to melt at one temperature but become completely liquid at a higher temperature.

4.3.3 Phase Diagrams

The temperatures at which phase transitions occur are functions of the pressure of the system. The behavior of a given substance over a wide range of temperature and pressure can be summarized in a phase diagram, such as the one shown for the water system (Fig. III.A.4.3).

The diagram is divided into three areas labelled **solid** (ice), **liquid** (water) and **vapor** in each of which only one phase exists. In these areas, P and T can be independently varied without a second phase appearing. These areas are bounded by curves AC, AD and AB. At any point on these curves, two phases are in equilibrium. Thus on AC, at a given T, the saturated vapor pressure of water has a fixed value. The boiling point of water (N) can be found on this curve, 100 °C at 760 mmHg pressure. The curve only extends as far as C, the critical point, where the vapor and liquid are indistinguishable.

GENERAL CHEMISTRY

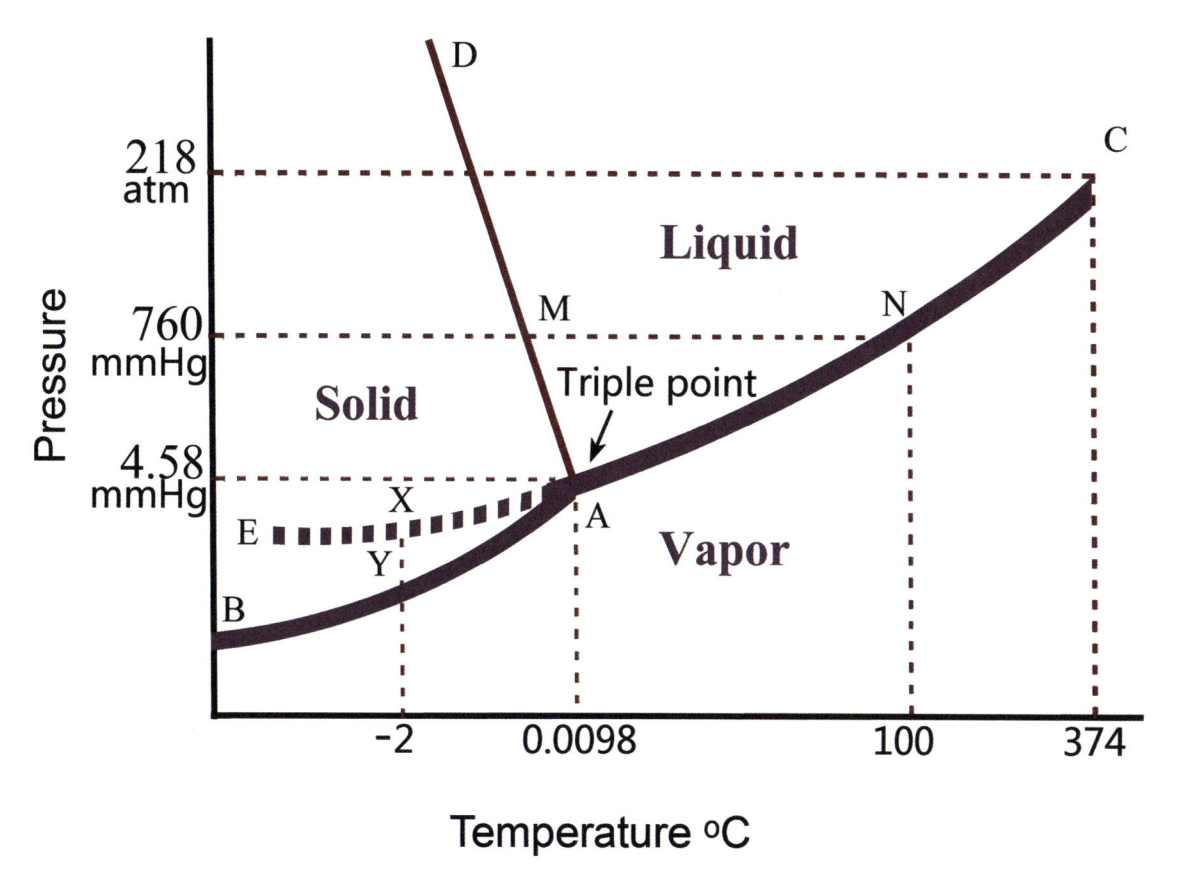

Figure III.A.4.3: Phase diagram for H$_2$O.

The extension of the curve CA to E represents the metastable equilibrium (*meta* = beyond) between supercooled water and its vapor. If the temperature is slightly raised at point X, a little of the liquid will vaporize until a new equilibrium is established at that higher temperature. Curve AB is the vapor pressure curve for ice. Its equilibria are of lower energy than those of AE and thus more stable.

The slope of line AD shows that an increase in P will lower the melting point of ice. This property is almost unique to water. Most substances *increase* their melting points with increased pressure. Thus the line AD slants to the right for almost all substances. Point M represents the true melting point of ice, 0.0023 °C at 760 mmHg of pressure. (The 0 °C standard refers to the freezing point of water saturated with air at 760 mmHg). At point A, solid, liquid and vapor are in equilibrium. At this one temperature, ice and water have the same fixed vapor pressure. This is the triple point, 0.0098 °C at 4.58 mmHg pressure.

THE PHYSICAL SCIENCES   CHM-45

GOLD NOTES

SOLUTION CHEMISTRY

Chapter 5

Memorize
- efine saturated, supersaturated,
- nvolatile
- ommon anions and cations in solution
- nits of concentration
- efine electrolytes with examples

Understand
* Colligative properties, Raoult's law
* Phase diagram change due to coll. properties
* Bp elevation, fp depression
* Osmotic press, equation
* Solubility product, common-ion effect

Not Required*
* Advanced level college info
* % solubility of glucose in water

GAMSAT-Prep.com

Introduction

A solution is a homogeneous mixture composed of two or more substances. For example, a solute (salt) dissolved in a solvent (water) making a solution (salt water). Solutions can involve gases in liquids (i.e. oxygen in water) or even solids in solids (i.e. alloys). Two substances are immiscible if they can't mix to make a solution. Solutions can be distinguished from non-homogeneous mixtures like colloids and suspensions.

Additional Resources

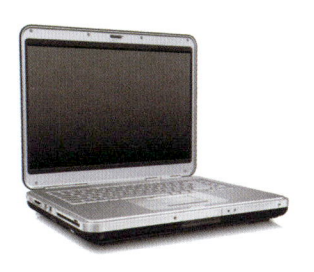

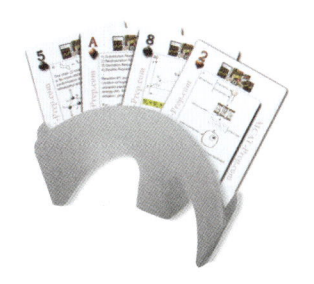

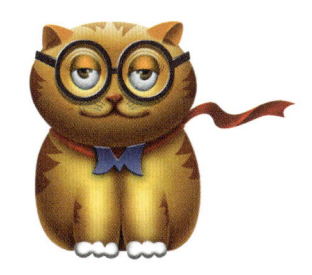

Free Online Q&A + Forum   Video: Online or DVD 2, 3   Flashcards   Special Guest

THE PHYSICAL SCIENCES   CHM-47

The real GAMSAT may have advanced level information presented (ie. in a passage) but previous knowledge of said information is not required to answer the questions that would follow. Practice ACER and GS practice GAMSATs can help you clarify this point.

5.1 Colligative Properties

The previous section refers to a one-component system, i.e. a pure substance, H₂O. Pure substances are often mixed together to form solutions. A solution is a sample of matter that is homogeneous but, unlike a pure substance, the composition of a solution can vary within relatively wide limits. Ethanol and water each have a fixed composition, C_2H_5OH and H_2O, but mixtures of the two can vary continuously in composition from almost 100% ethanol to almost 100% water. Solutions of sucrose in water, however, are limited to a maximum percentage of sucrose - the solubility - which is 67% at 20°C, thus the solution is saturated. If the solution is heated, a higher concentration of glucose can be achieved (i.e. 70%). Slowly cooling down to 20°C creates a supersaturated solution which may precipitate with any perturbation.

Generally the component of a solution that is stable in the same phase as the solution is called the solvent. If both components of a solution are in the same phase, the component present in the larger amount is called the solvent and the other is called the solute. Many properties of solutions are dependent only on the relative number of molecules (or ions) of the solute and of the solvent. Properties that depend **only** on the number of particles present are called colligative properties. The most important ones follow.

5.1.1 Vapor-Pressure Lowering (Raoult's Law)

The vapor pressure of the components of an ideal solution behaves as follows:

$$p_i = X_i (p_i)_{pure}$$

where p_i = vapor pressure of component *i* in equilibrium with the solution
$(p_i)_{pure}$ = vapor pressure of pure component *i* at the same T
X_i = mole fraction of component *i* in the liquid.

Thus the vapor pressure of any component of a mixture is lowered by the presence of the other components. Experimentally, it can be observed that when dissolving a solute which cannot evaporate (= *nonvolatile*) in a solvent, the vapor pressure of the resulting solution is lower than that of the pure solvent. The extent to which the vapor pressure is lowered is determined by the mole fraction of the solvent in solution (X):

$$P = P°X$$

where P = vapor pressure of solution
$P°$ = vapor pressure of pure solvent (at the same temperature as P).

When rearranged this way, Raoult's law states that the lowering of the vapor pressure of the solvent is proportional to the mole fraction of solvent and independent of the chemical nature of the solute.

5.1.2 Boiling-Point Elevation and Freezing-Point Depression

When the vapor-pressure curve of a dilute solution and the vapor-pressure curve of the pure solvent are plotted on a phase diagram, it can be seen that the freezing point and boiling point of a solution must be different from those of the pure liquid.

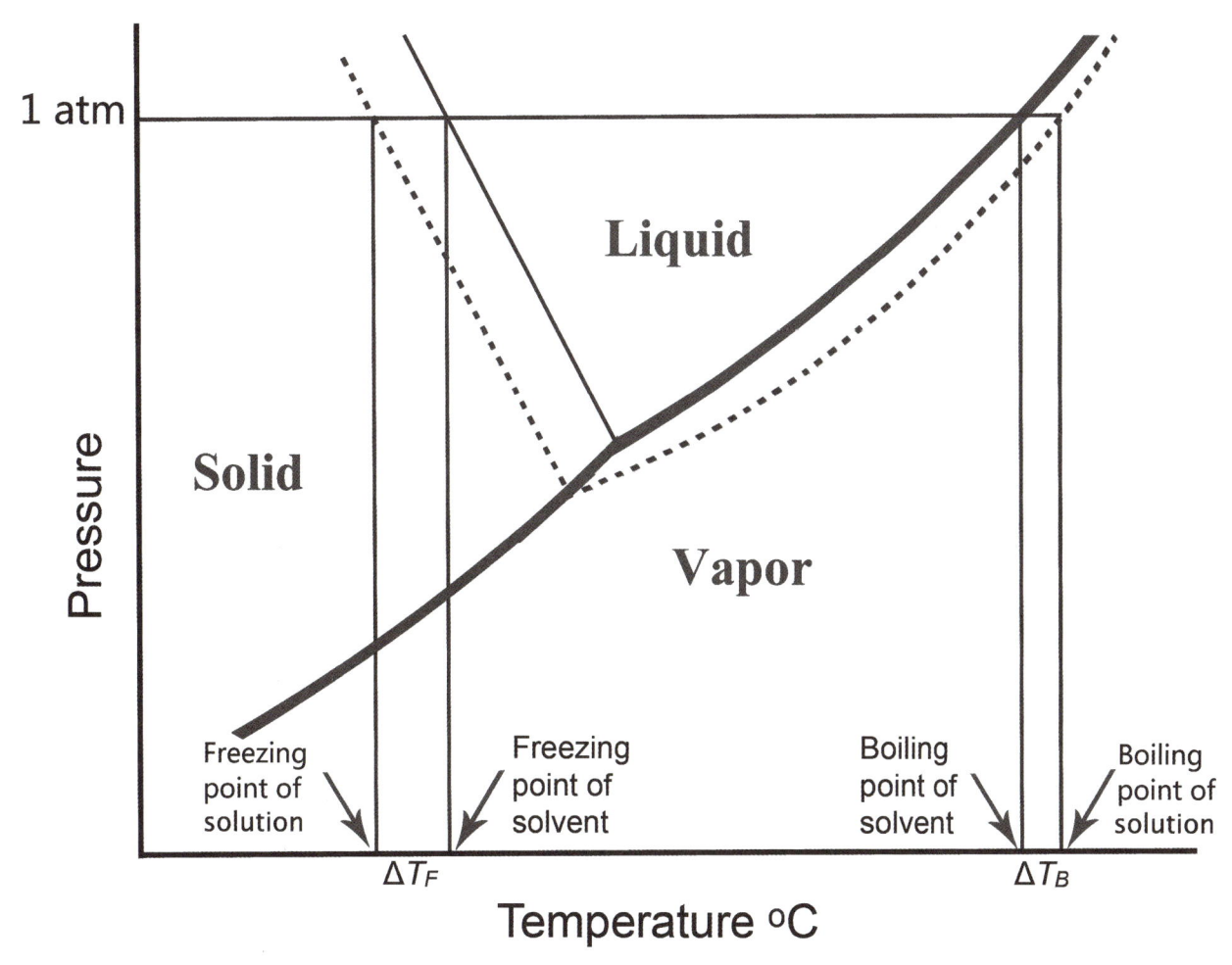

Figure III.A.5.1: Phase diagram of water demonstrating the effect of the addition of a solute.

The boiling point is higher for the solution than for the pure liquid. The freezing point is lower for the solution than for the pure liquid. Since the decrease in vapor pressure is proportional to the mole fraction of solute, the boiling point elevation (ΔT_B) is also proportional to the mole fraction of solute and:

$$\Delta T_B = K_B' X_B = K_B m$$

where K_B' = boiling point elevation constant for the solvent
X_B = mole fraction of solute
m = <u>molality</u> (moles solute per kilogram of solvent)

K_B is related to K_B' through a change of units.

Similarly, for the freezing point depression (ΔT_F):

$$\Delta T_F = K_F' X_B = K_F m$$

where K_F' = freezing point depression constant for the solvent.

If K_F or K_B is known, it is possible to determine the molality of a dilute solution simply by measuring the freezing point or the boiling point. These constants can be determined by measuring the freezing point and boiling point of a solution of known molality. If the mass concentration of a solute (in kg solute per kg of solvent) is known and the molality is determined from the freezing point of the solution, the mass of 1 mole of solute can be calculated.

It is important to note that for a solution of strong electrolyte such as NaCl which dissociates to give positive and negative ions, the right hand side is multiplied by a factor "n" equal to the number of ionic species generated per mole of solute. For NaCl n = 2 but for $MgCl_2$ n = 3. {Remember: colligative properties depend on the **number** of particles present}

5.1.3 Osmotic Pressure

The osmotic pressure (Π) of a solution describes the equilibrium distribution of solvent across membranes. When a solvent and solution are separated by a membrane permeable only to molecules of solvent (a <u>semipermeable</u> membrane), solvent spontaneously migrates into the solution. The semipermeable membrane allows the solvent to pass but not the solute. The solvent migrates into the solution across the membrane until a sufficient hydrostatic pressure develops to prevent further migration of solvent. The pressure required to prevent migration of the solvent is defined as the <u>osmotic pressure</u> of the solution and is equal to:

$$\Pi = CRT$$

where R = gas constant per mole,
T = temperature in degrees K and
C = concentration of solute (mole/liter).

GENERAL CHEMISTRY

5.2 Ions in Solution

An important area of solution chemistry involves aqueous solutions. Water has a property that causes many substances to split apart into charged species, that is, to dissociate and form ions. Ions that are positively charged are called cations and negatively charged ions are called anions. {Mnemonic: anions are negative ions} As a rule, highly charged species (i.e. AlPO$_4$, Al^{3+}/PO$_4^{3-}$) have a greater force of attraction thus are much less soluble in water than species with little charge (i.e. NaCl, Na$^+$/Cl$^-$). The word "aqueous" simply means containing or dissolved in water. All the following ions can form in water.

Common Anions

F$^-$	Fluoride	OH$^-$	Hydroxide
Cl$^-$	Chloride	NO$_3^-$	Nitrate
Br$^-$	Bromide	ClO$_4^-$	Perchlorate
I$^-$	Iodide	CO$_3^{2-}$	Carbonate
O^{2-}	Oxide	SO$_4^{2-}$	Sulfate
S^{2-}	Sulfide	PO$_4^{3-}$	Phosphate
N^{3-}	Nitride	CH$_3$CO$_2^-$	Acetate

Common Cations

Na$^+$	Sodium	H$^+$	Hydrogen
Li$^+$	Lithium	Ca^{2+}	Calcium
K$^+$	Potassium	Mg^{2+}	Magnesium
NH$_4^+$	Ammonium	Fe^{2+}	Iron (II)
H$_3$O$^+$	Hydronium	Fe^{3+}	Iron (III)

Table III.A.5.1: Common Anions and Cations. ACER does not normally ask Inorganic Chemistry nomenclature (= *naming*) questions but it may be useful to know the International Union of Pure and Applied Chemistry (IUPAC) standard suffixes: (1) Single atom anions are named with an *-ide* suffix (i.e. fluoride); (2) Oxyanions (*polyatomic* or "many atom" anions containing oxygen) are named with *-ite* or *-ate*, for a lesser or greater quantity of oxygen. For example, NO$_2^-$ is nitrite, while NO$_3^-$ is nitrate; (3) -ium is a very common ending of atoms in the periodic table (CHM 2.3) and it is also common among cations; (4) Compounds with cations: The name of the compound is simply the cation's name (usually the same as the element's), followed by the anion. For example, NaCl is *sodium chloride*.

5.3 Solubility

5.3.1 Units of Concentration

There are a number of ways in which solution concentrations may be expressed.

Molarity (*M*): A one-molar solution is defined as one mole of substance in each liter of solution: M = moles of solute/liter of solution.

Normality (*N*): A one-normal solution contains one equivalent per liter. An equivalent is a mole multiplied by the number of reacting units for each molecule or atom: the equivalent weight is the formula weight divided by the number of reacting units.

$$\begin{aligned}\text{\# of Equiv.} &= \text{mass (in g)/eq. wt. (in g/equiv.)} \\ &= \text{Normality (in equiv./liter)} \\ &\quad \times \text{Volume (in liters)}\end{aligned}$$

For example, sulfuric acid, H_2SO_4, has two reacting units of protons, that is, there are two equivalents of protons in each mole. Thus:

$$\begin{aligned}\text{eq. wt.} &= 98.08 \text{ g/mole}/2 \text{ equiv./mole} \\ &= 49.04 \text{ g/equiv.}\end{aligned}$$

and the normality of a sulfuric acid solution is twice its molarity. Generally speaking:

$$N = n\,M$$

where *N* is the normality,
       M the molarity,
       n the number of equivalents per unit formula.

Thus for 1.2 M H_2SO_4:

1.2 moles/L × 2 eq/mole = 2.4 eq/L = 2.4 N.

Molality (*m*): A one-molal solution contains one mole/1000g of solvent.

m = moles of solute/kg of solvent.

Molal concentrations are not temperature-dependent as molar and normal concentrations are (since the solvent volume is temperature-dependent).

Density (ρ): Mass per unit volume at the specified temperature, usually g/ml or g/cm³ at 20°C.

Osmole (*Osm*): The number of moles of particles (molecules or ions) that contribute to the osmotic pressure of a solution.

Osmolarity: A one-osmolar solution is defined as one osmole in each liter of solution. Osmolarity is measured in osmoles/liter of solution (Osm/L).

For example, a 0.001 *M* solution of sodium chloride has an osmolarity of 0.002 Osm/L (twice the molarity), because each NaCl molecule ionizes in water to form two ions (Na⁺ and Cl⁻) that both contribute to the osmotic pressure.

Osmolality: A one-osmolal solution is defined as one osmole in each kilogram of solution. Osmolality is measured in osmoles/kilogram of solution (Osm/kg).

For example, the osmolality of a 0.01 molal solution of Na_2SO_4 is 0.03 Osm/kg because each molecule of Na_2SO_4 ionizes in water to give three ions (2 Na^+ and 1 SO_4^{2-}) that contribute to the osmotic pressure.

5.3.2 Solubility Product Constant, the Equilibrium Expression

Any solute that dissolves in water to give a solution that contains ions, and thus can conduct electricity, is an *electrolyte*. The solid (s) that dissociates into separate ions surrounded by water is hydrated, thus the ions are aqueous (*aq*).

If dissociation is extensive, we have a strong electrolyte:

$$NaCl\ (s) \rightarrow Na^+\ (aq) + Cl^-\ (aq)$$

If dissociation is incomplete, we have a weak electrolyte:

$$CH_3COOH\ (aq) \rightleftharpoons CH_3COO^-\ (aq) + H^+\ (aq)$$

Strong electrolytes: salts (NaCl), strong acids (HCl), strong bases (NaOH).

Weak electrolytes: weak acids (CH_3COOH), weak bases (NH_3), complexes ($Fe[CN]_6$), water, soluble organic compounds (sugar), highly charged species (CHM 5.2; $AlPO_4$, $BaSO_4$, *exception*: AgCl).

When substances have limited solubility and their solubility is exceeded, the ions of the dissolved portion exist in equilibrium with the solid material. When a compound is referred to as insoluble, it is not completely insoluble, but is slightly soluble.

For example, if solid AgCl is added to water, a small portion will dissolve:

$$AgCl\ (s) \rightleftharpoons Ag^+\ (aq) + Cl^-\ (aq)$$

The precipitate will have a definite solubility (i.e. a definite amount in g/liter or moles/liter that will dissolve at a given temperature). An overall equilibrium constant can be written for the above equilibrium, called the solubility product, K_{sp}, given by the following equilibrium expression:

$$K_{sp} = [Ag^+][Cl^-]$$

The preceding relationship holds regardless of the presence of any undissociated intermediate. In general, each concentration must be raised to the power of that ion's coefficient in the dissolving equation (in our example = 1). A different example would be Ag_2S which would have the following solubility product expression: $K_{sp} = [Ag^+]^2[S^{2-}]$. The calculation of solubility s in mol/L for AgCl would simply be: $K_{sp} = [s][s] = s^2$. On the other hand, the expression for Ag_2S would become: $K_{sp} = [2s]^2[s] = 4s^3$. Knowing

GAMSAT-Prep.com
THE GOLD STANDARD

K_{sp} at a specified temperature, the solubility of compounds can be calculated under various conditions. The amount of slightly soluble salt that dissolves does not depend on the amount of the solid in equilibrium with the solution, as long as there is enough to saturate the solution. Rather, it depends on the volume of solvent. {Note: a low K_{sp} value means little product therefore low solubility and vice-versa}

5.3.3 Common-ion Effect

If there is an excess of one ion over the other, the concentration of the other is suppressed. This is called the <u>common ion effect</u>. The solubility of the precipitate is decreased and the concentration can still be calculated from the K_{sp}.

For example, Cl⁻ ion can be precipitated out of a solution of AgCl by adding a slight excess of $AgNO_3$. If a stoichiometric amount of $AgNO_3$ is added, [Ag⁺] = [Cl⁻]. If excess $AgNO_3$ is added, [Ag⁺] > [Cl⁻] but K_{sp} remains constant. Therefore, [Cl⁻] decreases if [Ag⁺] is increased. Because the K_{sp} product always holds, precipitation will not take place unless the product of [Ag⁺] and [Cl⁻] exceeds the K_{sp}. If the product is just equal to K_{sp}, all the Ag⁺ and Cl⁻ ions would remain in solution.

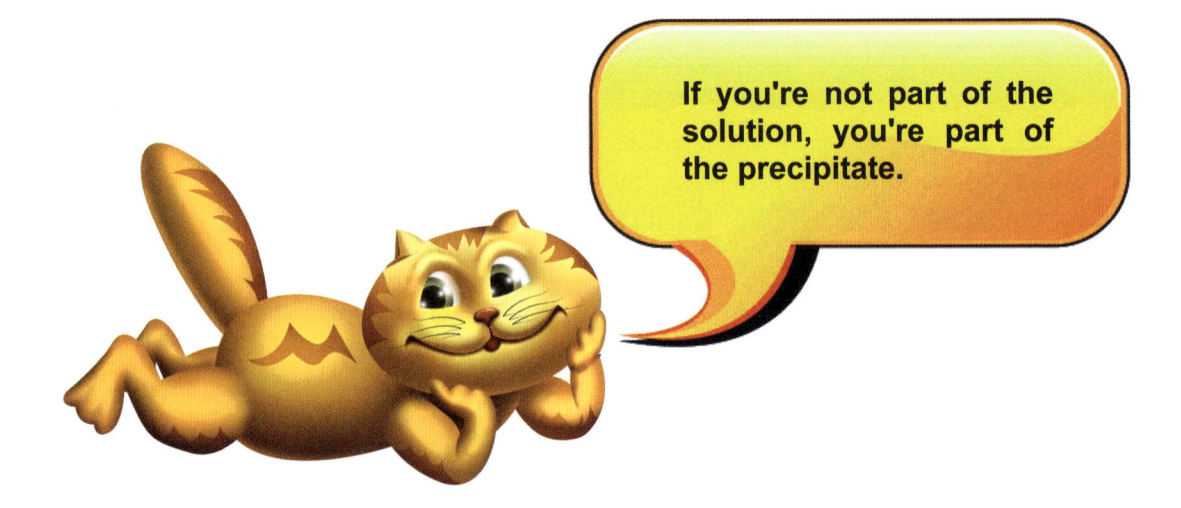

If you're not part of the solution, you're part of the precipitate.

CHM-54   SOLUTION CHEMISTRY

GOLD NOTES

GOLD NOTES

ACIDS AND BASES

Chapter 6

Memorize	Understand	Not Required*
ine: Bronsted acid, base, pH mples of strong/weak acids/bases at STP, neutral H₂O pH, conjugate d/base, zwitterions uations: K_a, K_b, pK_a, pK_b, K_w, pH, pOH uivalence point, indicator, rules of arithms	* Calculation of K_a, K_b, pK_a, pK_b, K_w, pH, pOH * Calculations involving strong/weak acids/bases * Salts of weak acids/bases, buffers; indicators * Acid-Base titration/curve, redox titration	* Advanced level college info * Specific values for K_a and/or K_b * Memorizing Henderson-Hasselback equation

GAMSAT-Prep.com

Introduction

Acids are compounds that, when dissolved in water, give a solution with a hydrogen ion concentration greater than that of pure water. Acids turn litmus paper (an indicator) red. Examples include acetic acid (in vinegar) and sulfuric acid (in car batteries). Bases may have [H⁺] less than pure water and turns litmus blue. Examples include sodium hydroxide (= lye, caustic soda) and ammonia (used in many cleaning products).

Additional Resources

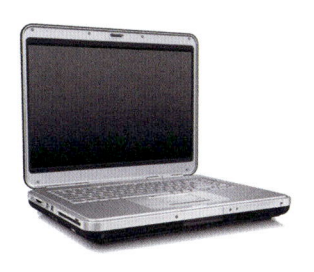

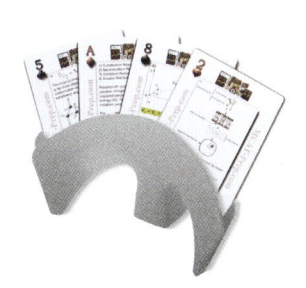

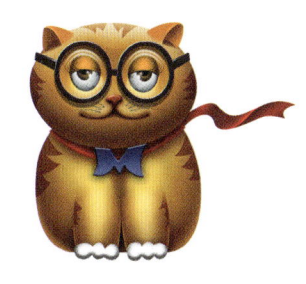

Free Online Q&A + Forum   Video: Online or DVD 3   Flashcards   Special Guest

THE PHYSICAL SCIENCES   CHM-57

* The real GAMSAT may have advanced level information presented (ie. in a passage) but previous knowledge of said information is not required to answer the questions that would follow. Practice ACER and GS practice GAMSATs can help you clarify this point.

6.1 Acids

A useful definition is given by Bronsted and Lowry: an acid is a proton (i.e. hydrogen ion) donor (cf. Lewis acids and bases, *see* CHM 3.4). A substance such as HF is an acid because it can donate a proton to a substance capable of accepting it. In aqueous solution, water is always available as a proton acceptor, so that the ionization of an acid, HA, can be written as:

$$HA + H_2O \rightleftharpoons H_3O^+ + A^-$$

or:

$$HA \rightleftharpoons H^+ + A^-$$

The equilibrium constant is:

$$K_a = [H^+][A^-]/[HA]$$

Examples of ionization of acids are:

$HCl \rightleftharpoons H^+ + Cl^-$ $K_a = $ infinity
$HF \rightleftharpoons H^+ + F^-$ $K_a = 6.7 \times 10^{-4}$
$HCN \rightleftharpoons H^+ + CN^-$ $K_a = 7.2 \times 10^{-10}$

Table III.A.6.1: Examples of strong and weak acids.

STRONG	WEAK
Perchloric $HClO_4$	Hydrocyanic HCN
Chloric $HClO_3$	Hypochlorous HClO
Nitric HNO_3	Nitrous HNO_2
Hydrochloric HCl	Hydrofluoric HF
Sulfuric H_2SO_4	Sulfurous H_2SO_3
Hydrobromic HBr	Hydrogen Sulfide H_2S
Hydriodic HI	Phosphoric H_3PO_4
Hydronium Ion H_3O^+	Benzoic, Acetic and other Carboxylic acids

Note that a diprotic acid (*two protons*, i.e. H_2SO_4) would have K_a values for each of its two ionizable protons: K_{a1} for the first and K_{a2} for the second.

GENERAL CHEMISTRY

6.2 Bases

A base is defined as a <u>proton acceptor</u>. In aqueous solution, water is always available to donate a proton to a base, so the ionization of a base B, can be written as:

$$B + H_2O \rightleftharpoons HB^+ + OH^-$$

The equilibrium constant is:

$$K_b = [HB^+][OH^-]/[B]$$

Examples of ionization of bases are:

$CN^- + H_2O \rightleftharpoons HCN + OH^-$ $\quad K_b = 1.4 \times 10^{-5}$

$NH_3 + H_2O \rightleftharpoons NH_4^+ + OH^-$ $\quad K_b = 1.8 \times 10^{-5}$

$F^- + H_2O \rightleftharpoons HF + OH^-$ $\quad K_b = 1.5 \times 10^{-11}$

Strong bases include any hydroxide of the group 1A metals. The most common weak bases are ammonia and any organic amine.

6.3 Conjugate Acid-Base Pairs

The <u>strength</u> of an acid or base is related to the extent that the dissociation proceeds to the right, or to the magnitude of K_a or K_b; the larger the dissociation constant, the stronger the acid or the base. From the preceding K_a values, we see that HCl is the strongest acid (almost 100% ionized), followed by HF and HCN. From the K_b's given, NH_3 is the strongest base listed, followed by CN^- and F^-. Clearly, when an acid ionizes, it produces a base. The acid, HA, and the base produced when it ionizes, A^-, are called a conjugate acid-base pair, so that the couples HF, F^- and HCN, CN^- are conjugate acids and bases.

Another example of conjugate acid-base pairs is amino acids. Amino acids bear at least 2 ionizable weak acid groups, a carboxyl (–COOH) and an amino (–NH_3^+) which act as follows:

$$R-COOH \rightleftharpoons R-COO^- + H^+$$
$$R-NH_3^+ \rightleftharpoons R-NH_2 + H^+$$

$R-COO^-$ and $R-NH_2$ are the conjugate bases (i.e. proton acceptors) of the corresponding acids. The carboxyl group is thousands of times more acidic than the amino group. Thus in blood plasma (pH ≈ 7.4) the predominant forms are the carboxylate anions ($R-COO^-$) and the protonated amino group ($R-NH_3^+$). This form is called a *zwitterion* as demonstrated by the amino acid alanine at a pH near 7:

CH_3-CH-COO$^-$
    |
   NH_3^+

The zwitterion bears no net charge.

GAMSAT-Prep.com
THE GOLD STANDARD

6.4 Water Dissociation

Water itself can ionize:

$$H_2O + H_2O \rightleftharpoons H_3O^+ + OH^-$$

or:

$$H_2O \rightleftharpoons H^+ + OH^-$$

At STP, $K_w = [H^+][OH^-] = 1.0 \times 10^{-14}$ = ion product constant for water. It increases with temperature and in a neutral solution, $[H^+] = [OH^-] = 10^{-7}$ M. Note that $[H_2O]$ is not included in the equilibrium expression because it is a large constant ($[H_2O]$ is incorporated in K_w).

6.5 The pH Scale

The pH of a solution is a convenient way of expressing the concentration of hydrogen ions $[H^+]$ in solution, to avoid the use of large negative powers of 10. It is defined as:

$$pH = -\log_{10}[H^+]$$

Thus, the pH of a neutral solution of pure water where $[H^+] = 10^{-7}$ is 7.

A similar definition is used for the hydroxyl ion concentration:

$$pOH = -\log_{10}[OH^-]$$

And $pH + pOH = pK_w$.

At 25 °C, $pH + pOH = 14$

A pH of 7 is neutral. Values of pH that are greater than 7 are alkaline (basic) and values that are lower are acidic. The pH can be measured precisely with a pH meter (quantitative) or globally with an indicator which will have a different color over different pH ranges (qualitative). For example, *litmus paper* (very common) becomes blue in basic solutions and red in acidic solutions; whereas, *phenolphthalein* is colorless in acid and pink in base.

We will see in CHM 6.9 that a weak acid or base can serve as a visual (qualitative) indicator of a pH range. Usually, only a small quantity (i.e. drops) of the indicator is added to the solution as to minimize the risk of any side reactions.

GENERAL CHEMISTRY

6.5.1 Properties of Logarithms

Many GAMSAT problems every year rely on a basic understanding of logarithms for pH problems, rate law (CHM 9.10) and sound intensity (PHY 8.3.1). Here are the rules you must know:

1) $\log_a a = 1$
2) $\log_a M^k = k \log_a M$
3) $\log_a(MN) = \log_a M + \log_a N$
4) $\log_a(M/N) = \log_a M - \log_a N$
5) $10^{\log_{10} M} = M$

For example, let us calculate the pH of 0.001 M HCl. Since HCl is a strong acid, it will completely dissociate into H^+ and Cl^-, thus:

$$[H^+] = 0.001$$
$$-\log[H^+] = -\log(0.001)$$
$$pH = -\log(10^{-3})$$
$$pH = 3 \log 10 \quad \text{(rule \#2)}$$
$$pH = 3 \quad \text{(rule \#1, } a = 10\text{)}$$

6.6 Weak Acids and Bases

Weak acids and bases are only <u>partially ionized</u>. The ionization constant can be used to calculate the amount ionized, and from this, the pH.

Example: Calculate the pH and pOH of a 10^{-3} M solution of acetic acid. K_a of acetic acid at 25°C = 1.75×10^{-5}.

$$HOAc \rightleftharpoons H^+ + OAc^-$$

The concentrations are:

	[HOAc]	[H⁺]	[OAc⁻]
Initial	10^{-3}	0	0
Change	$-x$	$+x$	$+x$
Equilibrium	$10^{-3}-x$	x	x

$$K_a = [H^+][OAc^-]/[HOAc] = 1.75 \times 10^{-5}$$
$$= (x)(x)/(10^{-3} - x)$$

The solution is a quadratic equation which may be simplified if <u>less than 15%</u> of the acid is ionized by neglecting x compared to the concentration (10^{-3} in this case). We then have:

$$x^2/10^{-3} = 1.75 \times 10^{-5}$$
$$x = 1.32 \times 10^{-4} \text{ M} = [H^+]$$
And $$pH = -\log 1.32 \times 10^{-4} = 3.88$$
$$pOH = 14.00 - 3.88 = 10.12$$

Similar calculations hold for weak bases. Note that all the preceding can be estimated without a calculator once you know the squares of all numbers between 1 and 15. The root of 1.69 (a fair estimate of 1.75) is thus 1.3 (also *see* CHM 6.6.1).

6.6.1 Determining pH with the Quadratic Formula

The solutions of the quadratic equation

$$ax^2 + bx + c = 0$$

are given by the formula

$$x = [-b \pm (b^2 - 4ac)^{1/2}]/2a$$

The problem in Section 6.6 reduced to

$$K_a = (x)(x)/(10^{-3} - x) = 1.75 \times 10^{-5}$$

or

$$x^2 + (1.75 \times 10^{-5})x + (-1.75 \times 10^{-8}) = 0.$$

Using the quadratic formula where $a = 1$, $b = 1.75 \times 10^{-5}$, $c = -1.75 \times 10^{-8}$, and doing the appropriate multiplications we get:

$$x = [-1.75 \times 10^{-5} \pm (3.06 \times 10^{-10} + 7.0 \times 10^{-8})^{1/2}]/2$$

thus

$$x = [-1.75 \times 10^{-5} \pm (7.03 \times 10^{-8})^{1/2}]/2$$
$$= [-1.75 \times 10^{-5} \pm 2.65 \times 10^{-4}]/2$$

hence the two possible solutions are

$$x = [-1.75 \times 10^{-5} - 2.65 \times 10^{-4}]/2$$
$$= -1.41 \times 10^{-4}$$

or

$$x = [-1.75 \times 10^{-5} + 2.65 \times 10^{-4}]/2$$
$$= 1.24 \times 10^{-4}.$$

The first solution is a negative number which is physically impossible for $[H^+]$, therefore

$$pH = -\log(1.24 \times 10^{-4}) = 3.91.$$

Our estimate in Section 6.6 (pH = 3.88) was valid as it is less than 1% different from the more precise calculation using the quadratic formula.

Given a multiple choice question with the following choices: 2.5, 3.9, 4.3 and 6.8 – the answer can be easily deduced.

$$-\log(1.24 \times 10^{-4}) = -\log 1.24 - \log 10^{-4}$$
$$= 4 - \log 1.24$$

however

$$0 = \log 10^0 = \log 1 < \log 1.24 \ll \log 10 = 1$$

Thus a number slightly greater than 0 but significantly less than 1 is substracted from 4. The answer could only be 3.9.

GENERAL CHEMISTRY

6.7 Salts of Weak Acids and Bases

A *salt* is an ionic compound in which the anion is not OH^- or O^{2-} and the cation is not H^+. Typically, an acid plus a base produces a salt and a neutral compound (i.e. CHM 6.9.1/2). The salt of a weak acid is a <u>Bronsted base</u>, which will accept protons. For example,

$$Na^+\,OAc^- + H_2O \rightleftharpoons HOAc + Na^+\,OH^-$$

The HOAc here is undissociated and therefore does not contribute to the pH. This ionization is known as <u>hydrolysis</u> of the salt ion. Because it hydrolyzes, sodium acetate is a weak base (the conjugate base of acetic acid). The ionization constant is equal to the basicity constant of the salt. ==The weaker the conjugate acid, the stronger the conjugate base==, that is, the more strongly the salt will combine with a proton.

$$K_H = K_b = [HOAc][OH^-]/[OAc^-]$$

K_H is the <u>hydrolysis constant</u> of the salt. The product of K_a of any weak acid and K_b of its conjugate base is always equal to K_w.

$$K_a \times K_b = K_w$$

For any salt of a weak acid, HA, that ionizes in water:

$$A^- + H_2O \rightleftharpoons HA + OH^-$$
$$[HA][OH^-]/[A^-] = K_w/K_a.$$

The pH of such a salt is calculated in the same manner as for any other weak base.

Similar equations are derived for the salts of weak bases. They hydrolyze in water as follows:

$$BH^+ + H_2O \rightleftharpoons B + H_3O^+$$

B is undissociated and does not contribute to the pH.

$$K_H = K_a = [B][H_3O^+]/[BH^+]$$

And

$$[B][H_3O^+]/[BH^+] = K_w/K_b.$$

6.8 Buffers

A <u>buffer</u> is defined as a solution that resists change in pH when a small amount of an acid or base is added or when a solution is diluted. A buffer solution consists of a <u>mixture of a weak acid and its salt or of a weak base and its salt</u>.

For example, consider the acetic acid-acetate buffer. The acid equilibrium that governs this system is:

$$HOAc \rightleftharpoons H^+ + OAc^-$$

If we were to add acetate ions into the system (i.e. from the salt), the H^+ ion concentration is no longer equal to the acetate ion concentration. The hydrogen ion concentration is:

$$[H^+] = K_a ([HOAc]/[OAc^-])$$

Taking the negative logarithm of each side, where $-\log K_a = pK_a$, yields:

$$pH = pK_a - \log ([HOAc]/[OAc^-])$$

or

$$pH = pK_a + \log([OAc^-]/[HOAc])$$

This equation is referred to as the <u>Henderson-Hasselbach</u> equation. It is useful for calculating the pH of a weak acid solution containing its salt. A general form can be written for a weak acid, HA, that dissociates into its salt, A^- and H^+:

$$HA \rightleftharpoons H^+ + A^-$$

$$pH = pK_a + \log([salt]/[acid])$$

The amount of acid or base that can be added without causing a large change in pH is governed by the <u>buffering capacity</u> of the solution. This is determined by the concentrations of HA and A^-. The higher their concentrations, the more acid or base the solution can tolerate. The buffering capacity is also governed by the ratios of HA to A^-. It is maximum when the ratio is equal to 1, i.e. when $pH = pK_a$.

Similar calculations can be made for mixtures of a weak base and its salt:

$$B + H_2O \rightleftharpoons BH^+ + OH^-$$

And

$$pOH = pK_b + \log ([salt]/[base])$$

Many biological reactions of interest occur between pH 6 and 8. One useful series of buffers is that of phosphate buffers. By choosing appropriate mixtures of $H_3PO_4/H_2PO_4^-$, $H_2PO_4^-/HPO_4^{2-}$ or HPO_4^{2-}/PO_4^{3-}, buffer solutions covering a wide pH range can be prepared. Another useful clinical buffer is the one prepared from tris(hydroxymethyl) aminomethane and its conjugate acid, abbreviated Tris buffer.

6.9 Acid-base Titrations

The purpose of a titration is usually the determination of concentration of a given sample of acid or base (the analyte) which is reacted with an equivalent amount of a strong base or acid of known concentration (the titrant). The end point or equivalence point is reached when a stoichiometric amount of titrant has been added. This end point is usually detected with the use of an indicator which changes color when this point is reached. The end point is determined precisely by measuring the pH at different points of the titration. The curve pH=f(V) where V is the volume of titrant added is called a titration curve. An indicator for an acid-base titration is a weak acid or base. The weak acid and its conjugate base should have two different colors in solution. Most indicators require a pH transition range during the titration of about two pH units. An indicator is chosen so that its pK_a is close to the pH of the equivalence point.

6.9.1 Strong Acid versus Strong Base

In the case of a strong acid versus a strong base, both the titrant and the analyte are completely ionized. For example, the titration of hydrochloric acid with sodium hydroxide:

$$H^+ + Cl^- + Na^+ + OH^- \rightarrow H_2O + Na^+ + Cl^-$$

The H^+ and OH^- combine to form H_2O and the other ions remain unchanged, so the net result is the conversion of the HCl to a neutral solution of NaCl. A typical strong-acid-strong base titration curve is shown in Fig. III.A.6.1 (case where the titrant is a base).

If the analyte is an acid the pH is initially acidic and increases very slowly. When the equivalent volume is reached the pH sharply increases. Midway between this transition jump is the equivalence point. In the case of strong acid-strong base titration the equivalence point corresponds to a neutral pH (because the salt formed does not react with water). If more titrant is added the pH increases and corresponds to the pH of a solution of gradually increasing concentration of the titrant base. This curve is simply reversed if the titrant is an acid.

There are more questions on acids-bases in ACER's GAMSAT practice materials than any other General Chemistry subject. Though this fact does not guarantee what could be emphasized on any 1 new exam, it does underline the relative importance of this chapter.

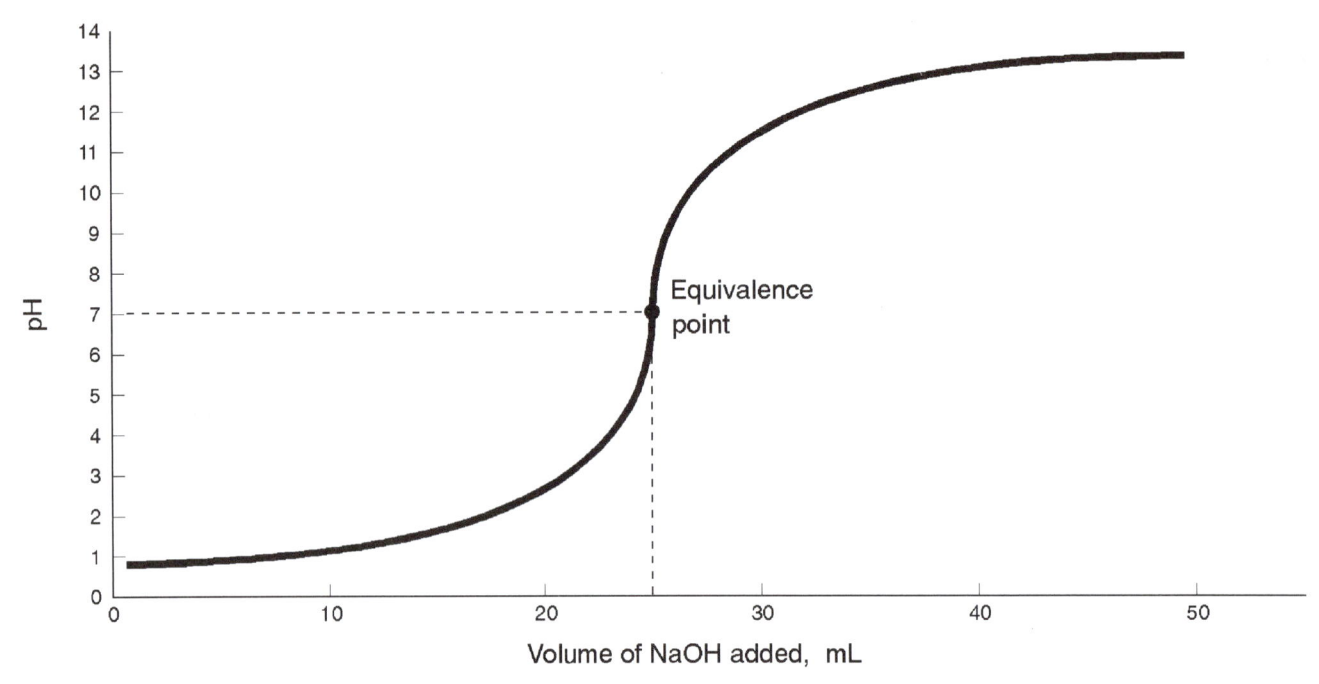

Figure III.A.6.1: Titration curve of a strong acid versus a strong base.

6.9.2 Weak Acid versus Strong Base

The titration of acetic acid with sodium hydroxide involves the following reaction:

$$HOAc + Na^+ + OH^- \rightarrow H_2O + Na^+ + OAc^-$$

The acetic acid is only a few percent ionized. It is neutralized to water and an equivalent amount of the salt, sodium acetate. Before the titration is started, the pH is calculated as described for weak acids. As soon as the titration is started, some of the HOAc is converted to NaOAc and a buffer system is set up. As the titration proceeds, the pH slowly increases as the ratio [OAc⁻]/[HOAc] changes. At the midpoint of the titration, [OAc⁻] = [HOAc] and the pH is equal to pK_a. At the equivalence point, we have a solution of NaOAc. Since it hydrolyzes, the pH at the equivalence point will be alkaline. The pH will depend on the concentration of NaOAc. The greater the concentration, the higher the pH. As excess NaOH is added, the ionization of the base, OAc⁻, is suppressed and the pH is determined only by the concentration of excess OH⁻. Therefore, the titration curve beyond the equivalence point follows that for the titration of a strong acid. The typical titration curve in this case is:

GENERAL CHEMISTRY

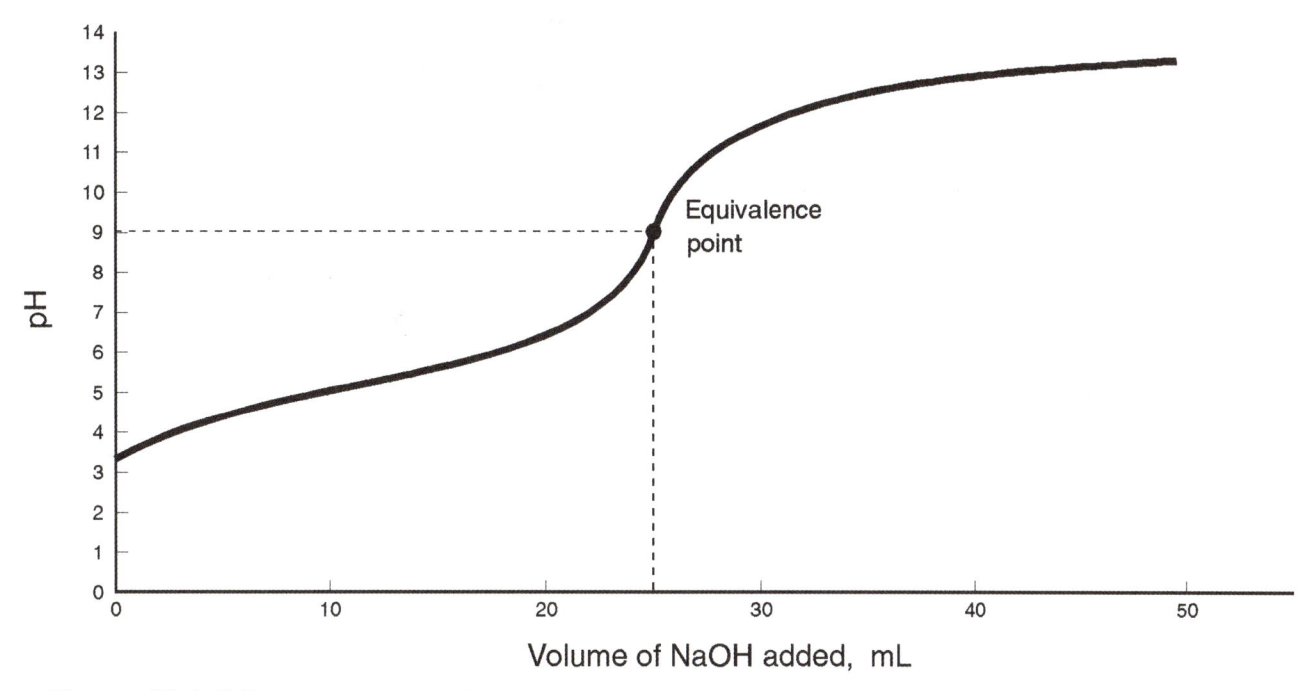

Figure III.A.6.2: Titration curve of a weak acid versus a strong base. N.B. the equivalence point is basic.

6.9.3 Weak Base versus Strong Acid

The titration of a weak base with a strong acid is analogous to the previous case except that the pH is initially basic and gradually decreases as the acid is added (curve in preceding diagram is reversed). Consider ammonia titrated with hydrochloric acid:

$$NH_3 + H^+ + Cl^- \rightarrow NH_4^+ + Cl^-$$

At the beginning, we have NH_3 and the pH is calculated as for weak bases. As soon as some acid is added, some of the NH_3 is converted to NH_4^+ and we are in the buffer region. At the midpoint of the titration, $[NH_4^+]$ = $[NH_3]$ and the pH is equal to $(14 - pK_b)$. At the equivalence point, we have a solution of NH_4Cl, a weak acid which hydrolyzes to give an acid solution. Again, the pH will depend on concentration: the greater the concentration, the lower the pH. Beyond the equivalence point, the free H^+ suppresses the ionization and the pH is determined by the concentration of H^+ added in excess. Therefore, the titration curve beyond the equivalence point will be similar to that of the titration of a strong base. {The midpoint of the titration is the equivalence point of the titration curve}

6.10 Redox Titrations

The most useful oxidizing agent for titrations is potassium permanganate - $KMnO_4$. Solutions of this salt are colorful since they contain the purple MnO_4^- ion. On the other hand, the more reduced form, Mn^{++}, is nearly colorless. So here is how this redox titration works: $KMnO_4$ is added to a reaction mixture with a reducing agent (i.e. Fe^{++}). MnO_4^- is quickly reduced to Mn^{++} so the color fades immediately. This will continue until there is no more reducing agent in the mixture. When the last bit of reducing agent has been oxidized (i.e. all the Fe^{++} is converted to Fe^{+3}), the next drop of $KMnO_4$ will make the solution colorful since the MnO_4^- will have nothing with which to react. Thus if the amount of reducing agent was unknown, it can be calculated using stoichiometry guided by the amount of potassium permanganate used in the reaction.

Little Jenny V. was a chemist Little Jenny V. is no more What she thought was H_2O Was H_2SO_4

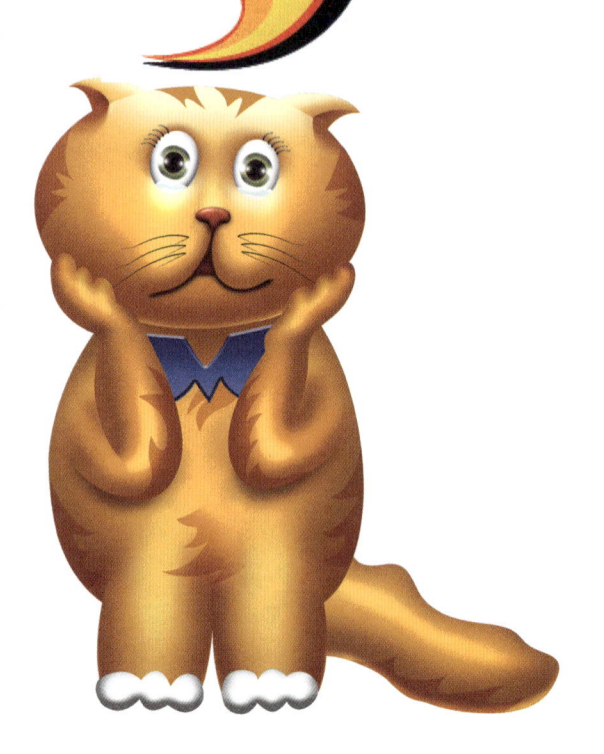

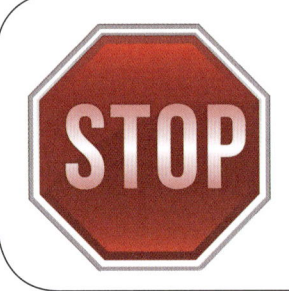

Reminder: when you register on gamsat-prep.com using your Online Access Card, you get free access to the features described on the book's cover. This includes chapter review practice questions in the Lessons section. This will help you understand what areas are emphasized on the GAMSAT and to solidify your overall understanding of this and other chapters in General Chemistry.

GOLD NOTES

GOLD NOTES

THERMODYNAMICS

Chapter 7

Memorize	Understand	Not Required*
Define: state function Conversion: thermal to mechanical E.	* System vs. surroundings * Law of conservation of energy * Heat transfer * Conduction, convection, radiation	* Advanced level college info * Memorizing: conversion between temperature scales or thermal units * Memorizing: 1st Law of Thermodynamics

GAMSAT-Prep.com

Introduction

Thermodynamics, in chemistry, refers to the relationship of heat with chemical reactions or with the physical state. Thermodynamic processes can be analyzed by studying energy and topics we will review in the next chapter including entropy, volume, temperature and pressure.

Additional Resources

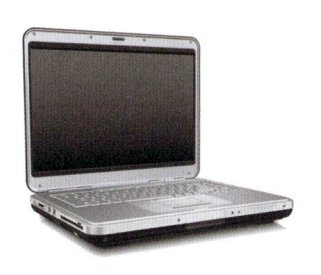

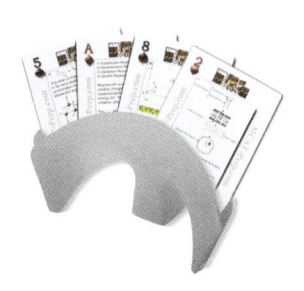

Free Online Q&A + Forum   Video: Online or DVD 4   Flashcards   Special Guest

THE PHYSICAL SCIENCES CHM-71

* The real GAMSAT may have advanced level information presented (ie. in a passage) but previous knowledge of said information is not required to answer the questions that would follow. Practice ACER and GS practice GAMSATs can help you clarify this point.

7.1 Generalities

Thermodynamics deals with fundamental questions concerning energy transfers. One difficulty you will have to overcome is the terminology used. For instance, remember that heat and temperature have more specific meanings than the ones attributed to them in every day life. A thermodynamic transformation can be as simple as a gas leaking out of a tank or a piece of metal melting at high temperature or as complicated as the synthesis of proteins by a biological cell. To solve some problems in thermodynamics we need to define a "system" and its "surroundings." The system is simply the object experiencing the thermodynamic transformation. The gas would be considered as the system in the first example of transformations. Once the system is defined any part of the universe in direct contact with the system is considered as its surroundings. For instance if the piece of metal is melted in a high temperature oven: the system is the piece of metal and the oven constitutes its surroundings. In other instances the limit between the system and its surroundings is more arbitrary, for example if one considers the energy exchanges when an ice cube melts in a thermos bottle filled with orange juice; the inside walls of the thermos bottle could be considered as part of "the system" or as part of the surroundings. In the first case one would carry out all calculations as though the entire system (ice cube + orange juice + inside walls) is isolated from its surroundings (rest of the universe) and all the energy exchanges take place within the system. In the second case the system (ice cube + orange juice) is not isolated from the surroundings (walls) unless we consider that the heat exchanges with the walls are negligible. There is also no need to include any other part of the universe in the latter case since all exchanges take place within the system or between the system and the inside walls of the thermos bottle.

7.2 The First Law of Thermodynamics

Heat, internal energy and work are the first concepts introduced in thermodynamics. Work should be a familiar concept from reading Physics section 5.1. Heat is thermal energy (a dynamic property defined during a transformation only), it is not to be confused with temperature (a static property defined for each state of the system). Internal energy is basically the average total mechanical energy (kinetic + potential) of the particles that make up the system. The first law of thermodynamics is often expressed as follows: when a system absorbs an amount of heat Q from the surroundings and does a quantity of work W on the the same surroundings its internal energy changes by the amount:

$$\Delta E = Q - W$$

This law is basically the law of conservation of energy for an isolated system. Indeed, it states that if a system does not exchange any energy with its surroundings its internal energy should not vary. If on the other hand a system does exchange energy with its surroundings, its internal energy should change by an amount corresponding to the energy it takes in from the surroundings.

The sign convention related to the previous mathematical expression of the first law of thermodynamics is:

- heat absorbed by the system: $Q > 0$
- heat released by the system: $Q < 0$
- work done by the system on its surroundings: $W > 0$
- work done by the surroundings on the system: $W < 0$

Caution: Some textbooks prefer a different sign convention: any energy (Q or W) flowing from the system to the surroundings (lost by the system) is negative and any energy flowing from the surroundings to the system (gained by the system) is positive. Within such a sign convention the first law is expressed as:

$$\Delta E = Q + W$$

i.e. the negative sign in the previous equation is incorporated in W.

7.3 Equivalence of Mechanical, Chemical and Thermal Energy Units

The previous equation does more than express mathematically the law of conservation of energy, it establishes a relationship between thermal energy and mechanical energy. Historically thermal energy was always expressed in calories (abbreviated as cal.) defined as the amount of thermal energy required to raise the temperature of water by 1 degree Celsius. The standard unit used for mechanical work is the "Joule" (J). This unit eventually became the standard unit for any form of energy. The conversion factor between the two units is:

$$1 \text{ cal} = 4.184 \text{ J}$$

Chemists often refer the amount of energies exchanged between the system and its surroundings to the mole, i.e., quantities of energy are expressed in J/mol or cal/mol. To obtain the energy per particle (atom or molecule), you should divide the energy expressed in J or cal/mol by Avogadro's number.

7.4 Temperature Scales

There are three temperature scales in use in science textbooks. The Celsius scale, the absolute temperature or Kelvin scale, and the Farenheit scale. In the Celsius scale the freezing point and the boiling point of water are arbitrarily defined as 0 °C and 100 °C, respectively. The scale is then divided into equal 1/100th intervals to define the degree Celsius or centigrade (from latin centi = 100). The absolute temperature or Kelvin scale is derived from the centigrade scale, i.e., an interval of 1 degree Celsius is equal to an interval of 1 degree Kelvin. The difference between the two scales is in their definitions of the zero point:

$$0 \text{ K} = -273.13 \text{ °C}.$$

Theoretically, this temperature can be approached but never achieved, it corresponds to the point where all motion is frozen out and matter is destroyed. The Farenheit scale used in English speaking countries has the disadvantage of not being divided into 100 degrees between its two reference points: the freezing point of water is 32 °F and its boiling point is 212 °F. To convert Farenheit degrees into Celsius degrees you have to perform the following transformation:

$$(X \text{ °F} - 32) \times 5/9 = Y \text{ °C}$$

or

$$\text{°F} = 9/5 \text{ °C} + 32.$$

7.5 Heat Transfer

There are three ways in which heat can be transferred between the system and its surroundings:

(a) heat transfer by conduction

(b) heat transfer by convection

(c) heat transfer by radiation

In the first case (a) there is an intimate contact between the system and its surroundings and heat propagates through the entire system from the heated part to the unheated parts. A good example is the heating of a metal rod on a flame. Heat is initially transmitted directly from the flame to one end of the rod through the contact between the metal and the flame. When carrying out such an experiment you would notice at some point that the part of the rod which is not in direct contact with the flame becomes hot as well.

In the second case (b), heat is transferred to the entire system by the circulation of a hot liquid or a gas through it. The difference between this mode of transfer and the previous one is that the entire system or a major part of it is heated up directly by the surroundings and not by propagation of the thermal energy from the parts of the system which are in direct contact with the heating source and the parts which are not.

In the third case (c) there is no contact between the heating source and the system. Heat is transported by radiation. The perfect example is the microwave oven where the water inside the food is heated by the microwave source. Most heat transfers are carried out by at least two of the above processes at the same time.

Note that when a metal is heated it expands at a rate which is proportional to the change in temperature it experiences. For a definition of the coefficient of expansion see Physics section 6.3.

7.6 State Functions

As we mentioned above, the first law of thermodynamics introduces three fundamental energy functions, i.e., the internal energy E, heat Q, and work W. Let us consider a transformation that takes the system from an initial state (I) to a final state (F) (which can differ by a number of variables such as temperature, pressure and volume). The change in the internal energy during this transformation depends only on the properties of the initial state (I) and the final state (F). In other words, suppose that to go from (I) to (F) the system is first subjected to an intermediate transformation that temporarily takes it from state (I) to an intermediate state (Int.) and then to another transformation that brings it from (Int.) to (F), the change in internal energy between the initial state (I) and the final state (F) are independent of the properties of the intermediate state (Int.). The internal energy is said to be a path-independent function or a state function. This is not the case for W and Q. In fact, this is quite conceivable since the amount of W or Q can be imposed by the external operator who subjects the system to a given transformation from (I) to (F). For instance, Q can be fixed at zero if the operator uses an appropriate thermal insulator between the system and its surroundings. In which case the change in the internal energy is due entirely to the work w ($\Delta E = -w$). It is easy to understand that the same result [transformation from (I) to (F)] could be achieved by supplying a small quantity of heat q while letting the system do more work W on the surroundings so that $q - W$ is equal to $-w$. In which case we have:

	Work	Heat	Change in internal energy
1st transf.	w	0	−w
2nd transf.	W = w + q	q	−w

and yet in both cases the system is going from (I) to (F).

W and Q are not state functions. They depend on the path taken to go from (I) to (F). If you remember the exact definition of the internal energy you will understand that a system changes its internal energy to respond to an input of Q and W. In other words, contrary to Q and W, the internal energy cannot be directly imposed on the system.

The fact that the internal energy is a state function can be used in two other equivalent ways:

(i) If the changes in the internal energy during the intermediate transformation are known, they can be used to calculate the change for the entire process from (I) to (F): the latter is equal to the sum of the changes in the internal energy for all the intermediate steps.

(ii) If the change in the internal energy to go from a state (I) to a state (F) is $E_{I \to F}$ the change in the internal energy for an opposite transformation that would take the system from (F) to (I) is:

$$\Delta E_{F \to I} = -\Delta E_{I \to F}$$

(iii) If we start from (I) and go back to (I) through a series of intermediate transformations the change in the internal energy for the entire process is zero.

W can be determined experimentally by calculating the area under a pressure-volume curve. The mathematical relation is presented in CHM 8.1.

GOLD NOTES

GOLD NOTES

ENTHALPY AND THERMOCHEMISTRY
Chapter 8

Memorize
* Define: endo/exothermic

Understand
* Area under curve: PV diagram
* Equations for enthalpy, Hess's law, free E.
* Calculation: Hess, calorimetry, Bond diss. E.
* 2nd law of thermodynamics
* Entropy, free E. and spontaneity

Not Required*
* Advanced level college info
* Memorizing constants for latent heats
* Memorizing equations

GAMSAT-Prep.com

Introduction

Thermochemistry is the study of energy absorbed or released in chemical reactions or in any physical transformation (i.e. phase change like melting and boiling). Thermochemistry for the GAMSAT includes understanding and/or calculating quantities such as enthalpy, heat capacity, heat of combustion, heat of formation, and free energy.

Additional Resources

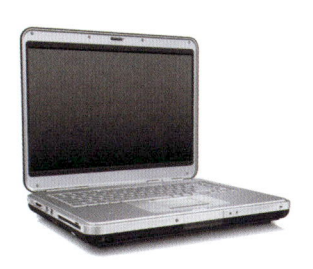

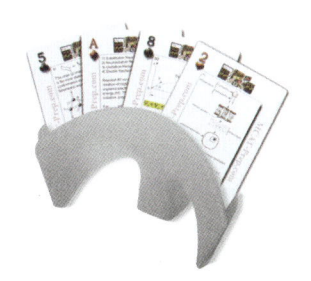

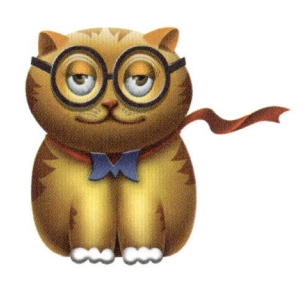

Free Online Q&A + Forum   Video: Online or DVD 4   Flashcards   Special Guest

* The real GAMSAT may have advanced level information presented (ie. in a passage) but previous knowledge of said information is not required to answer the questions that would follow. Practice ACER and GS practice GAMSATs can help you clarify this point.

8.1 Enthalpy as a Measure of Heat

The application of the general laws of thermodynamics to chemistry lead to some simplifications and adaptations because of the specificities of the problems that are dealt with in this field. For instance, in chemistry it is critical, if only for safety reasons, to know in advance what amounts of heat are going to be generated or absorbed during a reaction. In contrast, chemists are generally not interested in generating mechanical work and carry out most of their chemical reactions at constant pressure. For these reasons, although internal energy is a fundamental function its use is not very adequate in thermochemistry. Instead, chemists prefer to use another function derived from the internal energy: the enthalpy (H). This function is mathematically defined as:

$$\Delta H = \Delta E + P \times V$$

where P and V are respectively the pressure and the volume of the system. You may wonder about the use of artificially introducing another energy function when internal energy is well defined and directly related to kinetic and potential energy of the particles that make up the system. To answer this legitimate question you need to consider the case of the majority of the chemical reactions where P is constant and where the only type of work that can possibly be done by the system is of a mechanical nature. In this case, since $W = P \cdot V$ the change in enthalpy during a chemical reaction reduces to:

$$\Delta H = \Delta E + P \times V = (Q - W) + P \times V = Q$$

In other words, the change of enthalpy is a direct measure of the heat that evolves or is absorbed during a reaction carried out at constant pressure.

8.2 Heat of Reaction: Basic Principles

A reaction during which heat is released is said to be *exothermic* (ΔH is negative). If a reaction requires the supply of a certain amount of heat it is *endothermic* (ΔH is positive).

Besides the basic principle behind the introduction of enthalpy there is a more fundamental advantage for the use of this function in thermochemistry: it is a state function. This is a very practical property. For instance, consider two chemical reactions related in the following way:

reaction 1:   A + B → C
reaction 2:   C → D

If these two reactions are carried out consecutively they lead to the same result as the following reaction:

overall reaction: A + B → D

Because H is a state function we can apply the same arguments here as the ones we previously used for E. The initial state (I) corresponding to A + B , the intermediate state (Int.) to C, and the final state (F) to the final product D. If we know the changes in the enthalpy of the system for reactions 1 and 2, the change in the enthalpy during the overall reaction is:

$$\Delta H_{OVERALL} = \Delta H_1 + \Delta H_2$$

This is known as Hess's law. Remember that Hess's law is a simple application of the fact that H is a state function.

8.3 Hess's Law

Hess's law can be applied in several equivalent ways which we will illustrate with several examples:

Assume that we know the following enthalpy changes:

$$2H_2(g) + O_2(g) \to 2H_2O(l)$$
$$\Delta H_1 = -136.6 \text{ kcal} : R1$$

$$Ca(OH)_2(s) \to CaO(s) + H_2O(l)$$
$$\Delta H_2 = 15.3 \text{ kcal} : R2$$

$$2CaO(s) \to 2Ca(s) + O_2(g)$$
$$\Delta H_3 = +303.6 \text{ kcal} : R3$$

and are asked to compute the enthalpy change for the following reaction:

$$Ca(s) + H_2(g) + O_2(g) \to Ca(OH)_2(s) : R$$

It is easy to see that reaction (R) can be obtained by the combination of reactions (R_1), (R_2) and (R_3) in the following way:

$$
\begin{array}{ll}
-1/2\ (R3): & Ca(s) + 1/2\ O_2(g) \to CaO(s) \\
+1/2\ (R1): & H_2(g) + 1/2\ O_2(g) \to H_2O(l) \\
-\ \ \ \ (R2): & CaO(s) + H_2O(l) \to Ca(OH)_2(s) \\
\hline
& Ca(s) + H_2(g) + O_2(g) \to Ca(OH)_2(s)
\end{array}
$$

As we previously explained, since H is a state function the enthalpy change for (R) will be given by:

$$\Delta H = -1/2\Delta H_3 + 1/2\Delta H_1 - \Delta H_2$$

There are no general rules that would allow you to determine which reaction to use first and by what factor it needs to be multiplied. It is important to proceed systematically and follow some simple ground rules:

(i) For instance, you could start by writing the overall reaction that you want to obtain through a series of reaction additions.

(ii) Number all your reactions.

(iii) Keep in mind as you go along that the reactants of the overall reaction should always appear on the left-hand side and that the products should always appear on the right-hand side.

(iv) Circle or underline the first reactant of the overall reaction. Find a reaction in your list that involves this reactant (as a reactant or a product). Use that reaction first and write it in such a way that this reactant appears on the left-hand side with the appropriate stoichiometric coefficient (i.e., if this reactant appears as a product of a reaction on your list you should reverse the reaction).

(v) Suppose that in (iv) you had to use the second reaction on your list and that you had to reverse and multiply this reaction by a factor of 3 to satisfy the preceding rule. In your addition, next to this reaction or on top of the arrow write $-3 \times \Delta H_2$.

(vi) Repeat the process for the other reactants and products of the overall reaction until your addition yields the overall reaction. As you continue this process, make sure to cross out the compounds that appear on the right and left-hand sides at the same time.

8.4 Standard Enthalpies

Hess's law has a very practical use in chemistry. Indeed, the enthalpy change for a given chemical reaction can be computed from simple combinations of known enthalpy changes of other reactions. Because enthalpy changes depend on the conditions under which reactions are carried out it is important to define standard conditions:

(i) Standard pressure: 1 atmosphere pressure.

(ii) Standard temperature for the purposes of the calculation of the standard enthalpy change: generally 25 °C. The convention is that if the temperature of the standard state is not mentioned then it is assumed to be 25 °C, the standard temperature needs to be specified in all other instances.

(iii) Standard physical state of an element: it is defined as the "natural" physical state of an element under the above standard pressure and temperature. For instance, the standard physical state of water under the standard temperature and pressure of 1 atm and 25 °C is the liquid state. Under the same conditions oxygen is a gas.

Naturally, the standard enthalpy change (notation: $\Delta H°$) for a given reaction is defined as the enthalpy change that accompanies the reaction when it is carried out under standard pressure and temperature with all reactants and products in their standard physical state.

Note that the standard temperature defined here is different from the standard temperature for an ideal gas which is: 0 °C.

8.5 Enthalpies of Formation

The enthalpy of formation of a given compound is defined as the enthalpy change that accompanies the formation of the compound from its constituting elements. For instance, the enthalpy of formation of water is the $\Delta H_f°$ for the following reaction:

$$H_2 + 1/2\, O_2 \rightarrow H_2O$$

To be more specific the standard enthalpy of formation of water $\Delta H_f°$ is the enthalpy change during the reaction:

$$H_2(g) + 1/2 O_2(g) \xrightarrow[1\,atm]{25°C} H_2O(l)$$

where the reactants are in their natural physical state under standard temperature and pressure.

Note that according to these definitions, several of the reactions considered in the previous sections were in fact examples of reactions of formation. For instance, in section 8.3 on Hess's law, reaction (R1) is the reaction of formation of two moles of water, if reversed reaction (R3) would be the reaction of formation of two moles of CaO and the overall reaction (R) is the reaction of formation of 1 mole $Ca(OH)_2$. Also note that although one could use the reverse of reaction (R2) to form $Ca(OH)_2$, this reaction, even reversed, is not the reaction of formation of $Ca(OH)_2$. The reason is that the constitutive elements of this molecule are: calcium (Ca), hydrogen (H_2) and oxygen (O_2) and not CaO and H_2O. Enthalpies of formation are also referred to as heats of formation. As previously explained, if the reaction of formation is carried out at constant pressure, the change in the enthalpy represents the amount of heat released or absorbed during the reaction.

8.6 Bond Dissociation Energies and Heats of Formation

The bond dissociation energy (also called bond energy) is defined as the change in enthalpy when a particular bond is broken in the diatomic molecules of 1 mole of gas, i.e. it is the $\Delta H°$ which corresponds to the process:

homo-nuclear diatomic molecules:
$$X_2(g) \rightarrow 2\, X(g)$$

hetero-nuclear diatomic molecules:
$$XY(g) \rightarrow X(g) + Y(g)$$

The difficulty in defining bond dissociation energies in polyatomic molecules is that the amounts of energy required to break a given bond (say an O–H bond) in two different polyatomic molecules (H_2O and CH_3OH, for instance) are different. Bond dissociation energies in polyatomic molecules are approximated to an average value for molecules of the same nature. Within the framework of this commonly made approximation we can calculate the enthalpy change of any reaction using the *sum* of bond energies of the reactants and the products in the following way:

$$\Delta H° \text{ (reaction)} = \Sigma \text{ BE (reactants)} - \Sigma \text{ BE (products)}$$

where BE stands for bond energies.

Standard enthalpy changes of chemical reactions can also be computed using enthalpies of formation in the following way:

$$\Delta H° \text{ (reaction)} = \Sigma \Delta H°_{form.}\text{(products)} - \Sigma \Delta H°_{form.}\text{ (reactants)}$$

Note how this equation is similar but not identical to the one making use of bond energies. This comes from the fact that a bond energy is defined as the energy required to break (and not to form) a given bond. Also note that the standard enthalpy of formation of a mole of any **element** is zero.

8.7 Calorimetry

Measurements of changes of temperature within a reaction mixture allow the experimental determination of heat absorbed or released during the corresponding chemical reaction. Indeed the amount of heat required to change the temperature of any substance X from T_1 to T_2 is proportional to $(T_2 - T_1)$ and the quantity of X:

$$Q = mC(T_2 - T_1)$$

or

$$Q = nc(T_2 - T_1)$$

where m is the mass of X, n the number of moles. The constant C or c is called the heat capacity. The standard units for C and c are, respectively, the $Jkg^{-1}K^{-1}$ and the $Jmol^{-1}K^{-1}$. C which is the heat capacity per unit mass is also referred to as the specific heat capacity. If you refer back to the definition of the calorie (*see section 7.3*) you will understand that the specific heat of water is necessarily: 1 cal g^{-1} °C^{-1}.

Note that heat can be absorbed or released without a change in temperature. In fact this situation occurs whenever a phase change takes place for a pure compound. For instance, ice melts at a constant temperature of 0 °C in order to break the forces that keep the water molecules in a crystal of ice we need to supply an amount of heat of 6.01 kJ/mol. There is no direct way of calculating the heat corresponding to a phase change. Heats of phase changes (heat of fusion, heat of vaporization, heat of sublimation) are generally tabulated and indirectly determined in calorimetric experiment. For instance, if a block of ice is allowed to melt in a bucket of warm water, we can determine the heat of fusion of ice by measuring the temperature drop in the bucket of water and applying the law of conservation of energy. The relevant equation is:

$$Q = m\,L$$

where L is the latent heat which is a constant.

8.8 The Second Law of Thermodynamics

The first law of thermodynamics allows us to calculate energy transfers during a given transformation of the system. It does not allow us to predict whether a transformation can or cannot occur spontaneously. Yet our daily observations tell us that certain transformations always occur in a given direction. For instance, heat flows from a hot source to a cold source. We cannot spontaneously transfer heat in the other direction to make the hot source hotter and the cold source colder. The second law of thermodynamics allows the determination of the preferred direction of a given transformation. Transformations which require the smallest amount of energy and lead to the largest disorder of the system are the most spontaneous.

8.9 Entropy

Entropy S is the state function which measures the degree of "disorder" in a system. For instance, the entropy of ice is lower than the entropy of liquid water since ice corresponds to an organized crystalline structure (virtually no disorder). In fact generally speaking the entropy increases as we go from a solid to a liquid to a gas. For similar reasons: the entropy decreases when an elastic band is stretched. Indeed, in the "unstretched" elastic band the molecules of the rubber polymer are coiled up and form a disorganized structure. As the rubber is stretched these molecules will tend to line up with each other and adopt a more organized structure. The second law of thermodynamics can be expressed in the alternate form: a spontaneous transformation corresponds to an increase in the entropy of an isolated system. The stretching of an elastic band is not a spontaneous process, on the other hand if an elastic band is stretched it will spontaneously return to its normal length if no external force holds it back.

8.10 Free Energy

The Gibbs free energy G is another state function which can be used as a criterion for spontaneity. This function is defined as:

$$G = H - T \cdot S$$

where: H is the enthalpy of the system in a given state,

T is the temperature,

and S is the entropy of the system.

For a reaction carried out at constant temperature we can write that the change in the Gibbs free energy is:

$$\Delta G = \Delta H - T\Delta S$$

A reaction carried out at constant pressure is spontaneous if

$$\Delta G < 0$$

It is not spontaneous if:

$$\Delta G > 0$$

and it is in a state of equilibrium (reaction spontaneous in both directions) if:

$$\Delta G = 0.$$

Gibbs free energy questions appear frequently among ACER practice materials and exams.

GENERAL CHEMISTRY

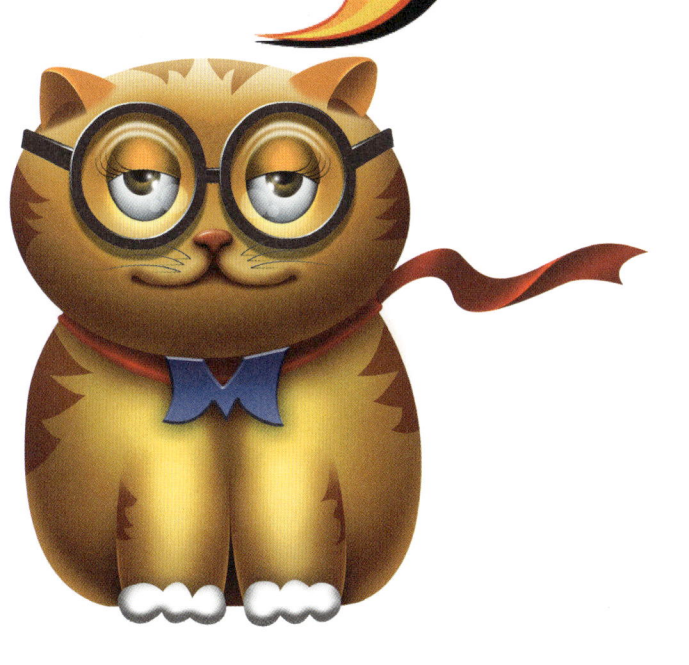

GOLD NOTES

RATE PROCESSES IN CHEMICAL REACTIONS
Chapter 9

Memorize	Understand	Not Required*
action order fine: rate determining step neralized potential energy diagrams fine: activation energy, catalysis fine: saturation kinetics, substrate	* Reaction rates, rate law, determine exponents * Reaction mechanism for free radicals * Rate constant equation; apply Le Chatelier's * Kinetic vs. thermodynamic control * Law of mass action, equations for Gibbs free E., saturation kinetics, Keq	* Advanced level college info * Memorizing the rate constant equation

GAMSAT-Prep.com

Introduction

Rate processes involve the study of the velocity (speed) and mechanisms of chemical reactions. **Reaction rate** (= *velocity*) tells us how fast the concentrations of reactants change with time. **Reaction mechanisms** show the sequence of steps to get to the overall change. Experiments show that 4 important factors generally influence reaction rates: (1) the nature of the reactants, (2) their concentration, (3) temperature, and (4) catalysis.

Additional Resources

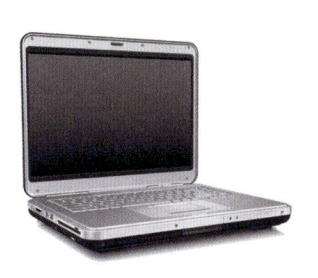

Free Online Q&A + Forum

Video: Online or DVD 4

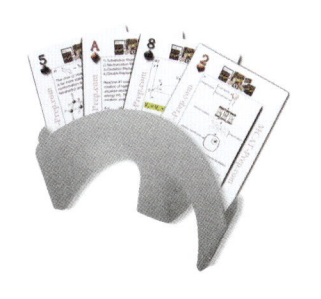

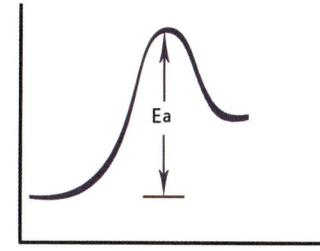

Flashcards

Special Guest

THE PHYSICAL SCIENCES   CHM-89

* The real GAMSAT may have advanced level information presented (ie. in a passage) but previous knowledge of said information is not required to answer the questions that would follow. Practice ACER and GS practice GAMSATs can help you clarify this point.

9.1 Reaction Rate

Consider a general reaction

$$2A + 3B \rightarrow C + D$$

The rate at which this reaction proceeds can be expressed by one of the following:

(i) rate of disappearance of A: $-\Delta[A]/\Delta t$

(ii) rate of disappearance of B: $-\Delta[B]/\Delta t$

(iii) rate of appearance or formation of C: $\Delta[C]/\Delta t$

(iv) rate of appearance or formation of D: $\Delta[D]/\Delta t$

Where [ ] denotes the concentration of a reactant or a product in moles/liter.

Since A and B are disappearing in this reaction, [A] and [B] are decreasing with time, i.e. $\Delta[A]/\Delta t$ and $\Delta[B]/\Delta t$ are negative quantities. On the other hand, the quantities $\Delta[C]/\Delta t$ and $\Delta[D]/\Delta t$ are positive since both C and D are being formed during the process of this reaction. By convention: rates of reactions are expressed as positive numbers; as a result, a negative sign is necessary in the first two expressions.

Suppose that A disappears at a rate of 6 (moles/liter)/s. In the same time interval (1s), in a total volume of 1L we have:

(3/2) × 6 = 9 moles of B disappearing
(1/2) × 6 = 3 moles of C being formed
(1/2) × 6 = 3 moles of D being formed

Therefore individual rates of formation or disappearance are not convenient ways to express the rate of a reaction. Indeed, depending on the reactant or product considered the rate will be given by a different numerical value unless the stoichiometric coefficients are equal (e.g. for C and D in our case). A more convenient expression of the rate of a reaction is the overall rate. This rate is simply obtained by dividing the rate of formation or disappearance of a given reactant or product by the corresponding stoichiometric coefficient, i.e.:

overall rate = $-(1/2) \Delta[A]/\Delta t$, or
$-(1/3) \Delta[B]/\Delta t$,

or $\Delta[C]/\Delta t$, or $\Delta[D]/\Delta t$.

A simple verification on our example will show you that these expressions all lead to the same numerical value for the overall rate: 3 (moles/L)/s.

Whenever the term "rate" is used (with no other specification) it refers to the "overall rate" unless individual and overall rates are equal.

GENERAL CHEMISTRY

9.2 Dependence of Reaction Rates on Concentration of Reactants

The rate of a reaction (given in moles per liter per second) can be expressed as a function of the concentration of the reactants. In the previous chemical reaction we would have:

$$\text{rate} = k\,[A]^m\,[B]^n$$

where [ ] is the concentration of the corresponding reactant in moles per liter

k is referred to as the rate constant
m is the order of the reaction with respect to A
n is the order of the reaction with respect to B
m+n is the overall reaction order.

According to the rate law above, the reaction is said to be an (m+n)th order reaction, or, an mth order reaction with respect to A, or, an nth order reaction with respect to B.

9.3 Determining Exponents of the Rate Law

The only way to determine the exponents with certainty is via experimentation. Consider the following five experiments varying the concentrations of reactants A and B with resulting rates of reaction:

$$A + B \rightarrow \text{products}$$

Exp. #	Initial Concentration [A]	Initial Concentration [B]	Initial Rate (mol L^{-1} s^{-1})
1	0.10	0.10	0.20
2	0.20	0.10	0.40
3	0.30	0.10	0.60
4	0.30	0.20	2.40
5	0.30	0.30	5.40

THE PHYSICAL SCIENCES CHM-91

In the first three experiments the concentration of A changes but B remains the same. Thus the resultant changes in rate only depend on the concentration of A. Note that when [A] doubles (exp. 1, 2) the reaction rate doubles, and when [A] triples (exp. 1, 3) the reaction rate triples. Because it is directly proportional, the exponent of [A] must be 1. Thus the rate of reaction is first order with respect to A.

In the final three sets of experiments, [B] changes while [A] remains the same. When [B] doubles (exp. 3,4) the rate increases by a factor of 4 (= 2^2). When [B] triples (exp. 3, 5) the rate increases by a factor of 9 (= 3^2). Thus the relation is exponential where the exponent of [B] is 2. The rate of reaction is second order with respect to B.

$$\text{rate} = k[A]^1[B]^2$$

The overall rate of reaction (n+m) is third order. The value of the rate constant k can be easily calculated by substituting the results from any of the five experiments. For example, using experiment #1:

$$k = \frac{\text{rate}}{[A]^1\,[B]^2}$$

$$k = \frac{0.20 \text{ mol } L^{-1}\, s^{-1}}{(0.10 \text{ mol } L^{-1})(0.10 \text{ mol } L^{-1})^2}$$

$$= 2.0 \times 10^2 \; L^2 mol^{-2} s^{-1}$$

k is the rate constant for the reaction which includes all five experiments.

9.4 Reaction Mechanism - Rate-determining Step

Chemical equations fail to describe the detailed process through which the reactants are transformed into the products. For instance, consider the reaction of formation of hydrogen chloride from hydrogen and chlorine:

$$Cl_2(g) + H_2(g) \rightarrow 2\; HCl(g)$$

The equation above fails to mention that in fact this reaction is the result of a chain of reactions proceeding in three steps:

Initiation step: formation of chlorine atoms (= *radicals*, the mechanism will be discussed in organic chemistry):

$$1/2\; Cl_2 \rightleftharpoons Cl\cdot$$

The double arrow indicates that in fact some of the Cl atoms recombine to form chlorine molecules, the whole process eventually reaches a state of equilibrium where the following ratio is constant:

$$K = [Cl\cdot]/[Cl_2]^{1/2}$$

The determination of such a constant will be dealt with in the sub-section on "equilibrium constants."

Propagation step: formation of reactive hydrogen atoms and reaction between hydrogen atoms and hydrogen molecules:

$$Cl\cdot + H_2 \rightarrow HCl + H\cdot$$

$$H\cdot + Cl_2 \rightarrow HCl + Cl\cdot$$

Termination step:

$$H\cdot + Cl\cdot \rightarrow HCl$$

The detailed chain reaction process above is called the mechanism of the reaction. Each individual reaction in a detailed mechanism is called an elementary process. Any reaction proceeds through some mechanism which is generally impossible to predict from its chemical equation. Such mechanisms are usually determined through an experimental procedure. Generally speaking each step proceeds at its own rate. The rate of the overall reaction is naturally limited by the the slowest step; therefore, the rate-determining step in the mechanism of a reaction is the slowest step. In other words, the overall rate law of a reaction is basically equal to the rate law of the slowest step. The faster processes have an indirect influence on the rate: they regulate the concentrations of the reactants and products. The chemical equation of an elementary step reflects the exact molecular process that transforms its reactants into its products. For this reason its rate law can be predicted from its chemical equation: in an elementary process, the orders with respect to the reactants are equal to the corresponding stoichiometric coefficients.

In our example experiments show that the rate-determining step is the reaction between chlorine atoms and hydrogen molecules, all the other steps are much faster. According to the principles above, the rate law of the overall reaction is equal to the rate law of this rate-determining step. Therefore, the rate of the overall reaction is proportional to the concentration of hydrogen molecules and chlorine atoms but is not directly proportional to the concentration of chlorine molecules. However since the ratio of concentrations Cl and Cl_2 is regulated by the initiation step concentration it can be shown that according to the mechanism above the rate law is:

$$\text{rate} = k[H_2] \cdot [Cl_2]^{1/2}$$

it is important to note that the individual orders of a reaction are generally not equal to the stoichiometric coefficients.

9.5 Dependence of Reaction Rates upon Temperature

From the collision theory of chemical kinetics it was established that the rate constant of a reaction can be expressed as follows:

$$k = A\,e^{-E_a/RT}$$

where: A is a constant related to the frequency of the collisions leading to a given reaction, it is referred to as Arrhenius' constant or the frequency factor,
e is the base of natural logarithms,
E_a is the activation energy, it is the energy required to get a reaction started, i.e., if two molecules of reactants have a total kinetic energy below E_a collide with each other, their collision will not lead to the formation of the product(s).
R is the ideal gas constant (1.99 cal mol^{-1}K^{-1})
T is the absolute temperature.

The species formed during an efficient collision, before the reactants transform into the final product(s) is called the activated complex or the transition state.

Within the framework of this theory, when a single step reaction proceeds the energy of the system varies according to Figure III.A.9.1.

The change in enthalpy (ΔH) during the reaction is the difference between the total energy of the products and the reactants. In the diagram on the left the total energy of the reactants is higher than the total energy of the products: this is obviously the case for an exothermic reaction. The diagram on the right shows the profile of an endothermic reaction. Also note than the bigger the difference between the total energy of the reactants and the activated complex, i.e. the activation energy E_a, the slower the reaction.

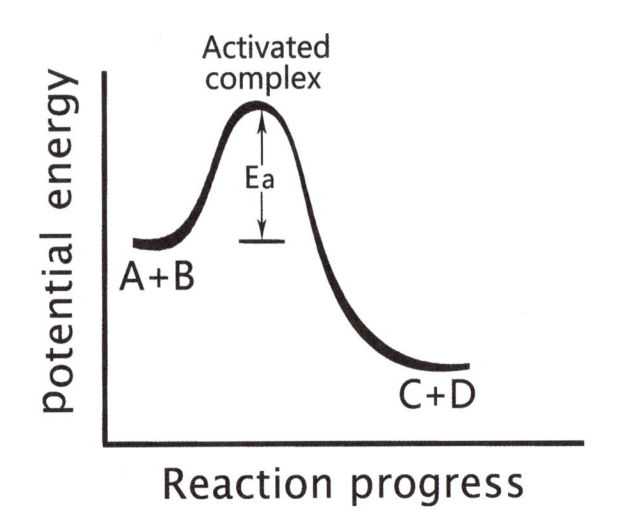

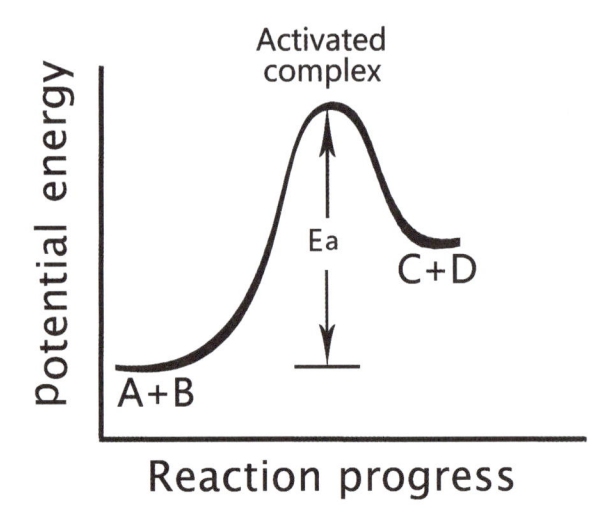

Figure III.A.9.1: Potential energy diagrams: exothermic vs. endothermic reactions.

If a reaction proceeds through several steps one can construct a diagram for each step and combine the single-step diagrams to obtain the energy profile of the overall reaction.

9.6 Kinetic Control vs. Thermodynamic Control

Consider the case where two molecules A and B can react to form either products C or D. Suppose that C has the lowest Gibbs free energy (i.e. the most thermodynamically stable product). Also suppose that product D requires the smallest activation energy and is therefore formed faster than C. If it is product C which is exclusively observed when the reaction is actually performed the reaction is said to be thermodynamically controlled (i.e. out of a list of possible pathways the reactants choose the one leading to the most stable product). If on the other hand the reactants choose the pathway leading to the product which is produced more quickly it is said to be kinetically controlled.

9.7 Catalysis

A catalyst is a compound that does not directly participate in a reaction (the initial number of moles of this compound in the reaction mixture is equal to the number of moles of this compound once the reaction is completed). Catalysts help lower the activation energy of a reaction and help the reaction to proceed. Enzymes are the typical biological catalysts. They are protein molecules with very large molar masses containing one or more active sites. Enzymes are very specialized catalysts. They are generally specific and operate only on certain biological reactants called substrates. They also generally increase the rate of reactions by large factors. The general mechanism of operation of enzymes is as follows:

Enzyme (E) + Substrate (S) → ES (complex)

ES → Product (P) + Enzyme (E)

If we were to compare the energy profile of a reaction performed with the appropriate enzyme to that of the same reaction performed in the absence of an enzyme we would obtain Figure III.A.9.2.

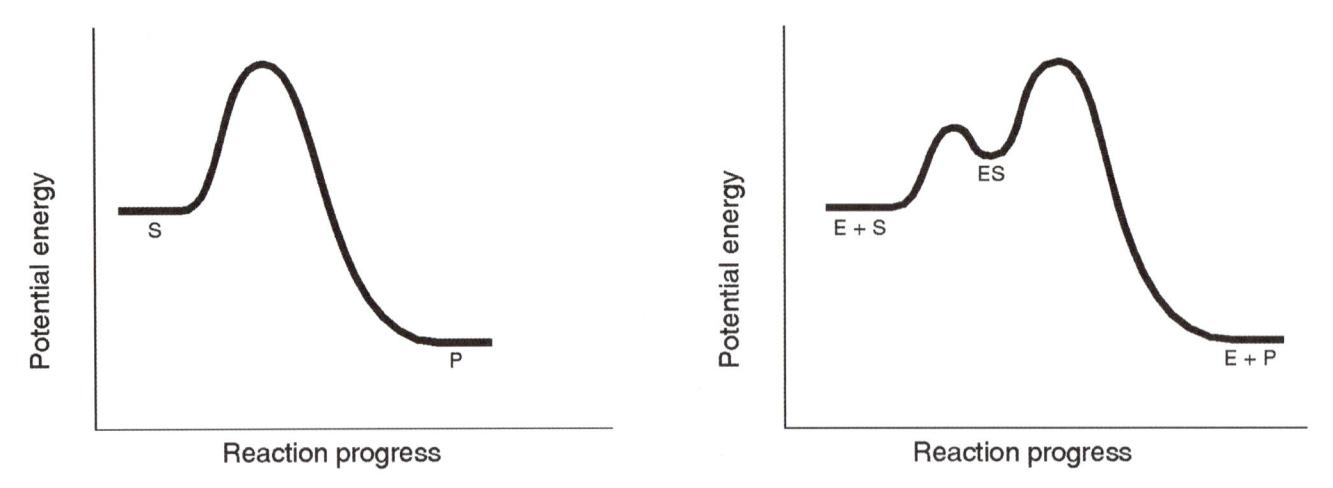

Figure III.A.9.2: Potential energy diagrams: with and without a catalyst.

As you can see from the diagram the reaction from the substrate to the product is facilitated by the presence of the enzyme because the reaction proceeds in two fast steps (low Ea's). Generally the rate of an enzyme-catalysed reaction is :

$$\text{rate} = k[ES]$$

The plot of the rate of formation of the product $\Delta [P]/\Delta t$ vs. the concentration of the substrate $[S]$ yields a plot as in Figure III.A.9.3.

When the concentration of the substrate is large enough for the substrate to occupy all the available active sites on the enzyme, any further increase would have no effect on the rate of the reaction. This is called *saturation kinetics*.

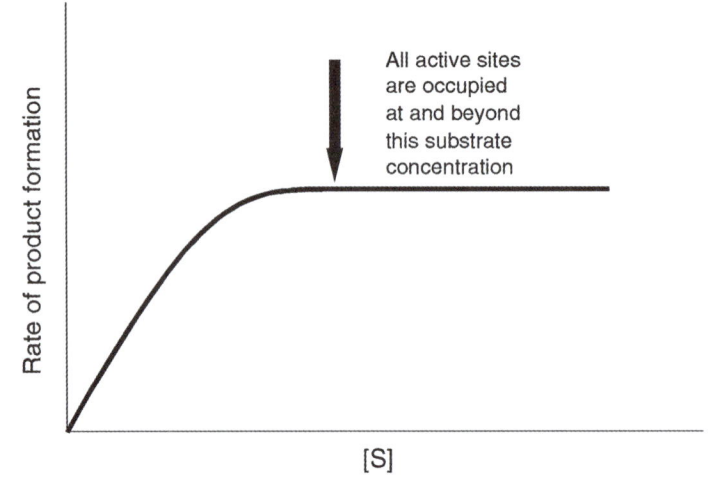

Figure III.A.9.3: Saturation kinetics.

GENERAL CHEMISTRY

9.8 Equilibrium in Reversible Chemical Reactions

In most chemical reactions once the product is formed it reacts in such a way to yield back the initial reactants. Eventually, the system reaches a state where there are as many molecules of products being formed as there are molecules of reactants being generated through the reverse reaction. This state is called a state of equilibrium. It is characterized by a constant K:

$$aA + bB \rightleftharpoons cC + dD$$

where a, b, c and d are the corresponding stoichiometric coefficients:

$$K = \frac{[C]^c [D]^d}{[A]^a [B]^b}$$

The equilibrium constant K (sometimes symbolized as K_{eq}) has a given value at a given temperature. If the temperature changes the value of K changes. At a given temperature, if we change the concentration of A, B, C or D, the system evolves in such a way as to re-establish the value of K. This is called the law of mass action. {Note: catalysts speed up the rate of reaction without affecting K_{eq}}

9.9 Le Chatelier's Principle

Le Chatelier's principle states that whenever a perturbation is applied to a system at equilibrium, the system evolves in such a way as to compensate for the applied perturbation. For instance, consider the following equilibrium:

$$N_2 + 3H_2 \rightleftharpoons 2NH_3$$

If we introduce some more hydrogen in the reaction mixture at equilibrium, i.e. if we increase the concentration of hydrogen, the system will evolve in the direction that will decrease the concentration of hydrogen (from left to right). If more ammonia is introduced the equilibrium shifts from the right-hand side to the left-hand side, while the removal of ammonia from the reaction vessel would do the opposite (i.e. shifts equilibrium from the left-hand side to the right-hand side).

In a similar fashion, an increase in total pressure (decrease in volume) favors the direction which decreases the total number of compressible (i.e. gases) moles (from the left-hand side where there are 4 moles to the right-hand side where there are 2 moles). It can also be said that when there are different forms of a substance, an increase in total pressure (decrease in volume) favors the form with the greatest density, and a decrease in total pressure (increase in volume) favors the form with the lowest density.

Finally, if the temperature of a reaction mixture at equilibrium is increased, the equilibrium evolves in the direction of the endothermic reaction. For instance, the forward reaction of the equilibrium:

$$N_2O_4(g) \rightleftharpoons 2NO_2(g)$$

is endothermic; therefore, an increase in temperature favors the forward reaction over the backward reaction. In other words, the dissociation of N_2O_4 increases with temperature.

9.10 Relationship between the Equilibrium Constant and the Change in the Gibbs Free Energy

In the "thermodynamics" section we defined the Gibbs free energy. The *standard* Gibbs free energy ($G°$) is determined at 25 °C (298 K) and 1 atm. The change in the standard Gibbs free energy for a given reaction can be calculated from the change in the standard enthalpy and entropy of the reaction using:

$$\Delta G° = \Delta H - T \Delta S°$$

where T is the temperature at which the reaction is carried out. If this reaction happens to be the forward reaction of an equilibrium, the equilibrium constant associated with this equilibrium is simply given by:

$$\Delta G° = -R\, T\, Ln\, K_{eq}$$

where R is the ideal gas constant (1.99 cal mol^{-1} K^{-1}) and Ln is the natural logarithm (i.e. log to the base *e*).

It is important to remember the sign for Gibbs free energy when the reaction is not spontaneous, spontaneous and at equilibrium (CHM 8.10).

Alert!

After acid-bases, questions based on the information provided in this chapter (Chapter 9) would be the 2nd most frequently tested amongst ACER's practice materials for General Chemistry.

GENERAL CHEMISTRY

GOLD NOTES

ELECTROCHEMISTRY

Chapter 10

Memorize
* Define: anode, cathode, anion, cation
* Define: standard half-cell potentials
* Define: strong/weak oxidizing/reducing agents

Understand
* Electrolytic cell, electrolysis
* Calculation involving Faraday's law
* Galvanic (voltaic) cell, purpose of salt bridge
* Half reaction, reduction potentials
* Direction of electron flow

Not Required*
* Advanced level college info
* Memorizing the value of a faraday
* Frost diagram

GAMSAT-Prep.com

Introduction

Electrochemistry links chemistry with electricity (the movement of electrons through a conductor). If a chemical reaction produces electricity (i.e. a battery or galvanic/voltaic cell) then it is an **electrochemical cell**. If electricity is applied externally to drive the chemical reaction then it is **electrolysis**. In general, oxidation/reduction reactions occur and are separated in space or time, connected by an external circuit.

Additional Resources

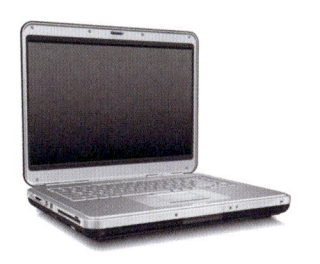

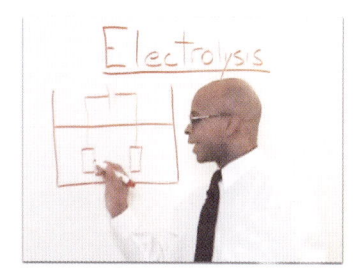

Free Online Q & A   Video: Online or DVD 4   Flashcards   Special Guest

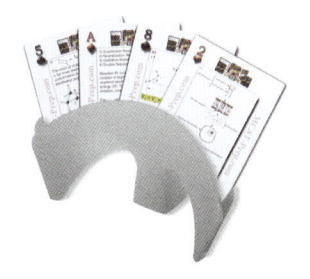

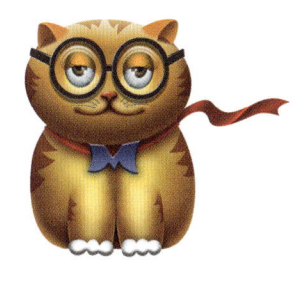

THE PHYSICAL SCIENCES   CHM-101

* The real GAMSAT may have advanced level information presented (ie. in a passage) but previous knowledge of said information is not required to answer the questions that would follow. Practice ACER and GS practice GAMSATs can help you clarify this point.

GAMSAT-Prep.com
THE GOLD STANDARD

10.1 Generalities

Electrochemistry is based on <u>oxidation-reduction or redox reactions</u> in which one or more electrons are transferred from one ionic species to another. Before you read this section you should review the rules that allow the determination of the oxidation state of an element in a polyatomic molecule or ion and the definition of oxidation and reduction processes. We had previously applied the rules for the determination of oxidation numbers in the case of the following overall reaction (see Section 1.6):

$$CuSO_4(aq) + Zn(s) \rightleftharpoons$$
Oxid.#:   +2   0
$$Cu(s) + ZnSO_4(aq)$$
Oxid.#:   0   +2

The reduction and oxidation half-reactions of the forward process are:

reduction half-reaction:
$Cu^{2+}(aq) + 2e^- \rightarrow Cu(s)$

oxidation half-reaction:
$Zn(s) \rightarrow Zn^{2+}(aq) + 2e^-$

To determine the number and the side on which to put the electrons one follows the simple rules:

(i) The <u>electrons</u> are always on the <u>left-hand</u> side of a <u>reduction</u> half-reaction.
(ii) The <u>electrons</u> are always on the <u>right-hand</u> side of an <u>oxidation</u> half-reaction.
(iii) For a reduction half-reaction:
    # of electrons required = initial oxidation #
                            − final oxidation #

(iv) For an oxidation half-reaction:
    # of electrons required = final oxidation #
                            − initial oxidation #

The next step is to balance each half-reaction, i.e. the charges and the number of atoms of all the elements involved have to be equal on both sides. The preceding example is very simple since the number of electrons required in the two half-reactions is the same. Consider the following more complicated example:

reduction: $Sn^{2+}(aq) + 2e^- \rightarrow Sn(s)$
oxidation: $Al(s) \rightarrow Al^{3+}(aq) + 3e^-$

to balance the overall reaction you need to multiply the first half-reaction by a factor of 3 and the second by a factor of 2.

The oxidization/reduction capabilitites of substances are measured by their standard <u>half-cell potentials</u> E°. These potentials are relative. The reference was chosen to correspond to the following half-reaction:

$2H^+(1\ molal) + 2e^- \rightarrow H_2(1\ atm)\quad E° = 0$

Standard half-cell potentials for other half-reactions have been tabulated. They are defined for standard conditions, i.e., concentration of all ionic species equal to 1 molal and pressure of all gases involved, if any, equal to 1 atm. The standard temperature is taken as 25 °C. In the case of the Cu²⁺/Zn reaction the relevant data is tabulated as reduction potentials as follows:

$Zn^{2+}(aq) + 2e^- \rightarrow Zn(s)\quad E° = -0.76\ volts$
$Cu^{2+}(aq) + 2e- \rightarrow Cu(s)\quad E° = +0.34\ volts$

CHM-102   ELECTROCHEMISTRY

The more positive the E° value, the more likely the reaction will occur spontaneously as written. The strongest reducing agents have large negative E° values. The strongest oxidizing agents have large positive E° values. Therefore, in our example Cu^{2+} is a stronger oxidizing agent than Zn^{2+}. This conclusion can be expressed in the following practical terms:

(i) If you put Zn in contact with a solution containing Cu^{2+} ions a spontaneous redox reaction will occur.

(ii) If you put Cu directly in contact with a solution containing Zn^{2+} ions, no reaction takes place spontaneously.

Thus for the spontaneous reaction:

$$E° = E°_{red} - E°_{ox} = +0.34 - (-0.76) = 1.1 \text{ V}.$$

The positive value confirms the spontaneous nature of the reaction. {A note about terminology: the oxidizing agent is *reduced*; the reducing agent is *oxidized*}

10.2 Galvanic Cells

Batteries are self-contained galvanic cells. A galvanic cell uses a spontaneous redox reaction to produce electricity. For instance, one can design a galvanic cell based on the spontaneous reaction:

$$Zn(s) + CuSO_4(aq) \rightarrow Cu(s) + ZnSO_4(aq)$$

The figure that follows shows the different parts of such a cell. Note that Zn is not in direct contact with the Cu^{2+} solution; otherwise electrons will be directly transferred from Zn to Cu^{2+} and no electricity will be produced to an external circuit.

The half-reaction occurring in the left-hand side compartment is the oxidation:

$$Zn(s) \rightarrow Zn^{2+}(aq) + 2e^-$$

The half-reaction occurring in the right-hand side compartment is the reduction:

$$Cu^{2+}(aq) + 2e^- \rightarrow Cu(s)$$

Therefore, electrons flow out of the compartment where the oxidation occurs to the compartment where the reduction takes place.

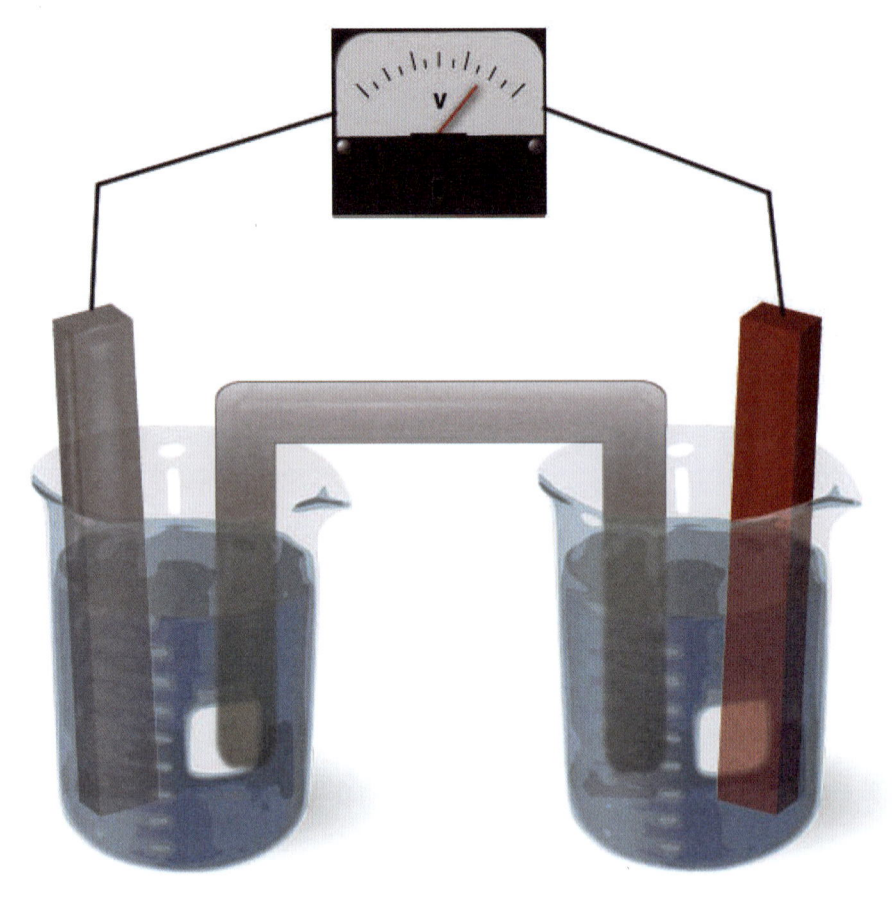

Figure III.A.10.1a: A galvanic (electrochemical) cell.

The metallic parts (Cu(s) and Zn(s) in our example) of the galvanic cell which allow its connection to an external circuit are called <u>electrodes</u>. The electrode <u>out</u> of which <u>electrons flow</u> is the <u>anode</u>, the electrode <u>receiving</u> these <u>electrons</u> is the <u>cathode</u>. In a galvanic cell the <u>oxidation</u> occurs in the <u>anodic compartment</u> and the <u>reduction</u> in the <u>cathodic compartment</u>. The voltage difference between the two electrodes is called the <u>electromotive force (emf)</u> of the cell, if the concentration of all the ions involved is 1 molal, the emf is simply:

$$\text{emf} = n \times E°(\text{reduction}) - m \times E°(\text{oxidation})$$

Where n and m are the stoichiometric factors by which each half-reaction needs to be multiplied to yield a balanced overall reaction. The stoichiometric factors are *not* used if one is simply calculating the E° of the cell. The voltage can be measured by the voltmeter. {Mnemonic: LEO is A GERC = <u>L</u>ose <u>E</u>lectrons <u>O</u>xidation is <u>A</u>node, <u>G</u>ain <u>E</u>lectrons <u>R</u>eduction at <u>C</u>athode}

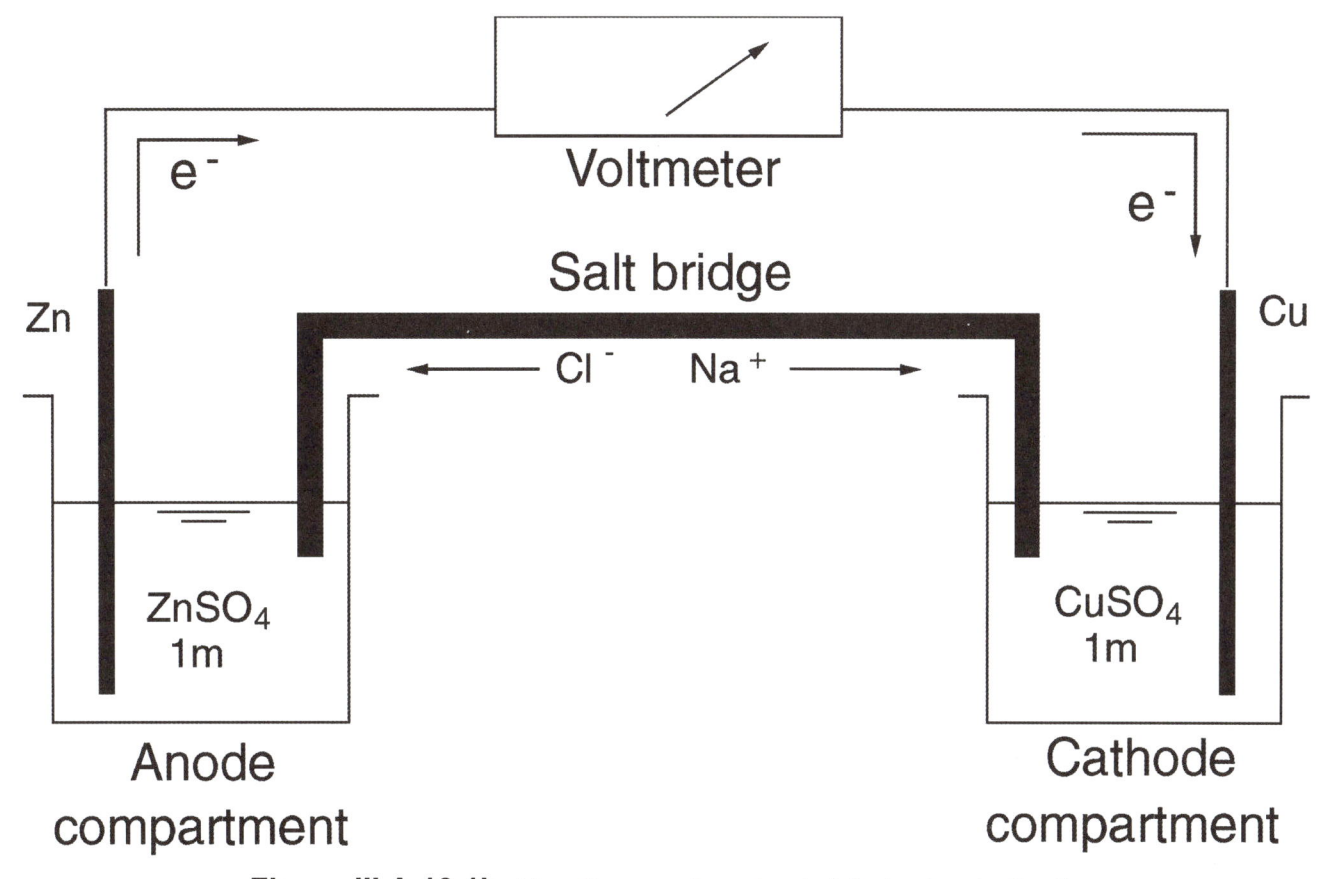

Figure III.A.10.1b: Line diagram of a galvanic (electrochemical) cell.

10.2.1 The Salt Bridge

The salt bridge connects the two compartments chemically (for example, with Na^+ and Cl^-). It has two important functions:

1) Maintenance of Neutrality: As Zn(s) becomes Zn^{2+}(aq), the net charge in the anode compartment becomes positive. To maintain neutrality, Cl^- ions migrate to the anode compartment. The reverse occurs in the cathode compartment: positive ions are lost (Cu^{2+}), therefore positive ions must be gained (Na^+).

2) Completing the Circuit: Imagine the galvanic cell as a circuit. Negative charge leaves the anode compartment via electrons in a wire and then returns via chemicals (i.e. Cl^-) in the salt bridge. Thus the galvanic cell is an electrochemical cell.

GAMSAT-Prep.com
THE GOLD STANDARD

As an alternative to a salt bridge, the solutions (i.e. ZnSO$_4$ and CuSO$_4$) can be placed in one container separated by a porous material which allows certain ions to cross (i.e. SO$_4^{2-}$, Zn^{2-}). Thus it would serve the same functions as the salt bridge.

10.3 Concentration Cell

If the concentration of the ions in one of the compartments of a galvanic cell is not 1 molal, the half-cell potential E is either higher or lower than E°. Therefore, in principle one could use the same substance in both compartments but with different concentrations to produce electricity. The emf is equal in this case to the difference between the two potentials E. Such a cell is called a concentration cell. To determine the direction of electron flow the same rules as above are used. The cathodic compartment, in which the reduction takes place is the one corresponding to the largest positive (smallest negative) E.

10.4 Electrolytic Cell

There is a fundamental difference between a galvanic cell or a concentration cell and an electrolytic cell: in the first type of electrochemical cell a spontaneous redox reaction is used to produce a current, in the second type a current is actually imposed on the system to drive a non-spontaneous redox reaction. A similarity between the two cells is that the cathode attracts cations, whereas the anode attracts anions.

Remember the following key concepts:
(i) generally a battery is used to produce a current which is imposed on the electrolytic cell.
(ii) the battery acts as an electron pump: electrons flow into the electrolytic cell at the cathode and flow out of it at the anode.
(iii) the half-reaction occurring at the cathode is a reduction since it requires electrons.
(iv) the half-reaction occurring at the anode is an oxidation since it produces electrons.

GENERAL CHEMISTRY

10.5 Faraday's Law

Faraday's law relates the amount of elements deposited or gas liberated at an electrode due to current.

We have seen that in a galvanic cell $Cu^{++}(aq)$ can accept electrons to become $Cu(s)$ which will actually plate onto the electrode. Faraday's Law allows us to calculate the amount of $Cu(s)$. In fact, the law states that the weight of product formed at an electrode is proportional to the amount of electricity transferred at the electrode and to the equivalent weight of the material. Thus we can conclude that 1 mole of $Cu^{++}(aq)$ + 2 moles of electrons will leave 1 mole of $Cu(s)$ at the electrode. One mole (= Avogadro's number) of electrons is called a *faraday* ($\mathfrak{F}$). A faraday is equivalent to 96 500 coulombs. As mentioned in Physics 10.1, a coulomb is the amount of electricity that is transferred when a current of one ampere flows for one second ($1C = 1A \cdot S$).

> The police stopped a driver who had NaCl and a 9 volt. He was booked for a salt and battery.

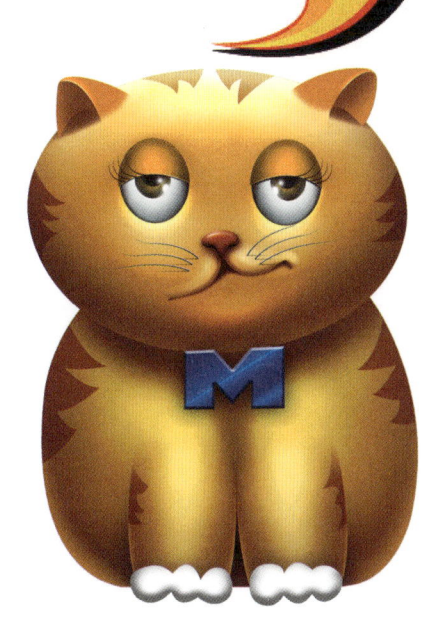

10.5.1 Electrolysis Problem

How many grams of copper would be deposited on the cathode of an electrolytic cell if, for a period of 20 minutes, a current of 2.0 amperes is run through a solution of $CuSO_4$? {The molecular weight of copper is 63.5.}

Calculate the number of coulombs:

$$Q = It = 2.0 \text{ A} \times 20 \text{ min} \times 60 \text{ sec/min}$$
$$= 2400 \text{ C}$$

Thus

$$\text{Faradays} = 2400 \text{ C} \times 1\mathcal{F}/96\,500 \text{ C}$$
$$= 0.025 \mathcal{F}$$

Faradays can be related to moles of copper since

$$Cu^{2+} + 2e^- \rightarrow Cu$$

Since 1 mol Cu : 2 mol e^- we can write

$$0.025\mathcal{F} \times (1 \text{ mol Cu}/2\mathcal{F}) \times (63.5\text{g Cu/mol Cu})$$
$$= 0.79\text{g Cu}$$

Electrolysis would deposit 0.79 g of copper at the cathode.

To do the previous problem, you must know the definition of current and charge (CHM 10.5; PHY 10.1) but the value of the constant (a faraday) would be given on the exam. You should be able to perform the preceding calculation quickly and efficiently because it involves dimensional analysis. Many questions on the GAMSAT are based on dimensional analysis (see Part II, Section 2.2, #16 of this book).

GOLD NOTES

GAMSAT-prep.com
PHYSICS
PART III.B: PHYSICAL SCIENCES

IMPORTANT: Before doing your science survey for the GAMSAT, be sure you have read the Preface, Introduction and Part II, Chapter 2. The beginning of each science chapter provides guidelines as to what you should Memorize, Understand and what is Not Required. These are guides to get you a top score without getting lost in the details. Our guides have been determined from an analysis of all ACER materials plus student surveys. Additionally, the original owner of this book gets a full year access to many online features described in the Preface and Introduction including an online Forum where each chapter can be discussed.

TRANSLATIONAL MOTION
Chapter 1

Memorize
* Trigonometric functions: definitions
* Pythagorean theorem
* Define: displacement, velocity, acceleration
* Equations: acceleration, kinematics

Understand
* Scalar vs. vector
* Add, subtract, resolve vectors
* Determine common values of functions
* Conversion of the angle to other units
* Displacement, velocity, acceleration (avg. and instant.) including graphs

Not Required*
* Advanced level college info
* Any derivatives with or without vectors
* Complex vector systems

GAMSAT-Prep.com

Introduction

Translational motion is the movement of an object (or particle) through space without turning (rotation). Displacement, velocity and acceleration are key vectors – specified by magnitude and direction - often used to describe translational motion. Being able to manipulate and resolve vectors is critical for problem solving in GAMSAT physics.

Additional Resources

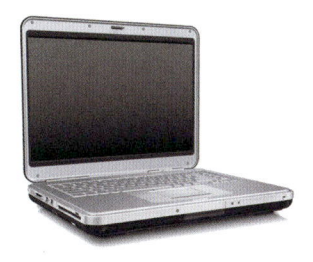

Free Online Q&A + Forum   Video: Online or DVD 3   Flashcards   Special Guest

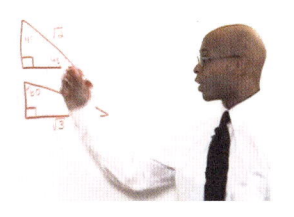

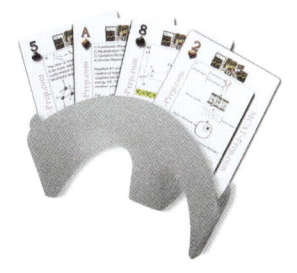

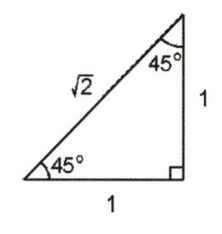

THE PHYSICAL SCIENCES   PHY-03

* The real GAMSAT may have advanced level information presented (ie. in a passage) but previous knowledge of said information is not required to answer the questions that would follow. Practice ACER and GS practice GAMSATs can help you clarify this point.

GAMSAT-Prep.com
THE GOLD STANDARD

1.1 Scalars and Vectors

Scalars, such as speed, have magnitude only and are specified by a number with a unit (55 miles/hour). Scalars obey the rules of ordinary algebra. *Vectors*, like velocity, have both magnitude **and** direction (100 km/hour, west). Vectors are represented by arrows where: i) the length of the arrow indicates the magnitude of the vector, and ii) the arrowhead indicates the direction of the vector. Vectors obey the special rules of vector algebra. Thus vectors can be moved in space but their orientation must be kept the same.

Addition of Vectors: Two vectors **a** and **b** can be added geometrically by drawing them to a common scale and placing them head to tail. The vector connecting the tail of **a** to the head of **b** is the sum or resultant vector **r**.

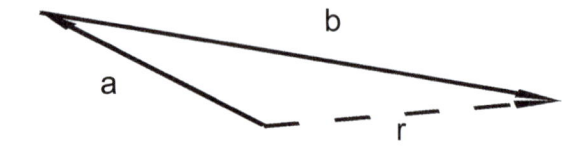

Figure III.B.1.1: The vector sum a + b = r.

Subtraction of Vectors: To subtract the vector **b** from **a**, reverse the direction of **b** then add to **a**.

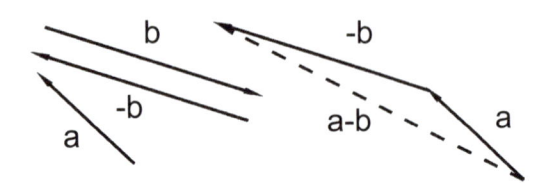

Figure III.B.1.2: The vector difference a - b = a + (-b).

Resolution of Vectors: Perpendicular projections of a vector can be made on a coordinate axis. Thus the vector **a** can be *resolved* into its x-component (a_x) and its y-component (a_y).

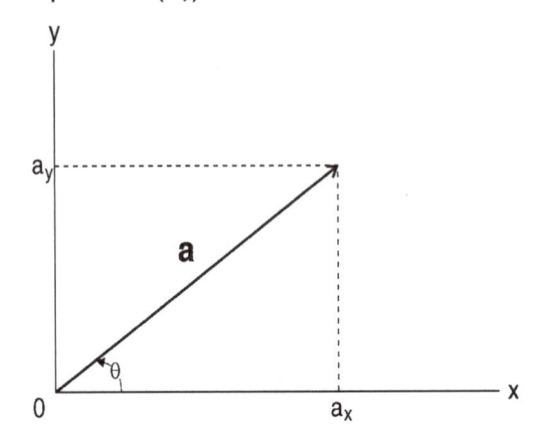

Figure III.B.1.3: The resolution of a vector into its scalar components in a coordinate system.

Analytically, the resolution of vector **a** is as follows:

$$a_x = \mathbf{a} \cos\theta \quad \text{and} \quad a_y = \mathbf{a} \sin\theta$$

Conversely, given the components, we can reconstruct vector **a**:

$$\mathbf{a} = \sqrt{a_x^2 + a_y^2} \quad \text{and} \quad \tan\theta = a_y / a_x$$

Another concept which is sometimes useful is the unit vector. It is a vector of one unit given the special symbols **i**, **j**, and **k** which represent a unit vector in the *x-*, *y-* and *z-*directions, respectively.

PHY-04 TRANSLATIONAL MOTION

Vector **a** can now be written in terms of its components and the unit vectors:

$$\mathbf{a} = \mathbf{i}a_x + \mathbf{j}a_y$$

Thus the vector **a** can be expressed using either scalar components (a_x, a_y) or vector components ($\mathbf{i}a_x$, $\mathbf{j}a_y$).

1.1.1 Trigonometric Functions

The power in trigonometric functions lies in their ability to relate an angle to the ratio of scalar components or *sides* of a triangle. These functions may be defined as follows:

$$\sin \theta = opp/hyp = y/r$$

$$\cos \theta = adj/hyp = x/r$$

[*opp* = the length of the side opposite angle θ, *adj* = the length of the side *adjacent* to angle θ, *hyp* = the length of the *hypotenuse*]

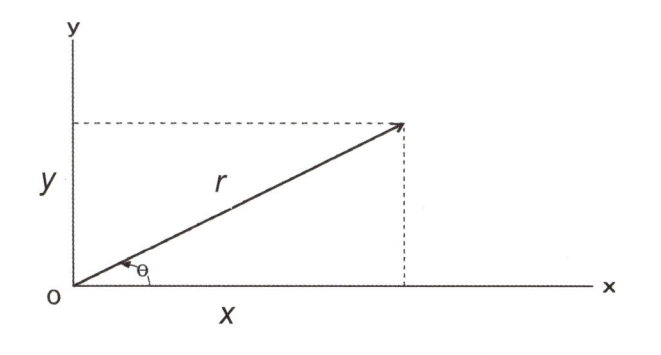

Thus sine ($r\sin \theta$) gives the *y*-component and cosine ($r\cos \theta$) gives the x-component of vector r. The tangent function ($\tan \theta$) and two important trigonometric identities relate sine and cosine:

$$\tan \theta = \sin \theta / \cos \theta = opp/adj = y/x$$

$$\sin^2 \theta + \cos^2 \theta = 1$$

and

$$\sin 2\theta = 2 \sin \theta \cos \theta$$

Other functions of very little importance for GAMSAT physics include: cotangent ($\cot \theta = x/y$), secant ($\sec \theta = r/x$) and cosecant ($\csc \theta = r/y$).

The Pythagorean Theorem relates the sides of the right angle triangle according to the following:

$$r^2 = x^2 + y^2.$$

THE PHYSICAL SCIENCES   PHY-05

1.1.2 Common Values of Trigonometric Functions

There are special angles which produce standard values of the trigonometric functions. These values should be memorized. Several of the values are derived from the following triangles:

θ	sin θ	cos θ	tan θ
0°	0	1	0
30°	1/2	√3/2	1/√3
45°	1/√2	1/√2	1
60°	√3/2	1/2	√3
90°	1	0	∞
180°	0	-1	0

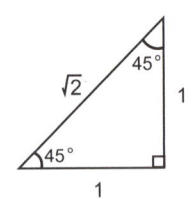

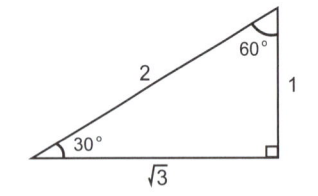

Table III.B.1.1:
Common values of trigonometric functions. The angle θ may be given in radians (R) where $2\pi^R$ = 360° = 1 revolution. Recall √3 ≈ 1.7, √2 ≈ 1.4.

Note that 1° = 60 arcminutes, 1 arcminute = 60 arcseconds.

Each trigonometric function (i.e. sine) contains an inverse function (i.e. $\sin^{-1}$), where if sin θ = x, θ = $\sin^{-1}$ x. Thus cos 60° = 1/2, and 60° = $\cos^{-1}$ (1/2). Some texts denote the inverse function with "arc" as a prefix. Thus arcsec (2) = $\sec^{-1}$ (2).

1.2 Distance and Displacement

Distance is the amount of separation between two points in space. It has a magnitude but no direction. It is a scalar quantity and is always positive. Another concept which is sometimes useful is the <u>unit vector</u>.

Displacement of an object between two points is the difference between the final position and the initial position of the object in a given referential system. Thus, a displacement has an origin, a direction and a magnitude. It is a vector.

The sign of the coordinates of the vector displacement depends on the system under study and the chosen referential system. The sign will be positive (+) if the system is moving towards the positive axis of the referential system and negative (-) if not.

The units of distance and displacement are expressed in length units such as *feet (ft)*, *meters (m)*, *miles* and *kilometers (km)*.

1.3 Speed and Velocity

Speed is the rate of change of distance with respect to time. It is a scalar quantity, it has a magnitude but no direction, like distance, and it is always positive.

Velocity is the rate of change of displacement with respect to time. It is a vector, and like the displacement, it has a direction and a magnitude. Its value depends on the position of the object. The sign of the coordinates of the vector velocity is the same as that of the displacement.

The instantaneous velocity of a system at a given time is the slope of the graph of the displacement of that system vs. time at that time. The magnitude of the velocity decreases if the vector velocity and the vector acceleration have opposite directions.

The units of speed and velocity are expressed in length divided by time such as *feet/sec., meters/sec. (m/s)* and *miles/hour.*

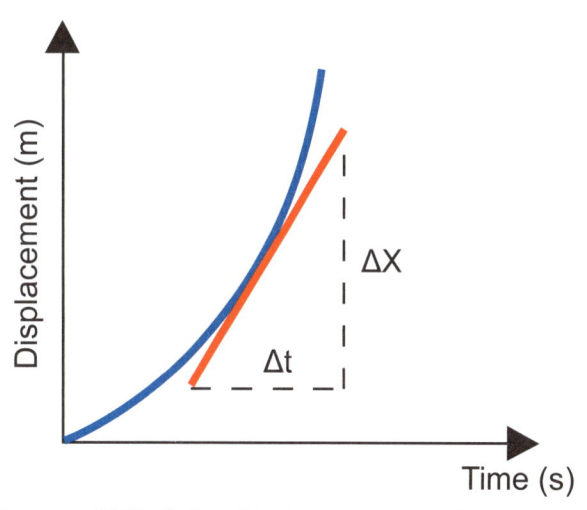

Figure III.B.1.4: Displacement vs. time. Please note that the capital letter X denotes displacement as opposed to referring to the x-axis (small letter x) which is time.

Dimensional Analysis: remember from High School math that a slope is "rise over run" meaning it is the change in the y-axis divided by the change in the x-axis (see Appendix A.3.1). This means when we pay attention to the units, we get, for example, m/s which is velocity.

1.4 Acceleration

Acceleration (a) is the rate of change of the velocity (v) with respect to time (t):

$$a = v/t$$

Like the velocity, it is a vector and it has a direction and a magnitude.

The sign of the vector acceleration depends on the net force applied to the system and the chosen referential system. The units of acceleration are expressed as velocity divided by time such as $meters/sec^2$. The term for negative acceleration is deceleration.

1.4.1 Average and Instantaneous Acceleration

The average acceleration av between two instants t and t' = t + Δt, measures the result of the increase in the speed divided by the time difference,

$$a_v = \frac{v' - v}{\Delta t}$$

The instantaneous acceleration can be determined either by calculating the **slope** (*see* Appendix A.3.1) of a velocity vs. time graph at any time, or by taking the limit when Δt approaches zero of the preceding expression.

$$a_v = \lim_{\Delta t \to 0} \frac{v' - v}{\Delta t}$$

Math involving "limits" does not exist on the GAMSAT. So let's discuss what this definition is describing in informal terms. The limit is the value of the change in velocity over the change in time as the time approaches 0. It's like saying that the change in velocity is happening in an instant. This allows us to talk about the acceleration in that incredibly fast moment: the instantaneous acceleration which can be determined graphically.

Consider the following events illustrated in the graph (Fig. III.B.1.4): your car starts at rest (0 velocity and time = 0); you steadily accelerate out of the parking lot (the change in velocity increases over time = acceleration); you are driving down the street at constant velocity (change in velocity = 0 and thus acceleration is 0 divided by the change in time which means: a = 0); you see a cat dart across the street safely which made you slow down temporarily (change in velocity is negative thus negative acceleration which, by definition, is deceleration); you now enter the on-ramp for the highway so your velocity is now increasing at a faster and faster rate (increasing acceleration). You can examine the instantaneous acceleration at any one point (or instant) during the period that your acceleration is increasing.

To determine the displacement (*not* distance), take the area under the graph or curve. To calculate area: a rectangle is base (b) times height (h); a triangle is ½b × h; and for a curve, they can use graph paper and expect you would count the boxes under the curve to estimate the area.

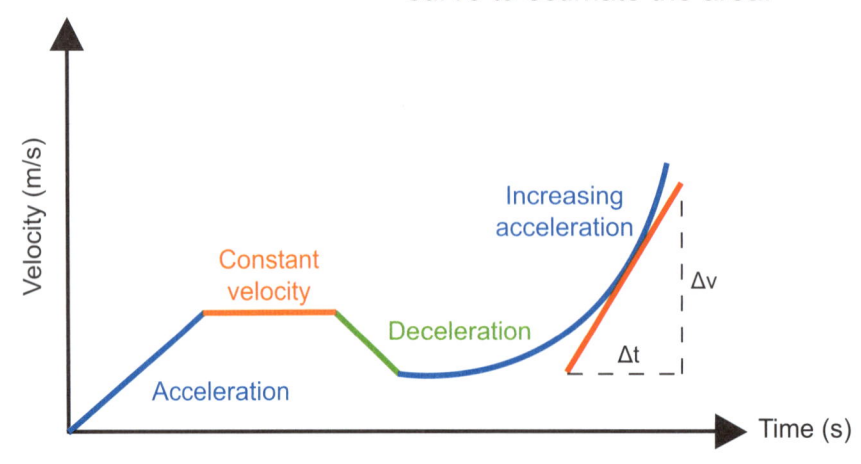

Figure III.B.1.4: Velocity vs. time. Note that at constant velocity, the slope and thus the acceleration are both equal to zero.

1.5 Uniformly Accelerated Motion

The magnitude and direction of the acceleration of a system are solely determined by the exterior forces acting upon the system. If the magnitude of these forces is constant, the magnitude of the acceleration will be constant and the resulting motion is a *uniformly accelerated motion*. The initial displacement, the velocity and the accelera-tion at any given time contribute to the over-all displacement of the system:

$x = x_0$ – displacement due to the initial displacement x_0.
$x = v_0 t$ – displacement due to the initial velocity v_0 at time t.
$x = \frac{1}{2} a t^2$ – displacement due the acceleration at time t.

The total displacement of the uniformly-accelerated motion is given by the following formula:

$$x = x_0 + v_0 t + \tfrac{1}{2} a t^2$$

The translational motion is the motion of the center of gravity of a system through space, illustrated by the above equation.

1.6 Equations of Kinematics

Kinematics is the study of objects in motion with respect to space and time. There are three related equations which must be memorized. The first is above (PHY 1.5), the others are:

$$v = v_0 + at \quad \text{and}$$
$$v^2 = v_0^2 + 2ax$$

where *v* is the final velocity; we will put these equations to use in PHY 2.6.

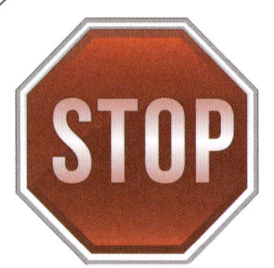

Reminder: Chapter review questions are available online for the original owner of this textbook. Doing practice questions will help clarify concepts and ensure that you study in a targeted way. First, register at gamsat-prep.com, then login and click on GAMSAT Textbook Owners in the right column so you can use your Online Access Card to have access to the Lessons section.

No science background? Consider watching the relevant videos at gamsat-prep.com and you have support at gamsat-prep.com/forum. Don't forget to check the Index at the beginning of this book to see which chapters are **HIGH**, **MEDIUM** and **LOW** relative importance for the GAMSAT.

Your online access continues for one full year from your online registration.

GOLD NOTES

FORCE, MOTION, AND GRAVITATION
Chapter 2

Memorize	Understand	Not Required*
Define with units: weight, mass Newton's laws, Law of Gravitation Equation for uniformly accelerated motion	* Mass, weight, center of gravity * Newton's laws * Law of Gravitation, free fall motion * Projectile motion equations and calculations	* Advanced level college info * Memorizing values for K,G

GAMSAT-Prep.com

Introduction

Force is a vector (often a push or pull) that can cause a mass to change velocity thus motion. Forces can be due to gravity, magnetism or anything that causes a mass to accelerate. Nuclear forces (strong) are far greater than electrostatic forces (opposite charges attract), which in turn are far greater than gravitational forces (one of the weakest forces in nature).

Additional Resources

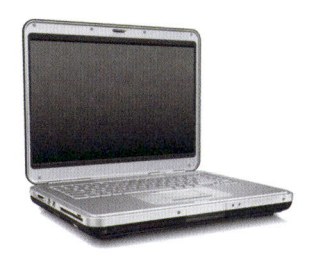

Free Online Q&A + Forum   Video: Online or DVD 1,3   Flashcards   Special Guest

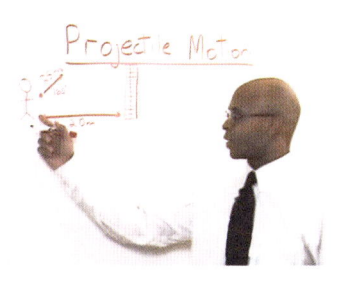

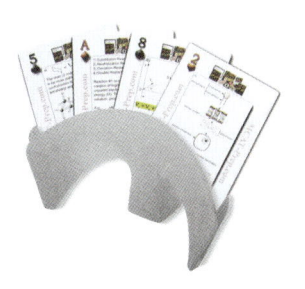

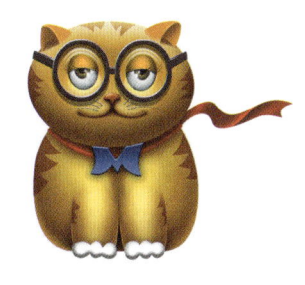

THE PHYSICAL SCIENCES   PHY-11

* The real GAMSAT may have advanced level information presented (ie. in a passage) but previous knowledge of said information is not required to answer the questions that would follow. Practice ACER and GS practice GAMSATs can help you clarify this point.

2.1 Mass, Center of Mass, Weight

The mass (m) of an object is its measure of inertia. It is the measure of the capacity of that object to remain motionless or to move with a constant velocity if the sum of the forces acting upon it is zero. This definition of inertia is derived from Newton's First Law.

The *center of mass* of an object is a point whose motion can be described like the motion of a particle through space. The center of mass of an object always has the simplest motion of all the points of that object.

The center of gravity (COG) is also the center of mass seen as the center of application of all the gravitational forces acting on the object. For example, for a uniform plank hanging horizontally, the COG is at half the length of the plank.

The COG can be determined experimentally by suspending an object by a string at different points and noting that the direction of the string passes through the COG. The intersection of the projected lines in the different suspensions is the COG.

An object is in *stable equilibrium* if the COG is as low as possible and any change in orientation will lead to an elevation of the COG. An object is in *unstable equilibrium* if the COG is high relative to the support point or surface and any change in orientation will lead to a lowering of the COG.

The *weight* is a force (i.e. newtons, pounds). It is a vector unlike the *mass* which is a scalar (i.e. kilograms, slugs). The weight is proportional to the mass. It is the product of the mass by the vector gravitational acceleration g.

$$W = m \times g$$

2.2 Newton's Second Law

Newton's Second Law, also called the fundamental dynamic relation, states that the sum of all the exterior forces acting upon the center of mass of a system is equal to the product of the mass of the system by the acceleration of its center of mass.

Therefore, if there is a net force, the object must accelerate. It is a vectorial equality which asserts that <u>a net force against an object *must* result in acceleration</u>:

$$\Sigma F = m \times a$$

It is important to note that for a system in complex motion, Newton's Second Law can only determine the acceleration of the center of mass. It does not give any indication about the motion of the other parts of the system.

Whereas, for a system in translational motion, Newton's Second Law gives the acceleration of the system.

In your daily life, you would already have the sense that objects with a greater mass (m) require a greater force (F) to get it to move with increasing speed (a). If you maintain a net force on an object, it will not only move, it must accelerate. We will be exploring more consequences of Newton's Second Law both in this and later chapters.

2.3 Newton's Third Law

For every action there is an equal and opposite reaction. If one object exerts a force, F, on a second object, the second object exerts a force, F', on the first object. F and F' have opposite direction but the same magnitude.

One conclusion would be that forces are found in pairs. Consider the time you sit in a chair. Your body exerts a force downward (mg) and that chair needs to exert an equal force upward (the normal force N) or the chair will collapse. There is symmetry. Acting forces encounter other forces in the opposite direction. Consider shooting a cannonball. When the explosion fires the cannonball through the air, the cannon is pushed backward. The force pushing the ball out is equal to the force pushing the cannon back, but the effect on the cannon is less noticeable because it has a much larger mass and it may be restrained. Similarly, a gun experiences a "kick" backwards when a bullet is fired forward.

2.4 The Law of Gravitation

The Law of Gravitation states that there is a force of attraction existing between any two bodies of masses m_1 and m_2. The force is proportional to the product of the masses and inversely proportional to the square of the distance between them.

$$F = K_G(m_1 m_2 / r_2)$$

r is the distance between the bodies; K_G is the universal constant of gravitation, and its value depends on the units being used.

2.5 Free Fall Motion

The free fall motion of an object is the upward or downward vertical motion of that object with reference to the earth.

The motion is always uniformly accelerated with the acceleration g: vertical, directed towards the center of the earth and the magnitude is considered constant during the free fall motion.

Also, during the free fall motion, the air resistance is considered negligible. The equation of the motion can easily be derived from Newton's Second Law.

$$\Sigma F = ma$$

Where ΣF represents all the forces acting on the object, m is the mass of the object and a is the acceleration of the center of mass of the object. Hence, a can be replaced by g since $a = g$ by definition. In the free fall motion, the only force acting on the object is the gravitational force, which gives the following equality:

$$K_G m_{object} \frac{M_{earth}}{r^2_{earth}} = m_{object}\, g$$

dividing both sides by m_{object} we get:

$$g = K_G \frac{M_{earth}}{r^2_{earth}}$$

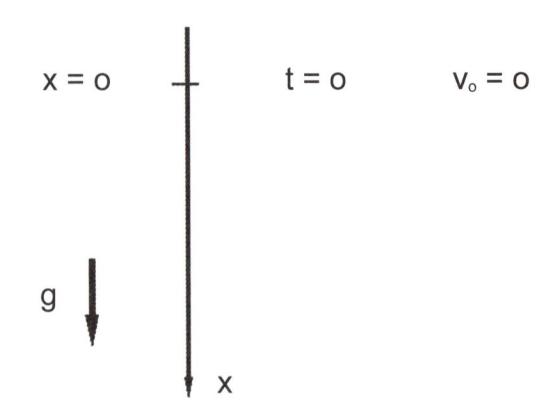

Figure III.B.2.1: Free fall motion.

The values of g are: 32 ft/s^2 (Imperial units), 980 cm/s^2 (CGS units), or 9.8 m/s^2 (**SI** units). The equation for uniformly accelerated motion is applicable by replacing a by g:

$$x = x_0 + v_0 t + 1/2 g t^2$$

$$v = gt$$

$$a = g$$

Before doing any calculation, the reference point and a positive direction must be chosen. In the free fall of an actual object, the value of g is modified by the buoyancy of air and resistance of air. This results in a *drag force* which depends on the location on earth, shape and size of the object, and the velocity of the object (as free fall velocity increases, the drag force increases). When the drag force reaches the force of gravity, the object reaches a final velocity called the terminal velocity and continues to fall at that velocity.

2.6 Projectile Motion

The projectile motion is the motion of any object fired or launched at some angle α from the horizontal. The motion defines a parabola (see Figure III.B.2.2) in the plane O-x-y that contains the initial (*original*) vector velocity v_o.

The motion can be decomposed into two distinct motions: a vertical component, affected by g, and a horizontal component, independent of g.

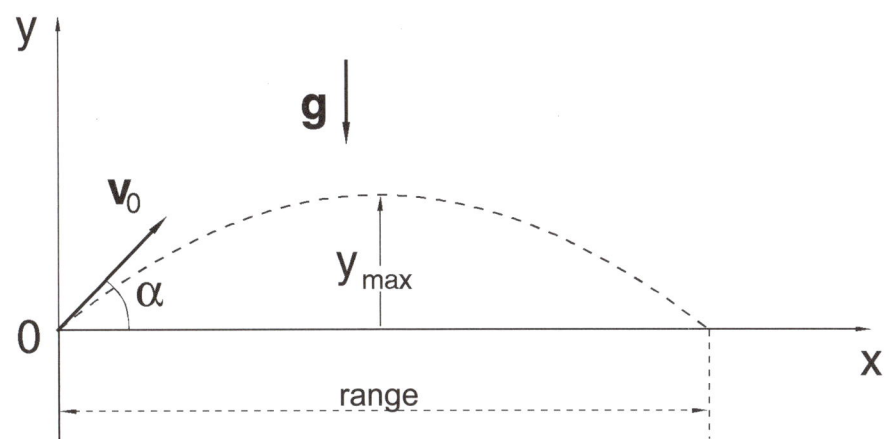

Figure III.B.2.2: Projectile motion.

Vertical component (free fall)
- initial speed : $V_{oy} = V_o \sin \alpha$
- displacement at time t: $y = V_{oy}t + 1/2gt^2$
- speed at any time t: $V_y = V_{oy} + gt$

Initial velocity
- magnitude: $|V_o| = \sqrt{V_{ox}^2 + V_{oy}^2}$
- direction: *alpha*: $\tan \alpha = V_{oy}/V_{ox}$

- important points to consider:
1) Neglecting air resistance, there is no acceleration in the horizontal direction: V_x is constant.
2) V_y is zero at Y_{max}, then $V_y = 0 = V_{oy} + gt_{up}$ or $-V_{oy} = gt_{up}$ can be solved for t.

Horizontal component (linear with constant speed)
- initial speed : $V_{ox} = V_o \cos \alpha$
- displacement at any time t: $x = V_{ox}t$
- speed at any time t: $V_x = V_{ox}$ (speed is constant)

3) Also, by eliminating the variables y and t in the equations, we can get the following equality :

$$x = \frac{V_o^2 \sin 2\alpha}{g}$$

The horizontal distance from the origin to where the object strikes the ground (= *the range*) is maximum for a given V_o when $\sin 2\alpha = 1$, hence for $2\alpha = (\pi/2)^R$ => $\alpha = (\pi/4)^R$ or α = 45 degrees.

2.6.1 Projectile Motion Problem (Imperial units)

In the Rugby World Cup, a player kicks the ball at an angle of 30° from the horizontal with an initial speed of 75 ft/s. Assume that the ball moves in a vertical plane and that air resistance is negligible.

(a) *Find the time at which the ball reaches the highest point of its trajectory.*
{key: height refers to the y-component; we can define gravity as a negative vector since it is directed downwards}

V_y is zero at Y_{max} (= the highest point), thus:

$V_y = 0$, $V_o = 75$ ft/s, $\alpha = 30°$, $g = -32$ ft/s²

$V_y = V_o \sin \alpha + gt_{up}$

Isolate t_{up}:

$$t_{up} = \frac{V_y - V_o \sin \alpha}{g} = \frac{-75(\sin 30°)}{-32}$$

$$= 1.2 \text{ seconds}$$

(b) *How high does the ball go?*

$Y_{max} = V_o (\sin \alpha) t_{up} + 1/2 g t_{up}^2$

$Y_{max} = 75(\sin 30°)1.2 + 1/2(-32)(1.2)^2 = 22$ feet

(c) *How long is the ball in the air and what is its range?*
{key: time is the same for x- and y-components, range = x-component}

Once the ball strikes the ground its vertical displacement y = 0, thus:

$y = 0 = V_o (\sin \alpha) t + 1/2 g t^2$

Divide through by t then isolate:

$t = 2V_o(\sin \alpha)/g = 2.4$ seconds.

Since $t = 2t_{up}$, we can conclude that the time required for the ball to go up to Y_{max} is the same as the time required to come back down: 1.2 seconds in either direction.

The range $x = V_o(\cos \alpha)t$

$x = 75(\cos 30°)2.4 \approx 150$ feet

or

$x \approx 150$ ft (1 yd/ 3 ft) = 50 yards

{Had the player kicked the ball at 45° from the horizontal he would have maximized his range. He should be benched for not having done his physics!}

PHY-16   FORCE, MOTION, AND GRAVITATION

(d) *What is the velocity of the ball as it strikes the ground?*

{*key:* velocity is the resultant vector of V_x and V_y - the final velocities in the *x* and *y* directions}

$V_x = V_o \cos \alpha = 75(\cos 30°) = 65$ ft/s

$V_y = V_o \sin \alpha + gt$

$= 75(\sin 30°) + (-32)(2.4) = -39$ ft/s

$V = \sqrt{V_x^2 + V_y^2} = \sqrt{(65)^2 + (-39)^2}$

$= \sqrt{(13 \times 5)^2 + (13 \times -3)^2}$

$V = 13\sqrt{(5)^2 + (-3)^2} = 13\sqrt{34}$

To estimate $\sqrt{34}$ we must first recognize that the answer must be at least 5 ($5^2 = 25$) but closer to 6 ($6^2 = 36$). Try squaring 5.7, 5.8, 5.9. Squaring 5.8 is the closest estimate (= *33.6*), thus

$V = 13(5.8) = 75$ ft/s.

Please note:
- With no air resistance and a symmetric problem (the ball is launched and returns to the same vertical point), the initial and final speeds are the same (75 ft/s).
- Usually ACER will use SI units in GAMSAT problems, but many problems are solved using dimensional analysis, with or without SI units.
- Please be sure you can do all the preceding calculations efficiently. To learn more about SI units, see Appendix B.

Dogs have owners. Cats have staff!

GOLD NOTES

PARTICLE DYNAMICS
Chapter 3

Memorize
* Centripetal force and acceleration
* Circumference and area of a circle

Understand
* Equations: f_{max}, μ_s
* Static vs. kinetic friction
* Resolving vectors, calculate for incline plane
* Uniform circular motion
* Solve pulley system, free body diagram

Not Required*
* Advanced level college info
* Memorizing values of μ

GAMSAT-Prep.com

Introduction

Particle dynamics is concerned with the physics of motion. Among other topics, particle dynamics includes Newton's laws, frictional forces, and problems dealing with incline planes, uniform circular motion and pulley systems.

Additional Resources

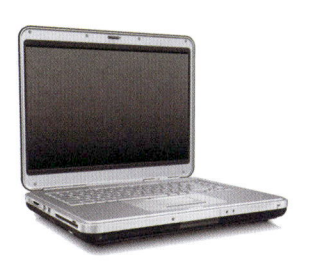

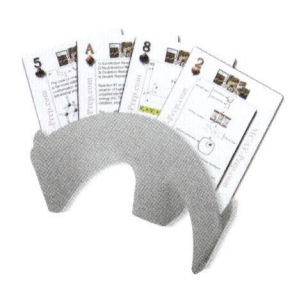

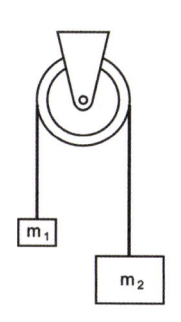

Free Online Q&A + Forum   Video: Online or DVD 3,4   Flashcards   Special Guest

THE PHYSICAL SCIENCES   PHY-19

* The real GAMSAT may have advanced level information presented (ie. in a passage) but previous knowledge of said information is not required to answer the questions that would follow. Practice ACER and GS practice GAMSATs can help you clarify this point.

GAMSAT-Prep.com
THE GOLD STANDARD

3.1 Overview

For the GAMSAT, particle dynamics is concerned with the physics of motion. Among other topics, particle dynamics includes Newton's laws, frictional forces, and problems dealing with incline planes, uniform circular motion and pulley systems.

3.2 Frictional Forces

Frictional forces are nonconservative (mechanical energy is not conserved) and are caused by molecular adhesion between tangential surfaces but are independent of the area of contact of the surfaces. Frictional forces always oppose the motion. The maximal frictional force has the following expression: $f_{max} = \mu N$, where μ is the coefficient of friction and N is the normal force to the surface on which the object rests, it is the reaction of that surface against the weight of the object. Thus N always acts perpendicular to the surface.

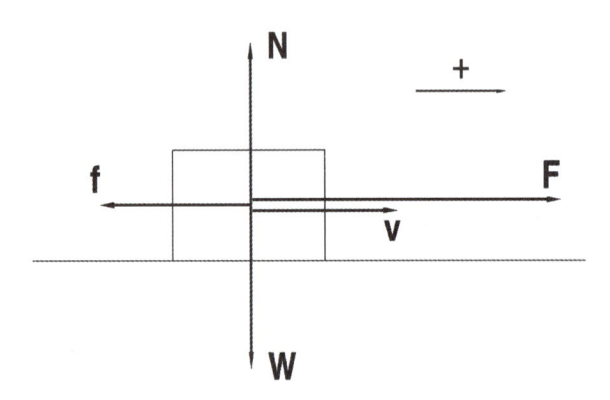

Figure III.B.3.1: Frictional force f and force normal N.

Static friction is when the object is not moving, and it must be overcome for motion to begin. The coefficient of static friction μ_s is given as :

$$\mu_s = \tan \alpha$$

where α is the angle at which the object first begins to move on an inclined plane as the angle is increased from 0 degrees to α degrees (see Figure III.B.3.2). There is also a coefficient of kinetic friction, μ_k, which exists when surfaces are in motion; $\mu_k < \mu_s$ always.

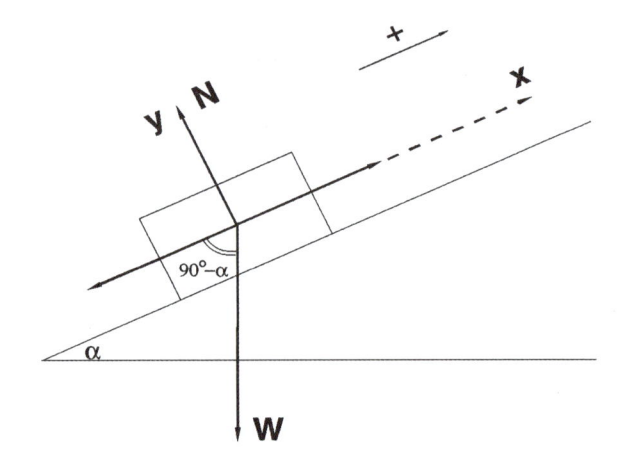

Figure III.B.3.2: Analysis of motion on an incline.

PARTICLE DYNAMICS

The weight (W) due to gravity (g) may be sufficient to cause motion if friction is overcome. The reference axes are usually chosen as shown such that one (the x) is along the surface of the incline.

Note that W is directed downward and N is directed upward but *perpendicular* to the surface of the incline (i.e. in the positive y direction).

3.2.1 Incline Plane Problem with Friction (SI units)

A 50 kilogram block is on an incline of 45°. The coefficient of sliding (= *kinetic*) friction between the block and the plane is 0.10.

Determine the acceleration of the block. {key: motion is along the plane, so only the x-components of the force is relevant to the acceleration}

Begin with Newton's Second Law:

$$F = m \times a$$

thus

$$F_x = f_k - W\sin\alpha = \mu_k N - W\sin\alpha = m \times a$$

The force normal (N) can be determined by summing the forces in the y direction where the acceleration is zero:

$$F_y = N - W\cos\alpha = m \times a = 0$$

Therefore,

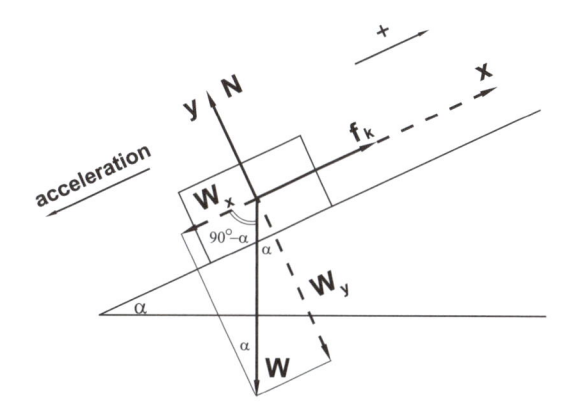

$$N = W\cos\alpha$$

Figure III.B.3.3: Resolving the weight W into its x-component (W sinα) and its y-component (W cosα).

Solving for a and combining our first and last equations we get (*recall:* W = mg):

$$a = (\mu_k W\cos\alpha - W\sin\alpha)/m$$
$$= mg(\mu_k\cos\alpha - \sin\alpha)/m = g(\mu_k\cos\alpha - \sin\alpha)$$

Substituting the values:

$$a = 9.8 \text{ m/s}^2(0.10\cos 45° - \sin 45°) = -6.2 \text{ m/s}^2$$

• Thus the block accelerates at 6.2 m/s² *down* the plane. Also note that the *mass* of the block is irrelevant.

3.3 Uniform Circular Motion

In Chapter 1 we saw that acceleration is due to a change in velocity (PHY 1.4). For a particle moving in a circle at constant speed (= *uniform circular motion*), the velocity vector changes continuously in direction but the magnitude remains the same.

The velocity is always tangent to the circle and since it is always changing (i.e. *direction*) it creates an acceleration directed radially inward called the *centripetal* acceleration (a_c). The magnitude of the acceleration a_c is given by v^2/r where r is the radius of the circle.

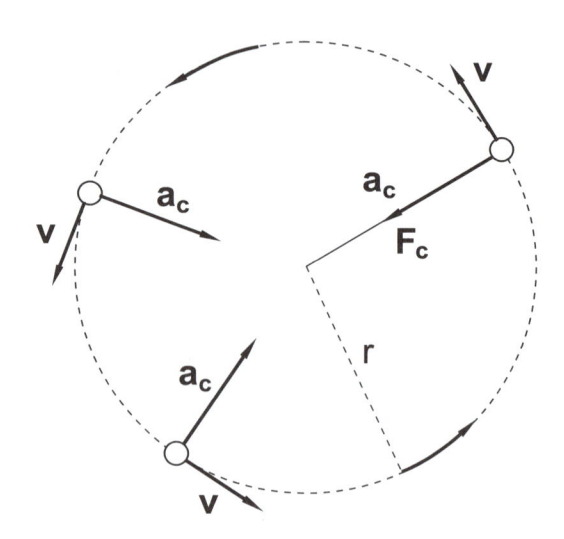

Figure III.B.3.4: Uniform Circular Motion.

Every accelerated particle must have a force acting on it according to Newton's Second Law. Thus we can calculate the *centripetal* force,

$$F_c = ma_c = mv^2/r.$$

The centripetal force can be produced in many ways: a taut string which is holding a ball at the end that is spinning in a circle; a radially directed frictional force like when a car drives around a curve on an unbanked road; a contact force exerted by another body like driving around a curve on a banked road or like the wall of an amusement park rotor.

Any particle moving in a circle with *non-uniform* speed will experience both centripetal and tangential forces and accelerations. {Reminder: the circumference of a circle is $2\pi r$ and the area is πr^2}

PHY-22 PARTICLE DYNAMICS

3.4 Pulley Systems

Consider two unequal masses connected by a string which passes over a frictionless, massless pulley (see Figure III.B.3.5). Let us determine the following parameters: i) the tension T in the string which is a force and ii) the acceleration of the masses given that m_2 is greater than m_1.

Always begin by drawing vector or *free-body* diagrams of a problem. The position of each mass will lie at the origin O of their respective axes. Now we assign positivity or negativity to the directions of motion. We can arbitrarily define the upward direction as positive. Thus if the acceleration of m_1 is a then the acceleration of m_2 must be $-a$.

Using Newton's Second Law we can derive the equation of motion for m_1:

$$F = T - m_1 g = m_1 a$$

and for m_2:

$$F = T - m_2 g = -m_2 a$$

Subtracting one equation from the other eliminates T then we can solve for a:

$$a = \frac{m_2 - m_1}{m_2 + m_1} g$$

Solve for a using the equations of motion, equate the formulas, then we can solve for T:

$$T = \frac{2 m_1 m_2}{m_1 + m_2} g$$

(a)   (b)

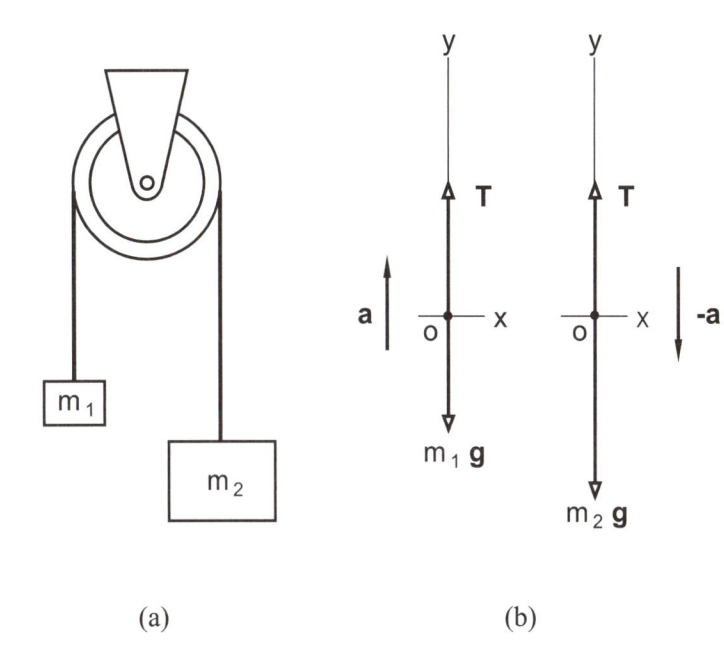

Figure III.B.3.5: A Pulley System. (a) Two unequal masses suspended by a string from a pulley (= Atwood's machine). (b) Free-body diagrams for m_1 and m_2.

Let us solve the problem using Imperial units where m_2 is 3.0 slugs ($W_2 = m_2 g$ = 96 pounds - lb) and m_1 is 1.0 slug ($W_1 = m_1 g$ = 32 lb):

$$a = \frac{3.0 - 1.0}{3.0 + 1.0} g = g/2 = 16 \text{ ft/s}^2$$

and

$$T = \frac{2\,(1.0)\,(3.0)}{1.0 + 3.0}(32) = 48 \text{ lb}.$$

- Note that T is always between the weight of mass m_1 and that of m_2. The reason is that T must exceed $m_1 g$ to give m_1 an upward acceleration, and $m_2 g$ must exceed T to give m_2 a downward acceleration.

GOLD NOTES

EQUILIBRIUM
Chapter 4

Memorize
Definitions and equations to solve torque problems
Newton's First Law, inertia
Equations for momentum, impulse

Understand
* Solve torque, collision problems
* Choosing an appropriate pivot point
* Create vector diagrams
* Elastic vs. inelastic vs. conservation of E.
* Solve momentum problem, significant figures

Not Required*
* Advanced level college info
* Complex torque or collision problems
* Torque as a function of time
* Machine torque

GAMSAT-Prep.com

Introduction

Equilibrium exists when a mass is at rest or moves with constant velocity. Translational (straight line) and rotational (turning) equilibria can be resolved using linear forces, torque forces, Newton's first law and inertia. Momentum is a vector that can be used to solve problems involving elastic (bouncy) or inelastic (sticky) collisions.

Additional Resources

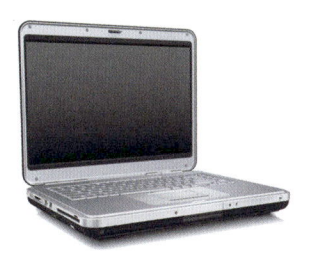

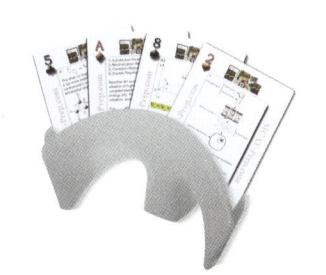

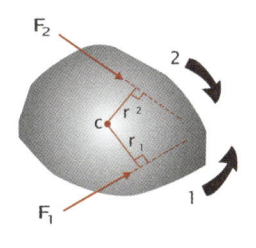

Free Online Q&A + Forum   Video: Online or DVD 4   Flashcards   Special Guest

THE PHYSICAL SCIENCES   PHY-25

* The real GAMSAT may have advanced level information presented (ie. in a passage) but previous knowledge of said information is not required to answer the questions that would follow. Practice ACER and GS practice GAMSATs can help you clarify this point.

4.1 Translational, Rotational and Complex Motion

When a force acts upon an object, the object will undergo translational, rotational or complex (translational and rotational) motion.

Rotational motion of an object about an axis is the rotation of that object around that axis caused by perpendicular forces to that axis. The effective force causing rotation about an axis is the torque (L).

The torque is like a *turning force*. Consider a hinged door. If you were to apply a force F at the pivot point (*the hinge*), the door would not turn ($L=0$). If you apply the *same* force further and further from the pivot point, the turning force multiplies and the acceleration of the door increases. Thus the torque can be defined as the force applied multiplied by the perpendicular distance from the pivot point (= *lever or moment arm = r*).

$$L = (\text{force}) \times (\text{lever arm})$$

Thus according to Figure III.B.4.1:

$$L_1 = F_1 \times r_1 = \text{counterclockwise torque (1)} = \text{positive}$$

and

$$L_2 = F_2 \times r_2 = \text{clockwise torque (2)} = \text{negative.}$$

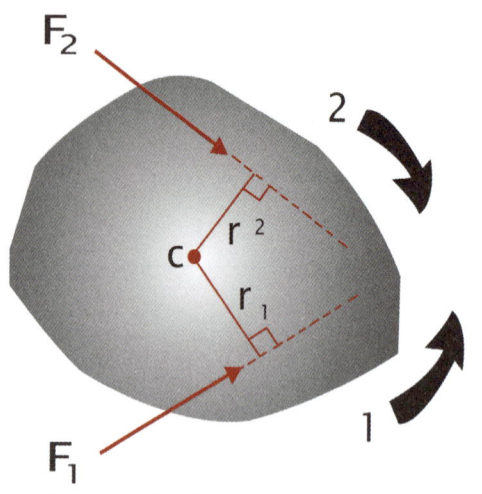

Figure III.B.4.1: Rotational Motion.

Positivity and negativity are arbitrary designations of the two opposite directions of motion. To determine the direction of rotation caused by the torque, imagine the direction the object would rotate if the force is pushing its moment arm at right angles. The net torques acting upon an object is obtained by summing the counterclockwise (+) and the clockwise (-) torques. An object is at equilibrium when the net forces and the net torques acting upon the object is zero. Thus, the object is either motionless or moving at a constant velocity due to its internal inertia.

The conditions of equilibrium are:

For translational equilibrium:

$$\Sigma F_x = 0 \text{ and } \Sigma F_y = 0$$

For rotational equilibrium:

$$\Sigma L = 0$$

If the torques sum to zero about one point in an object, they will sum to zero about any point in the object. If the point chosen as reference (= *pivot point or fulcrum*) includes the line of action of one of the forces, that force need not be included in calculating torques.

4.1.1 Torque Problem (SI units)

A 70 kg person sits 50 cm from the edge of a non-uniform plank which weighs 100 N and is 2.0 m long (*see Figure III.B.4.2*). The weight supported by point *B* is 250 N. Find the center of gravity (COG) of the plank.

{key: draw a vector diagram then choose an unknown value as the pivot point i.e. point A; see section 2.1 for a definition of COG}

(a)

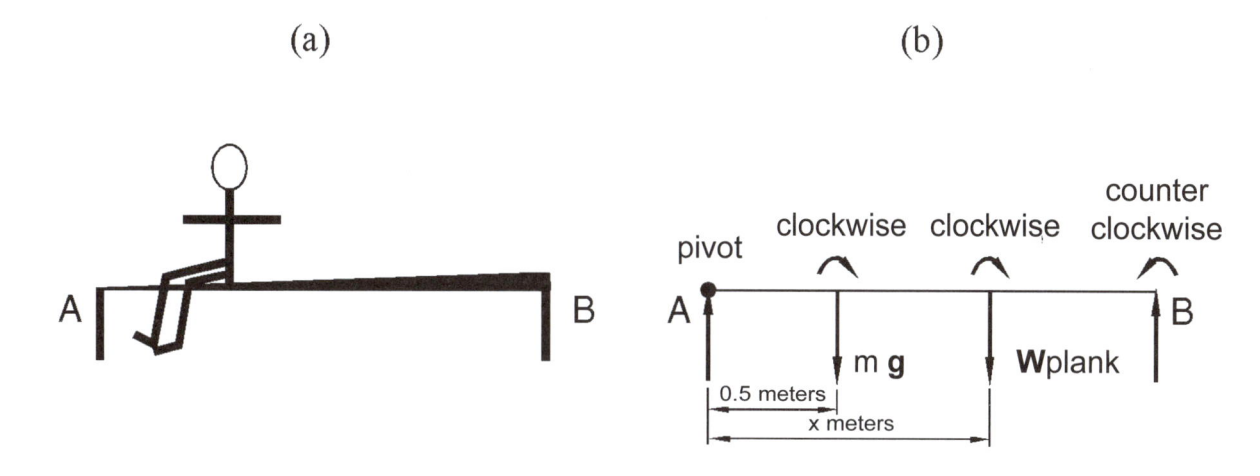

(b)

Figure III.B.4.2: Torque Problem.
(a) A person sitting on a non-uniform bench which is composed of a plank with two supports A and B. (b) Vector diagram with point A as the reference point. The torque force at point A is zero since its distance from itself is zero.

The counterclockwise torque (CCW) is given by the force at point B multiplied by its distance from the reference point A:

$$CCW = F_B r_B = 250(2.0) = 500 \text{ Nm}$$

The clockwise torques (CW) are given by the force exerted by the person (= the weight mg) multiplied by the distance from the pivot point (r = 50 cm = 0.5 m) *and* the force exerted by the plank (= the weight) multiplied by the distance from the pivot point where the weight of the plank acts (= COG):

$$CW = mgr + W(COG)$$
$$= 70(10)0.5 + 100(COG)$$
$$= 350 + 100(COG)$$

Gravity was estimated as 10 m/s². Now we have:

$$\Sigma L = CCW - CW = 500 - 350 - 100(COG) = 0$$

Isolate COG

$$COG = 150/100 = 1.5 \text{ m from point } A.$$

• Note that had the plank been uniform its COG would be at its center which is 1.0 m from either end.

• Had the problem requested the weight supported at point A, it would be easy to determine since $\Sigma F_y = 0$. If we define upward forces as positive, we get:

$$\Sigma F_y = F_A + F_B - mg - W_{plank} = 0$$

Isolate F_A

$$F_A = 70(10) + 100 - 250 = 550 \text{ N}.$$

4.2 Newton's First Law

Newton's First Law states that objects in motion or at rest tend to remain as such unless acted upon by an outside force. That is, objects have inertia (resistance to motion). For translational motion, the mass (m) is a measure of inertia.

For rotational motion, a quantity derived from the mass called the moment of inertia (I) is the measure of inertia. In general $I = \Sigma mr^2$ where r is the distance from the axis of rotation. However, the exact formulation depends on the structure of the object.

4.3 Momentum

The momentum (M) is a vector quantity. The momentum of an object is the product of its mass and its velocity.

$$M = m v$$

Linear momentum is a measure of the tendency of an object to maintain motion in a straight line. The greater the momentum (M), the greater the tendency of the object to remain moving along a straight line in the same direction. The momentum (M) is also a measure of the force needed to stop or change the direction of the object.

The impulse I is a measure of the change of the momentum of an object. It is the product of the force applied by the time during which the force was applied to change the momentum.

$$I = F \Delta t = \Delta M$$

where F is the acting force and Δt is the elapsed time during which the force was acting. The momentum is also conserved just like energy. The total linear momentum of a system is constant when the resultant external force acting on the system is zero.

4.4 Collisions

During motion, objects can collide. There are two kinds of collisions: *elastic* and *inelastic*. During an elastic collision (objects rebound off each other), there is a conservation of momentum and conservation of kinetic energy. Whereas, during an inelastic collision (objects stick together), there is conservation of momentum but not conservation of kinetic energy. Kinetic energy is lost as heat or sound, so total energy is conserved.

Examples of elastic collisions include 2 rubber balls colliding, particle collisions in ideal gases, and the slingshot type gravitational interactions between satellites and planets popularized in science fiction movies. Examples of inelastic collisions include 2 cars colliding at high speed becoming stuck together and a ballistic pendulum which can be a huge chunk of wood used to measure the speed of a moving object (i.e. bullet) which becomes completely embedded in the wood. If, however, the bullet were to emerge from the wood block, then it would be an elastic collision since the objects did not stick together.

Imagine two spheres with masses m_1 and m_2 and the velocity components before the collision v_{1i} and v_{2i} and after the collision v_{1f} and v_{2f}. If the momentum and the velocity are in the same directions, and we define that direction as positive, from the conservation of momentum we obtain:

$$m_1 v_{1i} + m_2 v_{2i} = m_1 v_{1f} + m_2 v_{2f} .$$

If the directions are not the same then each momentum must be resolved into x- and y-components as necessary.

• In the explosion of an object at rest, the total momentum of all the fragments must sum to zero because of the conservation of momentum and because the original momentum was zero.

• If one object collides with a second identical object that is at rest, there is a total transfer of kinetic energy, that is the first object comes to rest and the second object moves off with the momentum of the first one.

4.4.1 Collision Problem (CGS units)

A bullet of mass 10 g and a speed of 5.0×10^4 cm/s strikes a 700 g wooden block at rest on a very smooth surface. The bullet emerges with its speed reduced to 3.5×10^4 cm/s.

Find the resulting speed of the block. {CGS uses <u>c</u>entimeters, <u>g</u>rams, and <u>s</u>econds as units; the CGS unit of force is a <u>dyne</u>}

Let m_1 = the mass of the bullet (10 g), v_{1i} = the speed of the bullet before the collision (5.0×10^4 cm/s), m_2 = the mass of the wooden block (700 g), v_{2i} = the speed of the block before the collision (0 cm/s), v_{1f} = the speed of the bullet after the collision (3.5×10^4 cm/s), and v_{2f} = the speed of the block after the collision (*unknown*), now we have:

$$m_1 v_{1i} + m_2 v_{2i} = m_1 v_{1f} + m_2 v_{2f}$$

Solving for v_{2f}

$$v_{2f} = (m_1 v_{1i} - m_1 v_{1f})/m_2$$
$$= (5.0 \times 10^5 - 3.5 \times 10^5)/(700)$$
$$= 2.1 \times 10^2 \text{ cm/s}.$$

• Note: the least precise figures that we are given in the problem contain at least two digits or <u>significant figures</u>. Thus our answer can not be more precise than two significant figures. The exponent 10^x is not considered when counting significant figures unless you are *told* that the measurement was more precise than is evident {For more on significant figures *see* Appendix A.6 and PHY 8.5.1}.

• Note: you should be comfortable solving physics problems in Imperial, SI or CGS units (Appendix B).

GOLD NOTES

WORK AND ENERGY
Chapter 5

Memorize	Understand	Not Required*
define, equation, units: work equations and units: potential energy equations and units: kinetic energy, power	* Path independence of work done in a g field * Work-Energy Theorem * Conservation of E.; conservative forces * Solving Conservation of E. problems	* Advanced level college info

GAMSAT-Prep.com

Introduction

Work and energy are used to describe how bodies or masses interact with the environment or other bodies or masses. Conservation of energy, work and power describe the forms of energy and the changes between these forms.

Additional Resources

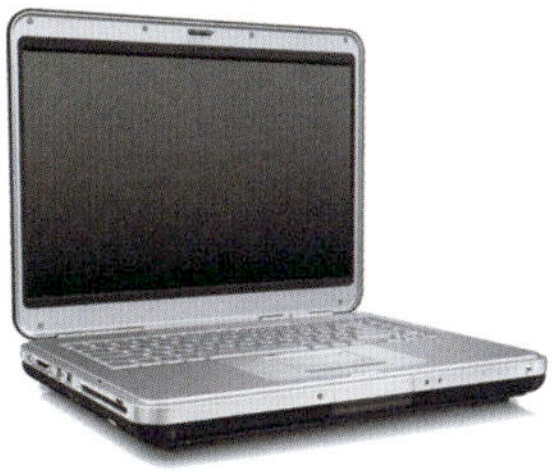

Free Online Q&A + Forum

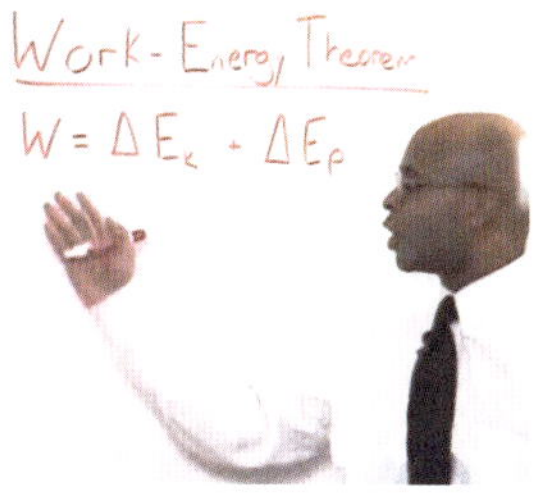

Video: Online or DVD 1, 3, 4

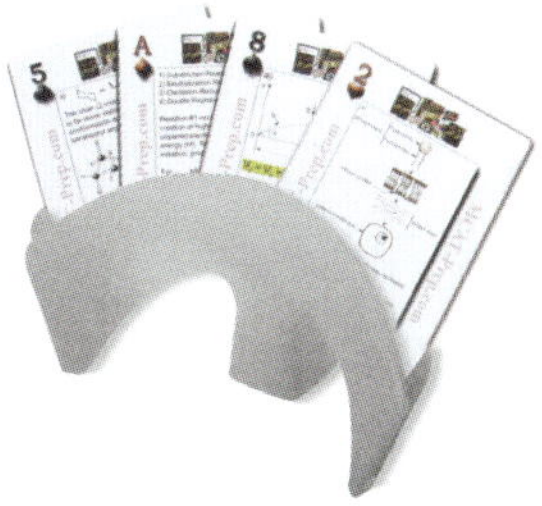

Flashcards

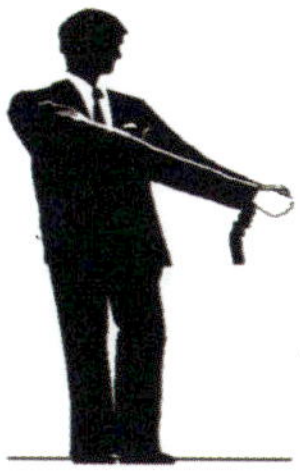

Special Guest

THE PHYSICAL SCIENCES   PHY-33

* The real GAMSAT may have advanced level information presented (ie. in a passage) but previous knowledge of said information is not required to answer the questions that would follow. Practice ACER and GS practice GAMSATs can help you clarify this point.

5.1 Work

The work of a force *F* on an object is the product of the force by the distance travelled by the object where the force is in the direction of the displacement.

- *Units*: both work and energy are measured in joules where 1 *joule (J)* = 1 N × 1 m. {Imperial units: the *foot-pound*, CGS units: the *dyne-centimeter* or *erg*}

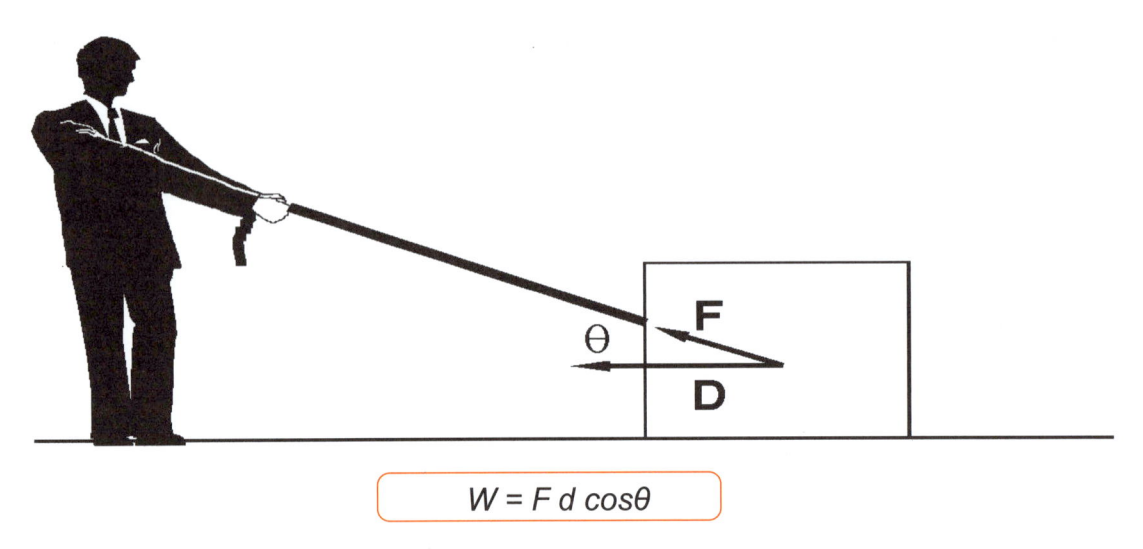

$$W = F\,d\,\cos\theta$$

Figure III.B.5.1: Work. The displacement depends on the final and initial positions of the object. The angle θ is necessary to determine the component of a constant force F in the same direction of the displacement. Note that if F acts perpendicular to the displacement then the work $W = F\,d\,\cos(90°) = 0$.

5.2 Energy

We usually speak of mechanical, electrical, chemical, potential, kinetic, atomic and nuclear energy, to name a few. In fact, these different kinds of energy are different forms or manifestations of the same energy. Energy is a scalar. It is defined as a physical quantity <u>capable of producing work</u>.

5.3 Kinetic Energy

1) Definition of kinetic energy

Kinetic energy (E_k) is the energy of motion which can produce work. It is proportional to the mass of the object and its velocity:

$$E_k = 1/2\, mv^2.$$

2) The Work-Energy Theorem

A net force is the sum of interior and exterior forces acting upon the system. The variation of the kinetic energy of a system is equal to the work of the net force applied to the system:

$$W \text{ (of the resultant force)} = \Delta E_k.$$

Consequently, if the speed of a particle is constant, $\Delta E_k = 0$, then the work done by the resultant force must be zero. For example, in uniform circular motion the speed of the particle remains constant thus the centripetal force does no work on the particle. A force at right angles to the direction of motion merely changes the direction of the velocity but not its magnitude.

5.4 Potential Energy

Potential energy (E_p) is referred to as potential because it is accumulated by the system that contained it. It varies with the configuration of the system, i.e., when distances between particles of the system vary, the interactions between these particles vary. The variation of the potential energy is equal to the work performed by the interior forces caused by the interaction between the particles of the system. The following are examples of potential energy:

a) potential energy (= electric potential = E_p) derived from the Coulomb force (r is the distance between point charges q_1 and q_2, PHY 9.1.4):

$$E_p = k\, q_1 q_2 / r$$

b) potential energy derived from the universal attraction force (r is the distance between the COG of masses m_1 and m_2):

$$E_p = G\, m_1 m_2 / r$$

c) potential energy derived from the gravitational force (h is the height):

$$E_p = mgh$$

d) potential energy derived from the elastic force (i.e. a compressed spring):

$$E_p = kx^2/2.$$

{k = the spring constant, x = displacement, cf. PHY 7.2.1}

5.5 Conservation of Energy

a) *Definition*

The mechanical energy (E_T) of a system is equal to the sum of its kinetic energy and its potential energy:

$$E_T = E_k + E_p.$$

b) *Theorem of mechanical energy*

The variation of the mechanical energy of a system is equal to the work of exterior forces acting on the system.

c) *Consequence*

An isolated system, i.e., which is not being acted upon by any exterior force, keeps a constant mechanical energy. The kinetic energy and the potential energy may vary separately but their sum remains constant. This makes conservation of energy a very simple way to solve many different types of physics problems.

5.5.1 Conservation of Energy Problem (SI units)

A 6.8×10^3 kg frictionless roller coaster car starts at rest 30 meters above ground level. Determine the speed of the car at (a) 20 m above ground level; (b) at ground level.

$$E_T = E_k + E_p = 1/2 mv^2 + mgh$$

Initially $v = 0$ since the car starts at rest, $h = 30$ m, and the constant $g \approx 10$ m/s², thus

$$E_T = 0 + m(10)(30) = 300m \text{ joules}.$$

Situation (a) where $h = 20$ m:

$$E_T = 300m = 1/2 mv^2 + mgh$$

m cancels, multiply through by 2, solve for v:

$$v = \sqrt{2(300) - 2(10)20} = \sqrt{2(100)}$$
$$= \sqrt{2}(10) = 14 \text{ m/s}$$

Situation (b) at ground level $h = 0$:

$$E_T = 300m = 1/2 mv^2 + 0$$

m cancels, multiply through by 2, solve for v:

$$v = \sqrt{600} = \sqrt{6(100)} = 10\sqrt{6} = 24 \text{ m/s}$$

- Note: the mass of the roller coaster is irrelevant!
- Note: you must be able to quickly estimate square roots (PHY 1.1.2, 2.6.1).

5.6 Conservative Forces

The three definitions of a conservative force are: i) after a round trip the kinetic energy of a particle on which a force acts must return to its initial value; ii) after a round trip the work done on a particle by a force must be zero; iii) the work done by the force on a particle depends on the initial and final positions of the particle and not on the path taken.

Examples: Friction disobeys all three of the preceding criteria thus it is a non-conservative force. The force $F_s = -kx$ (Hooke's Law, PHY 7.2.1) of an ideal spring on a frictionless surface is a conservative force. Gravity is a conservative force. If you throw a ball vertically upward, it will return with the same kinetic energy it had when it left your hand (*neglect air resistance*).

5.7 Power

The power *P* applied during the work *W* performed by a force *F* is equal to the work divided by the time necessary to do the work. In other words, power is the rate of doing work:

$$P = \Delta W/\Delta t.$$

• The SI unit for power is the *watt* (W) which equals one *joule per second* (J/s).

GOLD NOTES

FLUIDS AND SOLIDS
Chapter 6

Memorize	Understand	Not Required*
Equation: density Density of water Equations for pressure, pressure change	* Buoyancy force, SG and height immersed * Streamline, turbulent flow; continuity/ Bernouilli's equation * Fluid viscosity, Archimedes' principle, surface tension * Elastic properties of solids; effect of temperature	* Advanced level college info * Memorizing all the equations for solids * Memorizing equations: Continuity, hydrostatic pressure, Bernouilli's

GAMSAT-Prep.com

Introduction

A fluid is a substance that flows (*deforms*) under shear stress. This includes all gases and liquids. It is important to understand the properties without movement (hydrostatic pressure, Archimedes' principle) and with movement (continuity, Bernoulli's). On the other hand, a solid *resists* being deformed or submitting to changes in volume. A basic understanding of this *elastic* property of solids is required.

Additional Resources

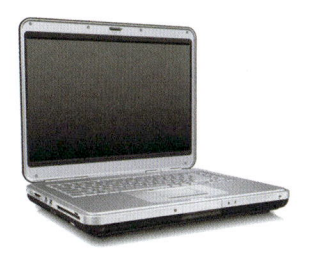

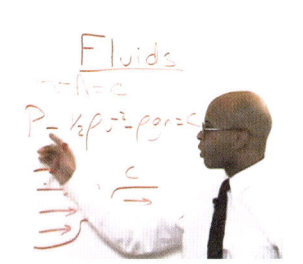

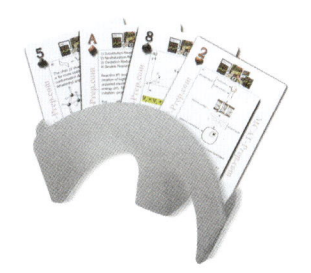

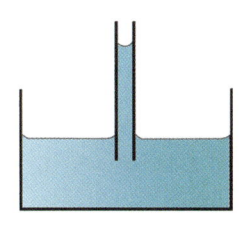

Free Online Q&A + Forum   Video: Online or DVD Disc 4   Flashcards   Special Guest

THE PHYSICAL SCIENCES PHY-39

* The real GAMSAT may have advanced level information presented (ie. in a passage) but previous knowledge of said information is not required to answer the questions that would follow. Practice ACER and GS practice GAMSATs can help you clarify this point.

GAMSAT-Prep.com
THE GOLD STANDARD

6.1 Fluids

6.1.1 Density, Specific Gravity

The *density* of an object is defined as the ratio of its mass to its volume.

$$\text{density} = \text{mass} / \text{volume}$$

This definition holds for solids, fluids and gases. From the definition, it is easy to see that solids are more dense than liquids which are in turn more dense than gases. This is true because for a given mass, the average distance between molecules of a given substance is bigger in the liquid state than in the solid state. Put simply, the substance occupies a bigger volume in the liquid state than in the solid state and a much bigger volume in gaseous state than in the liquid state.

At a given temperature, the *specific gravity* (SG) is defined as:

$$SG = \frac{\text{density of a substance}}{\text{density of water}}$$

The density of water is about 1 g/ml (= 1 g/cm^3 = 10^3 kg/m^3) over most common temperatures. So in most instances the specific gravity of a substance is the same as its density.

Note that the dimension of density is mass per unit volume, whereas the specific gravity is dimensionless. Density is one of the key properties of fluids (liquids or gases) and the other is pressure.

6.1.2 Hydrostatic Pressure, Buoyancy, Archimedes' Principle

Pressure (P) is defined as the force (F) per unit area (A):

$$P = F/A.$$

The force F is the normal (*perpendicular*) force to the area. The SI unit for pressure is the *pascal* (1 Pa = 1 N/m). Other units are: 1.00 atm = 1.01 × 10^5 Pa = 1.01 bar = 760 mmHg = 760 torr = 14.7 lb/in^2.

Pressure is also formulated as potential energy per unit volume as follows:

$$P = \frac{F}{A} = \frac{mg}{A} = \frac{(mg/a)}{(h/h)} = \frac{mgh}{v} = \rho gh$$

ρ = density and h = depth below surface; if the depth is changing we can write:

$$\Delta P = \rho g \Delta h.$$

PHY-40 FLUIDS AND SOLIDS

Characteristics of force and pressure of incompressible liquid fluids are:

1) Forces exerted by fluids are always perpendicular to the surface of the container.
2) The fluid pressure (*hydrostatic*) is directly proportional to the depth of the fluid and to its density.
3) At any particular depth, the pressure of the fluid is the same in all directions.
4) Fluid pressure is independent of the shape or area of its container.
5) An external pressure applied to an enclosed fluid is transmitted uniformly throughout the volume of the liquid (*Pascal's law*).
6) An object which is completely or partially submerged in a fluid experiences an upward force equal to the weight of the fluid displaced (*Archimedes' principle*).

This buoyant force F_b is:

$$F_b = V\rho g = mg$$

where ρ is the density of the fluid displaced. An object that floats must displace at most its own weight. Archimedes' principle can be used to calculate specific gravity.

And in turn, ==specific gravity is equivalent to the fraction of the *height* of a buoyant object below the surface of the fluid==. Thus if SG = 0.90, then 90% of the height of the object would be immersed in water.

Therefore, less dense objects float.

6.1.3 Fluids in Motion, Continuity Equation, Bernoulli's Equation

Fluids in motion are described by two equations, the continuity equation and Bernoulli's equation. Fluids are assumed to have <u>streamline</u> (= *laminar*) flow which means that the motion of every particle in the fluid follows the same path as the particle that preceded it. <u>Turbulent</u> flow occurs when that definition cannot be applied, resulting in molecular collisions, irregularly shaped whirlpools, energy is then dissipated and frictional drag is increased. The rate (R) of streamline flow is given by:

$$R = (\text{volume past a point})/\text{time} = Avt/t = Av$$

volume = (cross-sectional area) (length) = (A) (vt) = Avt

length = distance = (velocity) (time) = vt

cross-sectional area of a tube = ==area of a circle = πr^2== where π can be estimated as 3.14 and *r* is the radius of the circle.

- The equation can also be written as the **continuity equation**:

$$A_1 v_1 = A_2 v_2 = \text{constant}$$

where subscripts 1 and 2 refer to different points in the line of flow. The continuity equation can be used for an incompressible fluid flowing in an enclosed tube. For a compressible fluid:

$$\rho_1 A_1 v_1 = \rho_2 A_2 v_2 = \text{constant}$$

- **Bernoulli's equation** is an application of the law of conservation of energy and is:

$$P + \rho g h + 1/2\, \rho v^2 = \text{constant}$$

It follows:

$$P_1 + \rho g h_1 + 1/2\, \rho v_1^2 = P_2 + \rho g h_2 + 1/2\, \rho v_2^2$$

where subscripts 1 and 2 refer to different points in the flow.

A commonly encountered consequence of Bernoulli's equation is that where the height is relatively constant and the velocity of a fluid is high, the pressure is low, and vice versa.

{Various applications of the preceding equations will be explored in GS-1, the first practice test!}

6.1.4 Fluid Viscosity and Determining Turbulence

Viscosity is analogous to friction between moving solids. It may, therefore be viewed as the resistance to flow of layers of fluid (as in streamline or laminar flow) past each other. This also means that viscosity, as in friction, results in dissipation of mechanical energy. As one layer flows over another, its motion is transmitted to the second layer and causes this layer to be set in motion. Since a mass m of the second layer is set in motion and some of the energy of the first layer is lost, there is a transfer of momentum between the layers.

The greater the transfer of this momentum from one layer to another, the more energy that is lost and the slower the layers move.

The viscosity (η) is the measure of the efficiency of transfer of this momentum. Therefore the higher the viscosity coefficient, the greater the transfer of momentum and loss of mechanical energy, and thus loss of velocity. The reverse situation holds for a low viscosity coefficient.

Consequently, a high viscosity coefficient substance flows slowly (e.g. molasses), and a low viscosity coefficient substance flows relatively fast (e.g. water or, especially helium). Note that the transfer of momentum to adjacent layers is in essence, the exertion of a force upon these layers to set them in motion.

Whether flow is streamline or turbulent depends on a combination of factors already discussed. A convenient measure is Reynolds Number (R):

$$R = vd\rho / \eta$$

v = velocity of flow
d = diameter of the tube
ρ = density of the fluid
η = viscosity coefficient

In general, if R < 2000 the flow is streamline; if R > 2000 the flow is turbulent. Note that as v, d or ρ increases or η decreases, the flow becomes more turbulent.

6.1.5 Surface Tension

Molecules of a liquid exert attractive forces toward each other (cohesive forces), and exert attractive forces toward the surface they touch (adhesive forces). If a liquid is in a gravity free space without a surface, it will form a sphere (smallest area relative to volume).

If the liquid is lining an object, the liquid surface will contract (due to cohesive forces) to the lowest possible surface area. The forces between the molecules on this surface will create a membrane-like effect. Due to the contraction, a potential energy (PE) will present in the surface.

This PE is directly proportional to the surface area (A). An exact relation is formed as follows:

$$PE = \gamma A$$

γ = surface tension = PE/A = joules/m²

An alternative formulation for the surface tension (γ) is:

$$\gamma = F/l$$

F = force of contraction of surface
l = length along surface

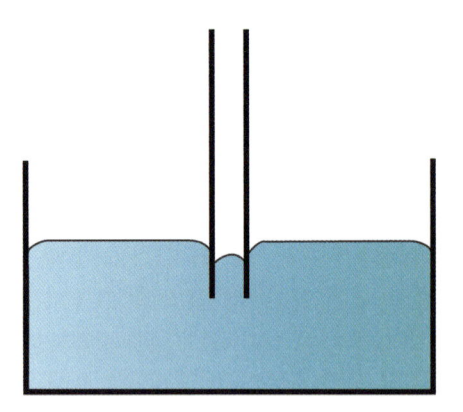

(a) cohesive > adhesive

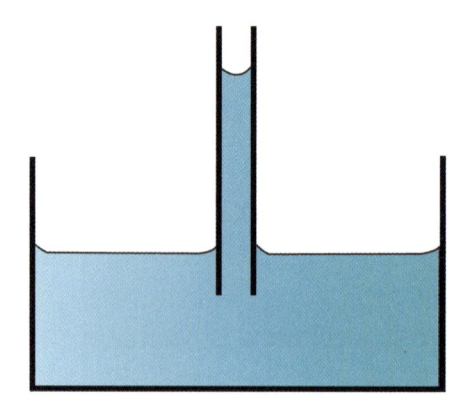

(b) adhesive > cohesive

Figure III.B.6.1: Effects of adhesive and cohesive forces. The distance the liquid rises or falls in the tube is directly proportional to the surface tension γ and inversely proportional to the liquid density and radius of the tube. Examples of 2 liquids consistent with the illustrations include: (a) mercury; (b) water.

Because of the contraction, a small object which would ordinarily sink in the liquid may float on the surface membrane. For example, a small insect like a "water strider."

The liquid will rise or fall on a wall or in a capillary tube if the adhesive forces are greater than cohesive or vice versa (*see* Figure III.B.6.1).

6.2 Solids

6.2.1 Elastic Properties of Solids

When a force acts on a solid, the solid is deformed. If the solid returns to its original shape, the solid is elastic. The effect of a force depends on the area over which it acts. Stress is defined as the ratio of the force to the area over which it acts. Strain is defined as the relative change in dimensions or shape of the object caused by the stress. This is embodied in the definition of the modulus of elasticity (ME) as:

$$ME = \frac{stress}{strain}$$

Some different types of stresses are tensile stress (equal and opposite forces directed away from each other), compressive stress (equal and opposite forces directed towards each other), and shearing stress (equal and opposite forces which do not have the same line of action). There are two commonly used moduli of elasticity:

1) Young's Modulus (Y) for compressive or tensile stress:

$$Y = \frac{longitudinal\ stress}{longitudinal\ strain}$$

$$Y = \frac{(F/A)}{(\Delta l/l)} = \frac{F \times l}{A \Delta l}$$

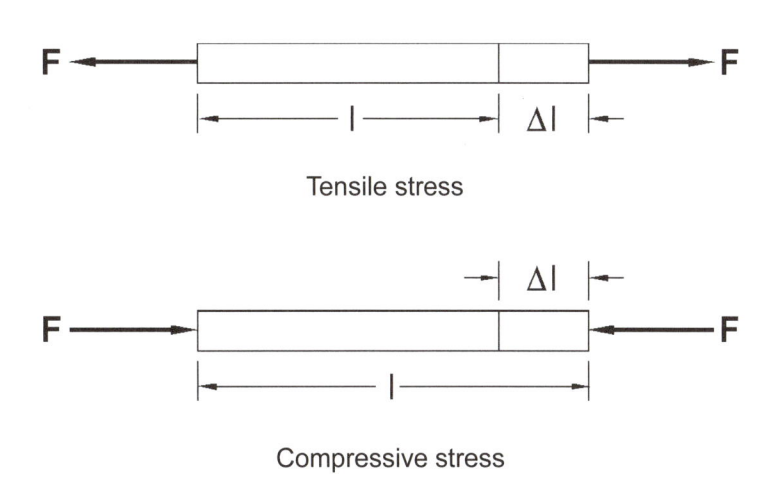

Figure III.B.6.2: Compressive and Tensile Stress.

2) Shear modulus (S) or the modulus of rigidity is:

S = shearing stress / shearing strain

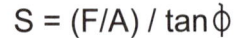

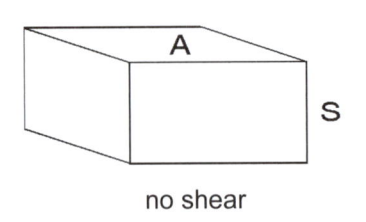

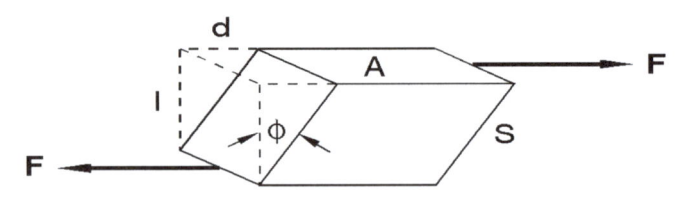

$$S = (F/A) / \tan\phi$$

Figure III.B.6.3: Shear Stress. A is the area tangential to the force F.

6.3 The Effect of Temperature on Solids and Liquids

When substances gain or lose heat they usually undergo expansion or contraction.

Expansion or contraction can be by linear dimension, by area or by volume.

Table III.B.6.1: Substance thermal expansion.

Type	Final	Original	Change caused by heat
(1) Linear	L $L = L_0 + \alpha \Delta T L_0$ $L = L_0(1 + \alpha \Delta T)$ α = coefficient of linear thermal expansion ΔT = change in temperature	L_0	$\alpha \Delta T L_0$
(2) Area	A $A = A_0 + \gamma \Delta T A_0$ $A = A_0(1 + \gamma \Delta T)$ γ = coefficient of area thermal expansion = 2α	A_0	$\gamma \Delta T A_0$
(3) Volume	V $V = V_0 + \beta \Delta T V_0$ $V = V_0(1 + \beta \Delta T)$ β = coefficient of volume thermal expansion = 3α	V_0	$\beta \Delta T V_0$

OLD NOTES

GOLD NOTES

WAVE CHARACTERISTICS AND PERIODIC MOTION

Chapter 7

Memorize	Understand	Not Required*
fine: wavelength, frequency, velocity, plitude fine: intensity, constructive/destructive erference, beat freq. ation: relating velocity to frequency, elength ation: Hooke's Law, work (periodic motion)	* SHM, transverse vs. longitudinal waves, phase * Resonance, nodes, antinodes, pipes (standing waves) * Harmonics, overtones * Periodic motion: force, accel., vel., diplace., period * The simple pendulum, theory and calculations	* Advanced level college info * Memorizing displacement/elementary vibration equations * Memorizing equation for harmonics, simple pendulum

GAMSAT-Prep.com

Introduction

Wave characteristics and periodic motion describe the motion of systems that vibrate. Topics include transverse and longitudinal waves, interference, resonance, Hooke's law and simple harmonic motion (SHM). Some basic equations must be memorized but for most of the material, you must seek a comfortable understanding.

Additional Resources

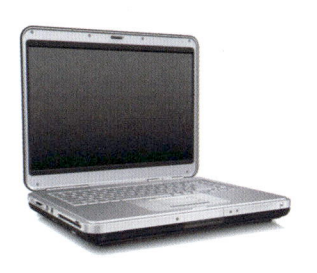

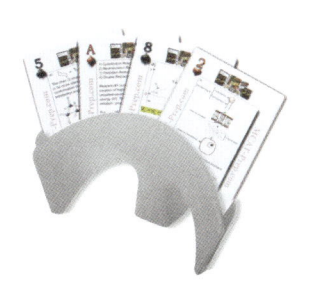

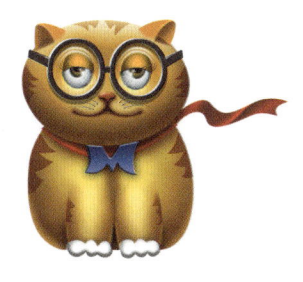

Free Online Q&A + Forum   Video: Online or DVD 2,4   Flashcards   Special Guest

THE PHYSICAL SCIENCES   PHY-49

* The real GAMSAT may have advanced level information presented (ie. in a passage) but previous knowledge of said information is not required to answer the questions that would follow. Practice ACER and GS practice GAMSATs can help you clarify this point.

7.1 Wave Characteristics

7.1.1 Transverse and Longitudinal Motion

A wave is a disturbance in a medium such that each particle in the medium vibrates about an equilibrium point in a simple harmonic (*periodic*) motion. If the direction of vibration is perpendicular to the direction of propagation of the wave, it is called a transverse wave (e.g. light or an oscillating string under tension).

If the direction of vibration is in the same direction as the propagation of the wave, it is called a longitudinal wave (e.g. sound). Longitudinal waves are characterized by condensations (regions of crowding of particles) and rarefactions (regions where particles are far apart) along the wave in the medium.

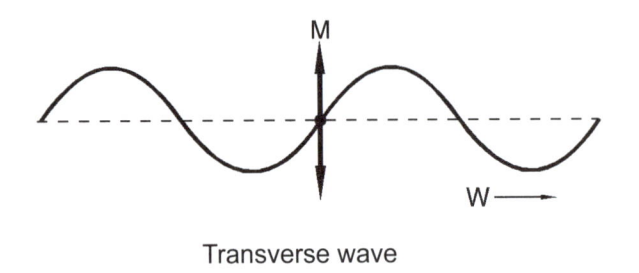

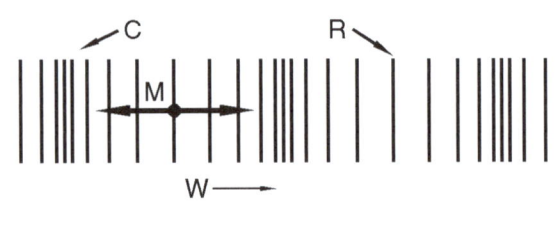

Figure III.B.7.1: Transverse and longitudinal waves.
W = wave propagation, R = rarefaction, C = condensation, M = motion of particle.

7.1.2 Wavelength, Frequency, Velocity, Amplitude, Intensity

The wavelength (λ) is the distance from crest to crest (or valley to valley) of a transverse wave. It may also be defined as the distance between two particles with the same displacement and direction of displacement. In a longitudinal wave, the wavelength is the distance from one rarefaction (or condensation) to another. The *amplitude* (A) is the maximum displacement of a particle in one direction from its equilibrium point. The *intensity* (I) of a wave is the square of the amplitude.

Frequency (f) is the number of cycles per unit time (per second). *Period (T)* is the duration of one cycle, it is the inverse of the frequency. The *velocity (v)* of a wave is the velocity of the propagation of the disturbance that forms the wave through the medium.

The velocity is inversely proportional to the inertia of the medium. The velocity can be calculated according to the following important equation:

$$v = \lambda f$$

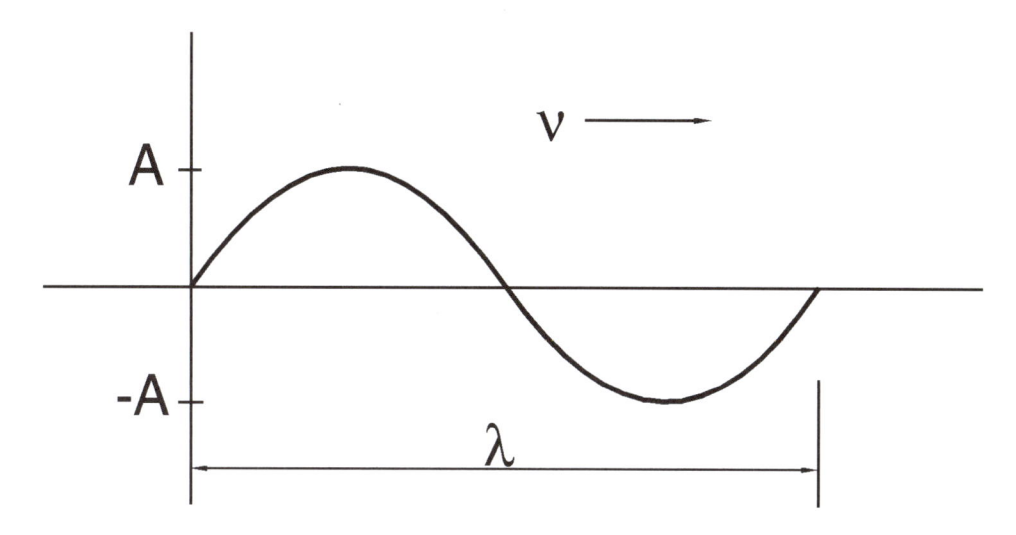

Figure III.B.7.2: Characteristics of waves.

7.1.3 Superposition of Waves, Phase, Interference, Addition

The superposition principle states that the effect of two or more waves on the displacement of a particle is independent. The final displacement of the particle is the resultant effect of all the waves added algebraically, thus the amplitude may increase or decrease. The *phase* of a particle under vibration is its displacement at the time of origin (t=0). The displacement can be calculated as follows:

$$x = A\sin(\omega t + \varphi)$$

where x is the displacement, A is the amplitude, ω is the angular velocity, t is the time, and φ is the phase.

Interference is the summation of the displacements of different waves in a medium. Certain criteria must first be established:

- *synchrony sources*: vibrations emitted by synchrony sources have the same phase.
- *coherent vibrations*: the phases of the vibrations are related, this means that the duration of the light impressions on the retina is much longer than the duration of a wave train between two emissions.
- *parallel vibrations*: the displacements of parallel vibrations keep parallel directions in space.

- *interference conditions*: two or more vibrations can interfere only when the are coherent, parallel and have the same period.
- *beat frequency*: the difference in frequency of two waves creates a new frequency (see Beats, PHY 8.4).

Given an elementary vibration $S_i = A_i \sin(w_t + \varphi_i)$ the composition of n vibrations that interfere is given by:

$S_1 + S_2 + S_3 + ... + S_n = a_1\sin(wt+\varphi_1) + a_2\sin(wt+\varphi_2) + ... + a_n\sin(wt+\varphi_n) = A\sin(wt+\Phi)$

where A is the resultant amplitude and Φ the resultant phase. Constructive interference (see Figure III.B.7.4) is when the waves add to a larger resultant wave than either original. This occurs maximally when the phase difference φ is a whole wavelength λ which corresponds to multiples of π.

This occurs at $\varphi = 0, 2\pi, 4\pi$, etc. Since $\varphi = 2\pi\Delta L/\lambda$, where ΔL equals the difference in path to a point of two waves of equal wavelength, these waves interfere constructively when $\Delta L = 0, \lambda, 2\lambda, 3\lambda$, etc. See Figure III.B.7.3 for the definition of ΔL.

Destructive interference (see Figure III.B.7.5) is when the waves add to a smaller resultant wave than either original wave. This occurs maximally when $\varphi = \pi, 3\pi, 5\pi$, etc., which are multiples of one-half of a wavelength where 180° = π which corresponds to ½λ. This occurs when $\Delta L = \lambda/2, 3\lambda/2, 5\lambda/2$, etc.

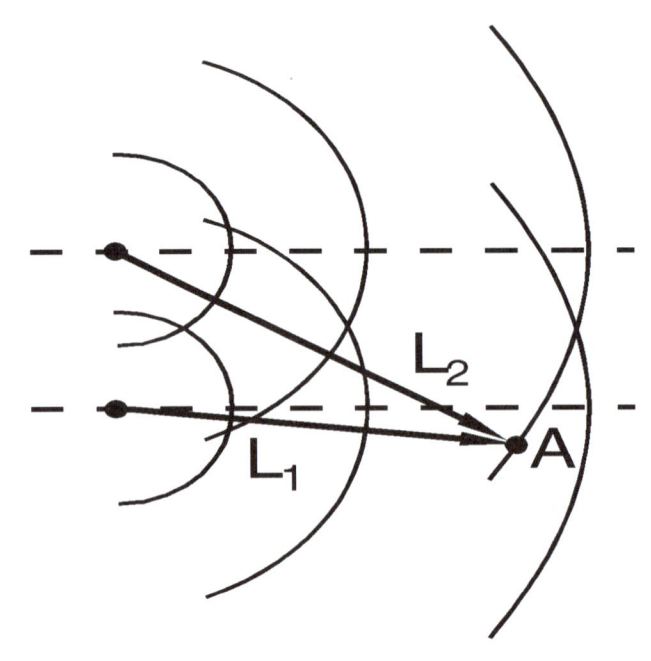

Figure III.B.7.3: Schematic for ΔL.
L_1 and L_2 are distances from the origins of the waves to point A. Thus $\Delta L = |L_2 - L_1|$ (absolute value).

($\Delta L = 0, \lambda, 2\lambda, etc.$)

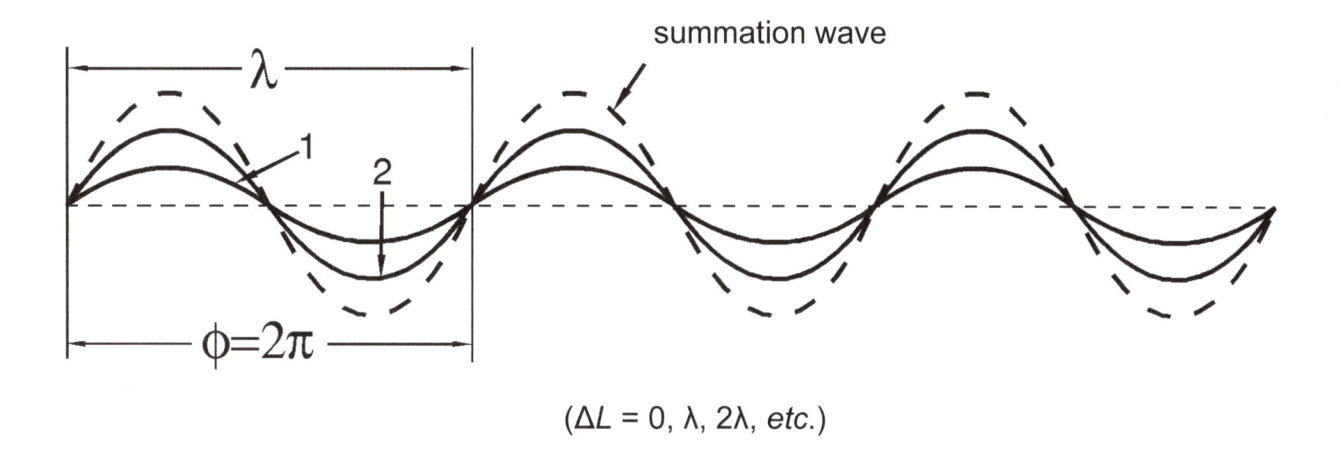

Figure III.B.7.4: Maximal constructive interference. Waves (1) and (2) begin at the points shown, have the same λ but different amplitudes. The summation wave is maximal (i.e. highest amplitude but same wavelength) since ΔL = λ *in this example.*

($\Delta L = \lambda/2, 3\lambda/2, 5\lambda/2, etc.$)

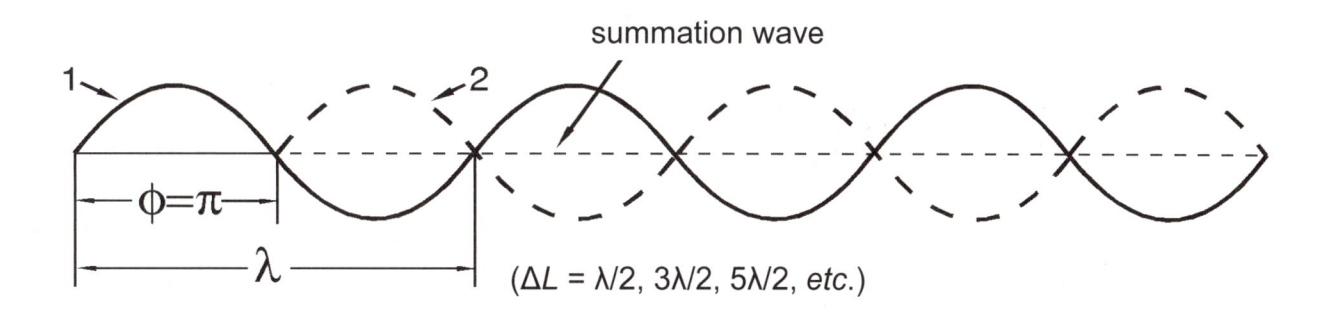

Figure III.B.7.5: Maximal destructive interference.

GAMSAT-Prep.com
THE GOLD STANDARD

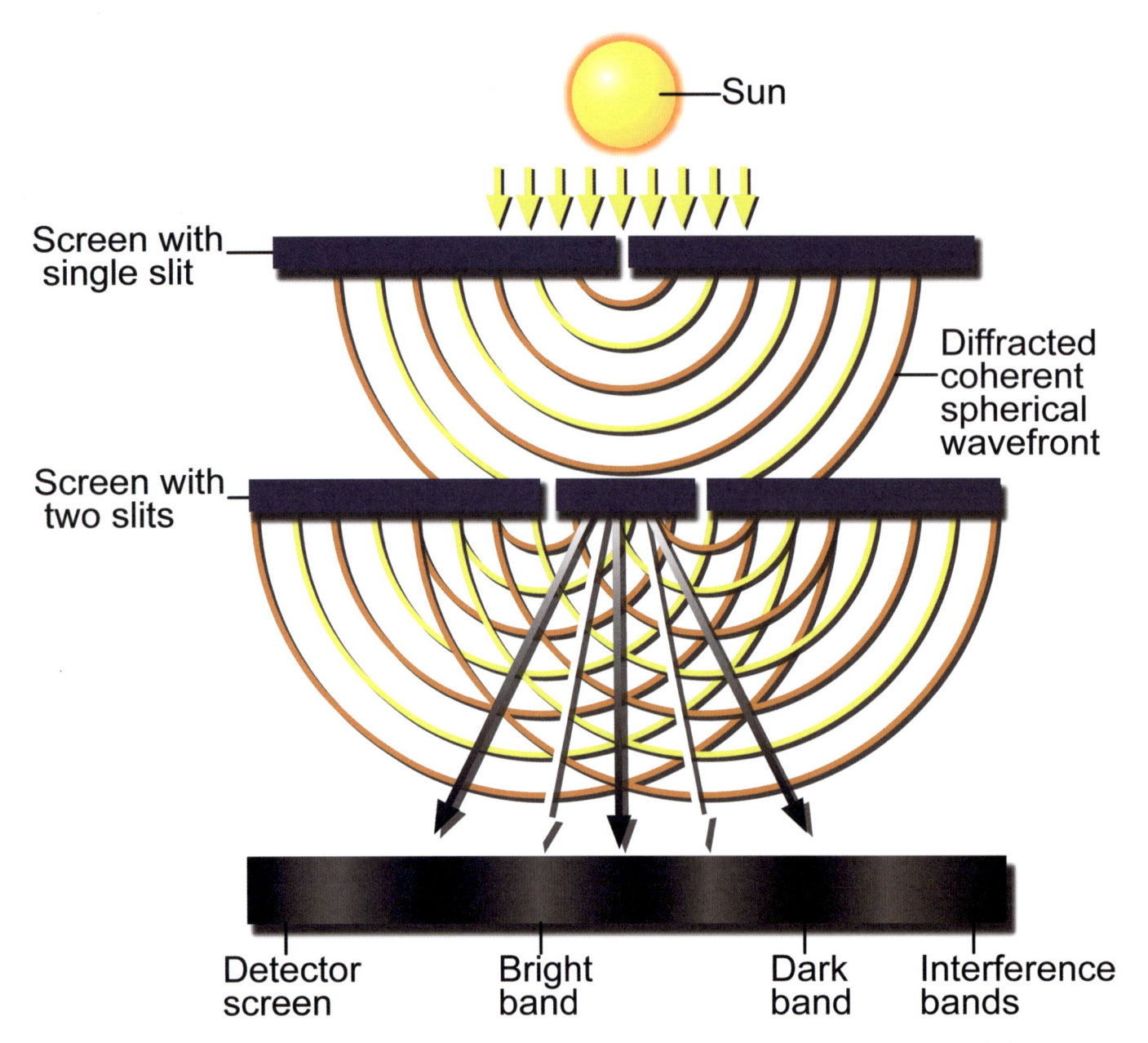

Figure III.B.7.5.1: Thomas Young's Double Slit Experiment Young's experiment demonstrates both the wave and particle natures of light. A coherent light source illuminates a thin plate with two parallel slits cut in it, and the light passing through the slits strikes a screen behind them. The wave nature of light causes the light waves passing through both slits to interfere, creating an interference pattern of bright and dark bands on the screen. However, at the screen, the light is always found to be absorbed as though it were made of discrete particles (photons). The double slit experiment can also be performed (using different apparatus) with particles of matter such as electrons with the same results. Again, this provides an additional circumstance demonstrating particle-wave duality. Diffraction is the apparent bending of a wave around a small obstacle. We see diffracted light waves through each of the slits above.

PHY-54   WAVE CHARACTERISTICS AND PERIODIC MOTION

7.1.4 Resonance

Forced vibrations occur when a series of waves impinge upon an object and cause it to vibrate. Natural frequencies are the intrinsic frequencies of vibration of a system. If the forced vibration causes the object to vibrate at one of its natural frequencies, the body will vibrate at maximal amplitude. This phenomenon is called *resonance*. Since energy and power are proportional to the amplitude squared, they also are at their maximum.

7.1.5 Standing Waves, Pipes and Strings

Standing waves result when waves are reflected off a stationary object back into the oncoming waves of the medium and superposition results. *Nodes* are points where there is no particle displacement, which are similar to points of maximal destructive interference.

Nodes occur at fixed end points (points that cannot vibrate). Antinodes are points that undergo maximal displacements and are similar to points of maximal constructive interference. Antinodes occur at open or free end points (*see Figure III.B.7.6*).

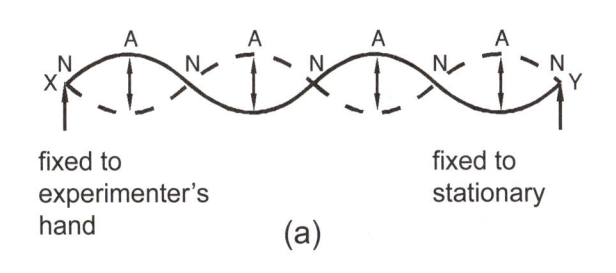

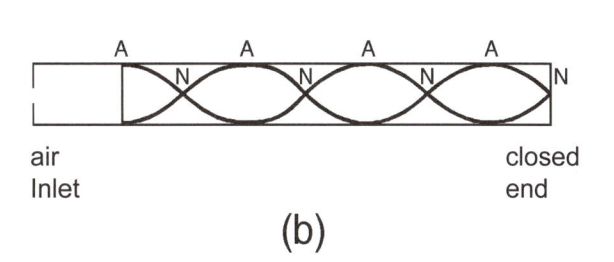

Figure III.B.7.6: Standing waves.
(a) <u>String</u>: Standing waves produced by an experimenter wiggling a string or rubber tube at point X towards a fixed point Y at the correct frequency. (b) <u>Pipe</u>: Standing wave produced in a pipe with a closed end point i.e. in a closed organ pipe where sound originates in a vibrating air column (A = antinode and N = node).

7.1.6 Harmonics

Consider a violin. A string is fixed at both ends and is bowed, transverse vibrations travel along the string; these disturbances are reflected at both ends producing a standing wave. The vibrations of the string give rise to longitudinal vibrations in the air which transmits the sound to our ears.

A string of length *l*, fixed at both ends, can resonate at frequencies *f* given by:

$$f_n = nv/(2l)$$

where the velocity *v* is the same for all frequencies and the number of antinodes $n = 1, 2, 3, ...$

The lowest frequency, $f_1 = v/(2l)$, is the *fundamental* frequency, and the others are called *overtones*. The fundamental is the first *harmonic*, the second harmonic $2f_1$ is the first overtone, the third harmonic $3f_1$ is the second overtone, etc. Overtones whose frequencies are integral multiples of the fundamental are called *harmonic series*.

7.2 Periodic Motion

7.2.1 Hooke's Law

The particles that are undergoing displacement when a wave passes through a medium undergo motion called simple harmonic motion (SHM) and are acted upon by a force described by Hooke's Law. SHM is caused by an inconstant force (called a *restoring force*) and as a result has an inconstant acceleration. The force is proportional to the displacement (*distance from the equilibrium point*) but opposite in direction,

$$F = -kx \text{ (Hooke's Law)}$$

where *k* = the spring constant, *x* = displacement from the equilibrium. The work *W* can be determined according to $W = \frac{1}{2}kx^2$.

What do physicists enjoy doing the most at football games? The 'wave'.

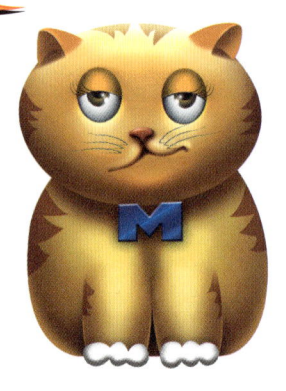

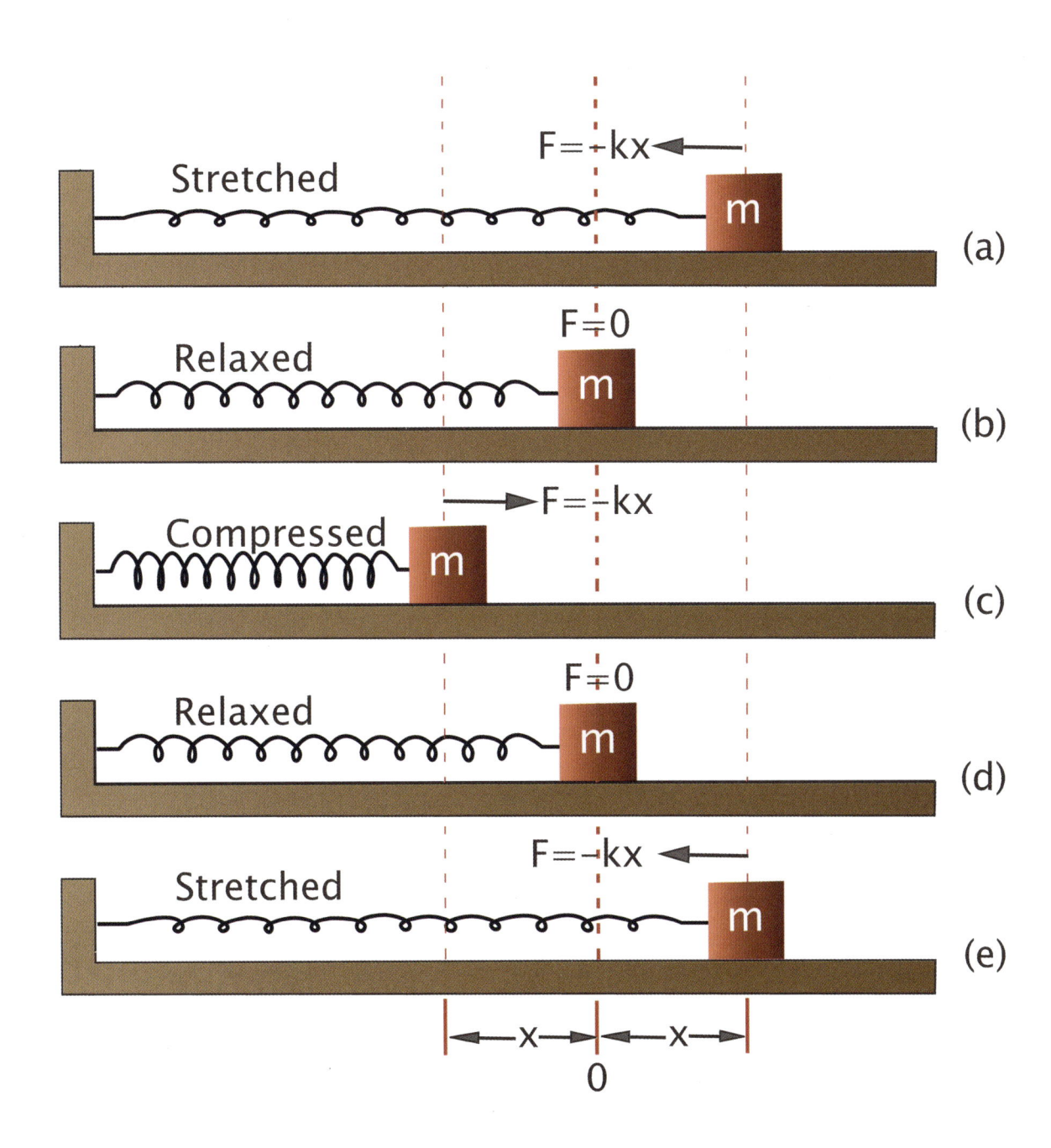

Figure III.B.7.7: Simple harmonic motion.
A block of mass m exhibiting SHM. The force F exerted by the spring on the block is shown in each case.

GAMSAT-Prep.com
THE GOLD STANDARD

7.2.2 Features of SHM and Hooke's Law

1) Force and acceleration are always in the same direction.
2) Force and acceleration are always in the opposite direction of the displacement (*this is why there is a negative sign in the equation for force*).
3) Force and acceleration have their maximal value at +A and -A; they are zero at the equilibrium point (*the amplitude A equals the maximum displacement x*).
4) Velocity direction has no constant relation to displacement and acceleration.
5) Velocity is maximum at equilibrium and zero at A and -A.
6) The period T can be calculated from the mass m of an oscillating particle:

$$T = 2\pi\sqrt{m/k}$$

where k is the spring constant. The frequency f is simply $1/T$.

7.2.3 SHM Problem: The Simple Pendulum

A simple pendulum consists of a point mass m suspended by a light inextensible cord of length l. When pulled to one side of its equilibrium position, the pendulum swings under the influence of gravity producing a periodic, oscillatory motion (= SHM). Given that the angle θ with the vertical is small, thus $\sin\theta \approx \theta$, determine the general equation for the period T.

The tangential component of mg is the restoring force since it returns the mass to its equilibrium position. Thus the restoring force is:

$$F = -mg\sin\theta.$$

Recall $\sin\theta \approx \theta$, $x = l\theta$, and for SHM $F = -kx$:

$$F = -mg\theta = -mgx/l = -(mg/l)x = -kx.$$

Hence $mg/l = k$, thus the equation for the period T becomes:

$$T = 2\pi\sqrt{\frac{m}{k}} = 2\pi\sqrt{\frac{m}{mg/l}} = 2\pi\sqrt{\frac{l}{g}}$$

The equation for the period in the simple pendulum is therefore independent of the mass of the particle.

WAVE CHARACTERISTICS AND PERIODIC MOTION

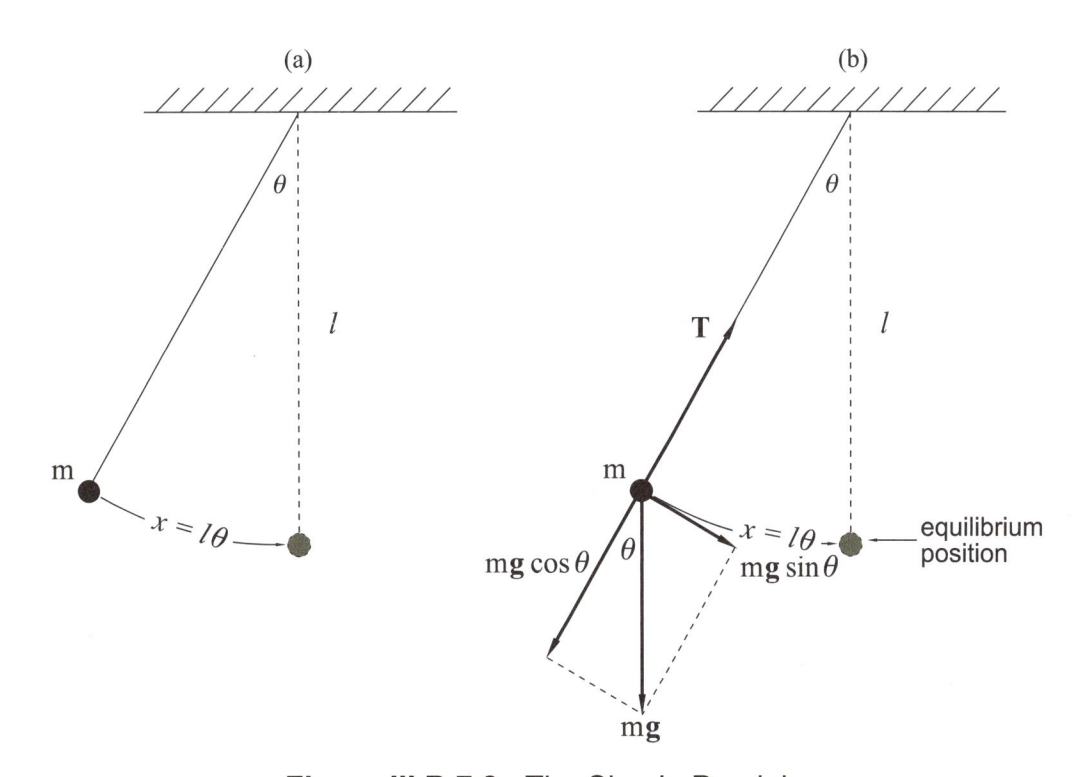

Figure III.B.7.8: The Simple Pendulum.
(a) The problem as it could be presented; the displacement x along the section of the circle (arc) is $l\theta$. (b) The vector components that should be drawn to solve the problem. The forces acting on a simple pendulum are the tension **T** in the string and the weight mg of the mass. The magnitude of the radial component of mg is mgcosθ and the tangential component is mgsinθ.

GOLD NOTES

SOUND
Chapter 8

Memorize	Understand	Not Required*
Sensory vs. physical correspondence of hearing	* Relative velocity of sound in solids, liquids and gases * The relation of intensity to P, area, f, amplitude * Calculation of the intensity level * Rules of logarithms * Doppler effect and calculations	* Advanced level college info * Memorizing specific frequencies, speed of sound, dB's

GAMSAT-Prep.com

Introduction

Sound waves are longitudinal waves which can only be transmitted in a material, elastic medium. Speed, intensity, resonance (Chapter 7) and the Doppler effect help to describe the behavior of sound in different media. If the equations for sound intensity or the Doppler effect are required for the GAMSAT, they will be provided.

Additional Resources

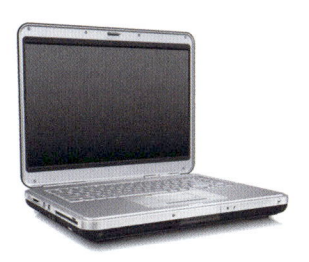

Free Online Q&A + Forum   Video: Online or DVD 2, 4   Flashcards   Special Guest

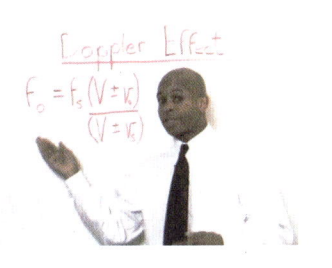

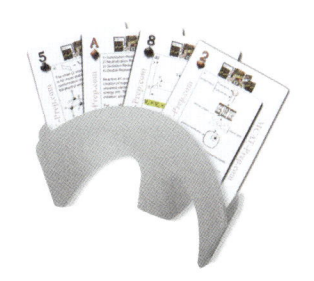

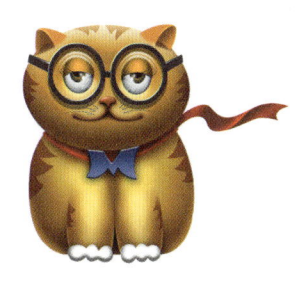

* The real GAMSAT may have advanced level information presented (ie. in a passage) but previous knowledge of said information is not required to answer the questions that would follow. Practice ACER and GS practice GAMSATs can help you clarify this point.

8.1 Production of Sound

Sound is a longitudinal mechanical wave which travels through an elastic medium. Sound is thus produced by vibrating matter. There is no sound in a *vacuum* because it contains no matter.

Compressions (condensations) are regions where particles of matter are close together; they are also high pressure regions. Rarefactions are regions where particles are sparse, they are low pressure regions of sound waves (PHY 7.1.1).

8.2 Relative Velocity of Sound in Solids, Liquids, and Gases

The velocity of sound is proportional to the square root of the elastic restoring force and inversely proportional to the square root of the inertia of the particles (e.g., density is a measure of inertia). Thus as a rule, the velocity of sound is higher in liquids as compared to gases, and highest in solids.

Furthermore, an increase in temperature increases the velocity of sound; conversely, a decrease in temperature decreases the velocity of sound in that medium.

8.3 Intensity, Pitch

Hearing is subjective but its characteristics are closely tied to physical characteristics of sound.

The quality depends on the number and relative intensity of the overtones of the waveform. Frequency, and therefore pitch are perceived by the ear from 20 to 20,000 Hz (hertz = cycles/second = s^{-1}). Frequencies below 20 Hz are called infrasonic. Frequencies above 20,000 Hz are called ultrasonic.

Sensory	Physical
loudness	intensity
pitch	frequency
quality	waveform

Table III.B.8.1:
Sensory and physical correspondence of hearing.

Sound intensity (I) is the rate of energy (power) propagation through space:

$I = $ (power/area) which is proportional to ($f^2 A^2$)

where f = frequency, A = amplitude.

The loudness varies with the frequency. The ears are most sensitive (hears sounds of lowest intensity) at approximately 2,000 to 4,000 Hz. I_o is taken to be 10^{-12} watts/cm², is barely audible and is assigned a value of 0 dB (zero *decibels*). Then intensity level (I) of a sound wave in dB is,

$$dB = 10 \log_{10}(I/I_o)$$

where dB = the sound level, I = the intensity at a given level, I_o = the threshold intensity. {To calculate a change in the sound level or volume ΔV in units of dB, given two values for sound intensity, the given equation can be modified thus: $\Delta V = 10\log(I_{new}/I_{old})$}

Examples of some values of dB's are: whisper (20), normal conversation (60), subway car (100), pain threshold (120), and jet engine (160). Continual exposure to sound greater than 90 dB can lead to hearing impairment.

8.3.1 Calculation of the Intensity Level

What is the loudness or intensity level of Mr. Yell Alot's voice when he generates a sound wave ten million times as intense as I_o?

$$I = (10,000,000) \quad I_o = (10^7) I_o$$

Thus
$$dB = 10 \log_{10}(10^7 I_o/I_o)$$
$$= 10 \log_{10} 10^7$$
$$= 70 \log_{10} 10 = 70$$

{See chemistry section 6.5.1 for rules of logarithms. Question types involving logs including acids-bases (CHM Chapter 6) and rate law (CHM Chapter 9) are common amongst ACER's GAMSAT materials.}

8.4 Beats

When sound of different frequencies are heard together, they interfere. Constructive interference results in beats. The number of beats per second is the absolute value of the difference of the frequencies ($|f_1 - f_2|$).

Hence, the new frequency heard includes the original frequencies and the absolute difference between them.

8.5 Doppler Effect

The Doppler effect is the effect upon the observed frequency caused by the relative motion of the observer (o) and the source (s). If the distance is decreasing between them, there is a shift to higher frequencies and shorter wavelengths (to higher pitch for sound and toward blue-violet for light, PHY 8.3 and 9.2.4). If the distance is increasing between them, there is a shift to longer wavelengths and lower frequencies (to lower pitch for sound and toward red for light). The summary equation of the above in terms of frequency (f) is :

$$f_o = f_s(V \pm v_o)/(V \pm v_s)$$

V = speed of the wave, v = speed of the observer (o) or the source (s).

Choose the sign such that the frequency varies consistently with the relative motion of the source and the observer. In other words, when the distance between the source and observer is *decreasing* use $+v_o$ and $-v_s$; if the distance is *increasing* use $-v_o$ and $+v_s$.

8.5.1 Doppler Effect Problem (SI units)

A car drives towards a bus stop with its car stereo playing opera. The opera singer sings the note middle C (= 262 Hz) loudly; however, the people waiting at the bus stop hear C sharp (= 277 Hz). Given that the speed of sound V in air is 331 m/s, how fast is the car moving?

{Remember the sign convention: since the distance between the source (the car) and the observer (people at the bus stop) is *decreasing* we use $+v_o$ and $-v_s$}

• the car (the *source* of the frequency) f_s = 262 Hz, v_s = unknown.

• the bus stop (where the *observers* are stationary) f_o = 277 Hz, v_o = 0 m/s.

$$f_o = f_s(V + v_o)/(V - v_s)$$

Thus

$$V - v_s = f_s(V + v_o)/f_o$$

Hence

$$v_s = -f_s(V + v_o)/f_o + V$$

Substitute

$$v_s = -262(331 + 0)/277 + 331 = 17.9 \text{ m/s}.$$

• Note that the answer contains three significant figures.

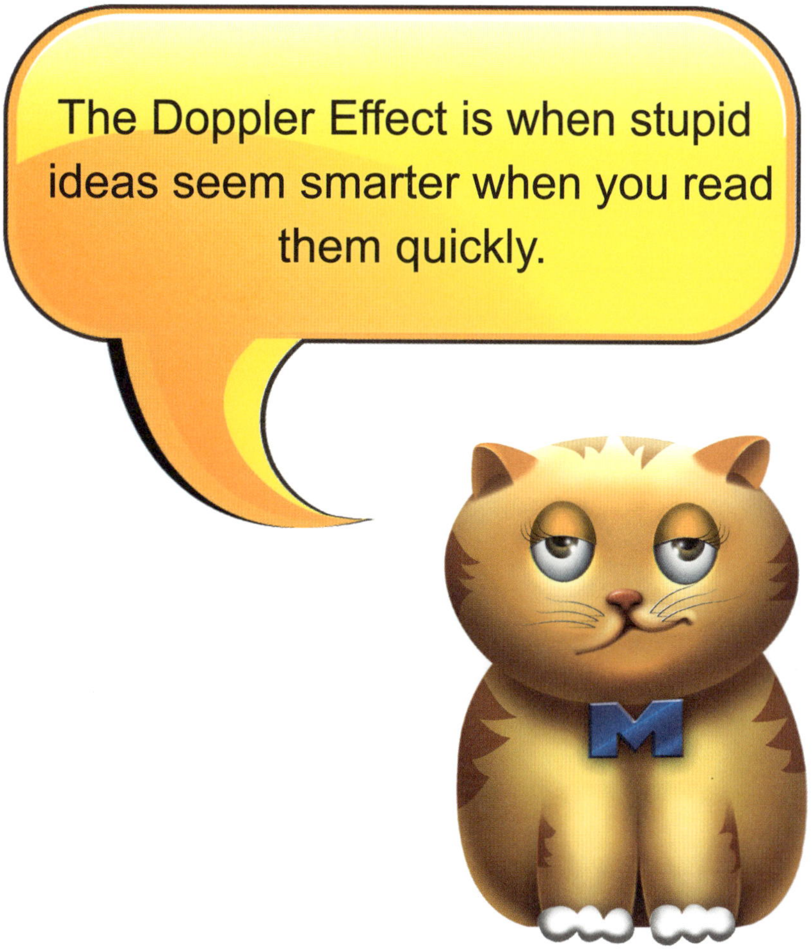

PHYSICS

> The Doppler Effect is when stupid ideas seem smarter when you read them quickly.

THE PHYSICAL SCIENCES PHY-65

GOLD NOTES

ELECTROSTATICS AND ELECTROMAGNETISM
Chapter 9

Memorize	Understand	Not Required*
...ations: for charge Q, Coulomb's law, ...tric field ...ations: potential energy, absolute potential ...ation relating energy, planck's constant, ...quency	* Conservation of charge, use of Coulomb's law * Graphs/theory: electric field/potential lines, mag. induction * Potential difference, electric dipoles, mag. induction * Laplace's law, the right hand rule, magnetic field * Direction of F in magn. field; electromagnetism	* Advanced level college info * Memorizing coulomb's, permittivity or planck's constants * Memorizing equation with permittivity constant or dF * Calculus, derivatives, integrals, speed of light

GAMSAT-Prep.com

Introduction

Electrostatics (statics = usu. at rest) refers to the science of stationary or slowly moving charges. Such charges can interact and behave in ways described by charge, electric force, electric field and potential difference. When a charge is in motion, it creates a magnetic field. Electromagnetism describes the relationship between electricity (moving electrical charge) and magnetism. The electromagnetic spectrum includes light and X-rays.

Additional Resources

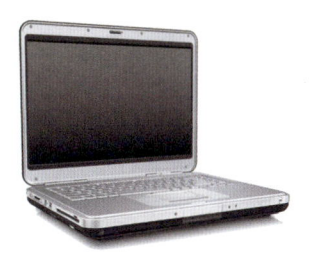

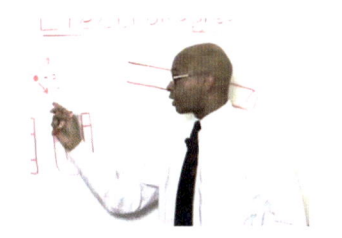

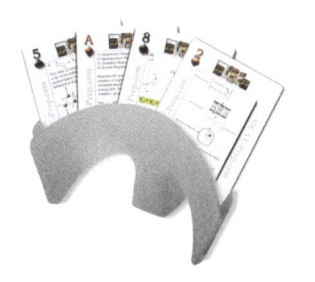

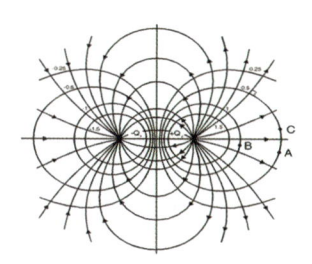

Free Online Q&A + Forum   Video: Online or DVD 1, 3, 4   Flashcards   Special Guest

* The real GAMSAT may have advanced level information presented (ie. in a passage) but previous knowledge of said information is not required to answer the questions that would follow. Practice ACER and GS practice GAMSATs can help you clarify this point.

9.1 Electrostatics

9.1.1 Charge, Conductors, Insulators

By friction of matter we create between substances repulsive or attractive electric forces. These forces are due to two kinds of electric charges, distinguished by positive (+) and negative (-) signs. Each has a charge of 1.6×10^{-19} coulombs (C) but differ in sign. The electron is the negative charge carrier, and the proton is the positive charge carrier. Substances with an excess of electrons have a net negative charge. Substances with a deficiency of electrons have a net positive charge. The total amount of charge Q of matter depends on the number of particles *n* and the charge *e* on each particle, thus $Q = ne$.

The conservation of charge states that a net charge cannot be created but that charge can be transfered from one object to another. One way of charging substances is by rubbing them (i.e., by contact).

For example, glass rubbed on fur becomes positive and rubber rubbed on fur becomes negative. Objects can also be charged by induction which occurs when one charged object is brought near to another uncharged object causing a charge redistribution in the latter to give net charge regions. Conductors transmit charge readily. Insulators resist the flow of charge.

9.1.2 Coulomb's Law, Electric Force

Charges exert forces upon each other. Like charges repel each other and unlike charges attract. For any two charges q_1 and q_2 the force *F* is given by Coulomb's Law:

$$F = k \frac{q_1 q_2}{r^2} = \frac{1}{4\pi\varepsilon_o}\left(\frac{q_1 q_2}{r^2}\right)$$

where k = coulomb's constant = 9.0×10^9 N-m²/C², ε_o = permittivity constant = 8.85×10^{-12} C²/N-m², and r = the distance between the charges. Note that the relationship of force and distance follows an inverse square law. Thus if the distance *r* is doubled [$(2r)^2 = 4r^2$], the new force is quartered ($F_{new} = F/4$). {cf. Law of Gravity: PHY 2.4}

9.1.3 Electric Field, Electric Field Lines

A charge generates an electric field (E) in the space around it. Fields (force fields) are vectors. A field is generated by an object and it is that region of space around the object that will exert a force on a second object brought into that field. The field exists independently of that second object and is not altered by its presence. The force exerted on the second object depends upon that object and the field. The electric field E is given by:

$$E = F/q = k\,Q/r^2$$

where E and F are vectors, Q = the charge generating the field, and q = the charge placed in the field.

Charges exert forces upon each other through fields. The direction of a field is the direction <u>a positive charge would move if placed in it</u>. *Electric field lines* are imaginary lines which are in the same direction as E at that point. The direction is away from positive charges and toward negative charges, or put another way, the electric field is directed toward the decreasing potentials.

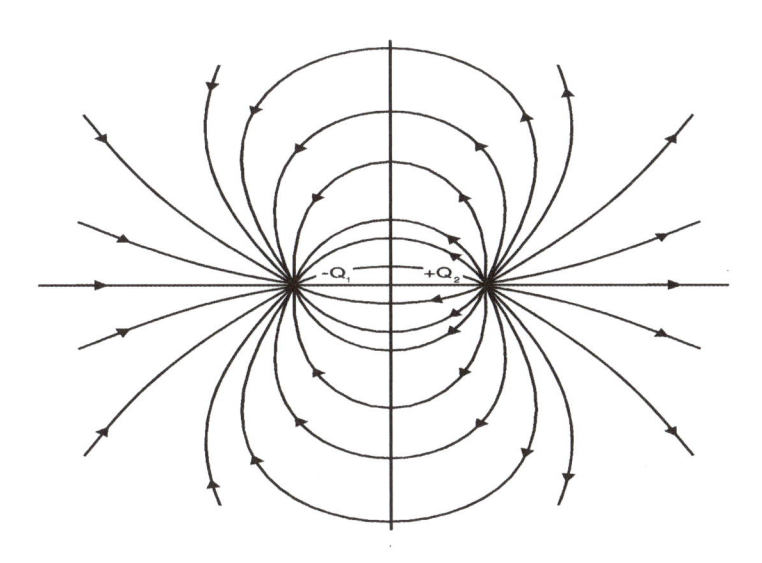

Figure III.B.9.1: Electric field lines. The electric field is generated by the charges $-Q_1$ and $+Q_2$. The arrowheads show the direction of the electric field.

If an electric potential is applied between two plates in a vacuum, and an electron is introduced, the electron will experience an attractive force to the positive plate (*see Figure III.B.9.2*).

The force will cause the electron to accelerate towards the positive plate in a straight line. It suffers no collisions because the area between the plates is *in vacuo*. This effect is used in thermoionic valves.

If the electron is given some motion, and the electric field is applied perpendicular to the motion, interesting things happen (see Figure III.B.9.3). For example, a beam of electrons is emitted from a device called an electron gun. These electrons are moving in the x direction.

As the electrons pass between the plates they are accelerated in the y direction, as explained before, but their velocity in the x direction is unaltered. The electron beam is thus deflected as shown.

By varying the potential applied to the plates, the angle of deflection can be controlled. This effect is the basis of the cathode ray oscilloscope.

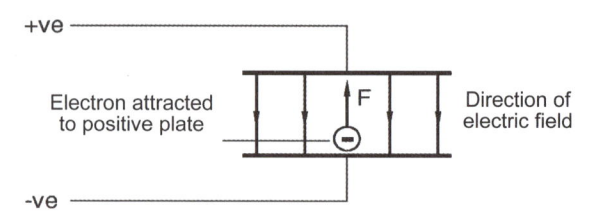

Figure III.B.9.2: Electric field between parallel plates.

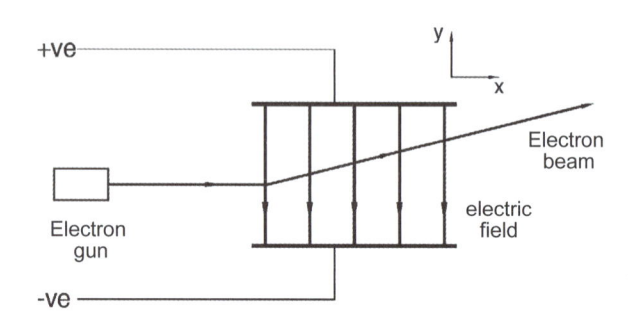

Figure III.B.9.3: Electrostatic deflection of an electron beam.

9.1.4 Potential Energy, Absolute Potential

The *potential energy* (E_p) of a charged object in a field equals the work done on that object to bring it from infinity to a distance (r) from the charge setting up the electric field,

$$E_p = \text{work} = Fr = (qE)r = kQq/r$$

where Q = the charge setting up field, and q = the charge brought in to a distance r.

When a +q moves against E, its E_p increases. When a -q moves against the electric field E, its E_p decreases. If two positive or negative charges were brought together, work would have to be done to the system (and E_p would increase), and vice versa for charges of opposite charges.

The *absolute potential* (V) is a scalar, and it is defined at each distance (r) from a charge (Q) generating an electric field. It represents the negative of the work per unit charge in bringing a +q from infinity to r:

• $V = E_p/q = kQ/r$ in volts where 1 volt = 1 joule/coulomb.

• $V = Ed$ for a parallel plate capacitor where d = distance between the plates (PHY 10.4).

9.1.5 Equipotential Lines, Potential Difference, Electric Dipoles

Equipotential lines are lines (and surfaces) of equal V and are *perpendicular* to electric field lines. Work can only be done when moving between surfaces of equal V and is, therefore, independent of the path taken. No work is done when a charge (q) is moved along an equal potential (*equipotential*) surface (or line), because the component of force is zero along it. Potential (V) is defined in terms of positive charges such that V is positive when due to a +Q and negative when due a -Q. Potential (V) is added algebraically at a point (because it is a scalar).

See Figure III.B.9.4:

1) V_1, V_2 are two potentials perpendicular to the electric field E and the force *F*;
2) $V_2 - V_1$ is the potential difference (PD);
3) charge (*q*) moved from A ($V_1 = 0.5$) to B ($V_2 = 1$) has work (*W*) done on it:

$$W = q(V_2 - V_1) = q(PD)$$

4) charge (*q*) moved from A to C has no work done on it because this is along an equipotential surface ($V = 0.5$) and the non-zero component of force (*F*) is perpendicular to it;
5) the lines of *F* are along the lines of *E*.

The *potential difference* (*PD*) is the difference in V between two points, or it is the work per unit positive charge done by electric forces moving a small test charge from the point of higher potential to the point of lower potential:

$$PD = V_a - V_b = \text{volts} = \text{work/charge}$$

$$\text{work} = q(V_a - V_b) = q(PD).$$

An *electric dipole* consists of two charges separated by some finite distance (d). Usually the charges are equal and opposite. The laws of forces, fields, etc., apply to dipoles. A dipole is characterized by its *dipole moment* which is the product of the charge (q) and d.

Dipoles tend to line up with the electric field (Fig. III.B.9.5). Motion of dipoles against an electric field requires energy as discussed above.

dipole moment = *(charge)(distance)* = *qd*

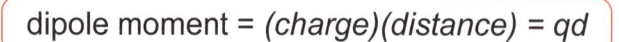

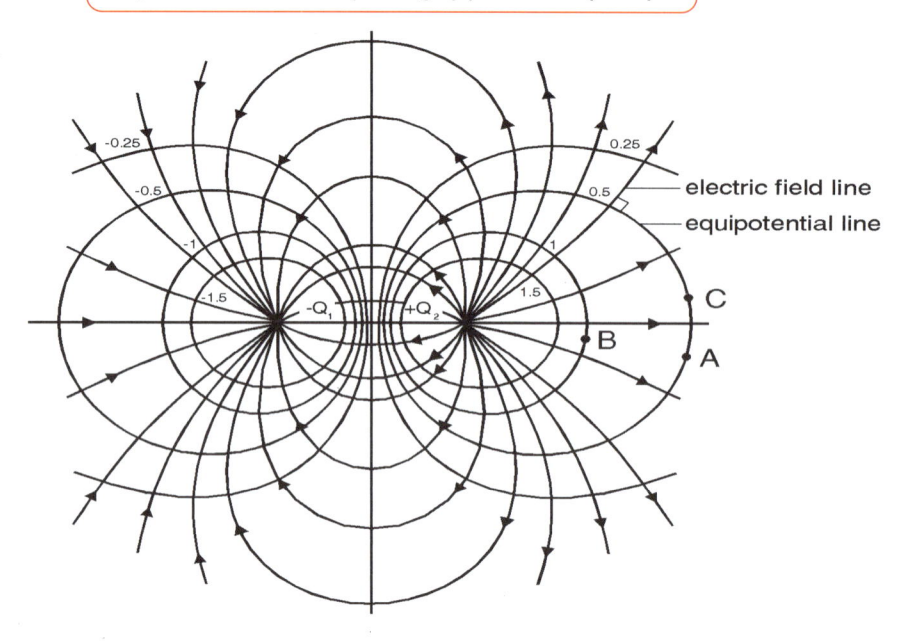

Figure III.B.9.4: Equipotential lines.
The circle-like curves around each charge $-Q_1$ and $+Q_2$ are the equipotential lines corresponding to each charge. The numbers represent the electric potential value (i.e. in millivolts) of the respective equipotential lines. Note the electric field lines as in Figure III.B.9.1.

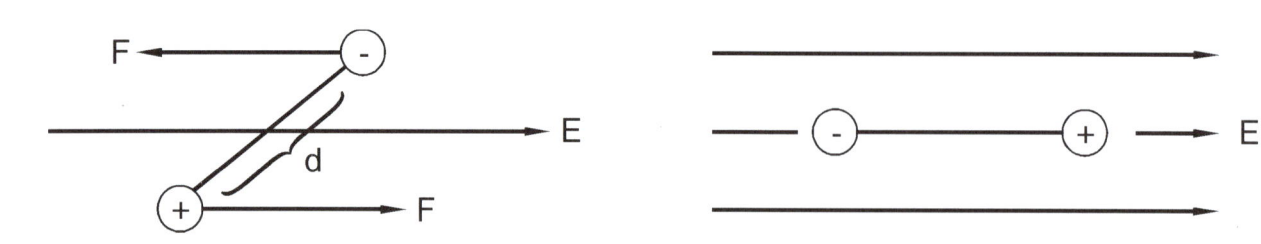

Dipole with equal and opposite charges

Alignment of dipole with E

Figure III.B.9.5: Dipole and electric field.
E = electric field, *F* = forces exerted by E on the dipole

PHY-72 ELECTROSTATICS AND ELECTROMAGNETISM

9.2 Electromagnetism

9.2.1 Notion of Electromagnetic Induction

Coulomb's Law in electrostatics gives the nature of the forces acting upon electric charges at rest, but when the charges are moving, new forces appear.

They are not of the same nature as the electrostatic forces and they act differently on the electric charges. They are called electromagnetic forces.

9.2.2 Magnetic Induction Vector

Experiments have shown that two straight conductors (e.g. copper wires) traversed by electric currents of intensities I and I' in the same direction are acted upon by an attractive force proportional to the product of the intensities and inversely proportional to the distance between the two conductors. It can be demonstrated that when the electric current in one of the conductors disappears, the force also disappears.

Therefore, the force is due to the motion of the electric charges in both conductors.

We decompose the phenomenon by introducing a new physical quantity: the magnetic induction vector B, also created by magnets.

The SI unit for B is the tesla where 1 T = 1 N/(A·m) = 10^4 gauss.

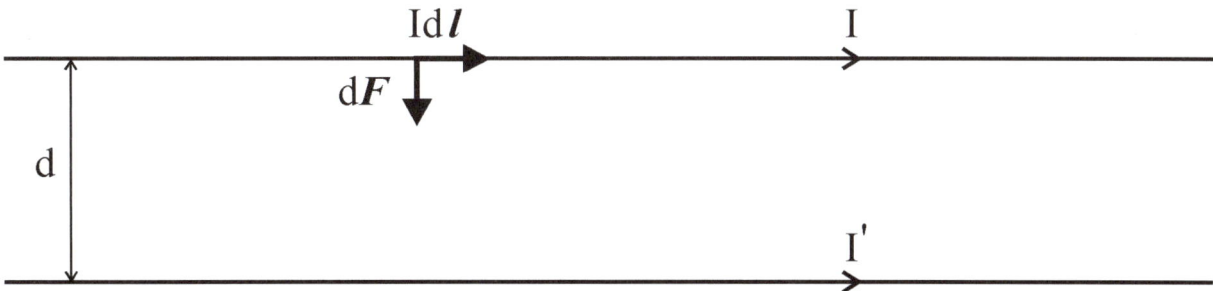

Figure III.B.9.6: Magnetic induction.
Two conductors a distance d apart; the current element Idl and the perpendicular force dF associated with the magnetic induction vector B are both shown. Vector B, which is not shown, has a direction perpendicular to both Idl and dF, pointing out of the page.

Thus, two effects have been shown by the preceding experiment:

1) a moving charge produces a magnetic induction.

2) a magnetic induction exerts a force on any nearby moving charge.

9.2.3 Laplace's Law

A test particle with charge dq moving at a velocity v in a magnetic induction field B is acted upon by a force dF given by the following formula:

$$dF = dq\, v \times B = dq\, v(B\sin \alpha)$$

where α is the angle formed by the direction of v with that of B (= the cross product).

The force dF is perpendicular to the magnetic induction vector and also to the displacement velocity vector of the charge (see Figure III.B.9.6).

When many charges are in motion so as to produce an electric current of intensity $I = dq/dt$ the force acting upon an elemental length of conductor dl traversed by that electric current is:

$$dF = I\, dl \times B = I\, dl(B \sin \alpha)$$

where α is the angle formed by the direction of the current element of conductor with that of B (= the cross product).

In order to determine the direction of a cross (= *vector*) product we can use the right-hand rule. If $c = a \times b$ then the right hand is held so that the curled fingers follow the rotation of a to b, the extended right thumb will point in the direction of c (dF in the preceding example). {Student's trick: "Grab the Wire!" Examine Fig. III.B.9.6. Turn the book around such that with your right hand open and thumb extended, the fingers point in the direction of dF and your thumb points in the direction Idl. As you begin to grab the wire, the initial direction of the tips of your fingers move perpendicular to both dF and Idl. Now the tips of your fingers make a circular motion around the wire. Those fingers have just described the direction of the magnetic induction vector B!}

9.2.4 Electromagnetic Spectrum, Radio, Infrared, X Rays

An electromagnetic field is described as having at every point of the field, two perpendicular vectors: *the electric field* vector E and the magnetic induction field vector B.

Radar (= *radio detection* and ranging) is an example of a radio wave.

Visible light can be broken down into colors remembered by the mnemonic (*from highest to lowest wavelength*), Roy G. BIV: Red, Orange, Yellow, Green, Blue, Indigo, Violet.

The separation of white light into these colors can occur as a result of refraction through a prism (PHY 11.4) or through water (i.e. mist or rain resulting in a rainbow).

Planck developed the relation between energy (E) and the frequency f of the electromagnetic radiation,

$$E = hf$$

where h = planck's constant. Thus high frequency or short wave length corresponds to high energy and vice versa.

{The preceding equation should be memorized in conjunction with the relationship between a wave's velocity, wavelength and frequency; PHY 7.1.2}

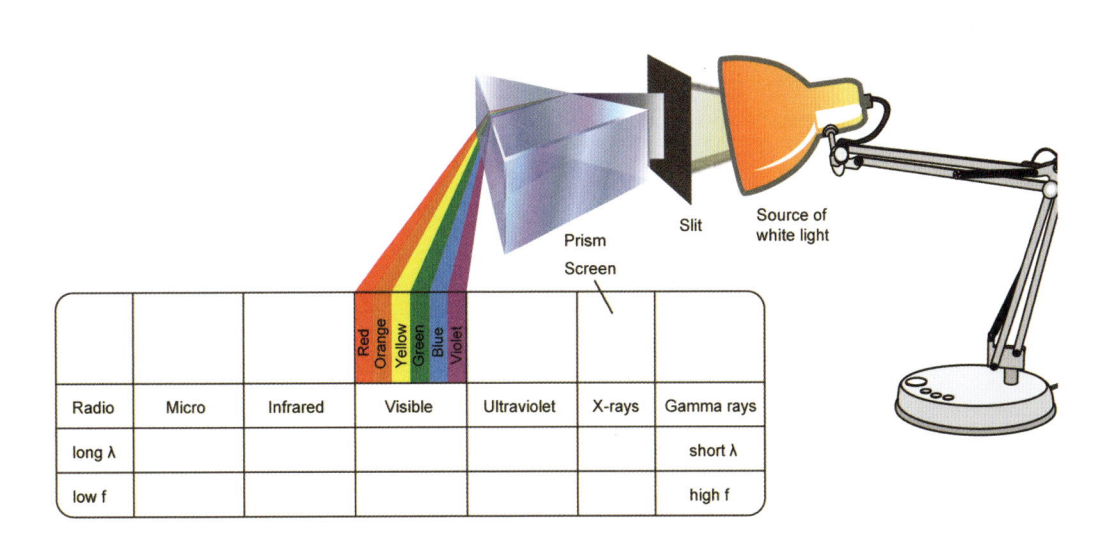

Figure III.B.9.7: The complete electromagnetic spectrum.

GOLD NOTES

ELECTRIC CIRCUITS
Chapter 10

Memorize	Understand	Not Required*
inition/equation/units: current, resistance m's law, resistors in series/parallel choff's laws	* Battery, emf, voltage, terminal potential * Internal resistance of the battery, resistivity * Ohm's law, resistors in series/parallel * Parallel plate capacitor, series, parallel * Conductivity, power in circuits, Kirchoff's laws	* Advanced level college info * Complex/discrete/digital circuits * Transistors, FPGAs, microprocessors

GAMSAT-Prep.com

Introduction

Electric circuits are closed paths which includes electronic components (i.e. resistors, capacitors, power supplies) through which a current can flow. There are 3 basic laws that govern the flow of current in an electrical circuit: Ohm's law and Kirchoff's first and second laws.

Additional Resources

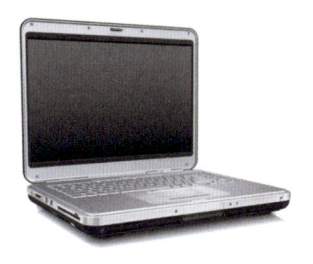

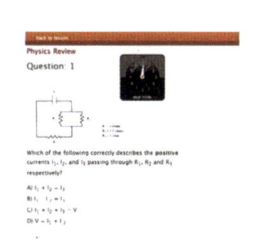

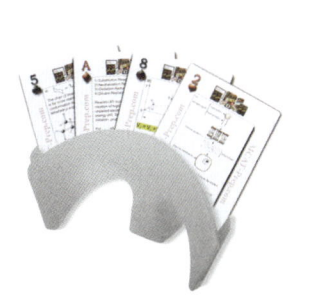

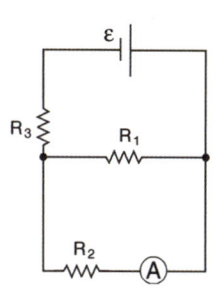

Free Online Q&A + Forum   Video: Online or DVD 1, 2, 4   Flashcards   Special Guest

THE PHYSICAL SCIENCES   PHY-77

*The real GAMSAT may have advanced level information presented (ie. in a passage) but previous knowledge of said information is not required to answer the questions that would follow. Practice ACER and GS practice GAMSATs can help you clarify this point.

10.1 Current

The current (*I*) is the amount of charge (*Q*) that flows past a point in a given amount of time (*t*),

$$I = Q/t = amperes = coulombs/sec.$$

Current is caused by the movement of electrons between two points of significant potential difference of an electric circuit. Free electrons will accelerate towards the positive connection. As they move they will collide with atoms in the substance, losing energy which we observe as heat. The net effect is a drift of electrons at a roughly constant speed towards the positive connection. The motion of electrons is an *electric current*. As electrons are removed by the electric potential source at the positive connection, electrons are being injected at the negative connection. The potential can be considered as a form of *electron pump*.

This model explains many observed effects.

If the magnitude of the electric potential is increased, the electrons will accelerate faster and their mean velocity will be higher, i.e., the current is increased. The collisions between electrons and atoms transfer energy to the atoms. The collisions manifest themselves as heat. This effect is known as *Joule heating*. Materials such as these are termed ohmic conductors, since they obey the well-known Ohm's Law:

$$V = IR$$

where *V* is the voltage, *I* is the current, and *R* is the resistance.

The potential difference is maintained by a voltage source (emf). The direction of current is taken as the direction of positive charge movement, by convention. It is represented on a circuit diagram by arrows. Ammeters are used to measure the flow of current and are symbolized as in Figure III.B.10.1.

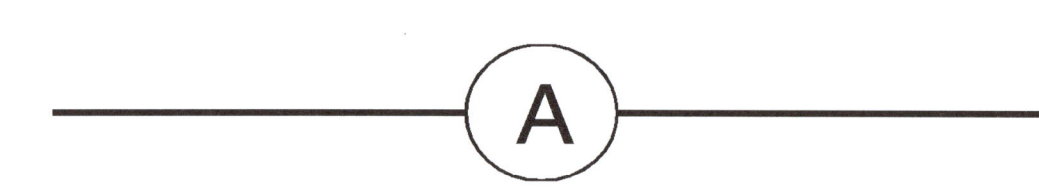

Figure III.B.10.1: Symbol of an ammeter.

10.2 Resistance, Resistivity, Series and Parallel Circuits

Resistance (R) is the measure of opposition to the flow of electrons in a substance. Resistivity (ρ) is an inherent property of a substance. It varies with temperature. For example, the resistivity of metals increases with increasing temperature.

Resistance is directly proportional to resistivity and length l but inversely proportional to the cross-sectional area A.

$$R = \rho l / A$$

Resistance increases with temperature because the thermal motion of molecules increases with temperature and results in more collisions between electrons which impede their flow.

The units of resistance are ohms, symbolized by Ω (omega). From Ohm's Law, 1 ohm = 1 volt/ampere.

When a positive current flows across a resistor, there is a voltage decrease and an energy loss:

$$\text{energy loss} = Vq = VIt = \text{joules}$$

$$\boxed{\text{power loss } (P) = VIt/t = VI = \text{watts}}$$

watts = volts × amperes = joules/sec.

The energy loss may be used to perform work. These relations hold for power (P),

$$P = VI = (IR)(I) = I^2R = V(V/R) = V^2/R.$$

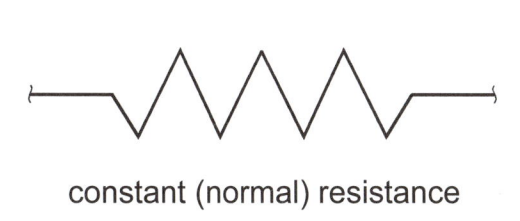

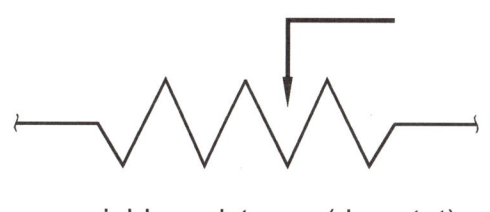

constant (normal) resistance

variable resistance (rheostat)

Figure III.B.10.2: Representation of two types of resistors.

Circuit elements are either in series or in parallel. Two components are in series when they have only one point in common; that is, the current travelling from one of them back to the emf source must pass through the other. In a complete series circuit, or for individual series loops of a larger mixed circuit, the current (*I*) is the same over each component and the total voltage drop in the circuit elements (resistors, capacitors, inductors, internal resistance of emf sources, etc.) is equal to the sum V_t of all the emf sources. The value of the equivalent resistance R_{eq} in a series circuit is:

$$R_{eq} = R_1 + R_2 + R_3 + \ldots$$

Two components are in parallel when they are connected to two common points in the circuit; that is, the current travelling from one such element back to the emf source need not pass through the second element because there is an alternate path.

In a parallel circuit, the total current is the sum of currents for each path and the voltage is the same for all paths in parallel. The equivalent resistance in a parallel circuit is:

$$1/R_{eq} = 1/R_1 + 1/R_2 + 1/R_3 + \ldots$$

10.2.1 Resistance Problem in Series and Parallel

Determine the equivalent resistance between points *A* and *B* in Figure III.B.10.3.

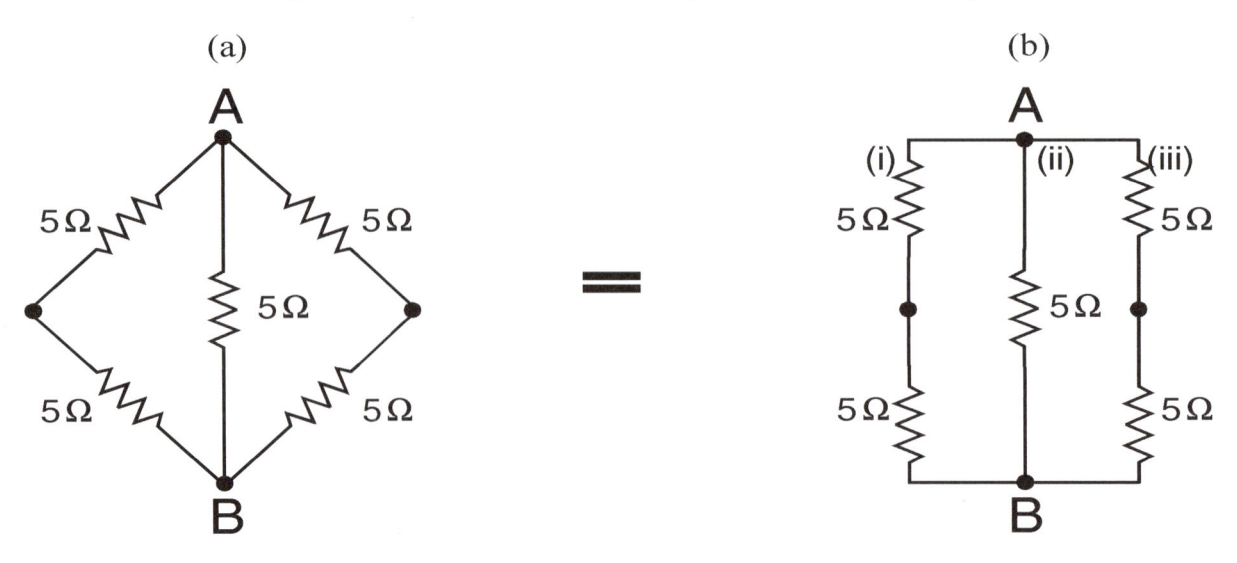

Figure III.B.10.3: Equivalent resistance.
(a) The problem as it could be presented; (b) the way you should interpret the problem.

- Wire (i) has two resistors in a row (*in series*): $R_{(i)} = 5 + 5 = 10\ \Omega$

- Wire (ii) has only one resistor: $R_{(ii)} = 5\ \Omega$

- Wire (iii) has two resistors in series: $R_{(iii)} = 5 + 5 = 10\ \Omega$

Between *A* and *B* we have three resistor systems in parallel: (i), (ii) and (iii), thus

$$1/R_{eq} = 1/R_{(i)} + 1/R_{(ii)} + 1/R_{(iii)}$$
$$= 1/10 + 1/5 + 1/10 = 4/10$$

multiply through by $10 R_{eq}$ to get: $10 = 4 R_{eq}$

thus $R_{eq} = 10/4 = 2.5\ \Omega.$

10.3 Batteries, Electromotive Force, Voltage, Internal Resistance

An *electromotive force (emf)* source maintains between its terminal points, a constant potential difference. The emf source replaces energy lost by moving electrons. Sources of emf are batteries (conversion of chemical energy to electrical energy) and generators (conversion of mechanical energy to electrical energy).

The source of emf does work on each charge to raise it from a lower potential to a higher potential.

Then as the charge flows around the circuit (naturally from higher to lower potential) it loses energy which is replaced by the emf source again.

energy supplied = energy lost

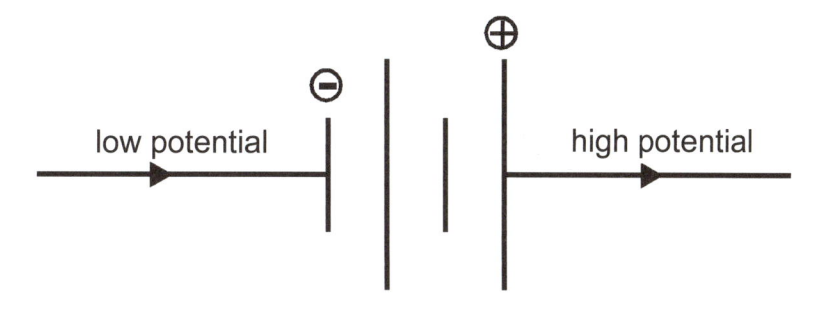

Figure III.B.10.4: Symbol of an emf source. Arrows show the normal direction of current.

Energy is lost whenever a charge (as current) passes through a resistor. The units of emf are volts. The actual voltage delivered to a circuit is not equal to the value of the source. This is reduced by an internal voltage lost which represents the voltage loss by the *internal resistance (r)* of the source itself. The net voltage is called the terminal voltage or *terminal potential V_t.*

Figure III.B.10.5:
Simplified symbol of an emf source.

$$V_t = V - Ir = IR_t$$

I, R_t = totals for the circuit; V = maximal voltage output of the emf source.

When two emf sources are connected in opposition, (positive pole to positive pole) the charge loses energy when passing in the second emf source.

Therefore, if there is more than one emf source in a circuit, the total emf is the sum of the individual emf sources not in opposition reduced by the sum of individual sources in opposition in a given direction.

10.3.1 Kirchoff's Laws and a Multiloop Circuit Problem

Given that the emf of the battery $\varepsilon = 12$ volts and the resistors $R_1 = 12\ \Omega$, $R_2 = 4.0\ \Omega$, and $R_3 = 6.0\ \Omega$, determine the reading in the ammeter (see Figure III.B.10.6).

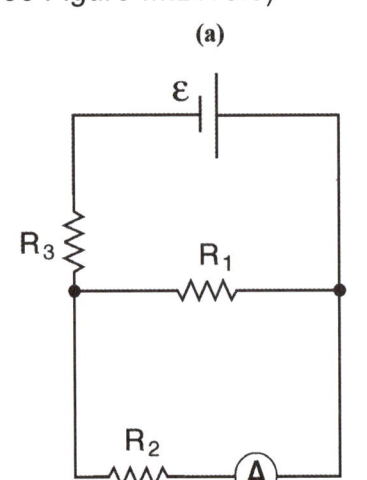

Ignore the internal resistance of the battery.

{The ammeter will read the current which flows through it which is i_2}

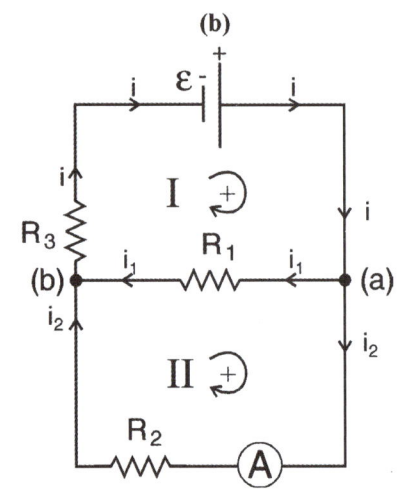

Figure III.B.10.6: A multiloop circuit.
(a) The problem as it could be presented; (b) the way you should label the diagram. Note that the current emanates from the positive terminal and is the same current i which returns to the emf source.

PHY-82 ELECTRIC CIRCUITS

Kirchoff's Law I (*the junctional theorem*): when different currents arrive at a point (= *junction*, as in points (*a*) and (*b*) in the labelled diagram) the sum of current equals zero.

We can arbitrarily define all current *arriving* at the junction as <u>positive</u> and all current *leaving* as <u>negative</u>.

Kirchoff's Law I $\Sigma i = 0$ at a junction

Thus at junction (a) $i - i_1 - i_2 = 0$

And for junction (b) $i_1 + i_2 - i = 0$

Both (a) and (b) reduce to equation (c):

$$i = i_1 + i_2$$

Kirchoff's Law II (*the loop theorem*): the sum of voltage changes in one continous loop of a circuit is zero. A single loop circuit is simple since the current is the same in all parts of the loop hence the loop theorem is applied only once.

In a multiloop circuit (loops *I* and *II* in the labelled diagram), there is more than one loop thus the current in general will not be the same in all parts of any given loop. We can arbitrarily define all voltage changes around the loop in the *clockwise* direction as <u>positive</u> and in the *counterclockwise* direction as <u>negative</u>.

Thus if by moving in the clockwise direction we can move from the battery's negative terminal (*low potential*) to its positive terminal (*high potential*), the value of the emf ε is negative.

Kirchoff's Law II $\Sigma \Delta V = 0$ in a loop

Thus in loop *I* (recall: $V = IR$)

$$i_1 R_1 + i R_3 - \varepsilon = 0$$

And in loop II

$$i_2 R_2 - i_1 R_1 = 0$$

We now have simultaneous equations. There are three unknowns (i, i_1, i_2) and three equations (c, loop *I*, and loop *II*). We need only solve for the current i_2 which runs through the ammeter.

Substitute (c) into loop I

$$i_1 R_1 + (i_1 + i_2) R_3 - \varepsilon = 0$$

Thus

$$i_1 R_1 + i_1 R_3 + i_2 R_3 - \varepsilon = 0$$

Substitute i_1 from loop *II* where $i_1 = i_2 R_2 / R_1$, hence

$$i_2 R_2 + i_2 R_2 R_3 / R_1 + i_2 R_3 = \varepsilon$$

Begin isolating i_2

$$i_2 (R_2 + R_2 R_3 / R_1 + R_3) = \varepsilon$$

Isolate i_2

$$i_2 = \varepsilon (R_2 + R_2 R_3 / R_1 + R_3)^{-1}$$

Substitute

$$i_2 = 12[4 + (4)(6)/(12) + 6]^{-1} = 12/12 = 1.0 \text{ ampere.}$$

10.4 Capacitors and Dielectrics

Capacitors can store and separate charge. Capacitors can be filled with dielectrics which are materials which can increase capacitance. The capacitance (C) is an inherent property of a conductor and is formulated as:

C = charge/electric potential = Q/V = farad = coulomb/volt

The capacitance is the number of coulombs that must be transferred to a conductor to raise its potential by one volt.

The amount of charge that can be stored depends on the shape, size, surroundings and type of the conductor.

The higher the dielectric strength (i.e., the electric field strength at which a substance ceases to be an insulator and becomes a conductor) of the medium, the greater the capacitance of the conductor.

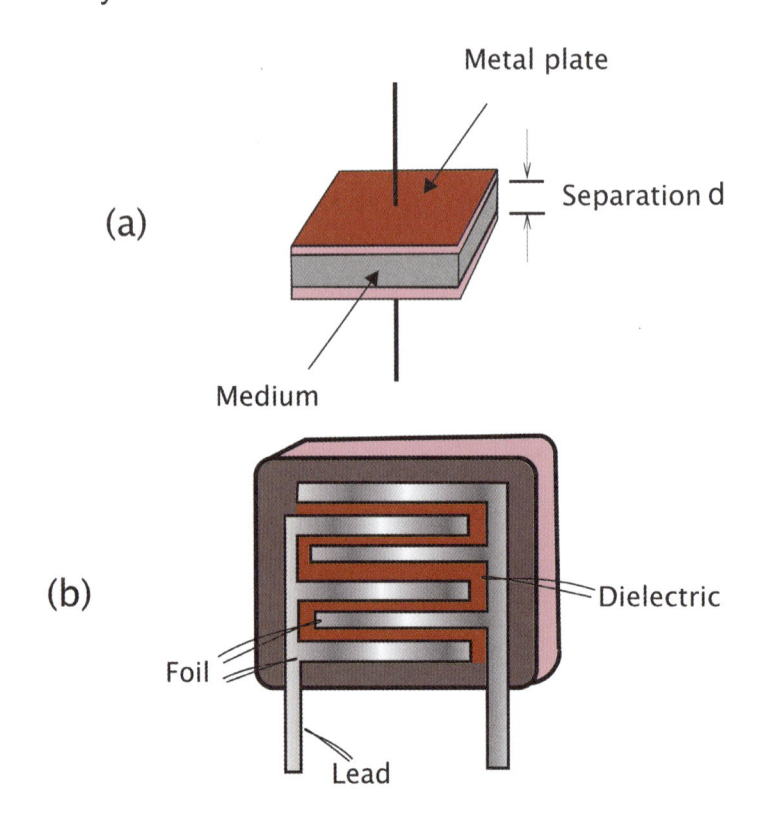

Figure III.B.10.7: (a) Parallel plate capacitor; (b) Ceramic capacitor.

A capacitor is made of two or more conductors with opposite but equal charges placed near each other.

A common example is the parallel plate capacitor. The important formulas for capacitors are:

1) $C = Q/V$ where V = the potential between the plates
2) $V = Ed$ where E = electric field strength, and d = distance between the plates
3) C is directly proportional to the surface area A of the plates and inversely proportional to the distance between the plates

$$C = \varepsilon_o A/d$$

for air as a medium between the plates. If the capacitor contains a dielectric, the above equation would by multiplied by the factor κ (= *dielectric constant*) whose value depends on the dielectric being used.

4) The equivalent capacitance C_{eq} for capacitors arranged in series and in parallel is:

Series: $1/C_{eq} = 1/C_1 + 1/C_2 + 1/C_3 \ldots$

Parallel: $C_{eq} = C_1 + C_2 + C_3 \ldots$

The dielectric substances set up an opposing electric field to that of the capacitor which decreases the net electric field and allows the capacitance of the capacitor to increase ($C = Q/Ed$). The molecules of the dielectric are dipoles which line up in the electric field.

{cf. Fig. III.B.9.5 from PHY 9.1.4 and Fig. III.B.10.8 in this section}

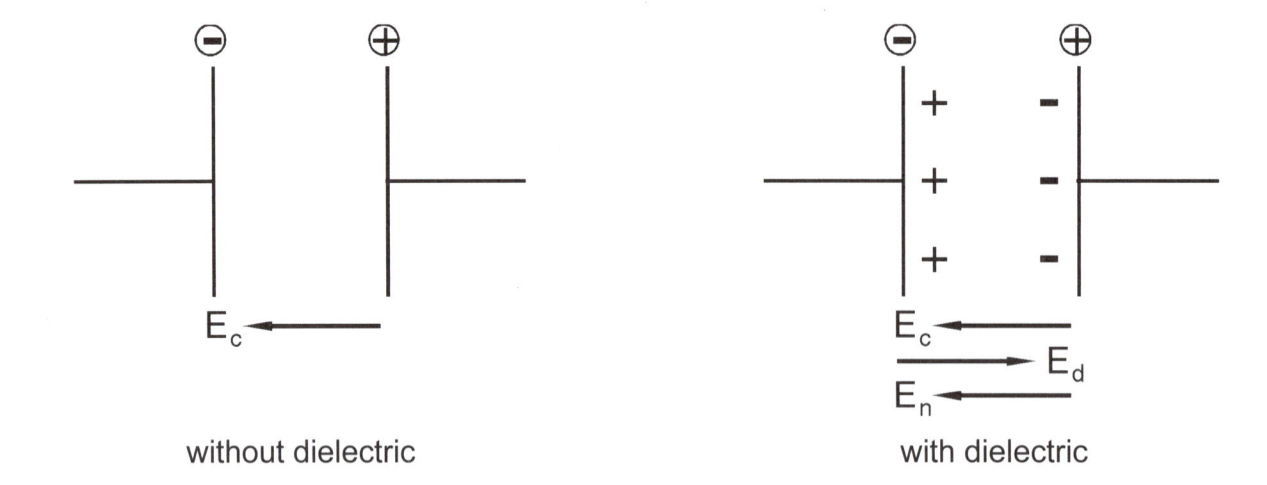

Figure III.B.10.8: Capacitors and dielectrics. Note that the capacitor is symbolized by two parallel lines of equal length. The electric fields: E_c generated by the capacitor, E_d generated by the dielectric, and E_n is the resultant electric field.

The energy associated with each charged capacitor is:

Potential Energy $(PE) = W = (1/2V)(Q) = 1/2QV$

also

and

$W = 1/2(CV)(V) = 1/2CV^2$

$W = 1/2Q(Q/C) = 1/2Q^2/C.$

10.5 Root-Mean-Square Current and Voltage

DC (*direct current*) circuits contain a continuous current. Thus calculating power output is quite simple using $P = I^2R = IV$. However, AC (*alternating current*) circuits pulsate; consequently, we must discuss the average power output P_{av} where

$$P_{av} = (I_{rms})^2 R = (I_{rms})(V_{rms})$$

which is true for a purely resistive load where the root-mean-square (*rms*) values are determined from their maximal (*max*) values:

$$I_{rms} = I_{max}/\sqrt{2} \quad \text{and} \quad V_{rms} = V_{max}/\sqrt{2}.$$

Thus by introducing the *rms* quantities the equations for DC and AC circuits have the same forms. AC circuit voltmeters and ammeters have their scales adjusted to read the *rms* values.

GOLD NOTES

GOLD NOTES

LIGHT AND GEOMETRICAL OPTICS

Chapter 11

Memorize	Understand	Not Required*
* Equations: PHY 11.3, 11.4, 11.5 * Rules for drawing ray diagrams	* Rules/equations: reflection, refraction, Snell's law * Dispersion, total internal reflection * Mirrors, lenses, real/virtual images * Ray diagrams * Lens strength, aberration	* Advanced level college info * Memorization of constants

GAMSAT-Prep.com

Introduction

Geometrical optics describes the propagation of light in terms of "rays." Rays are then bent at the interface of 2 rather different substances (i.e. air and glass) thus the ray may curve. A basic understanding of the equations and the geometry of light rays is necessary for solving problems in geometrical optics. Discrete questions regarding total internal reflection are frequent. Usually for the real GAMSAT, they will provide you with the optics equations to solve problems when needed. However, sometimes knowing the equation will give you an edge for "theoretical" questions and this is why we recommend that many optics equations be memorized.

Additional Resources

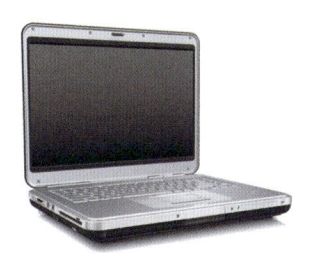

Free Online Q&A + Forum   Video: Online or DVD 2, 3   Flashcards   Special Guest

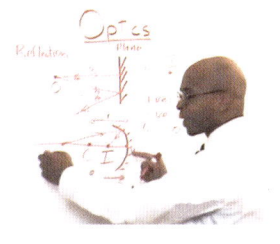

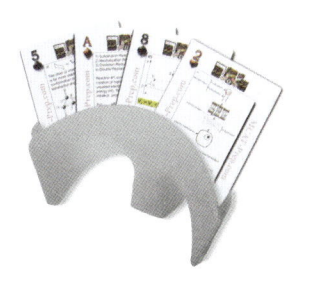

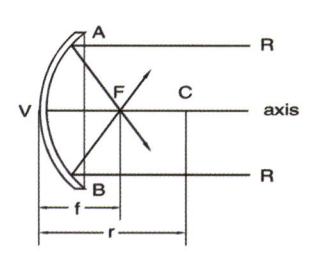

THE PHYSICAL SCIENCES   PHY-89

* The real GAMSAT may have advanced level information presented (ie. in a passage) but previous knowledge of said information is not required to answer the questions that would follow. Practice ACER and GS practice GAMSATs can help you clarify this point.

11.1 Visual Spectrum, Color

Geometrical optics is a first approximation of physical optics, which by its wavy nature, is part of the electromagnetic wave theory. The theory of light has a dualistic aspect:

• *particulate*: referring to a packet of energy called a photon when one wants, for example, to explain the photoelectric effect.

• *wavy* : when one wants to explain, for example, light interference and diffraction. Diffraction occurs when waves of light bend at the interface between two different media.

The optics domain of the electromagnetic wave theory corresponds to the following range of wavelengths of the electromagnetic spectrum (expressed in microns $1\mu = 10^{-6} m$):

$$0.4\mu < \lambda < 0.8\mu$$

or

$$0.4\mu < visible < 0.8\mu.$$

See PHY 9.2.4 for the colors in the visual spectrum.

11.2 Polarization

An electromagnetic field is described as having at every point of the field two perpendicular vectors: *the electric field vector E* and *the magnetic induction field vector B*.

The electromagnetic wave front is polarized in a straight line when *E* and *B* are fixed at all times. Thus polarized light is light that has waves in only one plane.

11.3 Reflection, Mirrors

Reflection is the process by which light rays (= *imaginary lines drawn perpendicular to the advancing wave fronts*) bounce back into a medium from a surface with another medium (*versus being refracted or absorbed*). The ray that arrives is the *incident* ray while the ray that bounces back is the *reflected* ray. The laws of reflection are:

1) the angle of incidence (I) equals the angle of reflection (R) at the normal (N, the line perpendicular to the surface)
2) the I, R, N all lie in the same plane.

After a ray strikes a mirror or a lens it forms an image. A virtual image has no light rays passing through it and cannot be projected upon a screen.

A <u>real image</u> has light rays passing through it and can be projected upon a screen.

Mirrors have a plane surface, like an ordinary household mirror, or a non-plane surface. For a plane mirror, all incident light is reflected in parallel off the mirror and therefore all images seen are virtual, erect, left-right reversed and appear to be just as far (perpendicular distance) behind the mirror as the object is in front of the mirror.

In other words, the object (o) and the image (i) distances have the same magnitudes but have opposite directions ($i = -o$).

Spherical mirrors are non-plane mirrors which may have the reflecting surface convex (*diverges light*) or concave (*converges light*). Note the images formed by a converging mirror (concave) are like those for a converging lens (convex); and diverging mirrors (convex) and a diverging lens (concave) also form similar images. The terminology for spherical mirrors is :

r = radius of curvature
C = center of curvature
F = focal point

V = vertex (center of the mirror itself)
axis = line through C and V
f = focal length (distance from F to V)

i = image distance (distance from V to image along the axis)
o = object distance (distance from V to object along the axis)
AB = linear aperture (cord connecting the ends of the mirror; the larger the aperture, the better the resolution).

As a rule, capital letters refer to a point (*or position*) and small case letters refer to a distance.

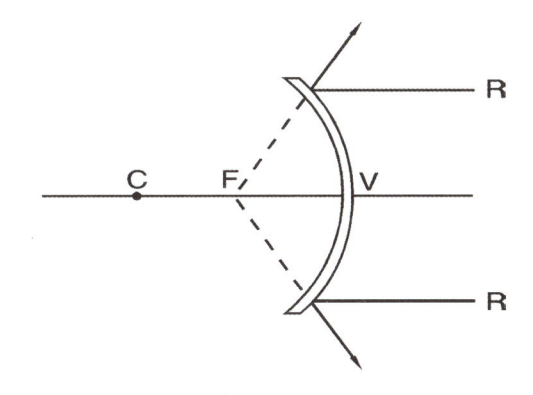

Concave (converging)   Convex (diverging)

Figure III.B.11.1: Reflection by spherical mirrors. R = the light rays.

With concave (spherical) mirrors the incident light is converged toward the axis. The path of light rays is as follows:

1)
if $o < f$, then the image is virtual and erect;
if $o > f$, then the image is real and inverted;
if $o = f$, then no image is formed;
2)
if $o < r$, then the image is enlarged in size;
if $o > r$, then the image is reduced in size;
if $o = r$, then the image is the same.

The relations are similar to those for a converging lens (convex). With convex (spherical) mirrors, the incident light is diverged from the axis after reflection. It is the backward extension (dotted lines in the diagram) that may pass through the focal point F. The path of light rays are as follows:

1) Incident rays parallel to the axis have backward extension of their reflections through F (see Figure III.B.11.1);
2) incident rays along a radius (that would pass C if extended) reflect back along themselves;
3) incident rays that pass through F (if extended) reflect parallel to the axis.

The image formed for a convex mirror is always virtual, erect and smaller than the object. The mirror equation and the derivations from it allow the above relations between object and image to be calculated instead of memorized. The equation is valid for convex and concave mirrors:

$$1/i + 1/o = 1/f$$

$$f = r/2$$

$$M = magnification = -i/o.$$

Convention :
• for i and o, *positive* values mean <u>real</u>, *negative* values mean <u>virtual</u>;
• for r and f, *positive* values mean <u>converging</u>, *negative* values mean <u>diverging</u>;
• for M, a *positive* value means <u>erect</u>, *negative* is <u>inverted</u>;
• for $M > 1$ the image is <u>enlarged</u>, $M < 1$ the image is <u>diminished</u>.

11.4 Refraction, Dispersion, Refractive Index, Snell's Law

Refraction is the bending of light as it passes from one transparent medium to another and is caused by the different speeds of light in the two media.

If θ_1 is taken as the angle (to the normal) of the incident light and θ_2 is the angle (to the normal) of the refracted light, where 1 and 2 represent the two different media, the following relations hold (Snell's Law):

where v = velocity and λ = wavelength.

$$\frac{\sin \theta_1}{\sin \theta_2} = \frac{v_1}{v_2} = \frac{n_2}{n_1} = \frac{\lambda_1}{\lambda_2}$$

$$n = \frac{\text{speed of light in vacuum}}{\text{speed of light in medium}} = \frac{c}{v}$$

$c = 3 \times 10^8$ *m/sec* or 181,000 *mi/sec*
n = 1.0 for air, n = 1.33 for H_2O
n = 1.5 for glass (at λ = 589 *nm*)
n = the refractive index which is a property of the medium
n_1 = refractive index of medium 1
n_2 = refractive index of medium 2
N = normal line to the surface
S = surface line, represents the separation between the two media
I = incident light
R = refracted light

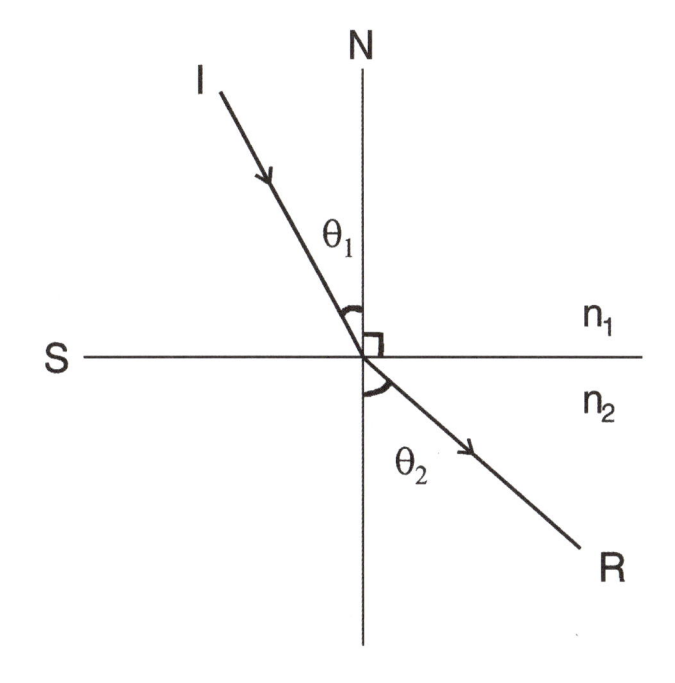

Figure III.B.11.2: Refraction.

The angle θ is smaller (closer to the normal, e.g. θ_1) in the more optically dense (higher n) medium.

Also the smaller wavelength of the incident light (i.e. toward the violet end), the closer θ_2 is to the normal (i.e. it is smaller than θ_1).

This means longer wavelengths travel faster in a medium than shorter wavelengths (i.e. longer wavelengths are more subject to refraction).

This leads to *dispersion* which is the separation of white light (= *all colors together*) into individual colors by this differential refraction. For example, a prism disperses white light.

The laws of refraction are:

1) The incident ray, the refracted ray and the normal ray all lie in the same plane.
2) The path of the ray (incident and refracted parts) is reversible.

When light passes from a more optically dense (higher n) medium into a less optically dense medium, there exists an angle of incidence such that the angle of refraction θ_2 is 90°.

This special angle of incidence is called the critical angle θ_c.

This is because when the angle of incidence is less then θ_c refraction occurs. If the angle of incidence is equal to θ_c, then neither refraction nor reflection occur.

And ==if $\theta_1 > \theta_c$, then total internal reflection (*ray is reflected back into the more optically dense medium*) occurs.== The θ_c is found from Snell's Law:

$n_1 \sin\theta_c = n_2 \sin\theta_2$

and $\theta_2 = 90° \Rightarrow \sin\theta_2 = 1$

giving $n_1 \sin\theta_c = n_2 \times 1$

finally $\sin\theta_c = n_2/n_1$

where $n_2 < n_1$.

When looking at an object under water from above the surface, the object appears closer than it actually is. This is due to refraction. In general:

apparent depth/actual depth = n_2/n_1

where n_2 = the medium of the observer, and n_1 = the medium of the object.

11.5 Thin Lens, Diopters

A lens is a transparent material which refracts light. Converging lenses refract toward the axis, and diverging lenses refract the light away from the axis.

A converging lens is wider at the middle than at the ends, and the diverging lens is thinner at the middle than at the ends.

Converging (convex) lens

Diverging (concave) lens

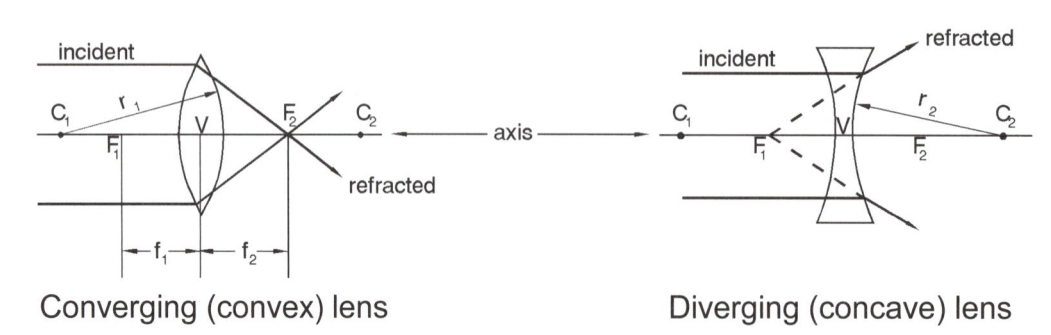

Figure III.B.11.3: Refraction by spherical lenses; *r* = the radius of curvature.

PHY-94 LIGHT AND GEOMETRICAL OPTICS

If the surface is convex, r is positive (e.g., r_1). If the surface is concave, r is negative (e.g., r_2).

Subscript 1 refers to the incident side, 2 refers to the refracted side.

C = center of curvature, F = focal point
V = the optical center of the lens or <u>v</u>ertex
axis = line through C and V

f = focal length is the distance between V and F
i = image distance (from V to the image)
o = object distance (from V to the object).

The path rays through a lens are:

1) incident rays parallel to the axis refract through F_2 of the converging lens, and appear to come from F_1 of a diverging lens (backward extensions of the refracted ray, see dotted line on diverging diagram);

2) an incident ray through F_1 of a converging lens or through F_2 of a diverging lens (if extended) are refracted parallel to the axis;

3) incident rays through V are deviated (refracted).

For a converging lens (e.g., convex) the image formed depends on the object distance relative to the focal length (f). The relations (note similarity with a converging mirror) are:

1)
if $o < f_1$, then image is virtual and erect;
if $o > f_1$, the image is real and inverted;
if $o = f_1$, then no image is formed;

2)
if $o < 2f_1$, then the image is enlarged is size;
if $o > 2f_1$, then the image is reduced in size;
if $o = 2f_1$, then the image is the same.
remember $2f_1 = r$.

For a diverging lens (e.g., concave), the image is always virtual, erect and reduced in size as for a diverging mirror.

The above relations can be calculated rather than memorized by use of the lens equation (similar to the mirror equation) and derivations from it,

1) $1/o + 1/i = 1/f$ (lens equation, same as mirror equation)

2) $D = 1/f = (n-1)(1/r_1 - 1/r_2)$, (lens maker's equation, n = index of refraction)

3) diopters (D) = 1/f where f is in meters, measures the refractive *power* of the lens; the larger the diopters, the stronger the lens. The diopters has a positive value for a converging lens and a negative value for a diverging lens.

To get the refractive power (D) of lenses in series just add the diopters which can then be converted into focal length:

$$D_T = D_1 + D_2 = 1/f_T \ (T = total).$$

4) Note that you can add only inverses of focal lengths:

$$1/f_T = 1/f_1 + 1/f_2 \ldots$$

5) M = Magnification = $-i/o = M_1 M_2$ for lenses in series.

Convention:
• for i and o, positive values mean real, negative values mean virtual;
• for r and f, positive values mean converging, negative values mean diverging;
• for M, a positive value means erect, negative is inverted.

The lens equation holds only for thin lenses (the thickness is small relative to other dimensions). For combination of lenses not in contact with each other, the image is found for the first lens (nearer the object) and then this image is used as the object of the second lens to find the image formed by it.

It should be noted that since concave lenses are concave on both sides they are sometimes called *biconcave*. Likewise, convex lenses may be called *biconvex*.

11.5.1 Lens Aberrations

In practice, the images formed by various refracting surfaces, as described in the previous section, fall short of theoretical perfection. Imperfections of image formation are due to several mechanisms or *aberrations*.

For example a nick or cut in a convex lens might create a microscopic area of concavity. Thus the light ray which strikes the aberration diverges instead of converging. Therefore the image will be less sharp or clear as the number or sizes of the aberrations increase.

PHYSICS

GOLD NOTES

ATOMIC AND NUCLEAR STRUCTURE
Chapter 12

Memorize
(Optional)
- quation relating energy and mass; half-life
- pha, beta, gamma particles
- quation for maximum number of electrons a shell
- quation relating energy to frequency
- quation for the total energy of the electrons an atom

Understand
* Basic atomic structure, amu
* Fission, fusion; the Bohr model of the atom
* Problem solving for half-life
* Quantized energy levels for electrons
* Fluorescence

Not Required*
* Advanced level college info
* Memorizing mass: neutrons/protons/electrons
* Memorizing constants, conversions

GAMSAT-Prep.com

Introduction

Atomic structure can be summarized as a nucleus orbited by electrons in different energy levels. Transition of electrons between energy levels and nuclear structure (i.e. protons, neutrons) are important characteristics of the atom. There is very little in this chapter that MUST be memorized for the GAMSAT. However, following our recommendations will give you an edge for many question types on this topic.

Additional Resources

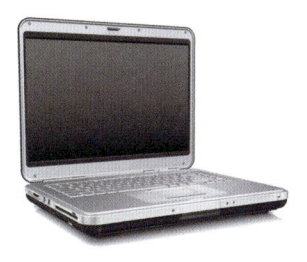

Free Online Q&A + Forum   Video: Online or DVD 1   Flashcards   Special Guest

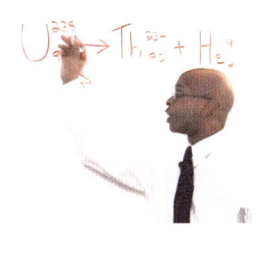

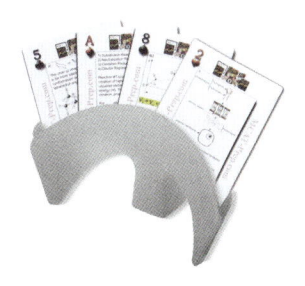

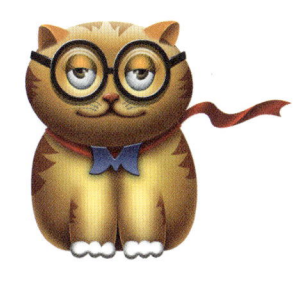

THE PHYSICAL SCIENCES

* The real GAMSAT may have advanced level information presented (ie. in a passage) but previous knowledge of said information is not required to answer the questions that would follow. Practice ACER and GS practice GAMSATs can help you clarify this point.

12.1 Protons, Neutrons, Electrons

Only recently, with high resolution electron microscopes, have large atoms been visualized. However, for years their existence and properties have been inferred by experiments. Experimental work on gas discharge effects suggested that an atom is not a single entity but is itself composed of smaller particles. These were termed elementary particles. The atom appears as a small solar system with a heavy nucleus composed of positive particles and neutral particles: *protons* and *neutrons*. Around this nucleus, there are clouds of negatively charged particles, called *electrons*. The mass of a neutron is slightly more than that of a proton (both ≈ 1.7×10^{-24} g); the mass of the electron is considerably less (9.1×10^{-28} g).

Since an atom is electrically neutral, the negative charge carried by the electrons must be equal in magnitude (but opposite in sign) to the positive charge carried by the protons.

Experiments with electrostatic charges have shown that opposite charges attract, so it can be considered that electrostatic forces hold an atom together. The difference between various atoms is therefore determined by their *composition*.

A hydrogen atom consists of one proton and one electron; a helium atom of two protons, two neutrons and two electrons. They are shown in diagram form in Figure III.B.12.1.

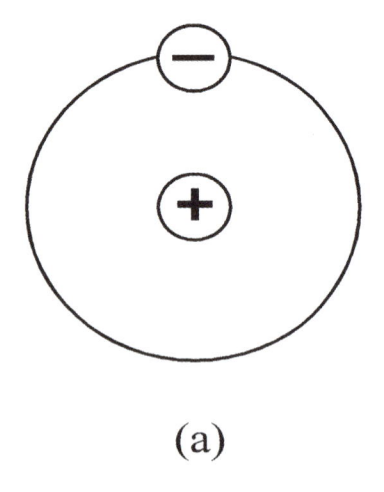

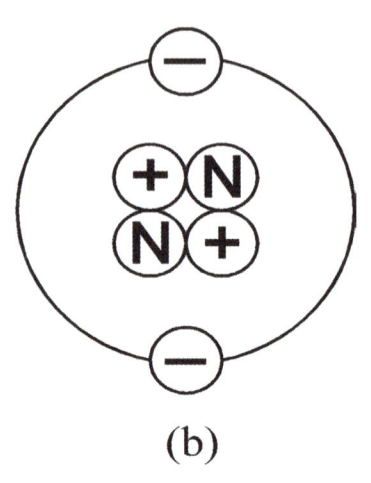

Figure III.B.12.1: Atomic structure simplified: (a) hydrogen atom; (b) helium atom.

12.2 Isotopes, Atomic Number, Atomic Weight

A proton has a mass of 1 a.m.u. (*atomic mass unit*) and a charge of +1, whereas, a neutron has a mass of 1 a.m.u. and no charge. The *atomic number* (*AN*) of an atom is the number of protons in the nucleus.

An *element* is a group of atoms with the same AN. *Isotopes* are elements which have the same AN (= protons) but different numbers of neutrons. It is the number of protons that distinguishes elements from each other.

The *mass number* (*MN*) of an atom is the number of protons and neutrons in an atom. The *atomic weight* (*AW*) is the weighted average of all naturally occurring isotopes of an element.

It is also important to note that as the number of protons distinguishes *elements* from each other, it is their electronic configuration (CHM 2.1, 2.2, 2.3) that determines their *reactivity*.

12.3 Nuclear Forces, Nuclear Binding Energy, Stability, Radioactivity

Coulomb repulsive force (between protons) in the nuclei are overcome by nuclear forces. The nuclear force is a non-electrical type of force that binds nuclei together and is equal for protons and neutrons. The nuclear binding energy (E_b) is a result of the relation between energy and mass changes associated with nuclear reactions,

$$\Delta E = \Delta mc^2$$

in ergs in the CGS system, i.e. m = grams and c = cm/sec; ΔE = energy released or absorbed; Δm = mass lost or gained, respectively; c = velocity of light = 3.0×10^{10} cm/sec.

Conversions:
1 *gram* = 9×10^{20} *ergs*
1 *a.m.u.* = 931.4 *MeV* (Mev = 10^6 electron volts)
1 *a.m.u.* = 1/12 the mass of $_6C^{12}$.

The preceding equation is a statement of the law of conservation of mass and energy. The value of E_b depends upon the mass number (MN) as follows, (*see Figure III.B.12.2*):

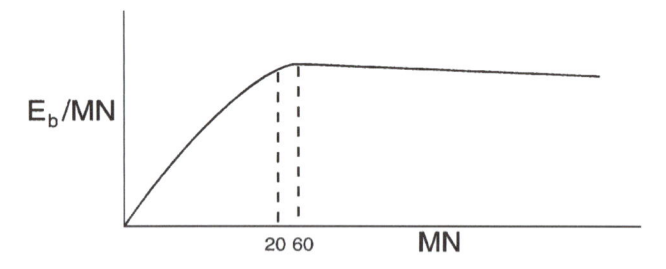

Figure III.B.12.2: Binding Energy per Nucleus. E_b/MN = binding energy per nucleus; this is the energy released by the formation of a nucleus.

Figure III.B.12.3: Stability of Atoms. AN = atomic number and N = number of neutrons.

The peak E_b/MN is at MN=60. Also, E_b/MN is relatively constant after MN=20. <u>Fission</u> is when a nucleus splits into smaller nuclei. <u>Fusion</u> is when smaller nuclei combine to form a larger nucleus. Energy is released from a nuclear reaction when nuclei with MN >> 60 undergo fission or nuclei with MN << 60 undergo fusion.

Not all combinations of protons are stable. The most stable nuclei are those with an even number of protons and an even number of neutrons. The least stable nuclei are those with an odd number of protons and an odd number of neutrons. Also, as the atomic number (AN) increases, there are more neutrons (N) needed for the nuclei to be stable.

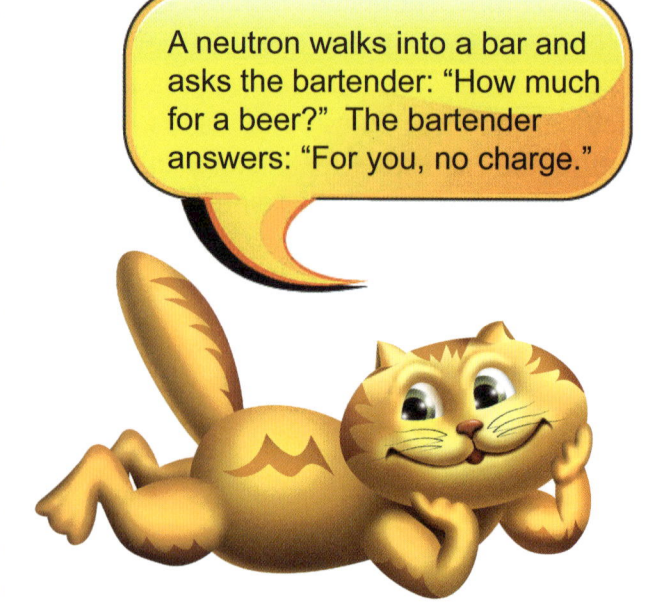

A neutron walks into a bar and asks the bartender: "How much for a beer?" The bartender answers: "For you, no charge."

Up to AN = 20 (Calcium) the number of protons is equal to the number of neutrons, after this there are more neutrons. If an atom is in region #1 in Figure III.B.12.3, it has too many protons or too few neutrons and must decrease its protons or increase its neutrons to become stable. The reverse is true for region #2. All nuclei after AN = 84 (Polonium) are unstable.

Unstable nuclei become stable by fission to smaller nuclei or by absorption or emission of small particles. Spontaneous fission is rare. Spontaneous radioactivity (emission of particles) is common. The common particles are:

1) alpha (α) particle = $_2He^4$ (helium nucleus);

2) beta (β) particle = $_{-1}e^0$ (an electron);

3) a positron $_{+1}e^0$ (same mass as an electron but opposite charge);

4) gamma (γ) ray = no mass and no charge, just electromagnetic energy;

5) orbital electron capture - nucleus takes electrons from K shell and converts a proton to a neutron. If there is a flux of particles such as neutrons ($_0n^1$), the nucleus can absorb these also.

12.4 Nuclear Reaction, Radioactive Decay, Half-Life

Nuclear reactions are reactions in which changes in nuclear composition occur. An example of a nuclear reaction which involves uranium and hydrogen:

$$_{92}U^{238} + _1H^2 \longrightarrow _{93}Np^{238} + 2\,_0n^1$$

for $_{92}U^{238}$: 238 = mass number, 92 = atomic number. The sum of the lower (or higher) numbers on one side of the equation equals the sum of the lower (or higher) numbers on the other side of the equation. Another way of writing the preceding reaction is: $_{92}U^{238}(_1H^2, 2\,_0n^1)_{93}Np^{238}$. {# neutrons (i.e. $_{92}U^{238}$) = superscript (238) - subscript (92) = 146}

Spontaneous radioactive decay is a first order process. This means that the rate of decay is *directly* proportional to the amount of material present:

$$\Delta m/\Delta t = \text{rate of decay}$$

where Δm = change in mass, Δt = change in time.

The preceding relation is equalized by adding a proportionality constant called the decay constant (k) as follows,

$$\Delta m/\Delta t = -km.$$

The minus sign indicates that the mass is decreasing. Also, $k = -(\Delta m/m)/\Delta t$ = fraction of the mass that decays with time.

The *half-life* ($T_{1/2}$) of a radioactive atom is the time required for one half of it to disintegrate. The half-life is related to k as follows,

$$T_{1/2} = 0.693/k.$$

If the number of half-lifes n are known we can calculate the percentage of a pure radioactive sample left after undergoing decay since the fraction remaining $= (1/2)^n$.

For example, given a pure radioactive substance X with $T_{1/2}$ = 9 years, calculating the percentage of substance X after 27 years is quite simple,

$$27 = 3 \times 9 = 3\, T_{1/2}$$

Thus

$$n = 3, (1/2)^n = (1/2)^3 = 1/8 \text{ or } 13\%.$$

After 27 years of disintegration, 13% of pure substance X remains. {Similarly, note that *doubling time* is given by $(2)^n$; see BIO 2.2}

12.5 Quantized Energy Levels For Electrons, Emission Spectrum

Work by Bohr and others in the early part of the present century demonstrated that the electron orbits are arranged in shells, and that each shell has a defined maximum number of electrons it can contain.

For example, the first shell can contain two electrons, the second eight electrons (*see* CHM 2.1, 2.2). The maximum number of electrons in each shell is given by:

$$N_{electrons} = 2n^2$$

$N_{electrons}$ designates the number of electrons in shell n.

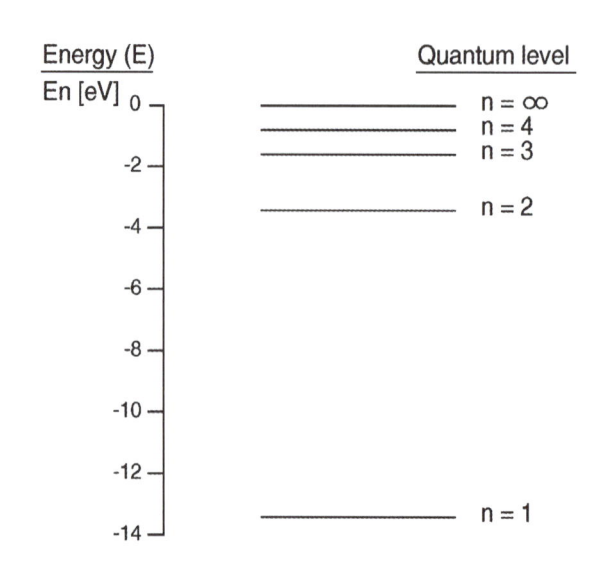

Figure III.B.12.4: Energy levels. The energy E_n in each shell n is measured in electron volts.

The state of each electron is determined by the four quantum numbers:

- *principal quantum number n* determines the number of shells, possible values are: 1 (K), 2 (L), 3 (M), etc...
- *angular momentum quantum number l*, determines the subshell, possible values are: 0 (s), 1 (p), 2 (d), 3 (f), n-1, etc...
- *magnetic momentum quantum number m_l*, possible values are: $\pm l, ... , 0$
- *spin quantum number m_s*, determines the direction of rotation of the electron, possible values are: $\pm 1/2$.

Chemical reactions and electrical effects are all concerned with the behavior of electrons in the outer shell of any particular atom. If a shell is full, for example, the atom is unlikely to react with any other atom and is, in fact, one of the noble (inert) gases such as helium.

The energy that an electron contains is not continuous over the entire range of possible energy. Rather, electrons in a atom may contain only discrete energies as they occupy certain orbits or shells. Electrons of each atom are restricted to these discrete energy levels. These levels have an energy below zero.

This means energy is released when an electron moves from infinity into these energy levels.

If there is one electron in an atom, its ground state is n = 1, the lowest energy level available. Any other energy level, n = 2, n = 3, etc., is considered an excited state for that electron. The difference in energy (E) between the levels gives the absorbed (or emitted) energy when an electron moves to a higher orbit (or lower orbit, respectively) and therefore, the frequency (f) of light necessary to cause excitation.

$$E_2 - E_1 = hf$$

where E_1 = energy level one, E_2 = energy level two, h = planck's constant, and f = the frequency of light absorbed or emitted.

Therefore, if light is passed through a substance (e.g., gas), certain wavelengths will be absorbed, which correspond to the energy needed for the electron transition. An *absorption* spectrum will result that has <u>dark lines</u> against a <u>light background</u>. Multiple lines result because there are possible transitions from all quantum levels occupied by electrons to any unoccupied levels.

An *emission* spectrum results when an electron is excited to a higher level by another particle or by an electric discharge, for example. Then, as the electron falls from the excited state to lower states, light is emitted that has a wavelength (which is related to frequency) corresponding to the energy difference between the levels since: $E_1 - E_2 = hf$.

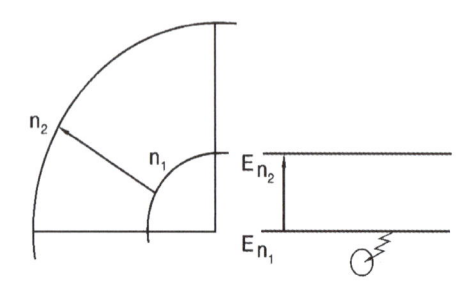

Step 1: light absorption

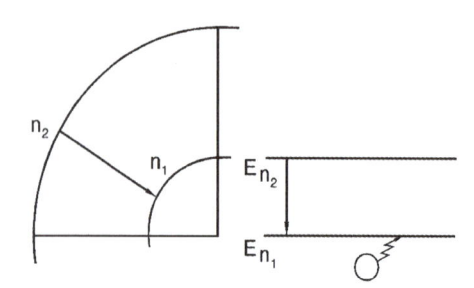

Step 3: light emission

Figure III.B.12.5: The fluorescence process. Represented is an atom with shells n_1, n_2 and their respective energy levels E_n.

The resulting spectrum will have <u>light lines</u> against a <u>dark background</u>. The absorption and emission spectrums should have the same number of lines but often will not. This is because in the absorption spectrum, there is a rapid radiation of the absorbed light in all directions, and transitions are generally from the ground state initially.

These factors result in fewer lines in the absorption than in the emission spectrum.

The total energy of the electrons in an atom can be given by:

$$E_{total} = E_{emission} \text{ (or } E_{ionization}) + KE$$

12.6 Fluorescence

Fluorescence is an <u>emission process</u> that occurs after light absorption excites electrons to higher electronic and vibrational levels. The electrons spontaneously lose excited vibrational energy to the electronic states. There are certain molecular types that possess this property, e.g., some amino acids (tryptophan).

The fluorescence process is as follows:
• step 1 - absorption of light;
• step 2 - spontaneous deactivation of vibrational levels to zero vibrational level for electronic state;
• step 3 - fluorescence with light emission (longer wavelength than absorption).

Figure III.B.12.5 shows diagrammatically the steps described above. Step 2 which is not shown in the figure is the intermediate step between light absorption and light emission.

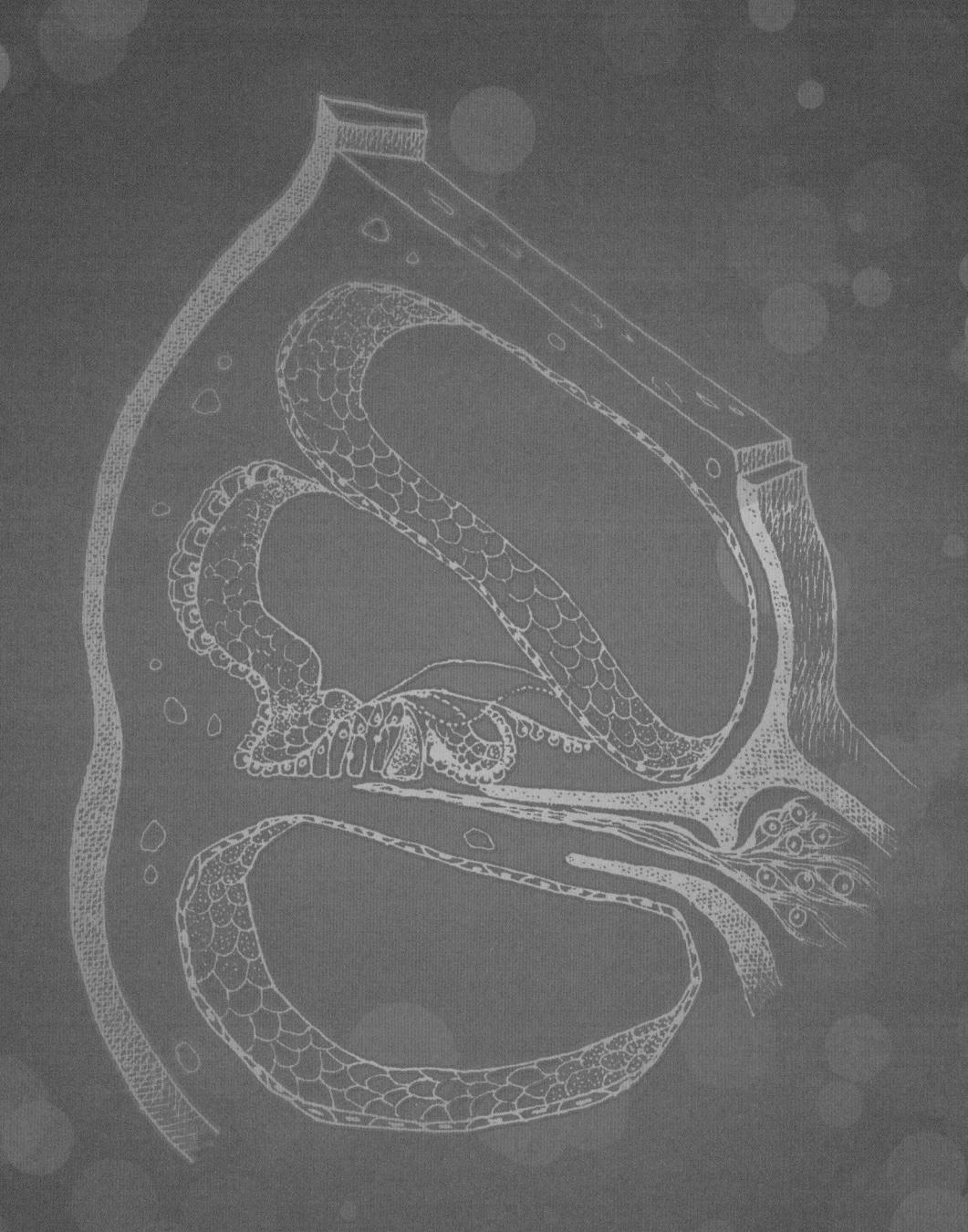

GAMSAT-Prep.com
BIOLOGY
PART IV.A: BIOLOGICAL SCIENCES

IMPORTANT: Before doing your science survey for the GAMSAT, be sure you have read the Preface, Introduction and Part II, Chapter 2. The beginning of each science chapter provides guidelines as to what you should Memorize, Understand and what is Not Required. These are guides to get you a top score without getting lost in the details. Our guides have been determined from an analysis of all ACER materials plus student surveys. Additionally, the original owner of this book gets a full year access to many online features described in the Preface and Introduction including an online Forum where each chapter can be discussed.

GENERALIZED EUKARYOTIC CELL
Chapter 1

Memorize	Understand	Not Required*
Structure/function: cell/components Components and function: cytoskeleton DNA structure and function Transmission of genetic information Mitosis, events of the cell cycle	* Intro level college info * Membrane transport * Hyper/hypotonic solutions * Saturation kinetics: graphs * Unique features of eukaryotes	* Advanced level college info * Molecular bio., detailed mechanisms * Plant cells, chloroplasts * Experiments in genetics * Specify polymerases or such details

GAMSAT-Prep.com

Introduction

Cells are the basic organizational unit of living organisms. They are contained by a plasma membrane and/or cell wall. Eukaryotic cells (*eu* = true; *karyote* refers to nucleus) are cells with a true nucleus found in all multicellular and nonbacterial unicellular organisms including animal, fungal and plant cells. The nucleus contains genetic information, DNA, which can divide into 2 cells by mitosis.

Additional Resources

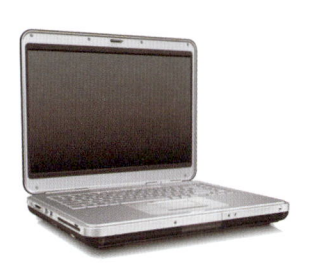

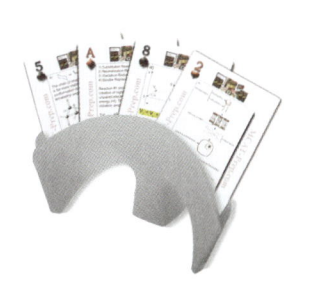

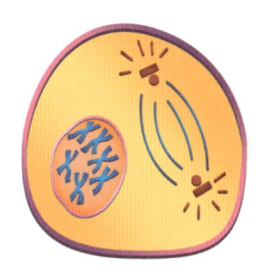

Free Online Q&A + Forum   Video: Online or DVD 3   Flashcards   Special Guest

THE BIOLOGICAL SCIENCES   BIO-03

* The real GAMSAT may have advanced level information presented (ie. in a passage) but previous knowledge of said information is not required to answer the questions that would follow. Practice ACER and GS practice GAMSATs can help you clarify this point.

GAMSAT-Prep.com
THE GOLD STANDARD

1.1 Plasma Membrane: Structure and Functions

The plasma membrane is a semipermeable barrier that defines the outer perimeter of the cell. It is composed of lipids (fats) and protein. The membrane is dynamic, selective, active, and fluid. It contains phospholipids which are amphipathic molecules. They are amphipathic because their tail end contains fatty acids which are insoluble in water (hydrophobic), the opposite end contains a charged phosphate head which is soluble in water (hydrophilic). The plasma membrane contains two layers of phospholipids thus it is called a bilipid layer.

The Fluid Mosaic Model tells us that the hydrophilic heads project to the outside and the hydrophobic tails project towards the inside of the membrane. Further, these phospholipids are fluid - thus they move freely from place to place in the membrane. Distributed throughout the membrane is a mosaic of proteins with limited mobility.

Proteins can be found associated with the outside of the membrane (extrinsic or peripheral) or may be found spanning the membrane (intrinsic or integral). Many intrinsic proteins represent channels through which specific molecules and ions can pass, or, receptors which hormones may activate.

The plasma membrane is semipermeable. In other words, it is permeable to small uncharged substances which can freely

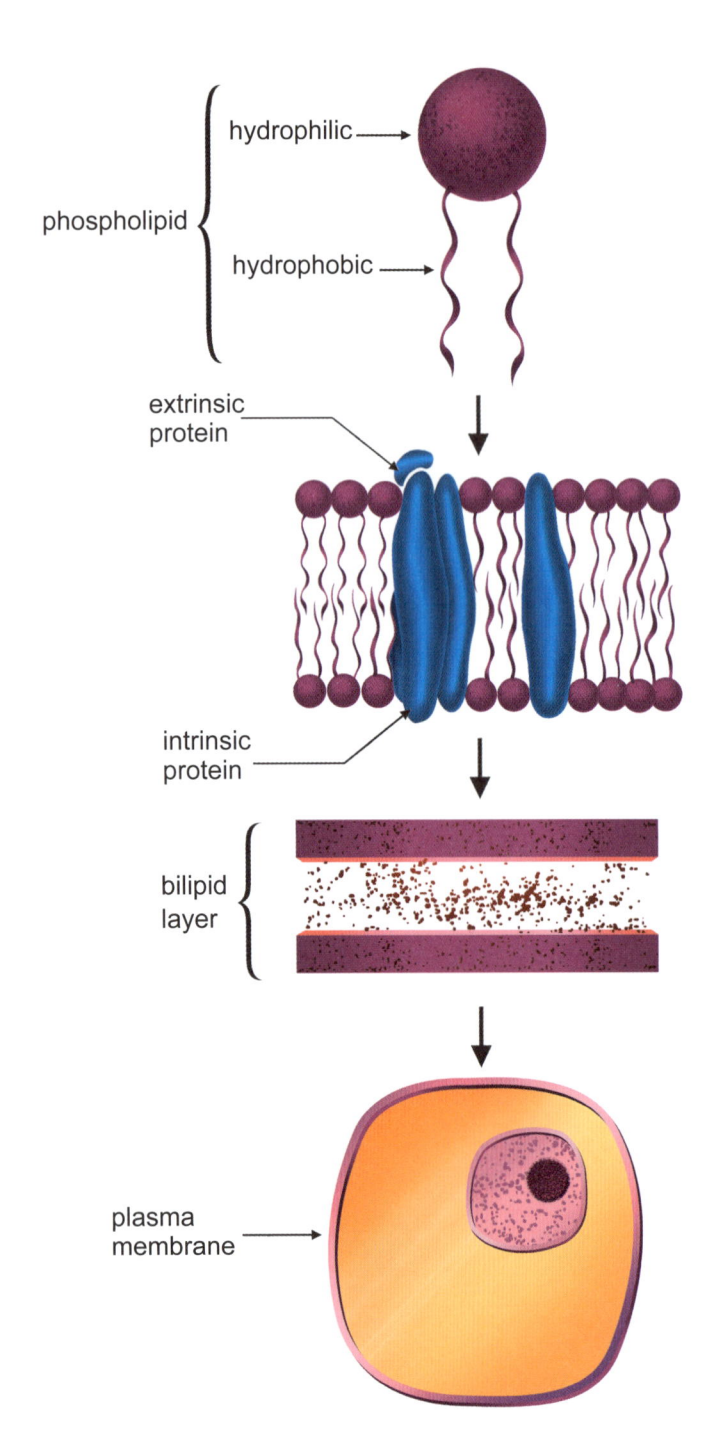

Figure IV.A.1.1: Structure of the plasma membrane.

BIO-04 GENERALIZED EUKARYOTIC CELL

diffuse across the membrane (i.e. O$_2$, CO$_2$, urea). On the other hand, it is relatively impermeable to charged or large substances which may require transport proteins to cross the membrane (i.e. ions, amino acids, sugars) or cannot cross the membrane at all (i.e. protein hormones, intracellular enzymes). Substances which can cross the membrane may do so by simple diffusion, carrier-mediated transport, or by endo/exocytosis.

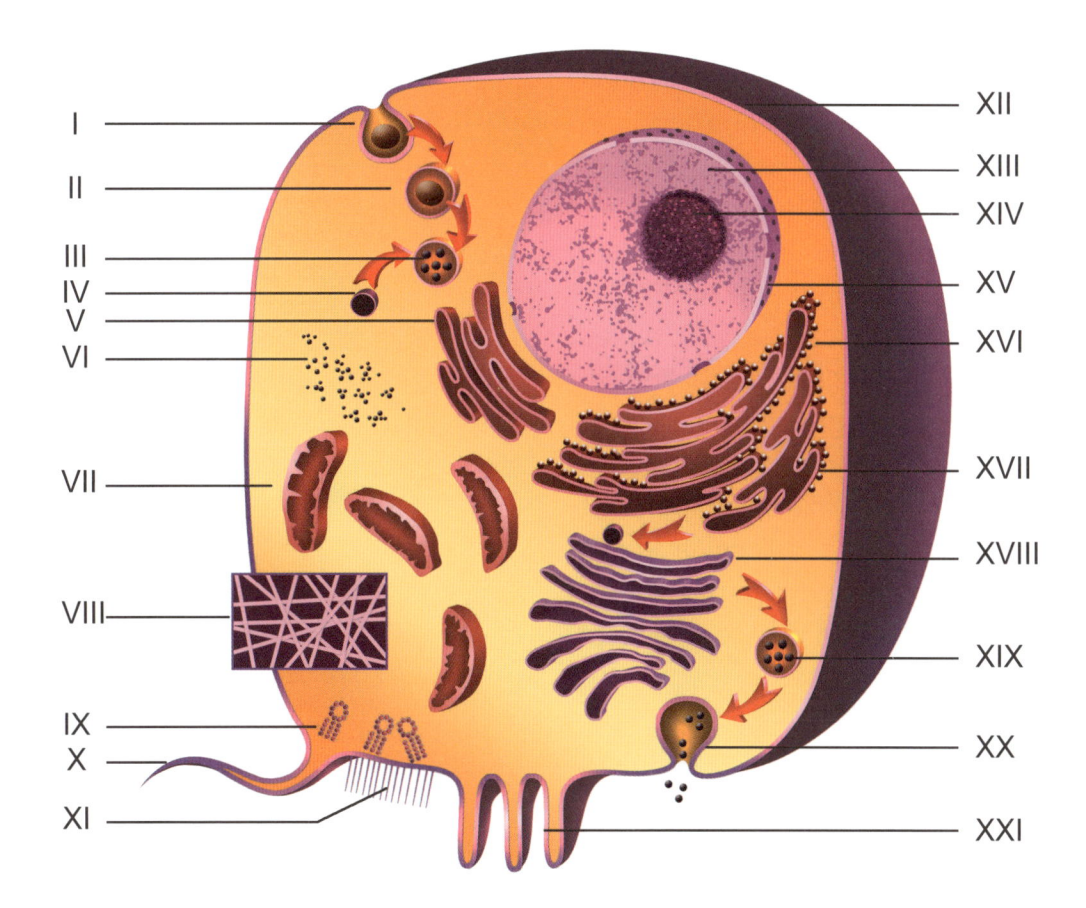

Figure IV.A.1.2: The generalized eukaryotic cell.

I	endocytosis	VIII	cytoskeleton (further magnified)	XV	nuclear envelope
II	endocytotic vesicle	IX	basal body (magnified)	XVI	cytosol
III	secondary lysosome	X	flagellum	XVII	rough endoplasmic reticulum
IV	primary lysosome	XI	cilia	XVIII	Golgi apparatus
V	smooth endoplasmic reticulum	XII	plasma membrane	XIX	exocytotic vesicle
VI	free ribosomes	XIII	nucleus	XX	exocytosis
VII	mitochondrion	XIV	nucleolus	XXI	microvillus

1.1.1 Simple Diffusion

Simple diffusion is the spontaneous spreading of a substance going from an area of higher concentration to an area of lower concentration (i.e. a concentration gradient exists). Gradients can be of a chemical or electrical nature. A chemical gradient arises as a result of an unequal distribution of molecules, and is often called a concentration gradient. In a chemical (or concentration) gradient, there is a higher concentration of molecules in one area than there is in another area, and molecules tend to diffuse from areas of high concentration to areas of lower concentration. An electrical gradient arises as a result of an unequal distribution of charge. In an electrical gradient, there is a higher concentration of charged molecules in one area than in another (this is independent of the concentration of all molecules in the area). Molecules tend to move from areas of higher concentration of charge to areas of lower concentration of charge.

Osmosis is the diffusion of water across a semipermeable membrane moving from an area of higher water concentration (i.e. lower solute concentration = hypotonic) to an area of lower water concentration (i.e. higher solute concentration = hypertonic). The hydrostatic pressure needed to oppose the movement of water is called the osmotic pressure. Thus, an isotonic solution (i.e. the concentration of solute on both sides of the membrane is equal), would have an osmotic pressure of zero.

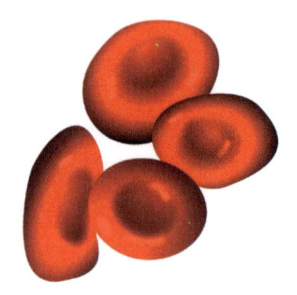

Figure IV.A.1.2.1a: Isotonic Solution.

The fluid bathing the cell (i.e. red blood cell or RBC in this case; see BIO 7.5) contains the same concentration of solute as the cell's inside or cytoplasm. When a cell is placed in an isotonic solution, the water diffuses into and out of the cell at the same rate.

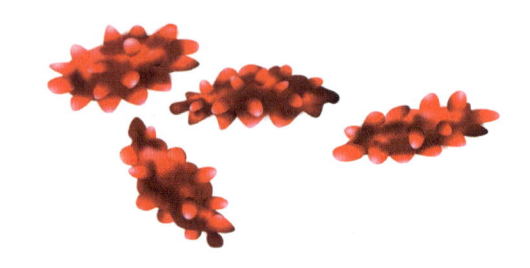

Figure IV.A.1.2.1b: Hypertonic Solution.

Here the fluid bathing the RBC contains a high concentration of solute relative to the cell's cytoplasm. When a cell is placed in a hypertonic solution, the water diffuses out of the cell, causing the cell to shrivel.

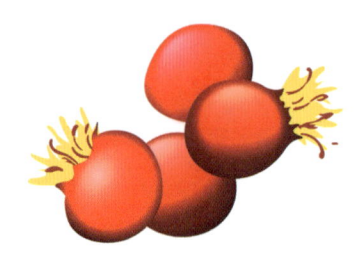

Figure IV.A.1.2.1c: Hypotonic Solution.

Here the surrounding fluid has a low concentration of solute relative to the cell's cytoplasm. When a cell is placed in a hypotonic solution, the water diffuses into the cell, causing the cell to swell and possibly explode.

{Memory guide: notice that the "O" in hyp-O-tonic looks like a swollen cell. The O is also a circle which makes you think of the word "around." So IF the environment is hypOtonic AROUND the cell, then fluid rushes in and the cell swells like the letter O}.

1.1.2 Carrier-Mediated Transport

Amino acids, sugars and other solutes need to reversibly bind to proteins (carriers) in the membrane in order to get across. Because there are a limited amount of carriers, if the concentration of solute is too high, the carriers would be saturated thus the rate of crossing the membrane would level off (= saturation kinetics).

The two carrier-mediated transport systems are:
i) facilitated transport where the carrier helps a solute diffuse across a membrane it could not otherwise penetrate, and ii) active transport where energy (i.e. ATP) is used to transport solutes against their concentration gradients. The Na^+- K^+ exchange pump uses ATP to actively pump Na^+ to where its concentration is highest (outside the cell) and K^+ is brought within the cell where its concentration is highest (see Neural Cells and Tissues, BIO 5.1.1).

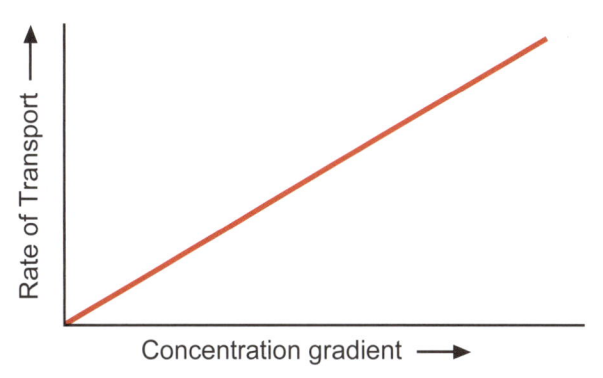

Simple Diffusion: the greater the concentration gradient, the greater the rate of transport across the plasma membrane.

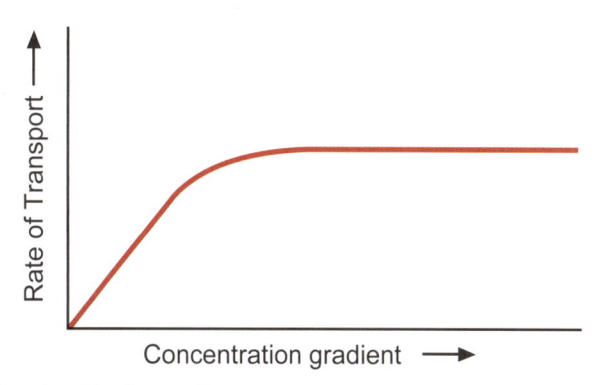

Carrier-Mediated Transport: increasing the concentration gradient increases the rate of transport until a maximum rate at which point all membrane carriers are saturated.

Figure IV.A.1.3: Simple diffusion versus carrier-mediated transport.

1.1.3 Endo/Exocytosis

Endocytosis is the process by which the cell membrane actually invaginates, pinches off and is released intracellularly (endocytotic vesicle). If a solid particle was ingested by the cell (i.e. a bacterium), it is called phagocytosis. If fluid was ingested, it is pinocytosis.

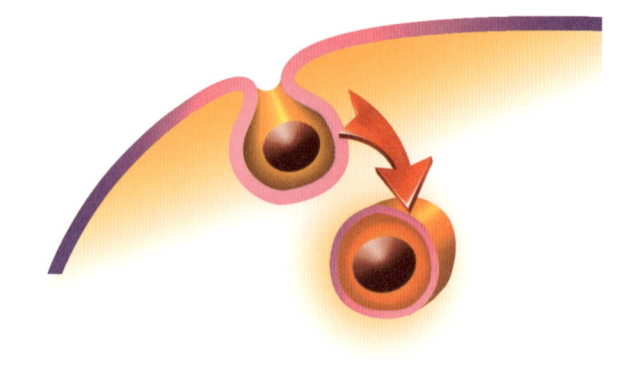

Figure IV.A.1.4: Endocytosis.

Exocytosis is, essentially, the reverse process. The cell directs an intracellular vesicle to fuse with the plasma membrane thus releasing its contents to the exterior (i.e. neurotransmitters, pancreatic enzymes, cell membrane proteins/lipids, etc.).

Figure IV.A.1.5: Exocytosis.

1.2 The Interior of a Eukaryotic Cell

Cytoplasm is the interior of the cell. It refers to all cell components enclosed by the cell's membrane which includes the cytosol, the cytoskeleton and the membrane bound organelles.

Cytosol is the solution which bathes the organelles and contains numerous solutes like amino acids, sugars, proteins, etc.

Cytoskeleton extends throughout the entire cell and has particular importance in shape and intracellular transportation. The cytoskeleton also makes extracellular complexes with other proteins forming a matrix so that cells can "stick" together. This is called cellular adhesion.

The components of the cytoskeleton in increasing order of size: microfilaments, intermediate filaments, and microtubules. Microfilaments are important for cell movement and contraction (i.e. actin and myosin, see Contractile Cells and Tissues, BIO 5.2).

Intermediate filaments and microtubules extend along axons and dendrites of neurons acting like railroad tracks so organelles or protein particles can shuttle to or from the cell body. Microtubules also form (i) the core of cilia and flagella; (ii) the mitotic spindles which we shall soon discuss; and (iii) centrioles.

A flagellum is a whiplike organelle of locomotion found in sperm and bacteria. Cilia are hair-like vibrating organelles which can be used to move particles along the surface of the cell (i.e. in the fallopian tubes cilia can help the egg move toward the uterus). Centrioles are cylinder-shaped complexes of microtubules associated with the mitotic spindle (MTOC, see later). At the base of flagella and cilia, two centrioles can be found at right angles to each other: this is called a basal body.

Microvilli are regularly arranged finger-like projections with a core of cytoplasm (*see* BIO 9.5). They are commonly found in the small intestine where they help to increase the absorptive and digestive surfaces (= brush border).

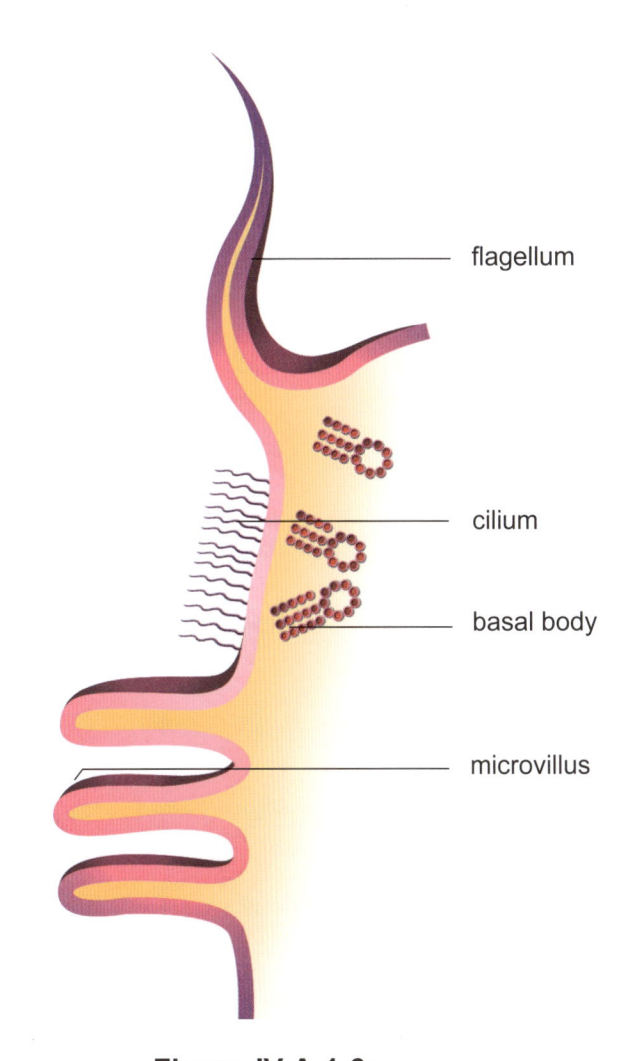

Figure IV.A.1.6:
Cytoskeletal elements and the plasma membrane.

1.2.1 Membrane Bound Organelles

Mitochondrion: The Power House

Mitochondria produce energy (i.e. ATP) for the cell through aerobic respiration. It is a double membraned organelle whose inner membrane has shelf-like folds and are called cristae. The matrix, the fluid within the inner membrane, contains the enzymes for the Krebs cycle (BIO 4.7) and circular DNA. The latter is the only cellular DNA found outside of the nucleus. There are numerous mitochondria in muscle cells.

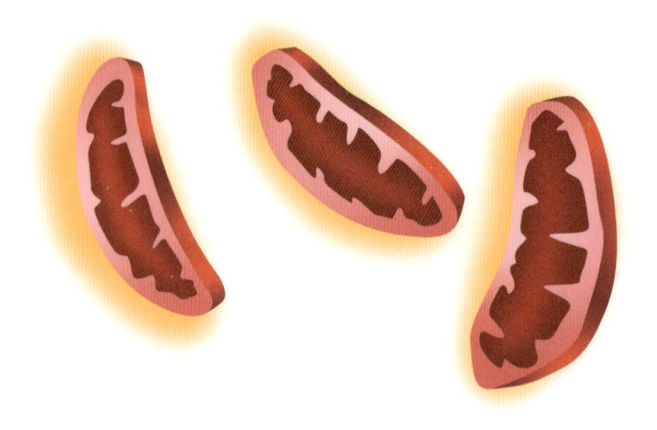

Figure IV.A.1.7: Mitochondria.

Lysosomes: Suicide Sacs

In a diseased cell, lysosomes may release their powerful acid hydrolases to digest away the cell (autolysis). In normal cells, a primary (normal) lysosome can fuse with an endocytotic vesicle to form a secondary lysosome where the phagocytosed particle (i.e. a bacterium) can be digested. This is called heterolysis. There are numerous lysosomes in phagocytic cells of the immune system (i.e. macrophages, neutrophils).

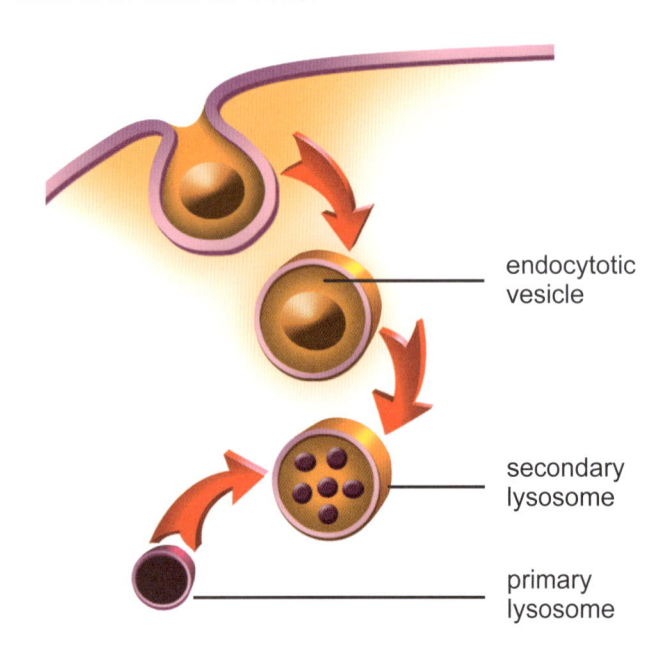

Figure IV.A.1.8: Heterolysis.

BIO-10   GENERALIZED EUKARYOTIC CELL

Endoplasmic Reticulum: Synthesis Center

The endoplasmic reticulum (ER) is an interconnected membraned system resembling flattened sacs. There are two kinds: (i) dotted with ribosomes on its surface which is called rough ER and (ii) without ribosomes which is smooth ER.

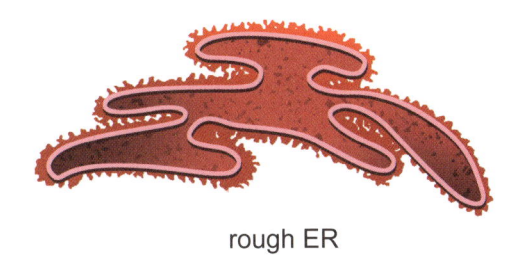

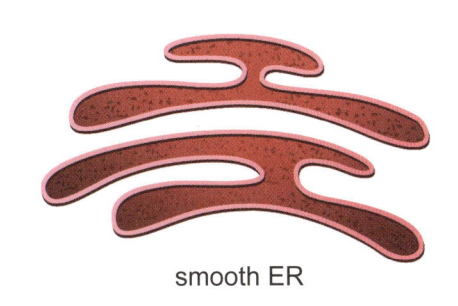

rough ER

smooth ER

Figure IV.A.1.9: The endoplasmic reticulum.

Rough ER is important in protein synthesis whereas smooth ER is a factor in phospholipid and fatty acid synthesis and metabolism. Smooth ER is also important in the liver to help detoxify many chemicals (i.e. carcinogens, pesticides).

Golgi Apparatus: The Export Department

The Golgi apparatus forms a stack of smooth membranous sacs or *cisternae* that function in protein modification like the addition of polysaccharides (i.e. glycosylation). The Golgi also packages secretory proteins in membrane bound vesicles which can be exocytosed.

An abundant amount of rER and Golgi is found in cells which produce and secrete protein. For example, *B-cells* of the immune system which secrete antibodies, *acinar cells* in the pancreas which secrete digestive enzymes into the intestines, and *goblet cells* of the intestine, which secrete mucus into the lumen.

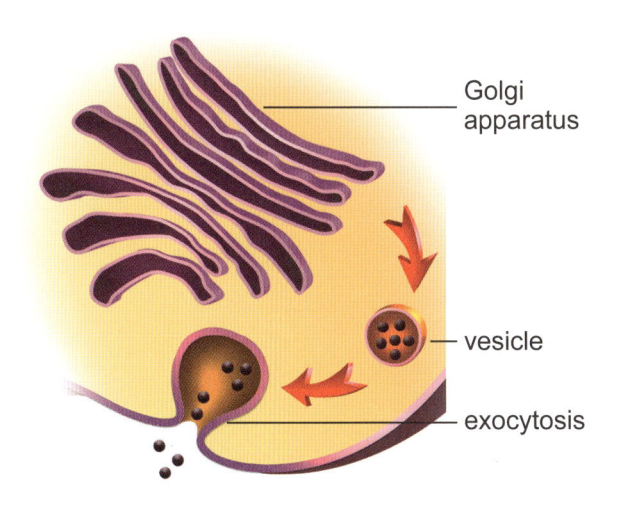

Figure IV.A.1.10: Golgi apparatus.

The Nucleus

The nucleus is surrounded by a double membrane called the nuclear envelope. Throughout the membrane are nuclear pores which selectively allow the transportation of large particles to and from the nucleus.

DNA can be found within the nucleus as chromatin (DNA complexed to proteins like *histones*) or as chromosomes which are more clearly visible in a light microscope. The nucleolus is not membrane bound. It contains the DNA necessary to synthesize ribosomal RNA.

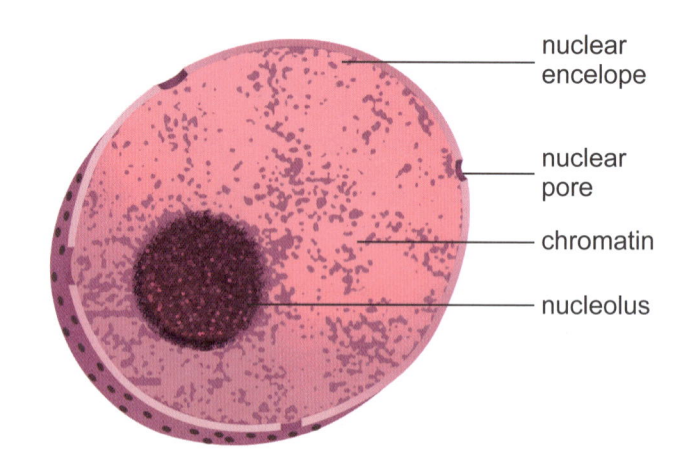

Figure IV.A.1.11: The nucleus.

1.2.2 DNA: The Cell's Architect

Deoxyribonucleic Acid (DNA) and ribonucleic acid (RNA) are essential components in constructing the proteins which act as the cytoskeleton, enzymes, membrane channels, antibodies, etc. It is the DNA which contains the genetic information of the cell.

DNA and RNA are both important nucleic acids. Nucleotides are the subunits which attach in sequence or in other words polymerize via phosphodiester bonds to form nucleic acids. A nucleotide (also called a *nucleoside phosphate*) is composed of a five carbon sugar, a nitrogen base, and an inorganic phosphate.

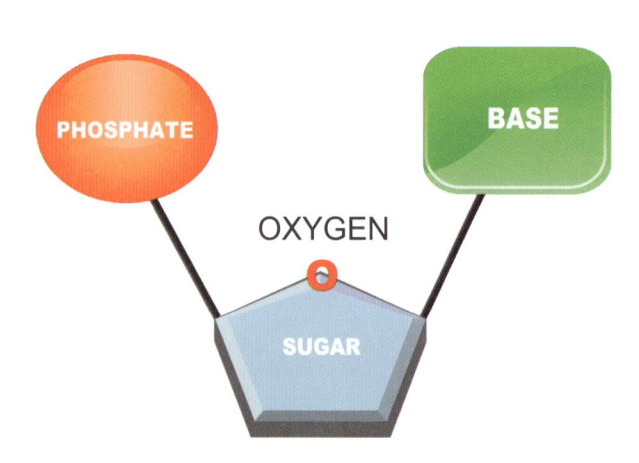

Figure IV.A.1.12: Nucleotide.

BIO-12   GENERALIZED EUKARYOTIC CELL

The sugar in RNA is ribose but for DNA an oxygen atom is missing in the second position thus it is 2-deoxyribose.

There are two categories of nitrogen bases: *purines* and *pyrimidines*. The purines have two rings and include adenine (A) and guanine (G). The pyrimidines contain one ring and include thymine (T), cytosine (C), and uracil (U).

DNA contains the following four bases: adenine, guanine, thymine, and cytosine. RNA contains the same bases except uracil is substituted for thymine.

Watson and Crick's model of DNA has allowed us to get insight into what takes shape as the nucleotides polymerize to form this special nucleic acid. The result is a double *helical* or *stranded* structure.

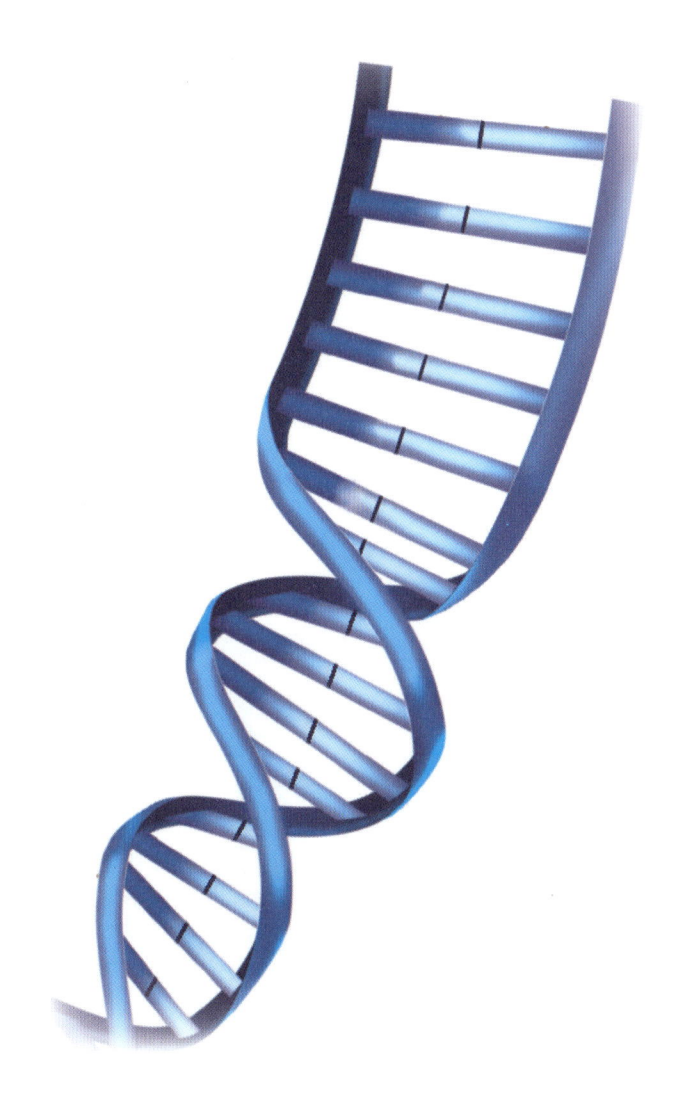

GAMSAT-Prep.com
THE GOLD STANDARD

The backbone of each helix is the 2-deoxyribose phosphates. The nitrogen bases project to the center of the double helix in order to hydrogen bond with each other (imagine the double helix as a winding staircase: each stair would represent a pair of bases binding to keep the shape of the double helix intact).

There is specificity in the binding of the bases: one purine binds one pyrimidine. In fact, adenine only binds thymine (through two hydrogen bonds) and guanine only binds cytosine (through three hydrogen bonds). The more the H-bonds (i.e. the more G-C), the more stable the helix will be.

The *replication* (duplication) of DNA is semi-conservative: thus each strand of the double helix can serve as a template to generate a complementary strand. Thus for each double helix there is one parent strand (*old*) and one daughter strand (*new*). The latter is synthesized using one nucleotide at a time, enzymes including DNA polymerase, and the parent strand as a template. The

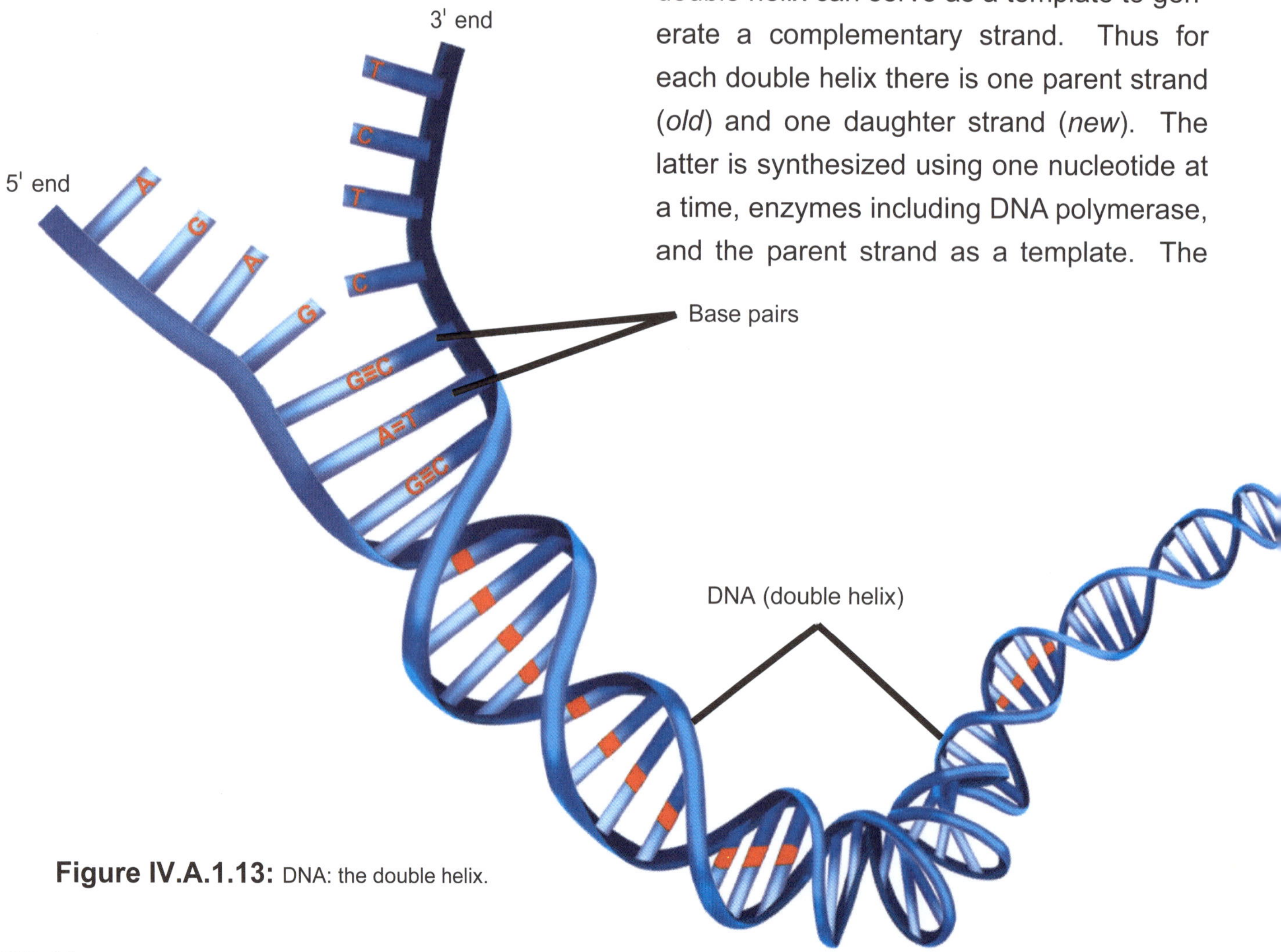

Figure IV.A.1.13: DNA: the double helix.

BIO-14   GENERALIZED EUKARYOTIC CELL

BIOLOGY

preceding is termed "DNA Synthesis" and occurs in the S stage of interphase during the cell cycle.

Each nucleotide has a hydroxyl or phosphate group at the 3rd and 5th carbons designated the 3' and 5' positions (see Organic Chemistry 12.3.2 and 12.5). Phosphodiester bonds can be formed between a free 3' hydroxyl group and a free 5' phosphate group. Thus the DNA strand has *polarity* since one end of the molecule will have a free 3' hydroxyl while the other terminal nucleotide will have a free 5' phosphate group. Polymerization of the two strands occurs in opposite directions (= *antiparallel*). In other words, one strand runs in the 5' - 3' direction, while its partner runs in the 3' - 5' direction.

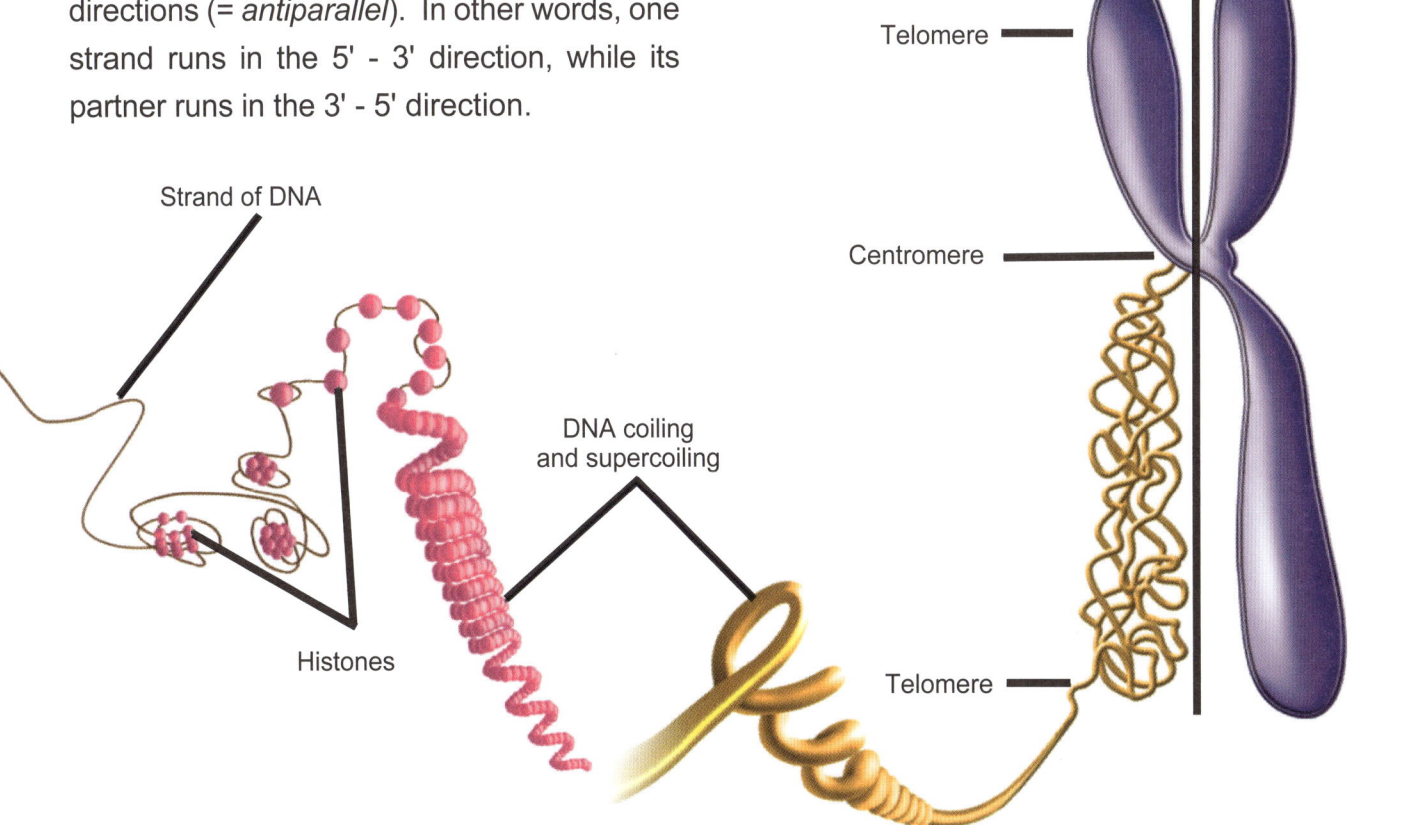

Nucleus

Cell

Chromosome

chromatid   chromatid

Telomere

Centromere

Strand of DNA

DNA coiling and supercoiling

Histones

Telomere

THE BIOLOGICAL SCIENCES   BIO-15

DNA replication is semi-discontinuous. DNA polymerase can only synthesize DNA in the 5' to 3' direction. As a result of the antiparallel nature of DNA, the 5' - 3' strand is replicated continuously (the *leading strand*), while the 3' - 5' strand is replicated discontinuously (the *lagging strand*) in the reverse direction. In this manner, DNA polymerase synthesizes only from 5' - 3'.

Previous knowledge of recombinant DNA techniques, restriction enzymes, hybridization, DNA repair mechanisms, etc., is not normally required for the GAMSAT. If you wish to get a "primer" in these areas, for background information, visit the Forum at www.GAMSAT-prep.com. The following is an overview regarding DNA repair.

Because of environmental factors including chemicals and UV radiation, any one of the trillions of cells in our bodies may undergo as many as 1 million individual molecular "injuries" per day. Structural damage to DNA may result and could have many effects including inducing mutation. Thus our DNA repair system is constantly active as it responds to damage in DNA structure.

A cell that has accumulated a large amount of DNA damage, or one that no longer effectively repairs damage to its DNA, can: (1) become permanently dormant; (2) exhibit unregulated cell division which could lead to cancer; (3) succumb to cell suicide, also known as *apoptosis* or programmed cell death.

1.3 The Cell Cycle

The cell cycle is a period of approximately 18 - 22 hours during which the cell can synthesize new DNA, partition the DNA equally, thus the cell can divide. These events are divided into a number of phases: interphase (G_1, S, G_2) and mitosis (prophase, metaphase, anaphase and telophase).

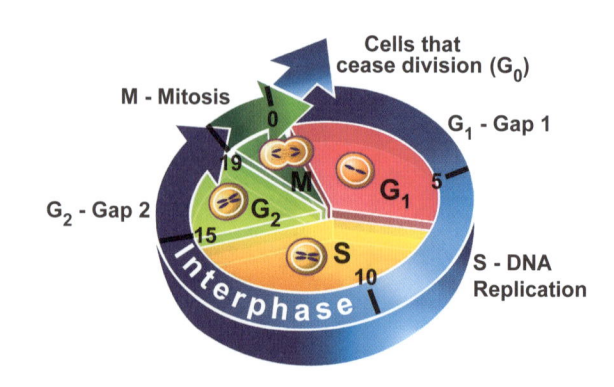

Figure IV.A.1.14: The cell cycle. The numbers represent time in hours. Note how mitosis (M) represents the shortest period of the cycle.

BIOLOGY

Interphase occupies about 90% of the cell cycle. During interphase, the cell prepares for DNA synthesis (G_1), synthesizes or replicates DNA (S), and ultimately begins preparing for mitosis (G_2). Mitosis begins with prophase.

<u>Prophase</u>: pairs of centrioles migrate away from each other while microtubules appear in between forming a spindle. Other microtubules emanating from the centrioles give a radiating star-like appearance; thus they are called *asters*. Therefore, centrioles form the core of the Microtubule Organizing Centers (MTOC).

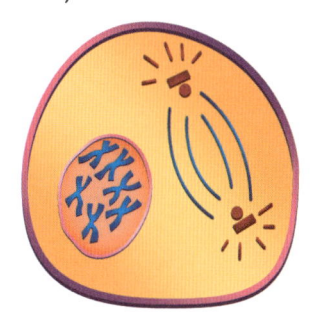

Figure IV.A.1.15: Prophase.

Simultaneously, the diffuse nuclear chromatin condenses into the visible chromosomes which consist of two identical sister chromatids. The area of constriction where the two chromatids are attached is the *centromere*. Just as centromere refers to the center, *telomere* refers to the ends of the chromosome. Ultimately, the nuclear envelope disappears at the end of prophase.

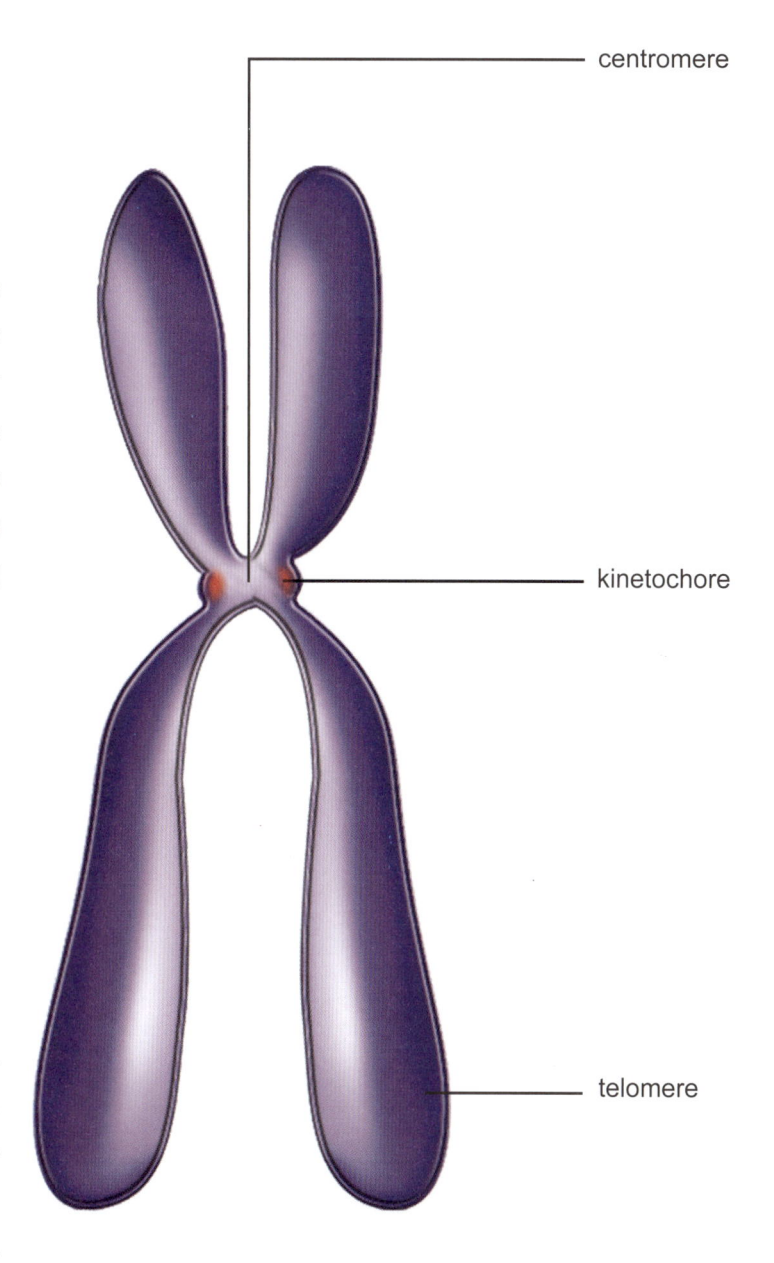

Figure IV.A.1.16: Chromosome.

THE BIOLOGICAL SCIENCES   BIO-17

Metaphase: centromeres line up along the equatorial plate. At or near the centromeres are the *kinetochores* which are proteins that face the spindle poles (asters). Microtubules, from the spindle, attach to the kinetochores of each chromosome.

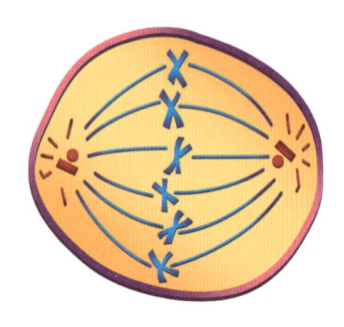

Figure IV.A.1.17: Metaphase.

Anaphase: sister chromatids are pulled apart such that each migrates to opposite poles being guided by spindle microtubules.

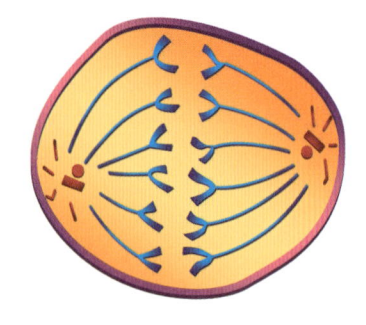

Figure IV.A.1.18: Anaphase.

Telophase: new membranes form around the daughter nuclei; nucleoli reappear; the chromosomes uncoil and become less distinct (decondense); and finally, *cytokinesis* (cell separation) occurs.

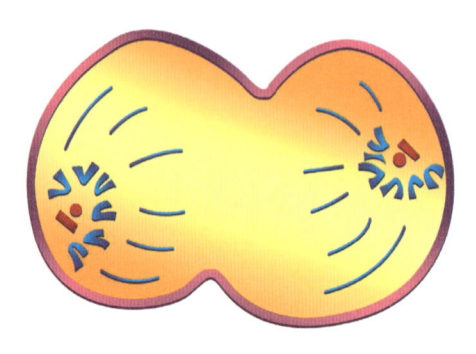

Figure IV.A.1.19: Telophase.

The cell cycle continues with the next interphase. {Mnemonic for the sequence of phases: P. MATI}

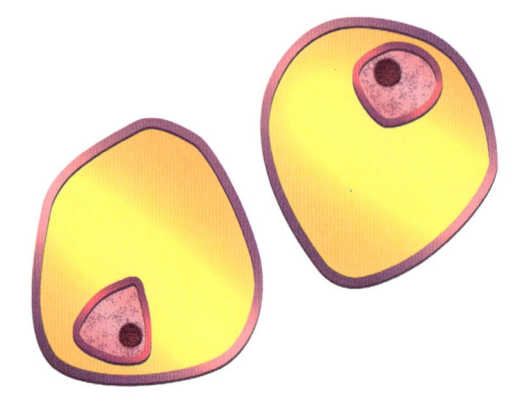

Figure IV.A.1.20: Interphase.

GOLD NOTES

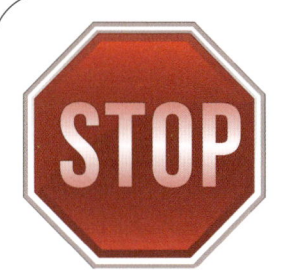

Reminder: Chapter review questions are available online for the original owner of this textbook. Doing practice questions will help clarify concepts and ensure that you study in a targeted way. First, register at gamsat-prep.com, then use your Online Access Card so that you can have access to the Lessons section.

No science background? Consider watching the relevant videos at gamsat-prep.com and you have support at gamsat-prep.com/forum. Don't forget to check the Index at the beginning of this book to see which chapters are HIGH, MEDIUM and LOW relative importance for the GAMSAT.

Your online access continues for one full year from your online registration.

GOLD NOTES

MICROBIOLOGY

Chapter 2

Memorize
* Structures, functions, life cycles
* Generalized viral life cycle
* Basic categories of bacteria
* Equation for bacterial doubling
* Differences, similtarities

Understand
* Eukaryotes vs. Prokaryotes
* General aspects of life cycles
* Gen. aspects of genetics/reproduction
* Calculation of exponential growth
* Scientific method (App. C) and microbiology

Not Required*
* Advanced level college info
* Evolutionary history, habitats
* Taxonomic (scientific) classification
* Role in infectious diseases

GAMSAT-Prep.com

Introduction

Microbiology is the study of microscopic organisms including viruses, bacteria and fungi. It is important to be able to focus on the differences and similarities between these microorganisms and the generalized eukaryotic cell you have just studied.

Additional Resources

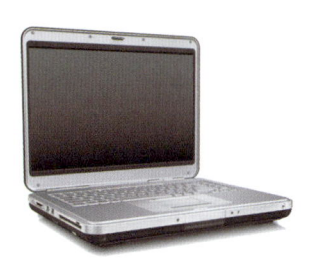

Free Online Q&A + Forum

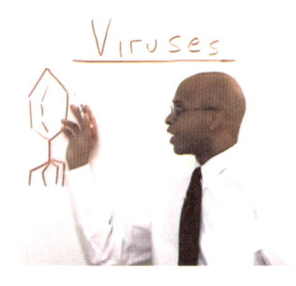

Video: Online or DVD 2

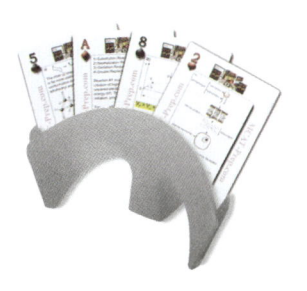

Flashcards

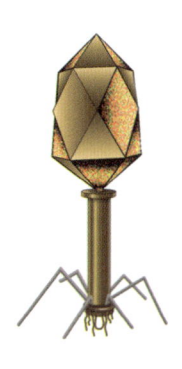

Special Guest

THE BIOLOGICAL SCIENCES   BIO-21

* The real GAMSAT may have advanced level information presented (ie. in a passage) but previous knowledge of said information is not required to answer the questions that would follow. Practice ACER and GS practice GAMSATs can help you clarify this point.

GAMSAT-Prep.com
THE GOLD STANDARD

2.1 Viruses

Unlike cells, viruses are too small to be vvseen directly with a light microscope. Viruses infect all types of organisms, from animals and plants to bacteria and archaea (BIO 2.2). Only a very basic and general understanding of viruses is required for the GAMSAT.

Viruses are obligate intracellular parasites; in other words, in order to replicate their genetic material and thus multiply, they must gain access to the inside of a cell. Viruses are often considered non-living for several reasons:

(i) they do not grow by increasing in size
(ii) they cannot carry out independent metabolism
(iii) they do not respond to external stimuli
(iv) they have no cellular structure.

The genetic material for viruses may be either DNA or RNA, never both. The nucleic acid core is encapsulated by a protein coat (capsid) which together forms the head region in some viruses. The tail region helps to anchor the virus to a cell. An extracellular viral particle is called a *virion*.

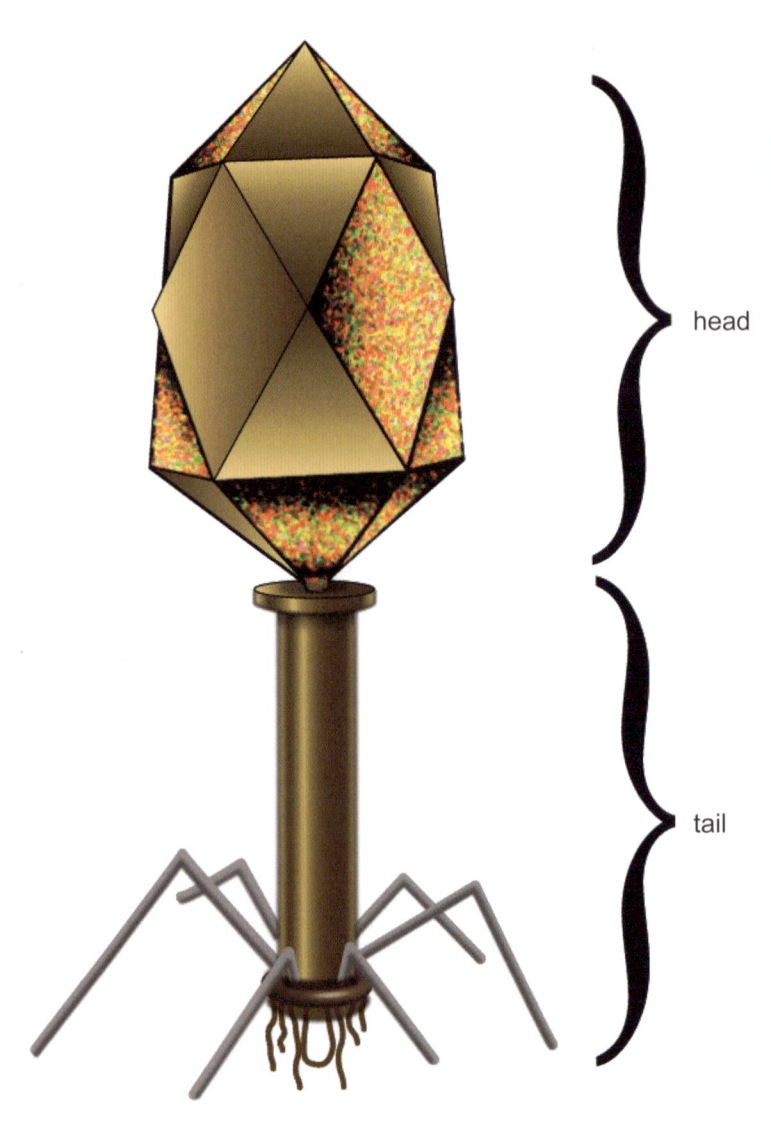

Figure IV.A.2.1: A virus.

BIOLOGY

Viruses are much smaller than prokaryotic cells (i.e. bacteria) which, in turn, are much smaller than eukaryotes (i.e. animal cells, fungi). A virus which infects bacteria is called a bacteriophage or simply a phage.

The life cycle of viruses has many variants; the following represents the main themes for GAMSAT purposes. A virus attaches to a specific receptor on a cell. Some viruses may now enter the cell; others, as in the diagram, will simply inject their nucleic acid. Either way, viral molecules induce the metabolic machinery of the host cell to produce more viruses.

The new viral particles may now exit the cell by lysing (bursting). The preceding is deemed lytic or virulent. Some viruses lie latent for long periods of time without lysing the host cell. These are called lysogenic or temperate viruses.

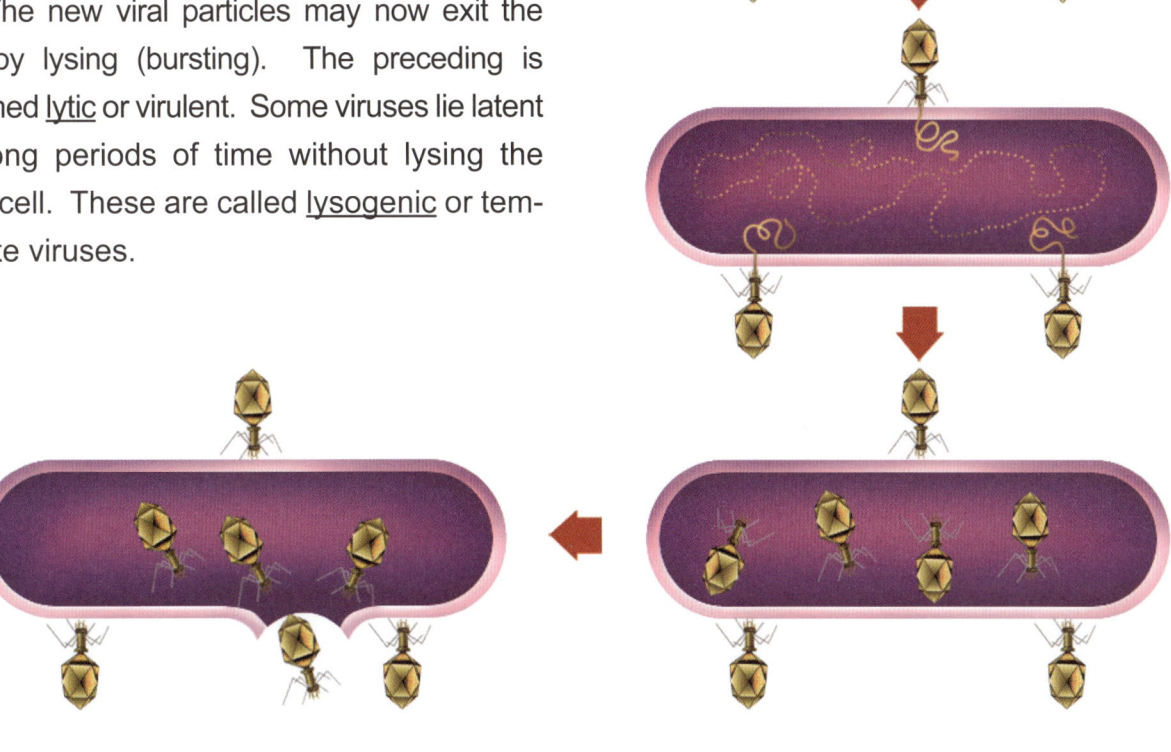

Figure IV.A.2.2: Lytic viral life cycle in a rod shaped bacterium (bacilli).

THE BIOLOGICAL SCIENCES BIO-23

2.1.1 Retroviruses

A retrovirus uses RNA as its genetic material. It is called a retrovirus because of an enzyme (reverse transcriptase) that gives these viruses the unique ability of transcribing RNA (their RNA) into DNA (see Biology Chapter 3 for the central dogma regarding protein synthesis). The retroviral DNA can then integrate into the chromosomal DNA of the host cell to be expressed there. The human immunodeficiency virus (HIV), the cause of AIDS, is a retrovirus.

Retroviruses are used, in genetics, to deliver DNA to a cell (= a vector); in medicine, they are used for gene therapy.

2.2 Prokaryotes

Prokaryotes (= pre-nucleus) are organisms without a membrane bound nucleus which includes 2 types of organisms: bacteria (= Eubacteria) and archaea (= bacteria-like organisms that live in extreme environments). For the purposes of the GAMSAT, we will focus on bacteria. They are haploid and have a long circular strand of DNA in a region called the nucleoid. Bacteria also have smaller circular DNA called plasmids which help to confer resistance to antibiotics.

Bacteria do not have mitochondria, Golgi apparatus, lysosomes, nor endoplasmic reticulum. Instead, metabolic processes can be carried out in the cytoplasm or associated with bacterial membranes. Bacteria have ribosomes (smaller than eukaryotes), plasma membrane, and a cell wall. The cell wall, made of peptidoglycans, helps to

Typical eukaryotic cell

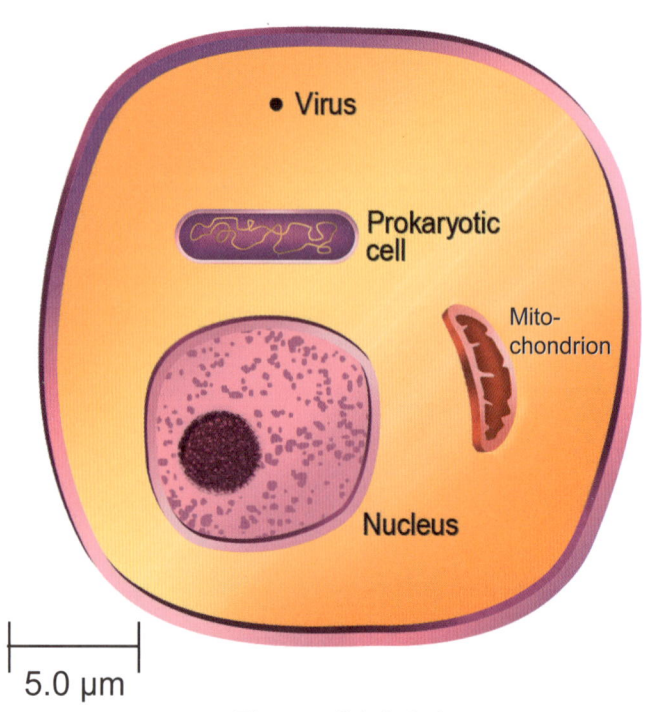

Figure IV.A.2.3
Comparing the size of a typical eukaryote, prokaryote and virus. Note that both the prokaryote and mitochondrion are similar in size and both contain circular DNA suggesting an evolutionary link.

prevent the hypertonic bacterium from bursting. Some bacteria have a slimy polysaccharide mucoid-like capsule on the outer surface for protection.

Bacteria can achieve movement with their whiplike flagella. The form and rotary engine of flagella are maintained by proteins (i.e. flagellin) which interact with the plasma

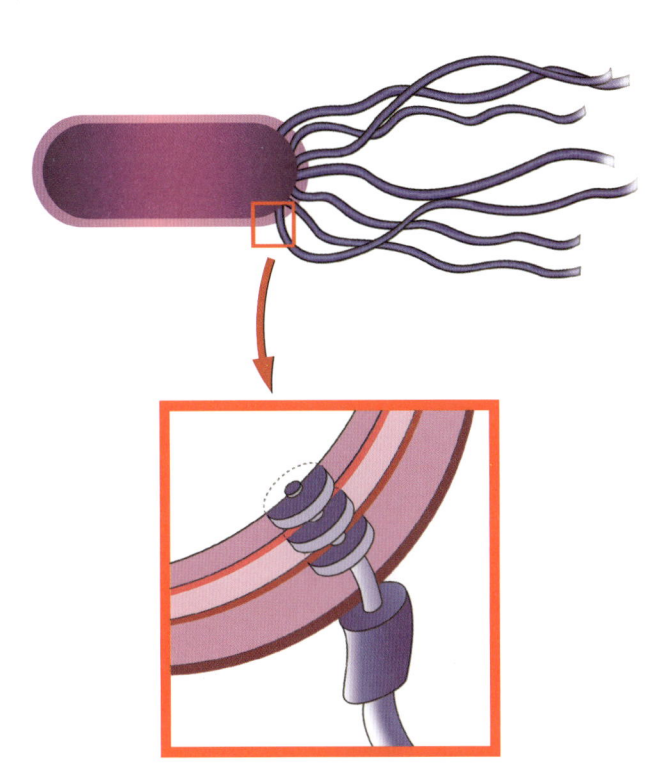

Figure IV.A.2.5
Schematic representation of bacteria colored for the purpose of identification: cocci (spherical, green), bacilli (cylindrical, purple) and spirilli (helical, orange).

membrane and the basal body (BIO 1.2). Power is generated by a proton motive force similar to the proton pump in metabolism (Biology, Chapter 4).

Bacteria are partially classified according to their shapes: cocci which are spherical or sometimes elliptical; bacilli which are rod shaped or cylindrical (Fig. IV.A.2.2 in BIO 2.1 showed phages attacking a bacillus bacterium); spirilli which are helical or spiral. They are also classified according to whether or not their cell wall reacts to a special dye called a Gram stain; thus they are gram-positive if they retain the stain and gram-negative if they do not.

Figure IV.A.2.4
Schematic representation of the basis for flagellar propulsion. The flagellum, similar to a flexible hook, is anchored to the membrane and cell wall by a series of protein rings forming a motor. Powered by the flow of protons, the motor can rotate the flagellum more than 100 revolutions per second.

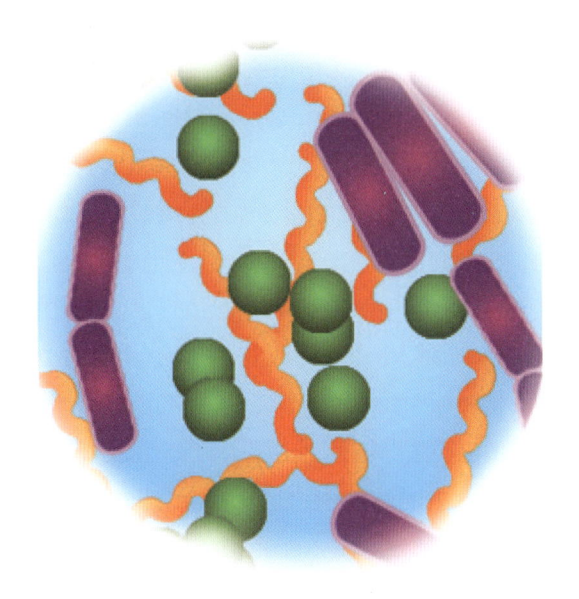

Most bacteria engage in a form of asexual reproduction called binary fission. Two identical DNA molecules migrate to opposite ends of a cell as a transverse wall forms, dividing the cell in two. The cells can now separate and enlarge to the original size. Under ideal conditions, a bacterium can undergo fission every 10-20 minutes producing over 10^{30} progeny in a day and a half. If resources are unlimited, exponential growth would be expected. The doubling time of bacterial populations can be calculated as follows:

$$b = B \times 2^n$$

where b is the number of bacteria at the end of the time interval, B is the number of bacteria at the beginning of the time interval and n is the number of generations. Thus if we start with 2 bacteria and follow for 3 generations then we get:

$b = B \times 2^n = 2 \times 2^3 = 2 \times 8 = 16$ bacteria after 3 generations.

{Note: bacterial doubling time is a relatively popular question type.}

Bacteria do not produce gametes nor zygotes, nor do they undergo meiosis; however, three forms of genetic recombination do occur: <u>transduction</u>, <u>transformation</u>, and <u>conjugation</u>. In transduction, phages act as a vector transferring DNA between bacteria. In transformation, bacteria incorporate free DNA from its immediate environment (i.e. from a dead cell which has released its DNA). In conjugation, part of the DNA strand may be passed from one mating type to another through a hollow tube (i.e. a pilus) while the two cells are in contact.

Most bacteria cannot synthesize their own food and thus depend on other organisms for it; such a bacterium is heterotrophic. Most heterotrophic bacteria obtain their food from dead organic matter; this is called saprophytic. Some bacteria are autotrophic meaning they can synthesize organic compounds from simple inorganic substances. Thus some are photosynthetic producing carbohydrate and releasing oxygen, while others are chemoautotrophic obtaining energy via chemical reactions including the oxidation of iron, sulfur, nitrogen, or hydrogen gas.

Bacteria can be either aerobic or anaerobic. The former refers to metabolism in the presence of oxygen and the latter in the absence of oxygen (i.e. fermentation). An obligate anaerobe would die in the presence of oxygen while a facultative anaerobe would survive.

Symbiosis generally refers to close and often long term interactions between different biological species. Bacteria have various symbiotic relationships with, for example, humans. These include mutualism (both benefit: GI tract bacteria, BIO 9.5), parasitism (parasite benefits over the host: tuberculosis, appendicitis) and commensalism (one benefits and the other is not significantly harmed or benefited: some skin bacteria).

2.3 Fungi

Fungi are eukaryotic (= true nucleus) organisms which absorb their food through their chitinous cell walls. They may either be unicellular (i.e. yeast) or filamentous (i.e. mushrooms, molds) with individual filaments called hyphae which collectively form a mycelium.

Fungi often reproduce asexually. Spores (i.e. conidia) can be produced and then liberated from outside of a sporangium; or, as in yeast, a simple asexual budding process may be used. Sexual reproduction can involve the fusion of opposite mating types to produce asci (singular: ascus), basidia (singular: basidium), or zygotes. All of the three preceding diploid structures must undergo meiosis to produce haploid spores. If resources are unlimited, exponential growth would be expected.

Fungi are relatively important for humans as a source of disease and a decomposer of both food and dead organic matter. On the lighter side, they also serve as food (mushrooms, truffles), for alcohol and food production (cheese molds, bread yeast) and they have given us the breakthrough antibiotic, penicillin (from penicillium molds).

2.4 Vectors

A vector can be a person, animal or microorganism that carries and transmits an infectious organism (i.e. bacteria, viruses, etc.) into another living organism. Examples: the mosquito is a vector for malaria; bats are vectors for rabies and a SARS-like virus.

GOLD NOTES

PROTEIN SYNTHESIS

Chapter 3

Memorize
* The genetic code (triplet)
* Central Dogma: DNA ➡ RNA ➡ protein
* Definitions: mRNA, tRNA, rRNA
* Codon-anticodon relationship
* Initiation, elongation and termination

Understand
* Mechanism of transcription
* Mechanism of translation
* Roles of mRNA, tRNA, rRNA
* Role and structure of ribosomes

Not Required*
* Advanced level college info
* Splicosomes, heterphil nuclear RNA
* Inhibitory, signal peptides
* Specific post translation changes
* Memorizing the ribosomal subunits in Svedberg units
* Memorizing stop or start codons

GAMSAT-Prep.com

Introduction

Protein synthesis is the creation of proteins using DNA and RNA. Individual amino acids are connected to each other in peptide linkages in a specific order given by the sequence of nucleotides in DNA. Thus the process occurs through a precise interplay directed by the genetic code and involving mRNA, tRNA and amino acids - all in an environment provided by a ribosome.

Additional Resources

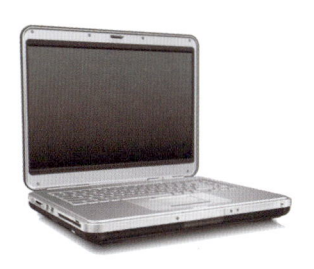

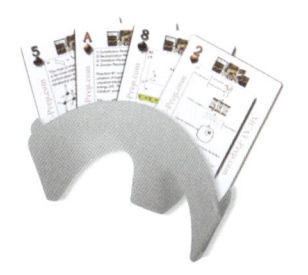

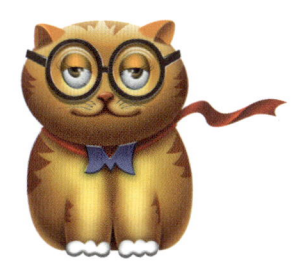

Free Online Q&A + Forum   Video: DVD Disc 1   Flashcards   Special Guest

THE BIOLOGICAL SCIENCES BIO-29

* The real GAMSAT may have advanced level information presented (ie. in a passage) but previous knowledge of said information is not required to answer the questions that would follow. Practice ACER and GS practice GAMSATs can help you clarify this point.

GAMSAT-Prep.com
THE GOLD STANDARD

Proteins (which comprise many hormones, all enzymes, antibodies, etc.) are long chains formed by peptide bonds between combinations of twenty amino acid subunits. Each amino acid is encoded in a sequence of three nucleotides (a triplet code = the genetic code). A gene is a conglomeration of such codes and thus is a section of DNA which encodes for a protein (or a polypeptide which is exactly like a protein but much smaller).

The information in DNA is rewritten (transcribed) into a messenger composed of RNA (= mRNA); the reaction is catalyzed by the enzyme RNA polymerase. The newly synthesized mRNA (the primary transcript) contains regions called introns that are not expressed in the synthesized protein. The introns are removed and the regions that are expressed (exons) are spliced together to form the final functional mRNA molecule. {EXons EXpressed; INtrons IN the garbage!} The messenger then leaves the nucleus with the information necessary to make a protein. It attaches to a small subunit of a ribosome which will then attach to a larger ribosomal subunit thus creating a full ribosome. A ribosome is composed of a complex of protein and ribosomal RNA (= rRNA).

Floating in the cytoplasm is yet another form of RNA; this RNA specializes in taking amino acids and transfering them onto other amino acids when contained within the environment of the ribosome. More specifically, this transfer RNA (tRNA) molecule can attach itself to a specific amino acid, enter

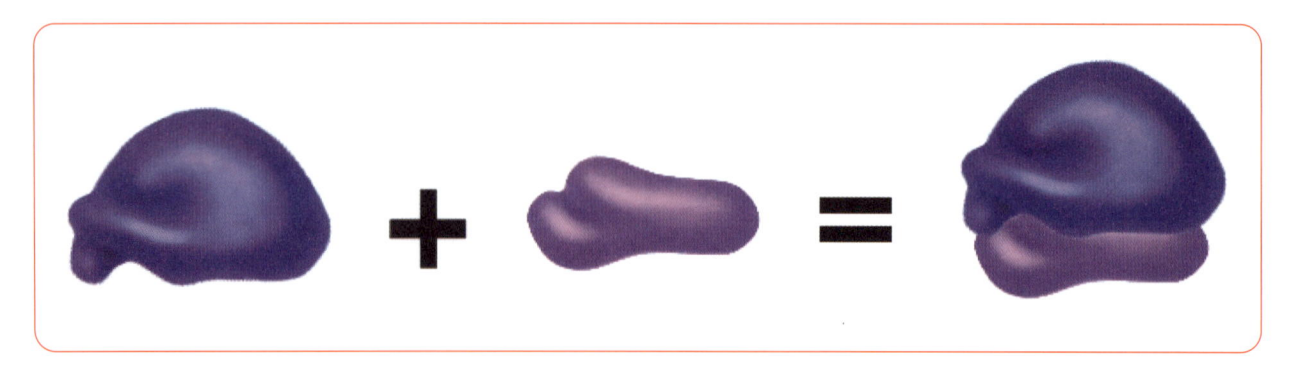

Figure IV.A.3.1: A ribosome provides the environment for protein synthesis. Ribosomes are composed of a large and a small subunit.

BIO-30 PROTEIN SYNTHESIS

BIOLOGY

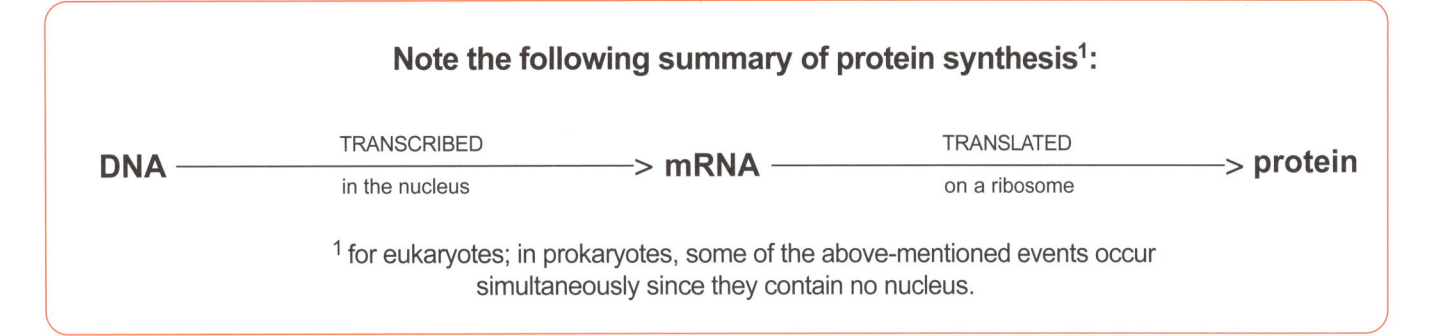

> **Note the following summary of protein synthesis[1]:**
>
> DNA —— TRANSCRIBED in the nucleus ——> mRNA —— TRANSLATED on a ribosome ——> protein
>
> [1] for eukaryotes; in prokaryotes, some of the above-mentioned events occur simultaneously since they contain no nucleus.

the environment of the ribosome, recognize the triplet code (= codon) on mRNA which codes for the amino acid tRNA is carrying (tRNA can do this since it has its own triplet code - an anticodon); and finally, tRNA can transfer its amino acid onto the preceding one thus elongating the polypeptide chain. In a way, tRNA translates the code that mRNA carries into a sequence of amino acids which can produce a protein. According to the base pair matching already discussed, if the codon on mRNA is AUG then the anticodon to match on tRNA would be UAC.

A nonsense mutation is a point mutation in a sequence of DNA that results in a premature stop codon (there are 3: UAA, UAG, UGA), or a nonsense codon in the transcribed mRNA. Either way, an incomplete, and usually nonfunctional protein is the result. A missense mutation is a point mutation where a single nucleotide is changed to cause substitution of a different

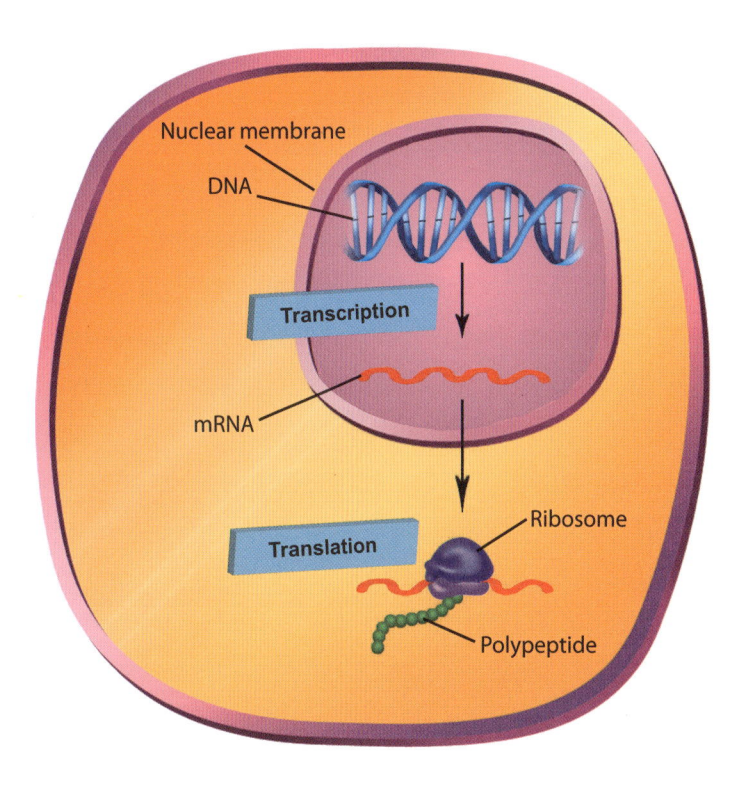

Figure IV.A.3.2: The central dogma of protein synthesis.

amino acid. Some genetic disorders (i.e. thalassemia) result from nonsense mutations.

Protein made on free ribosomes in the cytoplasm may be used for intracellular purposes (i.e. enzymes for glycolysis, etc.). Whereas proteins made on rER ribosomes are usually modified by both rER and the Golgi apparatus en route to the plasma membrane or exocytosis (i.e. antibodies, intestinal enzymes, etc.).

Note the following: i) the various kinds of RNA are single stranded molecules which are produced using DNA as a template; ii) hormones can have a potent regulatory effect on protein synthesis (esp. enzymes); iii) allosteric enzymes (= proteins with two different configurations - each with different biological properties) are important regulators of transcription; iv) there are many protein factors which trigger specific events in the initiation (using a start codon, AUG), elongation and termination (using a stop codon) of the synthesis of a protein; v) one end of the protein has an amino group (-NH$_2$, which projects from the first amino acid), while the other end has a carboxylic acid group (-COOH, which projects from the last amino acid). {Amino acids and protein structure will be explored in ORG 12.1 and 12.2}

> Peptide: the result of the moon pulling on the Pepsi.

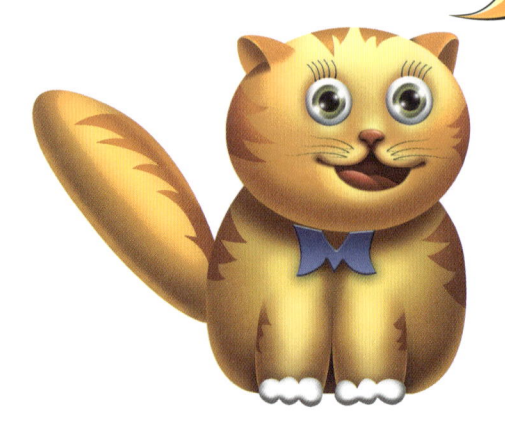

GOLD NOTES

GOLD NOTES

ENZYMES AND CELLULAR METABOLISM
Chapter 4

Memorize
* Define: catabolism, anabolism, activation energy
* Define: metabolism, active/ allosteric sites

Understand
* Feedback, competitive, non-competitive inhibition
* Krebs cycle, electron transport chain: main features
* Metabolism: carbohydrates (glucose), fats and proteins

Not Required*
* Advanced level college info
* Photosynthesis, gluconeogenesis, fatty acid oxidation
* Knowing the deficiencies in the theoretical yield (36 ATP) calculation

GAMSAT-Prep.com

Introduction

Cells require energy to grow, reproduce, maintain structure, respond to the environment, etc. Biochemical reactions and other energy producing processes that occur in cells, including cellular metabolism, are regulated in part by enzymes. GAMSAT tests almost always include multiple questions exploring your understanding of a cycle or biochemical mechanism with or without negative or positive feedback. The questions do not center on your memorizing details but rather having an understanding of how the presented cycle functions or how it can be stimulated or inhibited. The end of Chapter 6 will focus on feedback loops with respect to hormones.

Additional Resources

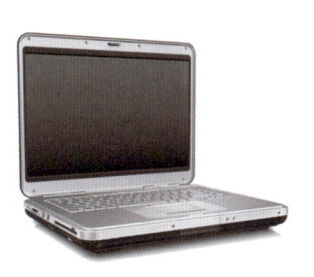

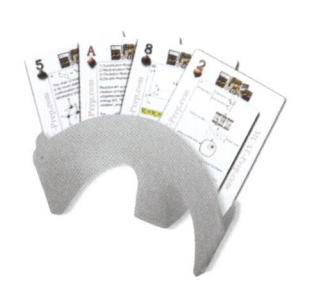

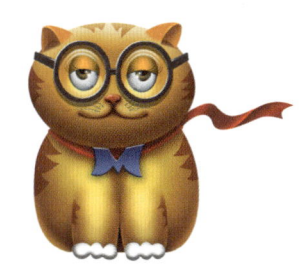

Free Online Q&A + Forum   Video: Online or DVD 2   Flashcards   Special Guest

THE BIOLOGICAL SCIENCES   BIO-35

* The real GAMSAT may have advanced level information presented (ie. in a passage) but previous knowledge of said information is not required to answer the questions that would follow. Practice ACER and GS practice GAMSATs can help you clarify this point.

4.1 Overview

In an organism or an individual many biochemical reactions take place. All these biochemical reactions are collectively termed metabolism. In general, metabolism can be broadly divided into two main categories. They are:

(a) <u>Catabolism</u> which is the breakdown of macromolecules (larger molecules) such as glycogen to micromolecules (smaller molecules) such as glucose.

(b) <u>Anabolism</u> which is the building up of macromolecules such as protein using micromolecules such as amino acids.

As we all know, chemical reactions in general involve great energy exchanges when they occur. Similarly both catabolic and anabolic reactions would involve massive amounts of energy if they were to occur in vitro (outside the cell). However, all these reactions could be carried out within a lower temperature range using substances called enzymes.

What is an enzyme?

An enzyme is a protein catalyst. A protein is a large polypeptide made up of amino acid subunits. A catalyst is a substance that alters the rate of a chemical reaction without itself being permanently changed into another compound. A catalyst accelerates a reaction by decreasing the <u>free energy of activation</u> (see Chemistry 9.7).

Enzymes fall into two general categories:

(a) Simple proteins which contain only amino acids like the digestive enzymes ribonuclease, trypsin and chymotrypsin.

(b) Complex proteins which contain amino acids and a non-amino acid cofactor. Thus the complete enzyme is called a holoenzyme and it is made up of a protein portion (apoenzyme) and a cofactor.

> Holoenzyme = Apoenzyme + Cofactor.

A metal may serve as a cofactor. Zinc, for example, is a cofactor for the enzymes carbonic anhydrase and carboxypeptidase. An organic molecule such as pyridoxal phosphate or biotin may serve as a cofactor. Cofactors such as biotin, which are covalently linked to the enzyme are called prosthetic groups or ligands.

In addition to their enormous catalytic power which accelerates reaction rates, enzymes exhibit exquisite specificity in the types of reactions that each catalyzes as well as specificity for the substrates upon which they act. Their specificity is linked to the concept of an active site. An active site is a cluster of amino acids within the tertiary (i.e. 3-dimensional) configuration of the enzyme where the actual catalytic event occurs. The active site is often similar to a pocket or groove with properties (chemical or structural) that accommodate the intended substrate with high specificity.

Examples of such specificity are as follows: Phosphofructokinase catalyzes a reaction between ATP and fructose-6-phosphate. The enzyme does not catalyze a reaction between other nucleoside triphosphates. It is worth mentioning the specificity of trypsin and chymotrypsin though both of them are proteolytic (i.e. they degrade or *hydrolyse* proteins). Trypsin catalyzes the hydrolysis of peptides and proteins only on the carboxyl side of polypeptidic amino acids lysine and arginine. Chymotrypsin catalyzes the hydrolysis of peptides and proteins on the carboxyl side of polypeptidic amino acids phenylalanine, tyrosine and tryptophan. The degree of specificity described in the previous examples originally led to the **Lock and Key Model** which has been generally replaced by the **Induced Fit Hypothesis.** While the former suggests that the molecular interaction is rigid, the latter describes a greater flexibility at the active site.

4.2 Enzyme Kinetics and Inhibition

There is an increase in reaction velocity with an increase in the concentration of substrate. At increasingly higher substrate concentrations the increase in activity is progressively smaller. From this, it could be inferred that enzymes exhibit saturation kinetics. The mechanism of the preceding lies largely with feedback inhibition. Feedback inhibition is when the product of the enzyme catalysed reaction returns (*feeds back*) to prevent or *inhibit* further reactions between the enzyme and its substrate.

Enzyme inhibitors are classified as reversible and irreversible. Irreversible inhibitors usually react covalently to render the enzyme inactive. Reversible inhibitors generally interact non-covalently and virtually instantaneously with an enzyme.

4.3 Regulation of Enzyme Activity

The activity of enzymes in the cell is subject to a variety of regulatory mechanisms. The amount of enzyme can be altered by increasing or decreasing its synthesis or degradation. Enzyme induction refers to an enhancement of its synthesis. Repression refers to a decrease in its biosynthesis.

Enzyme activity can also be altered by covalent modification. Phosphorylation of specific serine residues by protein kinases increases or decreases catalytic activity depending upon the enzyme. Proteolytic cleavage of proenzymes (e.g., chymotrypsinogen, trypsinogen, protease and clotting factors) converts an inactive form to an active form (e.g., chymotrypsin, trypsin, etc.).

Enzyme activity can be greatly influenced by its environment (esp. pH and temperature). For example, most enzymes exhibit optimal activity at a pH in the range 6.5 to 7.5. However, pepsin (an enzyme found in the stomach) has an optimum pH of ~ 2.0. Thus it cannot function adequately at a higher pH (i.e. in the small intestine). Likewise, enzymes function at an optimal temperature. When the temperature is lowered, kinetic energy decreases and thus the rate of reaction decreases. If the temperature is raised too much then the enzyme may become denatured and thus non-functional.

Enzyme activity can also be modified by non-covalent or allosteric mechanisms. Isocitrate dehydrogenase is an enzyme in the Krebs Tricarboxylic Acid Cycle, which is activated by ADP. ADP is not a substrate or substrate analogue. It is postulated to bind a site *distinct* from the active site called the *allosteric site*.

Some enzymes fail to behave by simple saturation kinetics. In such cases a phenomenon called positive co-operativity is explained in which binding of one substrate or ligand makes it easier for the second to bind.

4.4 Bioenergetics

Biological species must transform energy into readily available sources in order to survive. ATP (adenosine triphosphate) is the body's most important short term energy storage molecule. It can be produced by the breakdown or oxidation of protein, lipids (i.e. fat) or carbohydrates (esp. glucose). If the body is no longer ingesting sources of energy it can access its own stores: glucose is stored in the liver as glycogen, lipids are stored throughout the body as fat, and ultimately, muscle can be catabolized to release protein (esp. amino acids).

We will be examining four key processes that can lead to the production of ATP: glycolysis, Krebs Citric Acid Cycle, the electron transport chain (ETC), and oxidative phosphorylation. Figure IV.A.4.1 is a schematic summary.

BIOLOGY

Figure IV.A.4.1: Summary of ATP production.

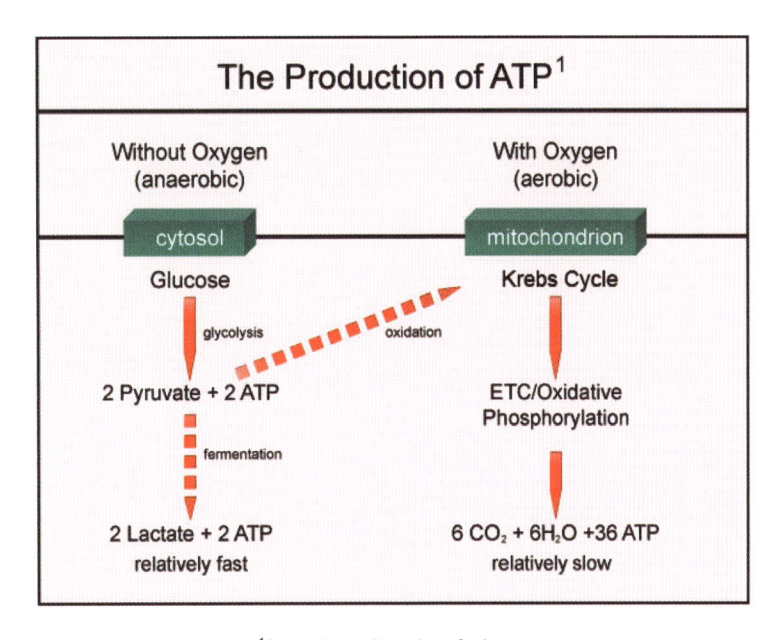

[1] from 1 molecule of glucose

4.5 Glycolysis

The initial steps in the catabolism or *lysis* of D-glucose constitute the Embden - Meyerhof glyco*lytic* pathway. This pathway can occur in the absence of oxygen (anaerobic). The enzymes for glycolysis are present in all human cells and are located in the cytosol. The overall reaction can be depicted as follows (ADP: adenosine diphosphate, NAD: nicotinamide adenine dinucleotide, Pi: inorganic phosphate):

$$\text{Glucose} + 2\text{ADP} + 2\text{NAD}^+ + 2P_i \longrightarrow 2\text{Pyruvate} + 2\text{ATP} + 2\text{NADH} + 2\text{H}^+$$

The first step in glycolysis involves the phosphorylation of glucose by ATP. The enzyme that catalyzes this irreversible reaction is either hexokinase or glucokinase. Phosphohexose isomerase then catalyzes the conversion of glucose-6-phosphate to fructose-6-phosphate. Phosphofructokinase (PFK) catalyzes the second phosphorylation. It is an irreversible reaction. This step, which produces fructose-1,6-diphosphate, is said to be the rate limiting or pacemaker step in glycolysis. Aldolase then catalyzes the cleavage of fructose-1,6-diphosphate to glyceraldehyde-3-phosphate and dihydroxyacetone phosphate (= 2 triose phosphates). Triose phosphate isomerase catalyzes the interconversion of the two preceding compounds. Glyceraldehyde-3-phosphate dehydrogenase mediates a reaction between the designated triose, NAD$^+$ and P$_i$ to yield 1,3-diphosphoglycerate. Next, phosphoglycerate kinase catalyzes the reaction of the latter, an energy rich compound, with ADP to yield ATP and phosphoglycerate. Phosphoglycerate mutase catalyzes the transfer of the phosphoryl group from carbon two to yield 2-phosphoglycerate. Enolase catalyzes an isogonic dehydration to yield phosphoenolpyruvate. The enzyme enolase is inhibited by fluoride at high, non-physiological concentrations. This is why blood samples that are drawn for estimation of glucose are added to fluoride to inhibit glycolysis. Phosphoenolpyruvate is then acted upon by pyruvate kinase to yield pyruvate which is a three carbon compound.

Under **aerobic** conditions (i.e. in the presence of oxygen) pyruvate is converted to Acetyl CoA which will enter the Krebs Cycle followed by oxidative phosphorylation producing a total of 38 ATP per molecule of glucose (i.e. 2 pyruvate). Under **anaerobic** conditions (i.e. absence of oxygen),

Glucose (C$_6$)
* ↓ Hexokinase or Glucokinase
Glucose-6-phosphate (C$_6$)
⇌ Phosphohexose isomerase
Fructose-6-phosphate (C$_6$)
* ↓ Phosphofructokinase (PFK) RATE LIMITING STEP
Fructose-1,6-diphosphate (C$_6$)
⇌ Aldolase
2 Triose-phosphate (C$_3$)
⇌
2 Phosphoenolpyruvate (C$_3$)
* ↓ Pyruvate kinase
2 Pyruvate (C$_3$)

The symbol in brackets represents the number of carbons in each compound. The asterix represents steps which are functionally irrecersible under physiologic conditions. PFK is involved in the rate limiting step which is activated by ADP and inhibited by ATP.

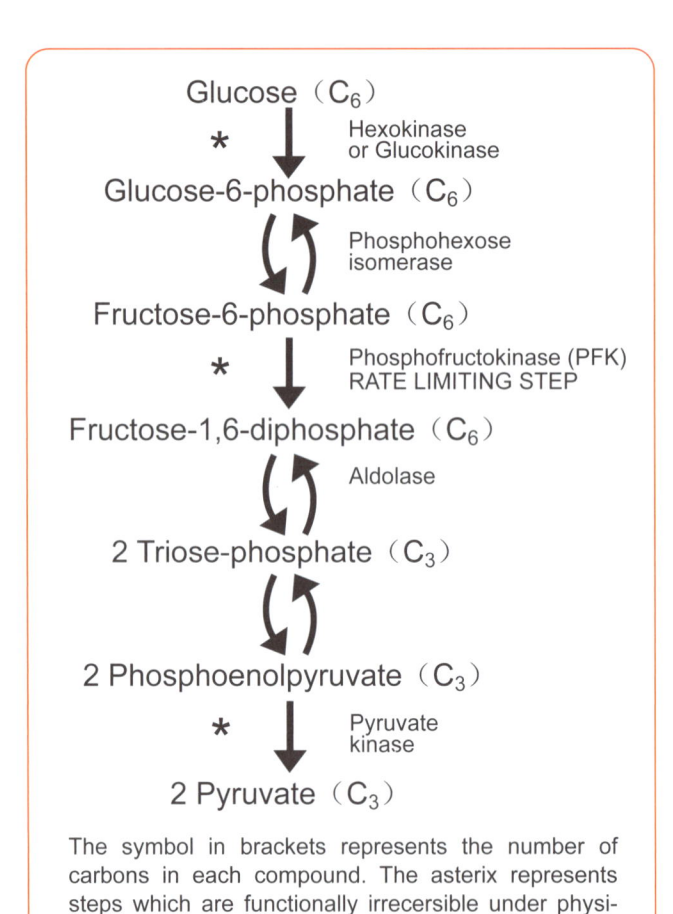

Figure IV.A.4.2: Summary of glycolysis.

pyruvate is quickly reduced by NADH to lactic acid using the enzyme lactate dehydrogenase. A net of only 2 ATP is produced per molecule of glucose (this process is called *fermentation*).

Oxygen Debt: after running a 100m dash you may find yourself gasping for air even if you have completely ceased activity. This is because during the race you could not get an adequate amount of oxygen to your muscles and your muscles needed energy quickly; thus the anaerobic pathway was used. The lactic acid which built up during the race will require you to *pay back* a certain amount of oxygen in order to oxidize lactate to pyruvate and continue along the more energy efficient aerobic pathway.

4.6 Glycolysis: A Negative Perspective

An interesting way to summarize the main events of glycolysis is to follow the fate of the phosphate group which contains a negative charge. Note that *kinases* and *phosphorylases* are enzymes that can add or subtract phosphate groups.

The first event in glycolysis is the phosphorylation of glucose. Thus glucose becomes negatively charged which prevents it from leaking out of the cell. Then glucose-6-phosphate becomes its isomer (= *same* molecular formula, *different* structure) fructose-6-phosphate which is further phosphorylated to fructose-1,6-diphosphate. Imagine that this six carbon sugar (fructose) now contains two large negatively charged ligands which repel each other! The six carbon sugar (*hexose*) sensibly breaks into two three-carbon compounds (*triose phosphates*).

A triose phosphate is ultimately converted to 1,3-diphosphoglycerate which is clearly an unstable compound (i.e. *two negative phosphate groups*). Thus it transfers a high energy phosphate group onto ADP to produce ATP. When ATP is produced from a substrate (i.e. 1,3-diphosphoglycerate), the reaction is called *substrate level phosphorylation*.

4.7 Krebs Citric Acid Cycle

Aerobic conditions: for further breakdown of pyruvate it has to enter the mitochondria where a series of reactions will cleave the molecule to water and carbon dioxide. All these reactions (which were discovered by Hans. A. Krebs) are collectively known as the Tricarboxylic Acid Cycle (TCA) or Krebs Citric Acid Cycle. Not only carbohydrates but also lipids and proteins use the TCA for channelling their metabolic pathways. This is why TCA is often called the final common pathway of metabolism.

The glycolysis of glucose (C_6) produces 2 pyruvate (C_3) which in turn produces 2 CO_2 and 2 acetyl CoA (C_2). The catabolism of both glucose and fatty acids yield acetyl CoA. Metabolism of amino acids yields acetyl CoA or actual intermediates of the TCA Cycle. The Citric Acid Cycle provides a pathway for the oxidation of acetyl CoA. The pathway includes eight discrete steps. Seven of the enzyme activities are found in the mitochondrial matrix; the eighth (succinate dehydrogenase) is associated with the Electron Transport Chain (ETC) within the inner mitochondrial membrane.

The following includes key points to remember about the TCA Cycle: i) glucose → 2 acetyl CoA → 2 turns around the TCA Cycle; ii) 2 CO_2 per turn is generated as a waste product which will eventually be blown off in the lungs; iii) one GTP (guanosine triphosphate) per turn is produced by substrate level phosphorylation; one GTP is equivalent to one ATP (*GTP + ADP → GDP + ATP*); iv) *reducing equivalents* are hydrogens which are carried by NAD^+ (→ NADH + H^+) three times per turn and FAD (→ $FADH_2$) once per turn; these reducing equivalents will eventually be oxidized to produce ATP (*oxidative phosphorylation*) and eventually produce H_2O as a waste product (the last step in the ETC); v) the hydrogens (*H*) which are reducing equivalents are not protons (*H^+*) - quite the contrary! Often the reducing equivalents are simply called electrons.

4.8 Oxidative Phosphorylation

The term oxidative phosphorylation refers to reactions associated with oxygen consumption and the phosphorylation of ADP to yield ATP. Oxidative phosphorylation is associated with an Electron Transport Chain or Respiratory Chain which is found in the inner mitochondrial membrane of eukaryotes. A similar process occurs within the plasma membrane of prokaryotes such as *E.coli*.

The importance of oxidative phosphorylation is that it accounts for the reoxidation of reducing equivalents generated in the reactions of the Krebs Cycle as well as in glycolysis. This process accounts for the preponderance of ATP production in humans. The ETC transfers electrons from reductants (hydrogens) to oxygen in a series of exergonic (exothermic) reactions thus producing H_2O. A schematic summary is in Figure IV.A.4.3.

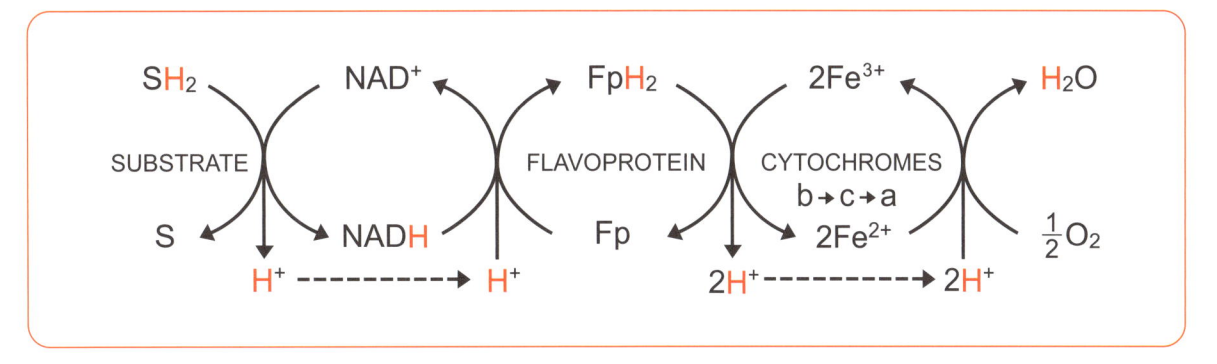

Figure IV.A.4.3: Transport of reducing equivalents through the respiratory chain. Examples of substrates (S) which provide reductants are isocitrate, malate, etc. Cytochromes contain iron (Fe).

4.9 Electron Transport Chain (ETC)

The following are the components of the ETC: iron - sulphur proteins, cytochromes c, b, a and coenzyme Q or *ubiquinone*. The respiratory chain proceeds from NAD-specific dehydrogenases through flavoprotein, ubiquinone, then cytochromes and ultimately molecular oxygen. Reducing equivalents can enter the chain at two locations. Electrons from NADH are transferred to NADH dehydrogenase. In reactions involving iron - sulphur proteins electrons are transferred to coenzyme Q; protons are translocated from the mitochondrial matrix to the exterior of the inner membrane during this process. This creates a proton gradient which is coupled to the production of ATP.

Electrons entering from succinate dehydrogenase (FADH$_2$) are donated directly to coenzyme Q. Electrons are transported from reduced coenzyme Q to cytochrome b and then cytochrome c. Electrons are then carried by cytochrome c to cytochrome a. Cytochrome a is also known as *cytochrome oxidase*. It catalyzes the reaction of electrons and protons with molecular oxygen to produce water. Cyanide is a powerful inhibitor of cytochrome oxidase.

4.10 Summary of Energy Production

Process of reaction	ATP yield
1. Glycolysis (Glucose → 2 Pyruvate)	2
2. Glycolysis (2NADH from glyceraldehyde-3-phosphate dehydrogenase)	6
3. Pyruvate dehydrogenase (2NADH)	6
4. Isocitrate dehydrogenase (2NADH)	6
5. Alpha-ketoglutarate dehydrogenase (2NADH)	6
6. Succinate thiokinase	2
7. Succinate dehydrogenase (2FADH$_2$)	4
8. Malate dehydrogenase (2NADH)	6
TOTAL	38 ATP yield per hexose.

Note the following: i) 1 NADH produces 3 ATP molecules while 1 FADH$_2$ produces only 2 ATP; ii) there is a *cost* of 2 ATP to get the two molecules of NADH generated in the cytoplasm (see the preceding point # 2.) to enter the mitochondrion, thus the *net yield for eukaryotes is 36 ATP*.

The efficiency of ATP production is far from 100%. Energy is lost from the system primarily in the form of heat. Under standard conditions, less than 40% of the energy generated from the complete oxidation of glucose is converted to the production of ATP. As a comparison, a gasoline engine fairs much worse with an efficiency rating generally less than 20%. Further inefficiencies reduce the net theoretical yield in the (non-GAMSAT!) real world.

I'm low on energy. What do you mean I can't have a CAT scan and a PET scan ?!!?

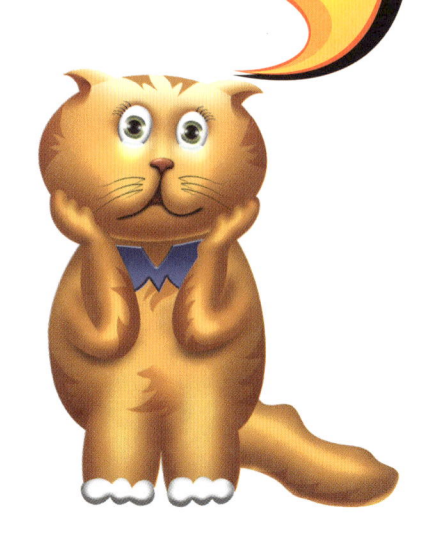

BIO-44   ENZYMES AND CELLULAR METABOLISM

BIOLOGY

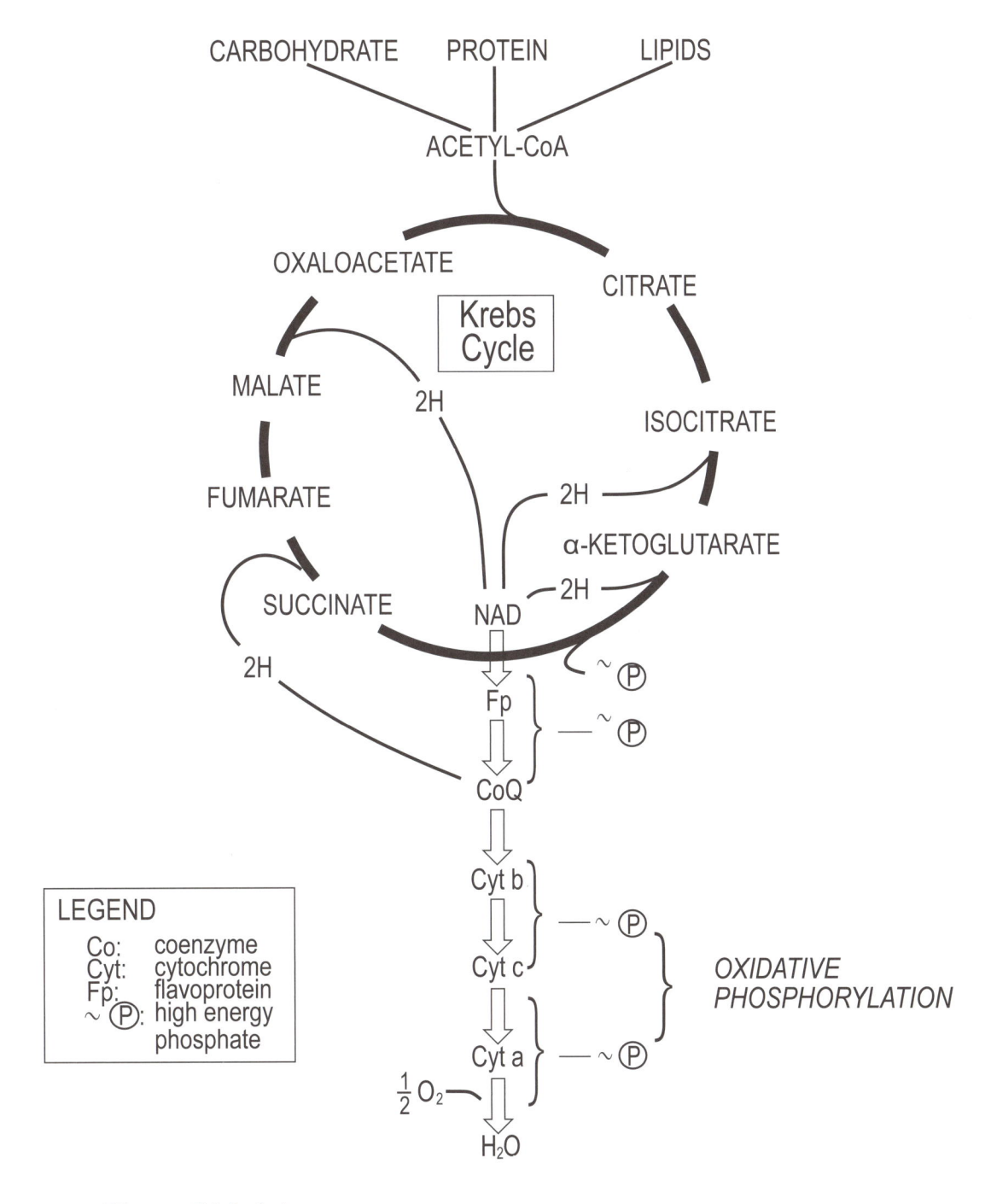

Figure IV.A.4.4: Summary of the Krebs Cycle and the Electron Transport Chain.
Note: Acetyl CoA can be the product of carbohydrate, protein, or lipid metabolism. Thick black arrows represent the Krebs Cycle while white arrows represent the Electron Transport Chain. High energy phosphate groups are transferred from ADP to produce ATP. Ultimately, oxygen accepts electrons and hydrogen from Cyt a to produce water.

THE BIOLOGICAL SCIENCES BIO-45

GOLD NOTES

SPECIALIZED EUKARYOTIC CELLS AND TISSUES
Chapter 5

Memorize	Understand	Not Required*
Neuron: basic structure and function Reasons for the membrane potential	* Resting potential: electrochemical gradient/action potential, graph * Excitatory and inhibitory nerve fibers: summation, frequency of firing * Organization of contractile elements: actin and myosin filaments * Cross bridges, sliding filament model; calcium regulation of contraction	* Advanced level college info * Memorizing details about epithelial cells, connective tissue

GAMSAT-Prep.com

Introduction

To build a living organism, with all the various tissues and organs, cells must specialize. Communication among cells and organs, movement, protection and support are achieved to a great degree by neurons, muscle cells, epithelial cells and the cells of connective tissue, respectively.

Additional Resources

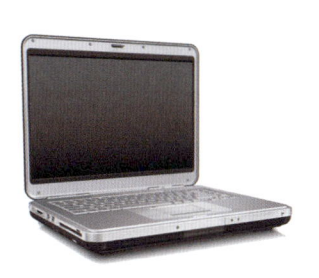

Free Online Q&A + Forum   Video: Online or DVD 2   Flashcards   Special Guest

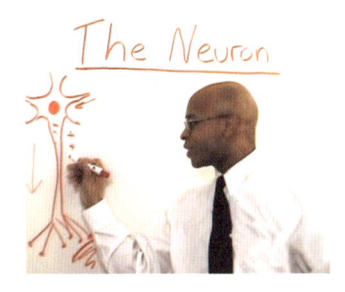

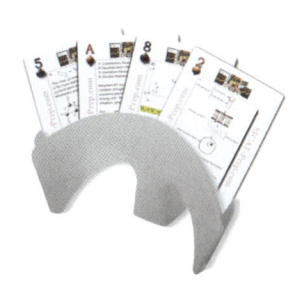

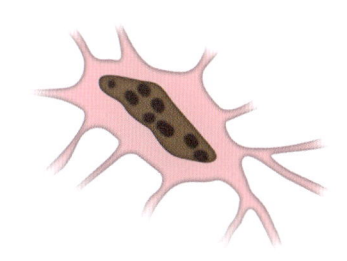

THE BIOLOGICAL SCIENCES   BIO-47

* The real GAMSAT may have advanced level information presented (ie. in a passage) but previous knowledge of said information is not required to answer the questions that would follow. Practice ACER and GS practice GAMSATs can help you clarify this point.

5.1 Neural Cells and Tissues

The brain, spinal cord and peripheral nervous system are composed of nerve tissue. The basic cell types of nerve tissue is the *neuron* and the *glial cell*. Glial cells support and protect neurons and participate in neural activity, nutrition and defense processes. Neurons, which we will examine in detail, conduct and transmit nerve impulses.

Each neuron consists of a nerve cell body (*perikaryon or soma*), and one or more nerve processes (*fibers*). The cell body of a typical neuron contains a nucleus, *Nissl* material which is rough endoplasmic reticulum, free ribosomes, Golgi apparatus, mitochondria, many neurotubules, neurofilaments and pigment inclusions. The cell processes of neurons occur as *axons* and *dendrites*. Dendrites contain most of the components of the cell body except the nucleus and Golgi apparatus whereas axons contain major structures found in dendrites except for the Nissl material. As a rule, dendrites conduct impulses *to* the cell body and ultimately through to the axon. At the synaptic (terminal) ends of axons the presynaptic process contains vesicles from which are elaborated excitatory or inhibitory substances.

The functional dendrites of some neurons, such as the sensory pseudounipolar neurons of spinal nerves, are structurally the same as axons. **Unmyelinated** fibers in peripheral nerves lie in grooves on the surface of the neurolemma (= plasma membrane) of a type of glial cell (*Schwann cell*). **Myelinated** peripheral neurons are invested by numerous layers of Schwann cell plasma membrane that constitute a *myelin sheath*. There are many Schwann cells along each myelinated fiber. In junctional areas between adjacent Schwann

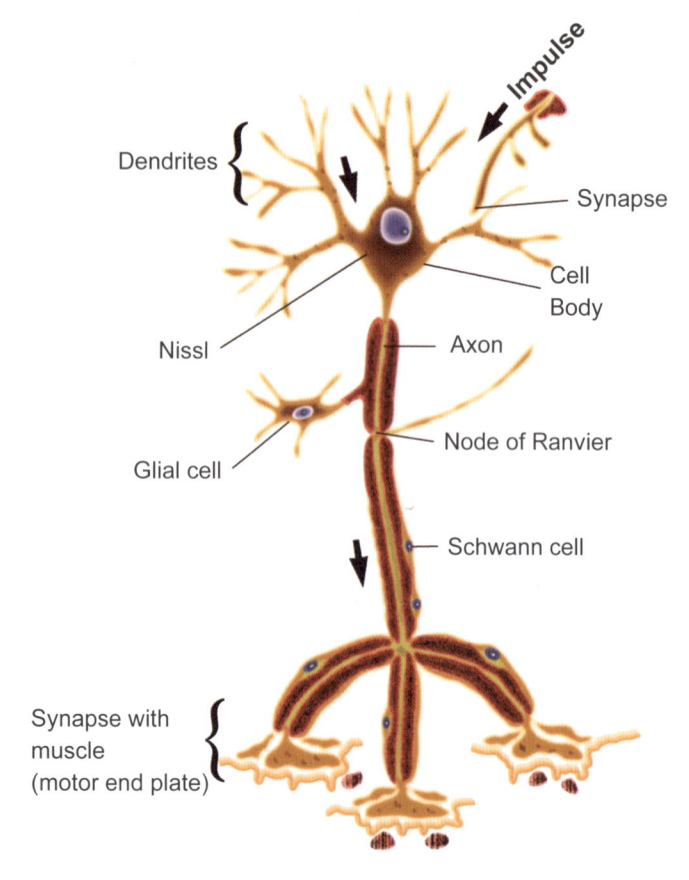

Figure IV.A.5.1: A neuron and other cells of nerve tissue, showing the neuromuscular junction, or motor end plate.

cells there is a lack of myelin. These junctional areas along the myelinated process constitute the nodes of Ranvier.

The neurons of the nervous system are arranged so that each neuron stimulates or inhibits other neurons and these in turn may stimulate or inhibit others until the functions of the nervous system are performed. The area between a neuron and the successive cell (i.e. another neuron, muscle fiber or gland) is called a *synapse*. When a neuron makes a synapse with muscle, it is called a *motor end plate* (*see* Fig. IV.A.5.1). The terminal endings of the nerve filament that synapse with the next cell are called presynaptic terminals, synaptic knobs, or more commonly - synaptic boutons.

At the synapse there is no physical contact between the two cells. The space between the dendrite of one neuron and the axon of another neuron is called the synaptic cleft and it measures about 200 - 300 angstroms (1 angstrom = 10^{-10} m). The chemical mediators which are housed in vesicles at the presynaptic terminal are exocytosed in response to an increase in intracellular calcium (Ca^{2+}) concentration. The mediators or *transmitters* diffuse through the synaptic cleft when an impulse reaches the terminal. This transmitter substance may either excite the *postsynaptic* neuron or inhibit it. They are therefore called either excitatory or inhibitory transmitters (examples include *acetylcholine* and *GABA*, respectively).

5.1.1 The Membrane Potential

A membrane or resting potential (V_m) occurs across the plasma membranes of all cells. In large nerve and muscle cells this potential amounts to about 90 millivolts with positivity outside the cell membrane and negativity inside (V_m = -90 mV). The development of this potential occurs as follows: every cell membrane contains a Na^+ - K^+ ATPase that pumps each ion to where its concentration is highest: Na^+ to the outside of the cell and K^+ to the inside. However, more Na^+ is pumped outward than K^+ inward ($3Na^+$ per $2K^+$). Also, the membrane is relatively permeable to K^+ so that it can leak out of the cell with relative ease. Therefore, the net effect is a loss of positive charges from inside the membrane and a gain of positive charges on the outside. The resulting membrane potential is the basis of all conduction of impulses by nerve and muscle fibers.

5.1.2 Action Potential

The action potential is a sequence of changes in the electric potential that occurs within a small fraction of a second when a nerve or muscle membrane impulse spreads over the surface of the cell. Any factor which makes the membrane suddenly permeable over and above a threshold potential (i.e. pinching a nerve fiber) will cause the membrane to become very permeable to sodium ions. As a result, the positive sodium ions on the outside of the membrane now flow rapidly to the more negative interior. Therefore, the membrane potential suddenly becomes reversed with positivity on the inside and negativity on the outside. This state is called *depolarization*.

Once a portion of a nerve fiber is depolarized the mechanisms in the nerve or muscle fiber function to achieve the previous polarity. This is called *repolarization*. The depolarized nerve goes on depolarizing the adjacent nerve membrane in a wavy manner which is called an impulse. In other words, an impulse is a wave of depolarization. The impulse is fastest in myelinated fibers since the wave of depolarization "jumps" from node to node of Ranvier: this is called *saltatory* conduction.

After depolarization the neuron will pass through three stages in the following order: a) it can no longer depolarize = *absolute refractory period*; b) it can depolarize but with difficulty = *relative refractory period*; c) it returns to its original resting potential and thus can depolarize as easily as it originally did.

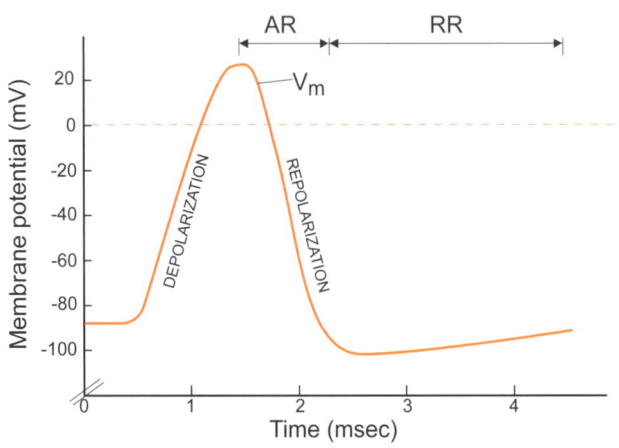

Action Potential: V_m is the membrane voltage or potential, AR is the absolute refractory period, RR is the relative refractory period.

Figure IV.A.5.2: Action potential.

The action potential is an all-or-none event. The magnitude or strength of the action potential is not graded according to the strength of the stimulus. It occurs with the same magnitude each time it occurs, or it does not occur at all.

5.1.3 Action Potential: A Positive Perspective

To better understand the action potential it is useful to take a closer look at what occurs to the positive ions Na$^+$ and K$^+$. To begin with, there are protein channels in the plasma membrane that act like gates which guard the passage of specific ions. Some gates open or close in response to V_m and are thus called *voltage gated channels*.

Once a threshold potential is reached, the voltage gated Na$^+$ channels open allowing the permeability or *conductance* of Na$^+$ to increase. The Na$^+$ ions can now diffuse across their chemical gradient: from an area of high concentration (*outside the membrane*) to an area of low concentration (*inside the membrane*). The Na$^+$ ions will also diffuse across their electrical gradient: from an area of relative positivity (*outside the membrane*) to an area of relative negativity (*inside the membrane*). Thus the inside becomes positive and the membrane is depolarized. Repolarization occurs as the Na$^+$ channels close and the voltage gated K$^+$ channels open. As K$^+$ conductance increases to the outside (where K$^+$ concentration is lowest), the membrane repolarizes to once again become relatively negative on the inside.

5.2 Contractile Cells and Tissues

There are three types of muscle tissue: smooth, skeletal and cardiac. All three types are composed of muscle cells (fibers) that contain myofibrils possessing contractile filaments of actin and myosin.

Smooth muscle:- Smooth muscle cells are spindle shaped and are organized chiefly into sheets or bands of smooth muscle tissue. This tissue is found in blood vessels and other tubular visceral structures (i.e. intestines). Smooth muscles contain both actin and myosin filaments but actin predominates. The filaments are not organized into patterns that give cross striations as in cardiac and skeletal muscle. Filaments course obliquely in the cells and attach to the plasma membrane.

Skeletal muscle:- Skeletal muscle fibers are characterised by their peripherally located multiple nuclei and striated myofibrils. The cross striations are due to the organization and distribution of actin and myosin filaments. These striations are organized within each muscle fiber into fundamental contractile units called sarcomeres which are joined end to end at the Z-lines. The striations in a sarcomere consists of an A-band (d<u>a</u>rk) bordered towards the Z-lines by I-bands (l<u>i</u>ght). The mid-region of the A-band contains a variable light H-band that is bisected by an M-line. The light I-band contains actin filaments that insert into the Z-line. The filaments interdigitate and are cross-bridged in the A-band with myosin filaments forming a hexagonal pattern of one myosin filament surrounded by six actin filaments. In the contraction of a muscle fiber a chemical reaction takes place in the region of the cross bridges causing the actin filaments of the I-bands to move deeper into the A-band thus resulting in a shortening of the I-bands.

Each skeletal muscle fiber is invested with a sarcolemma (= plasmalemma = plasma membrane) that extends into the fiber as numerous small transverse tubes called T-tubules. These tubules ring the myofibrils at the A-I junction and are bounded on each side by terminal cisternae of the endoplasmic (*sarcoplasmic*) reticulum. The sarcoplasmic reticulum is involved in catalysing the chemical reaction between the actin and myosin filaments in the region of the cross bridges.

The thin filaments within a myofibril are composed of actin and to a lesser degree two smaller proteins: *troponin and tropomyosin*. In muscle contraction, calcium is elaborated by the sarcoplasmic reticulum and attaches to a subunit of troponin resulting in the movement of tropomyosin and the uncovering of the active sites for the attachment of actin to the cross bridging heads of myosin. Due to this attachment, ATP in the

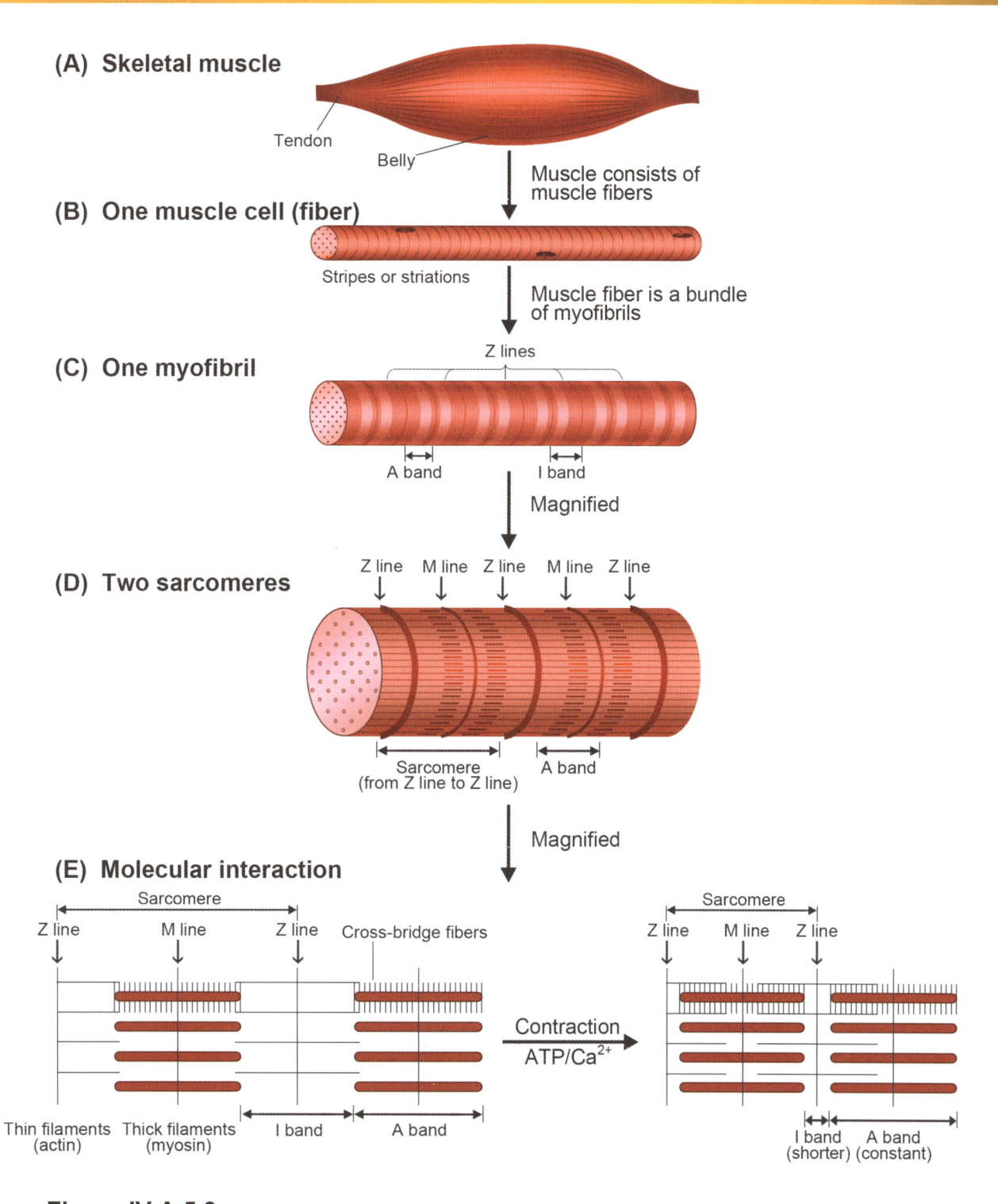

Figure IV.A.5.3: A schematic view of the molecular basis for muscle contraction. Note: the "H zone" is the central portion of an A band and is characterized by the presence of myosin filaments.

myosin head hydrolyses, producing energy, P_i and ADP which results in a bending of the myosin head and a pulling of the actin filament into the A-band. These actin-myosin bridges detach when myosin binds a new ATP molecule and when calcium returns to the terminal cisternae at the conclusion of neural stimulation.

There are three interesting consequences to the preceding:

i) neither actin nor myosin change length during muscle contraction; rather, shortening of the muscle fiber occurs as the filaments slide over each other increasing the area of overlap.

ii) initially a dead person is very stiff (*rigor mortis*) since they can no longer produce the ATP necessary to detach the actin-myosin bridges thus their muscles remain locked in position.

iii) Ca^{2+} is a critical ion both for muscle contraction and for transmitter release from presynaptic neurons.

Cardiac muscle:- Cardiac muscle contains striations and myofibrils that are similar to those of skeletal muscle. It differs from skeletal muscle in several major ways. Cardiac muscle fibers branch and contain centrally located nuclei (characteristically, one nucleus per cell) and large numbers of mitochondria. Individual cardiac muscle cells are attached to each other at their ends by *intercalated disks*. These disks contain several types of membrane junctional complexes, the most important of which is the *gap junction*.

The gap junction electrically couples one cell to its neighbor (= *syncytium*) so that electric depolarization is propagated throughout the heart by cell-to-cell contact rather than by nerve innervation to each cell. The sarcoplasmic reticulum - T-tubule system is arranged differently in cardiac muscle than in skeletal muscle. In cardiac muscle each T-tubule enters at the Z-line and forms a diad with only one terminal cisterna of sarcoplasmic reticulum.

5.3 Epithelial Cells and Tissues

Epithelia have the following characteristics:

1) they cover all body surfaces (i.e. skin, organs, etc.)
2) they are the principal tissues of glands
3) their cells are anchored by a non-living layer (= the *basement membrane*)
4) they lack blood vessels and are thus nourished by diffusion.

Epithelial tissues are classified according to the characteristics of their cells. Tissues with elongated cells are called *columnar*, those with thin flattened cells are *squamous*, and those with cube-like cells are *cuboidal*. They are further classified as **simple** if they have a single layer of cells and **stratified** if they have multiple layers of cells. As examples of the classification, skin is composed of a stratified squamous epithelium while various glands (i.e. thyroid, salivary, etc.) contain a simple cuboidal epithelium. The former epithelium serves to protect against microorganisms, loss of water or heat, while the latter epithelium functions to secrete glandular products.

5.4 Connective Cells and Tissues

Connective tissue connects and joins other body tissue and parts. It also carries substances for processing, nutrition, and waste release. Connective tissue is characterized by the presence of relatively few cells surrounded by an extensive network of material which is intercellular (*between cells*).

The adult connective tissues are: connective tissue proper, cartilage, bone and blood (see *The Circulatory System*, section 7.5). Connective tissue proper is further classified into loose irregular connective tissue and dense irregular connective tissue. These tissues contain cells and a preponderance of intercellular fibers and ground substance.

5.4.1 Loose Irregular Connective Tissue

Loose connective tissue is found in the superficial and deep *fascia*. It is generally considered as the *packaging material* of the body. Fascia helps to bind skin to underlying organs, to fill spaces between muscles, etc. Loose connective tissue contains most of the cell types and all the fiber types found in the other connective tissues. The most common cell types are the fibroblast, macrophage, adipose cell, mast cell, plasma cell and wandering cells from the blood (which include several types of white blood cells).

Fibroblasts contain the organelles that permit them to produce all of the fiber types and the intercellular material.

Macrophages are part of the *reticuloendothelial system* (tissue which predominately destroys foreign particles). They possess large lysosomes containing digestive enzymes which are necessary for the digestion of phagocytosed materials. Mast cells occur mostly along blood vessels and contain granules which contain *heparin* and *histamine*.

Heparin is a compound which prevents blood clotting while histamine is associated with allergic reactions. Plasma cells are part of the immune system in that they produce circulatory antibodies. They contain extensive amounts of rough endoplasmic reticulum (rER). Adipose cells are found in varying quantities, when they predominate, the tissue is called adipose (fat) tissue.

Collagenous reticular and elastic fibers are irregularly distributed in loose connective tissue. **Collagenous fibers** are usually found in bundles and provide **strength** to the tissue. Many different types of collagen are identified on the basis of their molecular structure.

Of the five most common types, collagen type I is the most abundant, being found in dermis, bone, dentine, tendons, organ capsules, fascia and sclera. Type II is located in hyaline and elastic cartilage. Type III is probably the collagenous component of reticular fibers. Type IV is found in a specific part (*the basal lamina*) of basement membranes. Type V is a component of placental basement membranes. **Reticular fibers** are smaller, more delicate fibers that form the basic framework of reticular connective tissue. **Elastic fibers** branch and provide elasticity and support to connective tissue.

Ground substance is the gelatinous material that fills most of the space between the cells and the fibers. It is composed of acid mucopolysaccharides and structural glycoproteins and its properties are important in determining the permeability and consistency of the connective tissue.

5.4.2 Dense Connective Tissue

Dense irregular connective tissue is found in the dermis, periosteum, perichondrium and capsules of some organs. All of the fiber types are present, but collagenous fibers predominate. Dense irregular connective tissue occurs as aponeuroses, ligaments and tendons. In most ligaments and tendons collagenous fibers are most prevalent and are oriented parallel to each other. Fibroblasts are practically the only cell type present.

5.4.3 Cartilage

Cartilage is composed of chondrocytes (= cartilage cells) embedded in an intercellular (= extracellular) matrix, consisting of fibers and an amorphous firm ground substance. In cases of injury, cartilage repairs slowly since it has no direct blood supply. Three types of cartilage are distinguished on the basis of the amount of ground substance and the relative abundance of collagenous and elastic fibers. They are hyaline, elastic and fibrous cartilage.

Hyaline Cartilage is found as costal (rib) cartilage, articular cartilage and cartilage of the nose, larynx, trachea and bronchi. The extracellular matrix consists primarily of collagenous fibers and a ground substance rich in chondromucoprotein, a copolymer of a protein and chondroitin sulphates.

Elastic Cartilage is found in the pinna of the ear, auditory tube and cartilage of the larynx. Elastic fibers predominate and thus provide greater flexibility. Calcification of this type of cartilage is rare.

Fibrous Cartilage occurs in the anchorage of tendons and ligaments, in intervertebral disks, in the symphysis pubis, and in some interarticular disks and in some ligaments. Chondrocytes occur singly or in rows between large bundles of collagenous fibers. Compared with hyaline cartilage, only small amounts of hyaline matrix surround the chondrocytes of fibrous cartilage.

5.4.4 Bone

Bone tissue consists of three **cell types** and an **extracellular matrix** that contains organic and inorganic components. The three cell types are: *osteocytes* which are embedded in cavities (lacunae) within the matrix; *osteoblasts* which synthesize the organic components of the matrix; and *osteoclasts* which help to resorb and remodel bone.

The organic matrix consists of dense collagenous fibers and an osteomucoid substance containing chondroitin sulphate which is important in providing flexibility and tensile strength to bone. The inorganic component is responsible for the *rigidity* of the bone and is composed chiefly of calcium phosphate and calcium carbonate with small amounts of magnesium, fluoride, hydroxide, sulphate and hydroxyapatite.

Compact bone contains haversian systems (osteons), interstitial lamellae and circumferential lamellae. Lamellae are usually a concentric deposit (*circumferential*) of bone matrix around tiny tubes called Haversian canals. Haversian systems are the structural units for bone. Haversian systems consist of extensively branching haversian canals that are oriented chiefly longitudinally in long bones. Each canal contains blood vessels and is surrounded by 8 to 15 concentric lamellae and osteocytes.

Nutrients from blood vessels in the haversian canals pass through canaliculi and lacunae to reach all osteocytes in the system. Volkmann's canals traverse the bone transversely and interconnect the haversian systems. They enter through the outer circumferential lamellae and carry blood vessels and nerves which are continuous with those of the haversian canals and the periosteum. The periosteum is the connective tissue layer which envelopes bone.

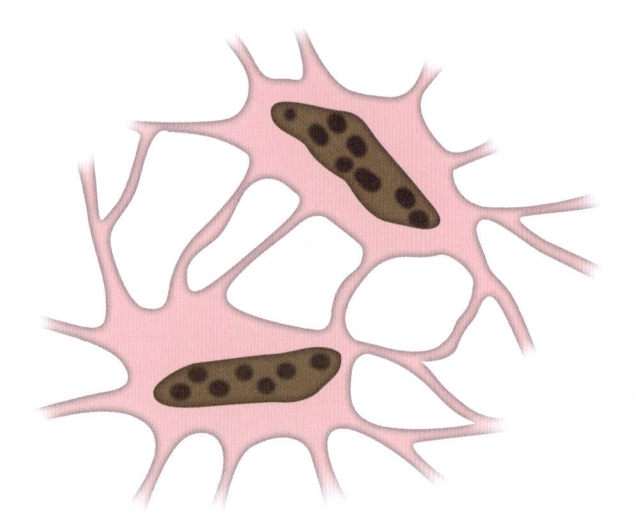

Figure IV.A.5.4: Osteocytes.

BIOLOGY

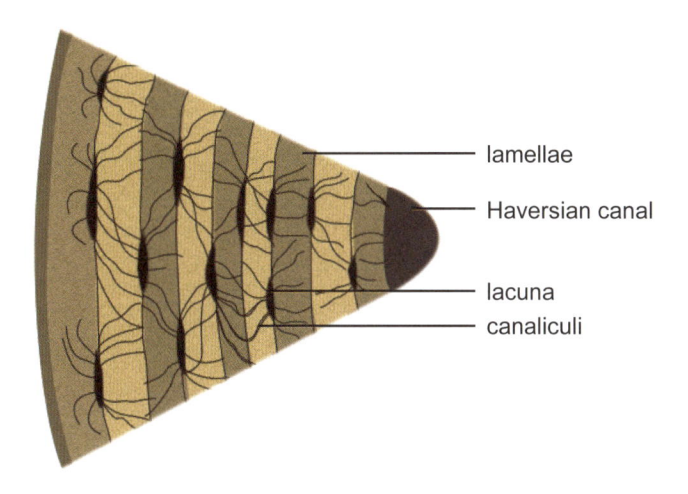

Figure IV.A.5.5: Schematic drawing of part of a haversian system.

Bones are supplied by a loop of blood vessels that enter from the periosteal region, penetrate the cortical bone, and enter the medulla before returning to the periphery of the bone. Long bones are specifically supplied by arteries which pass to the marrow through diaphyseal, metaphyseal and epiphyseal arteries.

Bone undergoes extensive remodelling, and harvesian systems may break down or be resorbed in order that calcium can be made available to other parts of the body. Bone resorption occurs by osteocytes engaging in osteolysis or by osteoclastic activity.

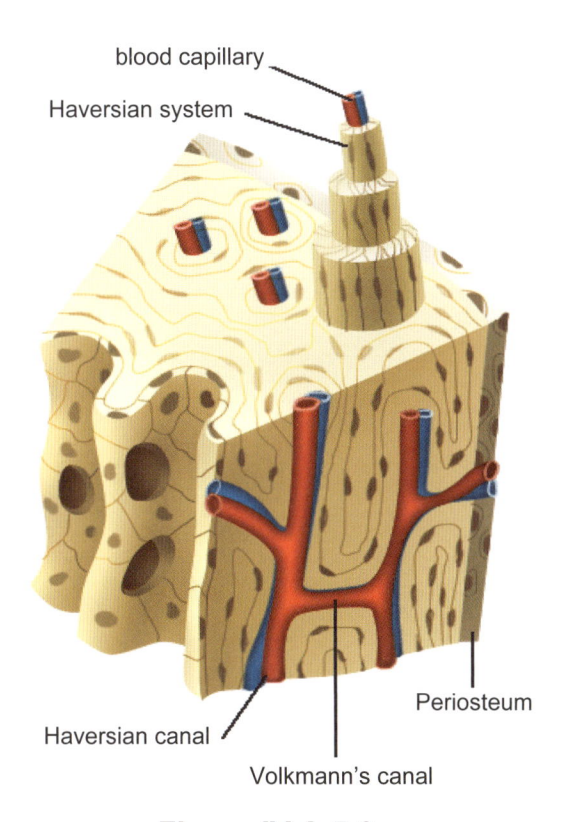

Figure IV.A.5.6
Schematic drawing of the wall of a long bone.

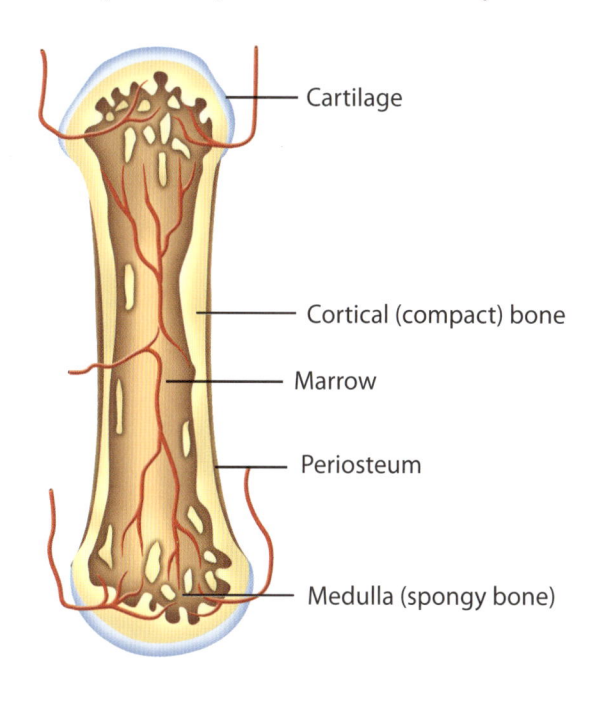

Figure IV.A.5.7
Schematic drawing of adult bone structure.

THE BIOLOGICAL SCIENCES

GOLD NOTES

NERVOUS AND ENDOCRINE SYSTEMS
Chapter 6

Memorize	Understand	Not Required*
Nervous system: basic structure, major functions Basic sensory reception and processing Define: endocrine gland, hormone	* Organization of the nervous system; sensor and effector neurons * Feedback loop, reflex arc: role of spinal cord, brain * Endocrine system: specific chemical control at cell, tissue, and organ level * Cellular mechanisms of hormone action, transport of hormones * Integration with nervous system: feedback control	* Advanced level college info * Memorizing all cranial nerves * Details regarding ear, eye: structure and function * Details regarding endocrine glands: names

GAMSAT-Prep.com

Introduction

The nervous and endocrine systems are composed of a network of highly specialized cells that can communicate information about an organism's surroundings and itself. Thus together, these two systems can process incoming information and then regulate and coordinate responses in other parts of the body.

Additional Resources

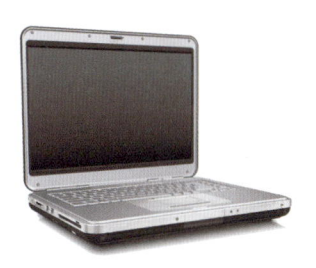

Free Online Q&A + Forum   Video: Online or DVD 2   Flashcards   Special Guest

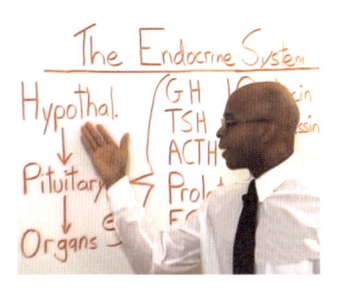

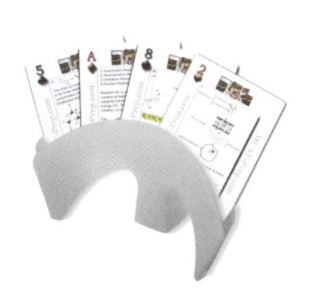

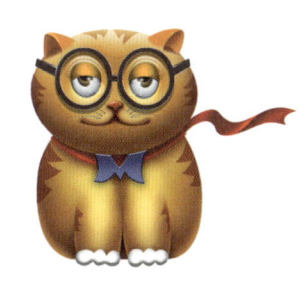

* The real GAMSAT may have advanced level information presented (ie. in a passage) but previous knowledge of said information is not required to answer the questions that would follow. Practice ACER and GS practice GAMSATs can help you clarify this point.

6.1 Organisation of the Vertebrate Nervous System

The role of the nervous system is to control and coordinate body activities in a rapid and precise mode of action. The nervous system is composed of central and peripheral nervous systems.

The **central nervous system** (CNS) is enclosed within the cranium (skull) and vertebral (spinal) canal and consists respectively of the brain and spinal cord. The **peripheral nervous system** (PNS) is outside the bony encasement and is composed of peripheral nerves, which are branches or continuations of the spinal or cranial nerves. The PNS can be divided into the **somatic nervous system** and the **autonomic nervous system** which are *anatomically* a portion of both the central and peripheral nervous systems. As a rule, a collection of nerve cell bodies in the CNS is called a *nucleus* and outside the CNS it is called a *ganglion*.

The spinal cord is a long cylindrical structure whose hollow core is called the *central canal*. The central canal is surrounded by a gray matter which is in turn surrounded by a white matter (the reverse is true for the brain: outer gray matter and inner white matter). Basically, the gray matter consists of the cell bodies of neurons whereas the white matter consists of the nerve fibers (axons and dendrites). There are 31 pairs of spinal nerves each leaving the spinal cord at various levels: 8 cervical (neck), 12 thoracic (chest), 5 lumbar (abdomen), 5 sacral and 1 coccygeal (these latter 6 are from the pelvic region). The lower end of the spinal cord is cone shaped and is called the *conus medullaris*.

The brain can be divided into three main regions: the forebrain which contains the telencephalon and the diencephalon; the midbrain; and the hindbrain which contains the cerebellum, the pons and the medulla. The **brain stem** includes the latter two structures and the midbrain.

The telencephalon is the **cerebral hemispheres** (cerebrum) which contain an outer surface (cortex) of gray matter. Its function is in higher order processes (i.e. learning, memory, emotions, voluntary motor activity, processing sensory input, etc.). For most people, the *l*eft hemisphere specializes in *l*anguage, while the right hemisphere specializes in patterns and spatial relationships. Each hemisphere is subdivided into four lobes: *occipital* which receives input from the optic nerve for vision; *temporal* which receives auditory signals for hearing; *parietal* which receives somatosensory information from the opposite side of the body (= heat, cold, touch, pain, and the sense of body movement); and *frontal* which is involved in problem solving and controls voluntary movements for the opposite side of the body.

BIOLOGY

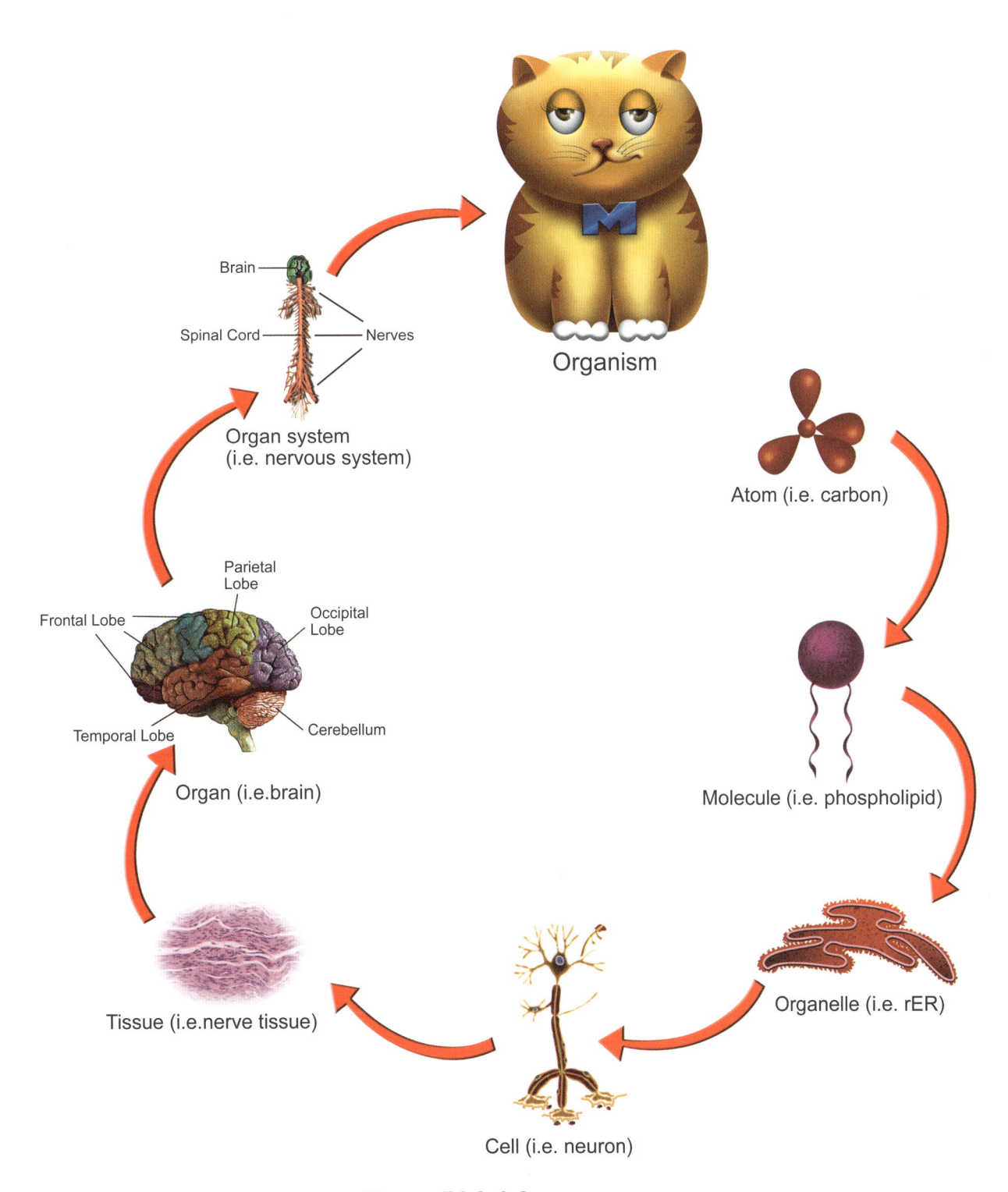

Figure IV.A.6.0: Levels of organization.

The diencephalon contains the **thalamus** which is a relay center for sensory input, and the **hypothalamus** which is crucial for homeostatic controls (heart rate, body temperature, thirst, sex drive, hunger, etc.). Protruding from its base and greatly influenced by the hypothalamus is the **pituitary** which is an endocrine gland. The limbic system, which functions to produce emotions, is composed of the diencephalon and deep structures of the cerebrum (esp. basal ganglia). The **cerebellum** plays an important role in coordination and the control of muscle tone. The **medulla** contains many vital centers (i.e. for breathing, heart rate, arteriole blood pressure, etc.).

There are 12 pairs of cranial nerves which emerge from the base of the brain (esp. the brain stem): *olfactory* (I) for smell; *optic* (II) for vision; *oculomotor* (III), *trochlear* (IV) and *abducens* (VI) for eye movements; *trigeminal* (V) for motor (i.e. *mastication* which is chewing) and sensory activities (i.e. pain, temperature, and pressure for the head and face); *facial* (VII) for taste (sensory) and facial expression (motor); *vestibulo-cochlear* (VIII) for the senses of equilibrium (vestibular branch) and hearing (cochlear branch); *glosso-pharyngeal* (IX) for taste and swallowing; ***vagus (X)*** for speech, swallowing, slowing the heart rate, and many sensory and motor innervations to smooth muscles of the viscera (internal organs) of the thorax and abdomen; *accessory* (XI) for head rotation and shoulder movement; and *hypoglossal* (XII) for tongue movement.

Both the brain and the spinal cord are surrounded by three membranes (= meninges). The outermost covering is called the dura mater, the innermost is called the pia mater (which is in direct contact with nervous tissue), while the middle layer is called the arachnoid mater. {DAP = **d**ura - **a**rachnoid - **p**ia, repectively, from out to in}

6.1.1 The Sensory Receptors

The sensory receptors include any type of nerve ending in the body that can be stimulated by some physical or chemical stimulus either outside or within the body. These receptors include the rods and cones of the eye, the cochlear nerve endings of the ear, the taste endings of the mouth, the olfactory endings in the nose, sensory nerve endings in the skin, etc. Afferent neurons carry sense signals to the central nervous system.

6.1.2 The Effector Receptors

These include every organ that can be stimulated by nerve impulses. An important effetor system is skeletal muscle. Smooth muscles of the body and the glandular cells are among the important effector organs. Efferent neurons carry motor signals from the CNS to effector receptors.

6.1.3 Reflex Arc

One basic means by which the nervous system controls the functions in the body is the reflex arc, in which a stimulus excites a receptor, appropriate impulses are transmitted into the CNS where various nervous reactions take place, and then appropriate effector impulses are transmitted to an effector organ to cause a reflex effect (i.e. removal of one's hand from a hot object, the knee jerk reflex, etc.). The preceding can be processed at the level of the spinal cord.

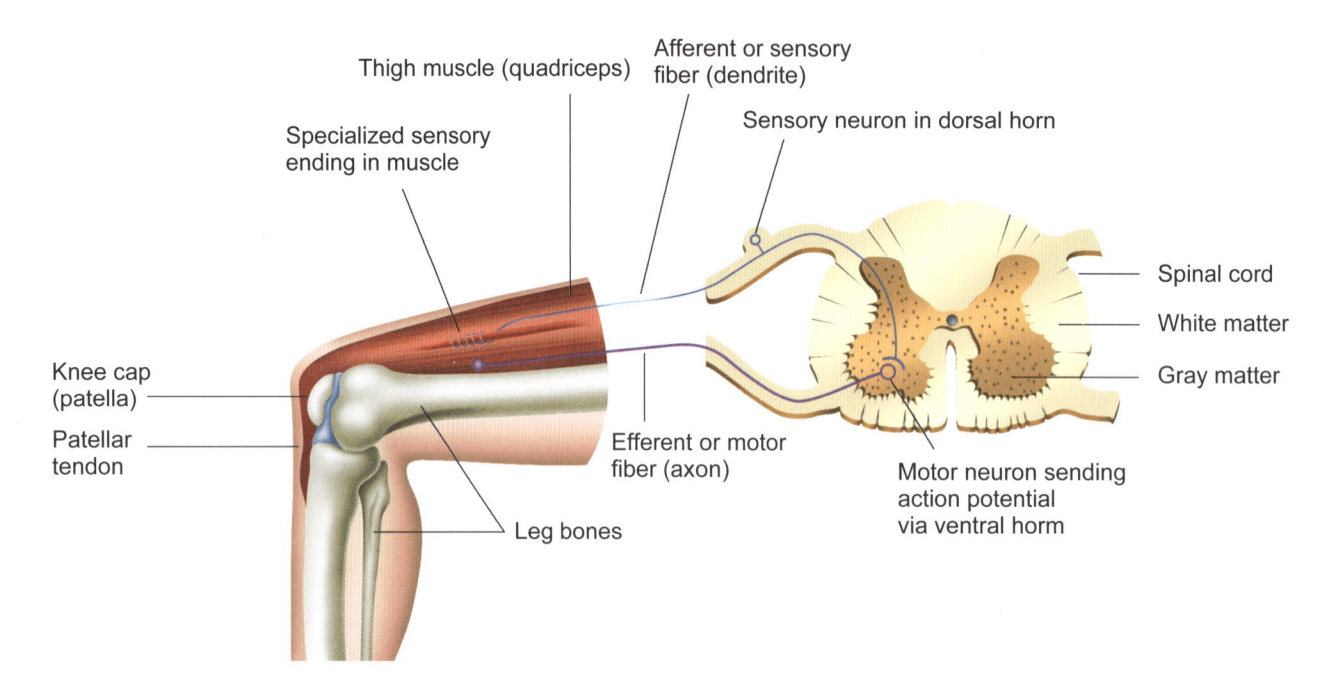

Figure IV.A.6.1: Schematic representation of the basis of the knee jerk reflex.

6.1.4 Autonomic Nervous System

While the Somatic Nervous System controls voluntary activities (i.e. innervates skeletal muscle), the Autonomic Nervous System (ANS) controls involuntary activities. The ANS consists of two components which often antagonize each other: the sympathetic and parasympathetic nervous systems.

The **Sympathetic Nervous System** originates in neurons located in the lateral horns of the gray matter of the spinal cord. Nerve fibers pass by way of anterior (ventral) nerve roots first into the spinal nerves and then immediately into the sympathetic chain. From here fiber pathways are transmitted to all portions of the body, especially to the different visceral organs and to the blood vessels.

This division of the nervous system is crucial in the "fight, fright, or flight" responses (i.e. pupillary dilation, increase in breathing and heart rates, increase of blood flow to skeletal muscle, etc.).

Parasympathetic Nervous System: The parasympathetic fibers pass mainly through the *vagus nerves*, though a few fibers pass through several of the other cranial nerves and through the anterior roots of the sacral segments of the spinal cord. Parasympathetic fibers do not spread as extensively through the body as do sympathetic fibers, but they do innervate some of the thoracic and abdominal organs, as well as the pupillary sphincter and ciliary muscles of the eye and the salivary glands.

This division of the nervous system is crucial for "vegetative" responses (i.e. pupillary constriction, decrease in breathing and heart rates, increase in blood flow to the gastro-intestinal tract, etc.).

6.1.5 Autonomic Nerve Fibers

The nerve fibers from the ANS are primarily motor fibers. Unlike the motor pathways of the somatic nervous system, which usually include a single neuron between the CNS and an effector, those of the ANS involve *two* neurons. The first neuron has its cell body in the brain or spinal cord but its axon (= *preganglionic fiber*) extends outside of the CNS. The axon synapses with the cell body of a second neuron in an autonomic ganglion (*recall: a ganglion is a collection of nerve cell bodies outside the CNS*). The axon of the second neuron (= *postganglionic fiber*) extends to a visceral effector.

The sympathetic ganglia form chains which, for example, may extend longitudinally along each side of the vertebral column. Conversely, the parasympathetic ganglia are located *near* or *within* various visceral organs (i.e. bladder, intestine, etc.) thus requiring relatively short postganglionic fibers.

Both divisions of the ANS secrete *acetylcholine* from their preganglionic fibers. Most sympathetic postganglionic fibers secrete *norepinephrine* (= nor*adren*alin), and for this reason they are called **adren**ergic fibers. The parasympathetic postganglionic fibers secrete acetyl**choline** and are called **cholin**ergic fibers.

6.2 Sensory Reception and Processing

Each modality of sensation is detected by a particular nerve ending. The most common nerve ending is the free nerve ending. Different types of free nerve endings result in different types of sensations such as pain, warmth, pressure, touch, etc. In addition to free nerve endings, skin contains a number of specialized endings that are adapted to respond to some specific type of physical stimulus.

Sensory endings deep in the body are capable of detecting *proprioceptive sensations* such as joint receptors, which detect the degree of angulation of a joint, Golgi tendon organs which detect the degree of tension in the tendons, and muscle spindles which detect the degree of stretch of a muscle fiber.

6.2.1 Olfaction

Olfaction (the sense of smell) is perceived by the brain following the stimulation of the olfactory epithelium located in the nostrils. The olfactory epithelium contain large numbers of neurons with chemoreceptors called *olfactory cells* which are responsible for the detection of different types of smell. It is believed that there might be seven or more primary sensations of smell which combine to give various types of smell that we perceive in life.

6.2.2 Taste

Taste buds in combination with olfaction give humans the taste sensation. Taste buds are primarily located on the surface of the tongue with smaller numbers found in the roof of the mouth and the walls of the pharynx (throat). Taste buds contain chemoreceptors which are activated once the chemical is dissolved in saliva which is secreted by the salivary glands.

Four different types of taste buds are known to exist, each of these responding principally to saltiness, sweetness, sourness and bitterness.

When a stimulus is received by either a taste bud or an olfactory cell for the second time, the intensity of the response is diminished. This is called *sensory adaptation*.

BIOLOGY

6.2.3 Ears: Structure and Function

Ears function in both hearing and balance. The external ear is composed of the external cartilaginous portion, the pinna or *auricle*, and the external auditory meatus or canal. The external auditory meatus connects the auricle and the middle ear or *tympanic cavity*. The tympanic cavity is bordered on the outside by the tympanic membrane, and inside the air-filled cavity are the <u>auditory ossicles</u> - the *malleus* (hammer), *incus* (anvil), and *stapes* (stirrup). The stapes is held by ligaments to a part of inner ear called the *oval window*.

The inner ear or *labyrinth* consists of an osseous labyrinth containing a membranous labyrinth. Three semicircular canals, which are oriented at right angles to each other, and the cochlea are the important structures of the inner ear. The semicircular canals function in providing a sense of equilibrium (balance).

The eustachian tube connects the middle ear to the pharynx. This tube is important in maintaining equal pressure on both sides of the tympanic membrane.

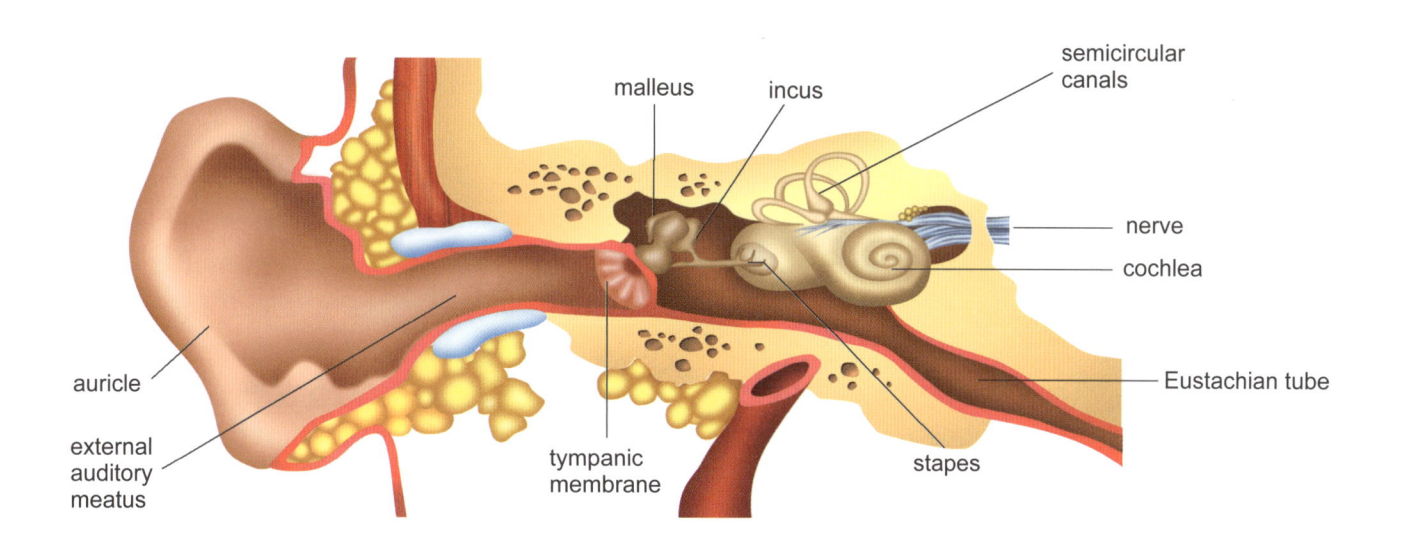

Figure IV.A.6.2: Structure of the external, middle and inner ear.

THE BIOLOGICAL SCIENCES BIO-69

Mechanism of hearing: Sound is caused by compression of waves that travel through the air. Each compression wave is funneled by the external ear to strike the tympanic membrane (ear drum). Thus the sound vibrations are transmitted through the osseous system which consists of three tiny bones (the malleus, incus, and stapes) into the cochlea at the oval window. The sound waves then travel through the lymph of the cochlea and stimulate the hairy cells found in the **basilar membrane** which is called the *organ of Corti*. From here the auditory nerves carry the impulses to the auditory area of the brain (*temporal lobe*) where it is interpreted as sound.

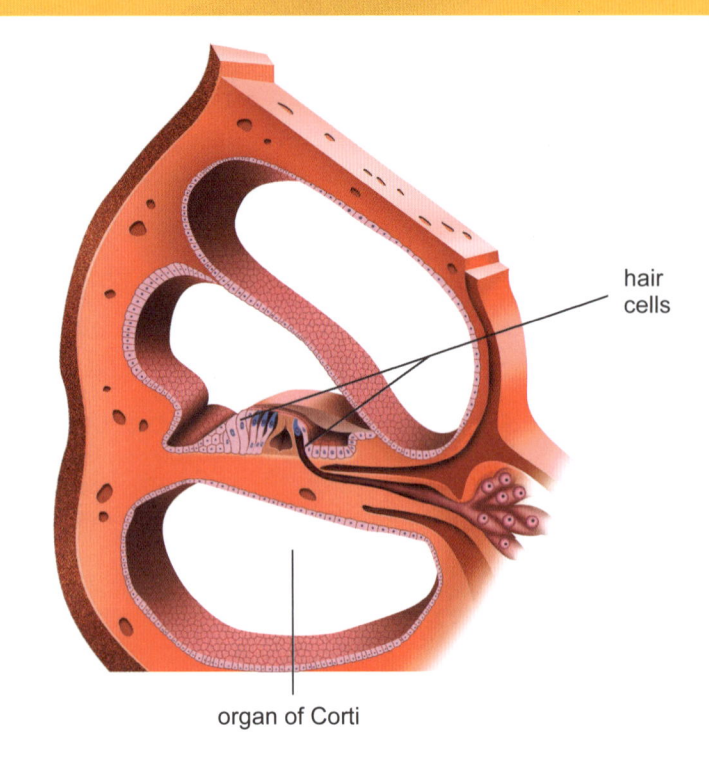

Figure IV.A.6.3: Cross-section of the cochlea.

6.2.4 Vision: Eye Structure and Function

The eyeball consists of three layers: i) an outer fibrous tunic composed of the sclera and cornea; ii) a vascular coat (*uvea*) of choroid, the ciliary body and iris; and iii) the retina formed of pigment and sensory (nervous) layers. The anterior chamber lies between the cornea anteriorly (in front) and the iris and pupil posteriorly (behind); the posterior chamber lies between the iris anteriorly and the ciliary processes and the lens posteriorly.

The cornea constitutes the anterior one sixth of the eye. The sclera forms the posterior five sixths of the fibrous tunic and is composed of dense fibrous connective tissue. The choroid layer consists of vascular loose connective tissue. The lens can focus light on the retina by the contraction or relaxation of muscles in the ciliary body which transmit tension along *suspensory ligaments* to the lens. The iris helps to control the intensity of light impinging on the retina by alternating the diameter of the pupil.

The retina is divisible into ten layers. Layers two to five contain the rod and cone receptors of the light pathway.

BIOLOGY

Rods and Cones: The light sensitive receptors (*photoreceptors*) of the retina are millions of minute cells called rods and cones. The rods ("*night vision*") distinguish only the black and white aspects of an image while the cones ("*day vision*") are capable of distinguishing three colors: red, green and blue. From different combinations of these three colors, all colors can be seen.

Photoreceptors contain photosensitive pigments. For example, rods contain the membrane protein *rhodopsin* which is covalently linked to a form of vitamin A. Light causes an isomerization of the pigment which can affect Na^+ channels in a manner as to start an action potential.

The central portion of the retina which is called the *fovea centralis* has only cones, which allows this portion to have very sharp vision, while the peripheral areas, which contain progressively more and more rods, have progressively more diffuse vision.

Each point of the retina connects with a discrete point in the visual cortex which is in the back of the brain (i.e. the *occipital lobe*). The image that is formed on the retina is upside down and reversed from left to right. This information leaves the eye via the optic nerve en route to the visual cortex which corrects the image.

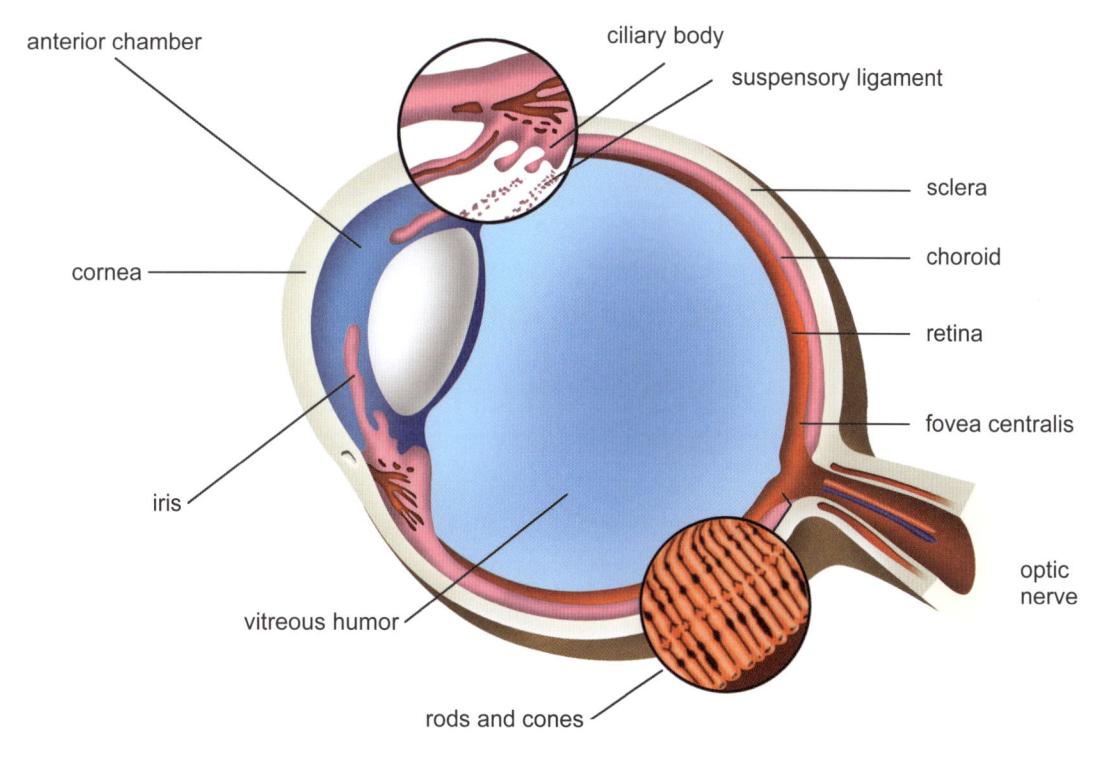

Figure IV.A.6.4: Structure of the eye.

Defects of vision

1. **Myopia** (short-sighted or nearsighted): In this condition, an image is formed in front of the retina because the lens converges light too much since the eyeballs are long. A diverging (concave) lens helps focus the image on the retina and it is used for the correction of myopia.

2. **Hyperopia** (long-sighted or farsighted): In this condition, an image is formed behind the retina since the eyeballs are too short. A converging (convex) lens helps focus the image on the retina.

3. **Astigmatism**: In this condition, the curvatures of either the cornea or the lens are different at different angles. A cylindrical lens helps to improve this condition.

4. **Presbyopia**: This condition is characterized by the inability to focus (especially objects which are closer). This condition, which is often seen in the elderly, is corrected by using a converging lens.

6.3 Endocrine Systems

The endocrine system is the set of glands, tissues and cells that secrete hormones directly into bodily fluids (usu. blood). The hormones are transported by the blood system, sometimes bound to plasma proteins, en route to having an effect on the cells of a target organ. Hormones control many of the body's functions. Hormones function in three major ways:

1. By controlling transport of substances through cell membranes
2. By controlling the activity of some of the specific genes, which in turn determine the formation of specific enzymes
3. By controlling directly some metabolic systems of cells.

Steroid hormones can diffuse across the plasma membrane thus they tend to have a direct intracellular effect (i.e. on DNA; ORG 12.4.1). Non-steroid hormones do not diffuse across the membrane. They tend to bind plasma membrane receptors which increase intracellular *cyclic AMP* concentration which, in turn, brings about cellular changes which are recognized as the hormone's actions.

Of the following hormones, if there is no mention as to its chemical nature, then it is a non-steroidal hormone (i.e. protein, polypeptide, etc.).

6.3.1 Pituitary Hormones

The **pituitary gland** secretes hormones that regulate a wide variety of functions in the body. This gland is divided into two major divisions: the *anterior* and the *posterior* pituitary gland. Six hormones are secreted by the anterior pituitary gland whereas two hormones are secreted by the posterior gland. The **hypothalamus** influences the secretion of hormones from both parts of the pituitary in different ways: i) it secretes specific *releasing factors* into special blood vessels (*a portal system*) which carries these factors (hormones) which affect the cells in the anterior pituitary; ii) the hypothalamus contains neurosecretory cells that secrete their products (esp. the two hormones oxytocin and vasopressin) directly <u>into</u> the posterior pituitary where they can be released.

The hormones secreted by the anterior pituitary gland are as follows:

1. Growth hormone (GH)
2. Thyroid Stimulating Hormone (TSH)
3. Adrenocorticotropic hormone (ACTH)
4. Prolactin
5. Follicle Stimulating Hormone (FSH) or Interstitial Cell Stimulating Hormone (ICSH)
6. Luteinizing Hormone (LH)

[N.B. these latter two hormones will be discussed in the section on "Reproduction"]

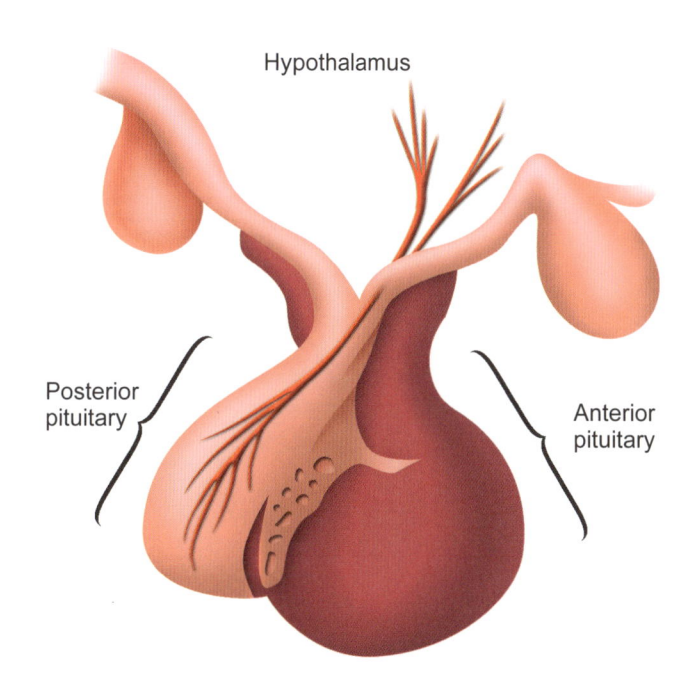

Figure IV.A.6.5: The pituitary gland.

The hormones secreted by the posterior pituitary are:

1. Vasopressin or Anti-diuretic Hormone (ADH)
2. Oxytocin

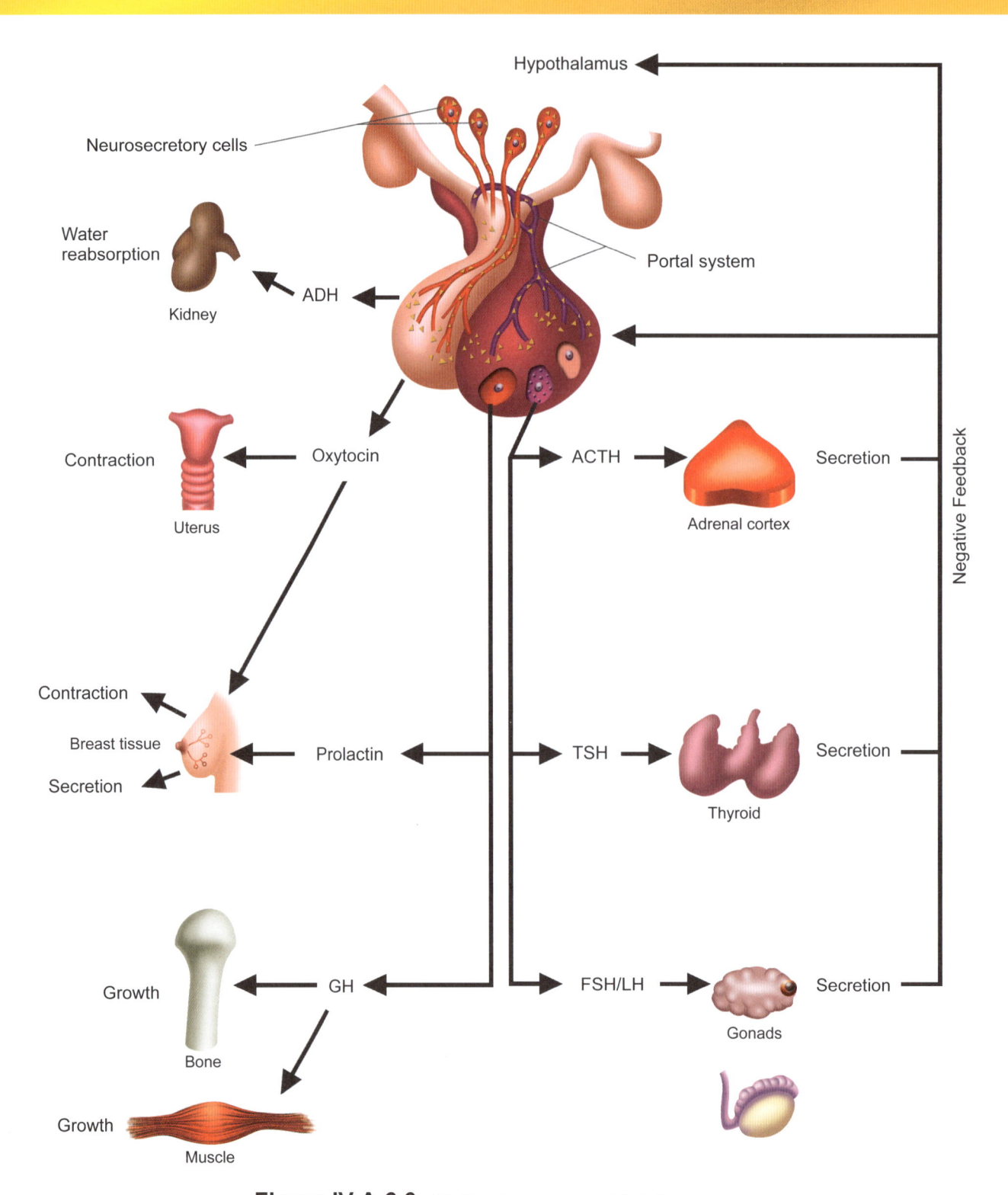

Figure IV.A.6.6: Pituitary hormones and their target organs.

Growth Hormone causes growth of the body. It causes enlargement and proliferation of cells in all parts of the body. Ultimately, the epiphyses of the long bones unite with the shaft of the bones. After adolescence growth hormone continues to be secreted lower than the pre-adolescent rate. Though most of the growth in the body stops at this stage primarily because of the loss of growth potential in long bones following the fusion of epiphyses with the shaft, the metabolic roles of the growth hormone continues, such as enhancement of protein synthesis, increasing the blood glucose concentration, etc.

Abnormal increase in the secretion of growth hormone at a young age results in a condition called gigantism, while a reduction in the production of growth hormone leads to dwarfism.

Thyroid Stimulating Hormone stimulates the thyroid gland. The hormones produced by the thyroid gland (*thyroxine*: T_4, *triiodothyronine*: T_3) contain four and three iodine atoms, respectively. They increase the basal metabolic rate of the body (BMR). Therefore, indirectly, TSH increases the overall rate of metabolism of the body.

Adrenocorticotropic hormone strongly stimulates the production of cortisol by the adrenal cortex, and it also stimulates the production of the other adrenocortical hormones, but to a lesser extent.

Prolactin plays an important role in the development of the breast during pregnancy and promotes milk secretion after childbirth.

Antidiuretic hormone enhances the rate of water reabsorption from the renal tubules. ADH also constricts the arterioles and causes a rise in arterial pressure and hence it is also called *vasopressin*.

Oxytocin causes contraction of the uterus and to a lesser extent the other smooth muscles of the body. It also stimulates the myoepithelial cells of the breast in a manner that makes the milk flow into the ducts. This is termed milk ejection or milk *let-down*.

6.3.2 Adrenocortical Hormones

On the top of each kidney lies an adrenal gland which contains an inner region (*medulla*) and an outer region (*cortex*). The adrenal cortex secretes three different types of steroid hormones that are similar chemically but vary widely in a physiological manner.

These are:
1. Mineralocorticoids - e.g., Aldosterone
2. Glucocorticoids - e.g., Cortisol, Cortisone
3. Sex Hormones e.g., Androgens, Estrogens

Mineralocorticoids - Aldosterone

The mineralocorticoids influence the electrolyte balance of the body. Aldosterone is a mineralocorticoid which is secreted and then enhances sodium transport from the renal tubules into the peritubular fluids, and at the same time enhances potassium transport from the peritubular fluids into the tubules. In other words, aldosterone causes conservation of sodium in the body and excretion of potassium in the urine. As a result of sodium retention, there is an increased passive reabsorption of chloride ions and water from the tubules.

Glucocorticoids - Cortisol

Several different glucocorticoids are secreted by the adrenal cortex, but almost all of the glucocorticoid activity is caused by cortisol, also called hydrocortisone. Glucocorticoids affect the metabolism of carbohydrates, proteins and lipids. It causes an increase in the blood concentration of glucose by decreasing the uptake of glucose into cells. It causes degradation of proteins and causes increased use of fat for energy.

Sex hormones

Androgens (i.e. testosterone) are the masculinizing hormones in the body. They are responsible for the development of the secondary sexual characteristics in a male (i.e. increased body hair). On the contrary estrogens have a feminizing effect in the body and they are responsible for the development of the secondary sexual characteristics in a female (i.e. breast development). The proceeding hormones supplement secretions from the gonads which will be discussed later (see "*Reproduction*").

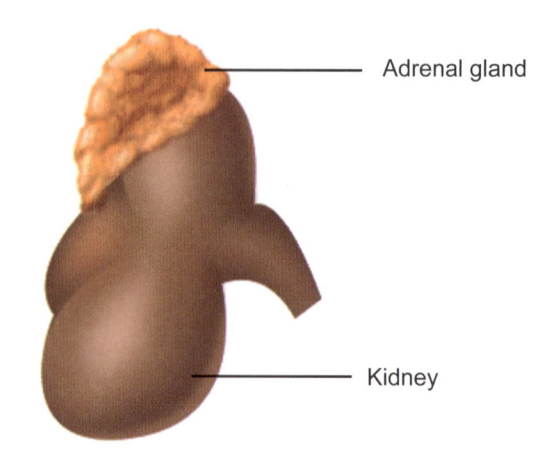

Figure IV.A.6.7: The adrenal gland sits on top of the kidney.

The Adrenal Medulla

The <u>adrenal medulla</u> synthesizes epinephrine (= *adrenal*ine) and norepinephrine which: i) are non-steroidal stimulants of the sympathetic nervous system and ii) raise blood glucose concentrations.

6.3.3 Thyroid Hormones

The thyroid gland is located anteriorly in the neck and is composed of follicles lined with thyroid glandular cells. These cells secrete a glycoprotein called *thyroglobulin*. Thyroxine, which is a thyroid hormone, is formed within the thyroglobulin molecule. The rate of synthesis of thyroid hormone is influenced by TSH from the pituitary.

Once thyroid hormones have been released into the blood stream they combine with several different plasma proteins. Then they are released into the cells from the blood stream. They increase the rate of synthesis of proteins in most cells. They also increase the size and numbers of mitochondria and these in turn increase the rate of production of ATP, which is a factor that promotes <u>cellular metabolism</u>.

<u>Hyperthyroidism</u> is an excess of thyroid hormone secretion above that needed for normal function. Basically, an increased rate of metabolism throughout the body is observed.

<u>Hypothyroidism</u> is an inadequate amount of thyroid hormone secreted into the blood stream. Generally it slows down the metabolic rate and enhances the collection of mucinous fluid in the tissue spaces, creating an edematous (fluid filled) state called myxedema.

The thyroid and parathyroid glands affect blood calcium concentration in different ways. The thyroid produces *calcitonin* which inhibits osteoclast activity and stimulates osteoblasts to form bone tissue; thus blood [Ca^{2+}] decreases. The parathyroid glands produce parathormone (= parathyroid hormone = PTH), which stimulates osteoclasts to break down bone, thus raising [Ca^{2+}] and [PO_4^{3-}] in the blood.

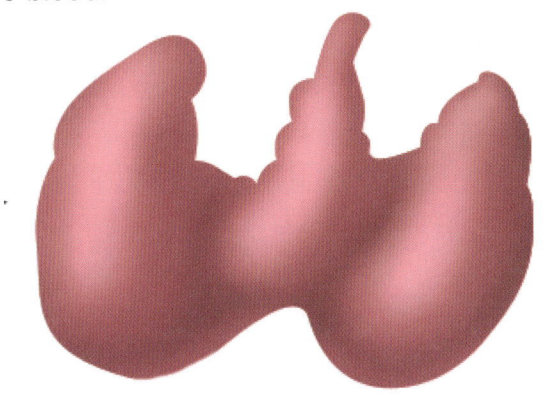

Figure IV.A.6.8: The thyroid gland.

6.3.4 Pancreatic Hormones

The pancreas contains clusters of cells (= *islets of Langerhans*) closely associated with blood vessels. The islets of Langerhans contain alpha cells which secrete *glucagon* and beta cells which secrete *insulin*. Glucagon increases blood glucose concentration by promoting the following events in the liver: the conversion of glycogen to glucose (*glycogenolysis*) and the production of glucose from amino acids (*gluconeogenesis*). Insulin decreases blood glucose by increasing cellular uptake of glucose. A deficiency in insulin results in *diabetes mellitus*.

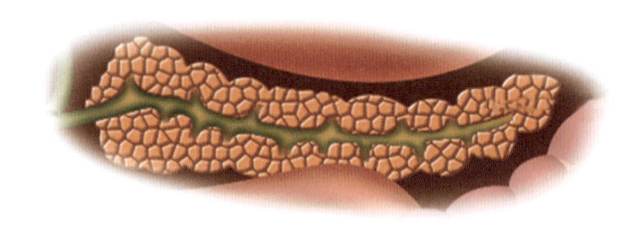

Figure IV.A.6.9: The pancreas.

6.3.5 Kidney Hormones

The kidney produces and secretes *renin, erythropoietin* and it helps in the activation of vitamin D. Renin increases water resorption and blood pressure through the activation of the **Renin-Angiotensin System** which produces angiotensin II from angiotensin I. Angiotensin II acts on the adrenal cortex to increase the synthesis and release of aldosterone and it constricts blood vessels. Erythropoietin increases the production of erythrocytes by acting on red bone marrow. Vitamin D is a steroid which is critical for the proper absorption of calcium from the small intestine; thus it is essential for the normal growth and development of bone and teeth. Vitamin D can either be ingested or produced from a precursor by the activity of ultraviolet light on skin cells. It must be further activated in the liver and kidney by hydroxylation.

BIOLOGY

6.3.6 A Negative Feedback Loop

In order to maintain the internal environment of the body in equilibrium (= *homeostasis*), our hormones engage in various negative feedback loops.

For example, if the body is exposed to extreme cold, the hypothalamus will activate systems to conserve heat (see *Skin as an Organ System*, BIO 13.1) and to produce heat. Heat production can be attained by increasing the basal metabolic rate. To achieve this, the hypothalamus secretes a releasing factor (thyrotropin releasing factor - TRF) which stimulates the anterior pituitary to secrete TSH. Thus the thyroid gland is stimulated to secrete the thyroid hormones.

Body temperature begins to return to normal. The high levels of circulating thyroid hormones begin to *inhibit* the production of TRF and TSH (= *negative feedback*) which in turn ensures the reduction in the levels of the thyroid hormones. Thus homeostasis is maintained.

6.3.7 A Positive Feedback Loop

As opposed to negative feedback, a positive feedback loop is where the body senses a change and activates mechanisms that accelerate or increase that change. Occasionally this may help homeostasis by working in conjunction with a larger negative feedback loop, but unfortunately it often produces the opposite effect and can be life-threatening.

An example of a beneficial positive feedback loop is seen in childbirth, where stretching of the uterus triggers the secretion of oxytocin (BIO 6.3.1), which stimulates uterine contractions and speeds up labor. Of course, once the baby is out of the mother's body, the loop is broken.

Often, however, positive feedback produces the very opposite of homeostasis: a rapid loss of internal stability with potentially fatal consequences. For example, most human deaths from SARS and the bird flu (H5N1) epidemic were caused by a "cytokine storm" which is a positive feedback loop between immune cells and cytokines (signalling molecules similar to hormones). Thus, in many cases, it is the body's exaggerated response to infection that is the cause of death rather than the direct action of the original infecting agent. Many diseases involve dangerous positive feedback loops.

GOLD NOTES

THE CIRCULATORY SYSTEM
Chapter 7

Memorize

Circ. and lymphatic systems: basic structures and functions
Composition of blood, lymph, purpose of lymph nodes
RBC production and destruction; spleen, bone marrow

Understand

* Circ: structure/function; 4 chambered heart: systolic/diastolic pressure
* Oxygen transport; hemoglobin, oxygen content/affinity
* Substances transported by blood, lymph
* Source of lymph: diffusion from capillaries by differential pressure

Not Required*

* Advanced level college info
* Memorizing names of small to medium arteries, veins
* Memorizing Starling's equation

GAMSAT-Prep.com

Introduction

The circulatory system is concerned with the movement of nutrients, gases and wastes to and from cells. The circulatory or cardiovascular system (closed) distributes blood while the lymphatic system (open) distributes lymph.

Additional Resources

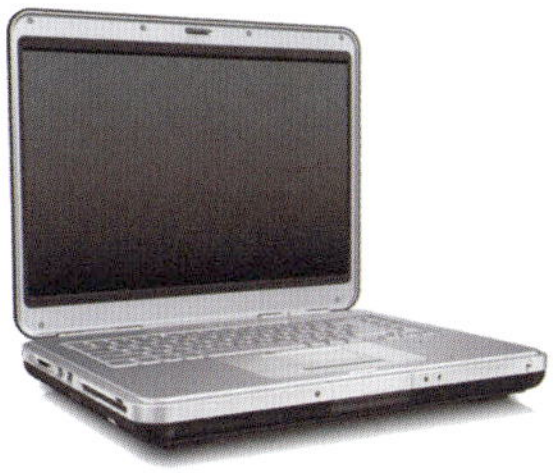

Free Online Q&A + Forum

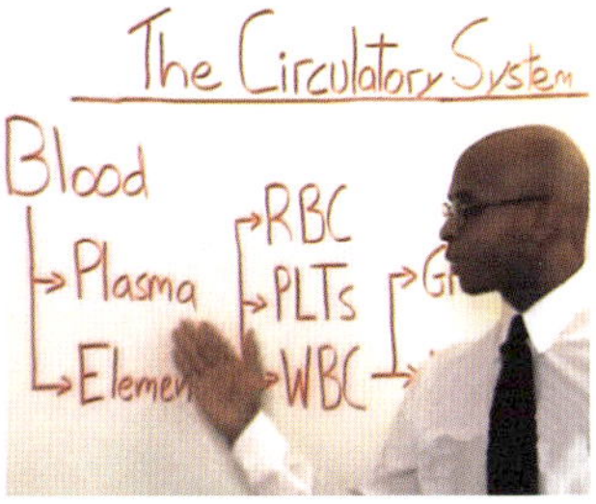

Video: Online or DVD 3

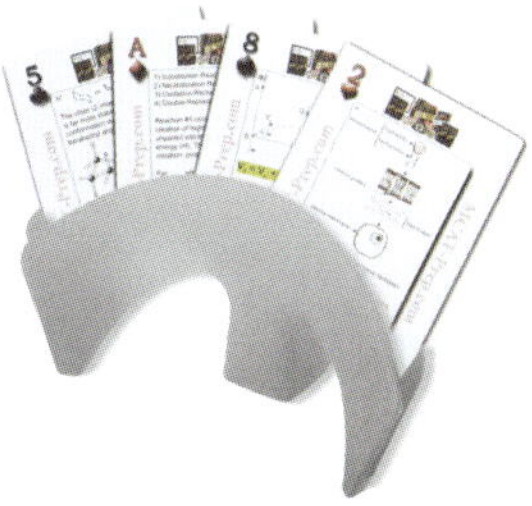

Flashcards

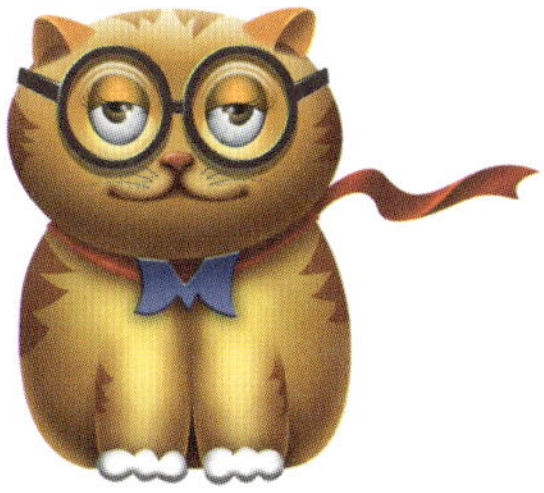

Special Guest

THE BIOLOGICAL SCIENCES BIO-81

* The real GAMSAT may have advanced level information presented (ie. in a passage) but previous knowledge of said information is not required to answer the questions that would follow. Practice ACER and GS practice GAMSATs can help you clarify this point.

7.1 Generalities

The circulatory system is composed of the heart, blood, and blood vessels. The heart (which acts like a pump) and its blood vessels (which act like a closed system of ducts) are called the *cardiovascular system* which moves the blood throughout the body. The following represents some important functions of blood within the circulatory system.

* It transports:
   - hormones from endocrine glands to target tissues
   - molecules and cells which are components of the immune system
   - nutrients from the digestive tract (usu. to the liver)
   - oxygen from the respiratory system to body cells
   - waste from the body cells to the respiratory and excretory systems.

* It aids in temperature control (*thermoregulation*) by:
   - distributing heat from skeletal muscle and other active organs to the rest of the body
   - being directed to or away from the skin depending on whether or not the body wants to release or conserve heat, respectively.

7.2 The Heart

The heart is a muscular, cone-shaped organ about the size of a fist. The heart contains four chambers: two thick muscular walled *ventricles* and two thinner walled *atria*. An inner wall or *septum* separates the heart (and therefore the preceding chambers) into left and right sides. The atria contract or *pump* blood more or less simultaneously and so do the ventricles.

Deoxygenated blood returning to the heart from all body tissues except the lungs (= *systemic circulation*) enters the right atrium through large veins (= *venae cavae*). The blood is then pumped into the right ventricle through the tricuspid valve (which is one of

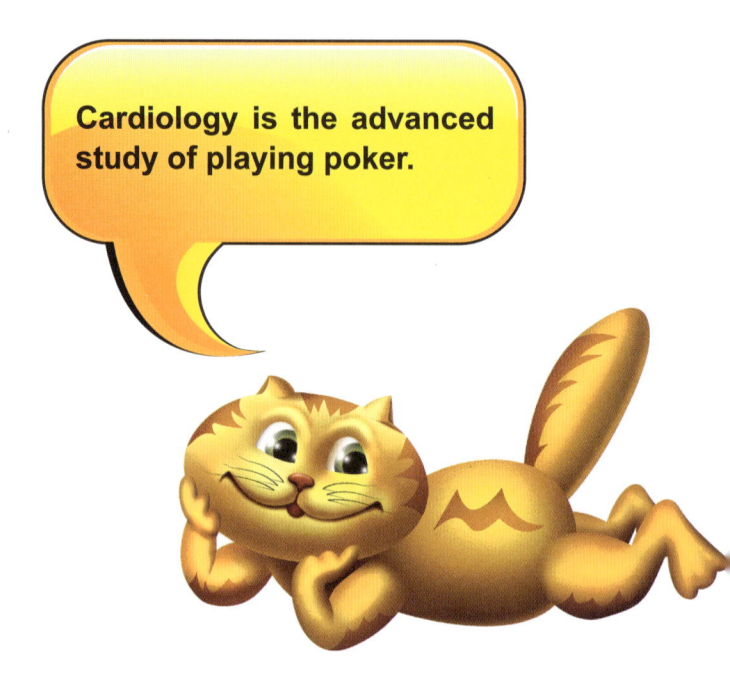

Cardiology is the advanced study of playing poker.

many one-way valves in the cardiovascular system). Next the blood is pumped to the lungs (= *pulmonary circulation*) through semilunar valves and pulmonary arteries {remember: blood in arteries goes away from the heart}.

The blood loses CO_2 and is **oxygenated** in the lungs and returns through pulmonary veins to the left atrium. Now the blood is pumped through the mitral (= bicuspid) valve into the largest chamber of the heart: the left ventricle. This ventricle's task is to return blood into the systemic circulation by pumping into a huge artery: the *aorta* (its valve is the aortic valve).

The mitral (= bicuspid = 2 leaflets) and tricuspid (tri = 3 leaflets) valves are prevented from everting into the atria by strong fibrous cords (*chordae tendineae*) which are attached to small mounds of muscle (*papillary muscles*) in their respective ventricles. A major cause of heart murmurs is the inadequate functioning of these valves.

7.3 Blood Vessels

Blood vessels include arteries, arterioles, capillaries, venules and veins. Whereas arteries tend to have smooth muscular walls and contain blood at high pressure, veins have thinner walls and lower blood pressures. The wall of a blood vessel is composed of an outer adventitia, an inner intima and a *m*iddle *m*uscle layer, the media.

Oxygenated blood entering the systemic circulation must get to all the body's tissues. The aorta must divide into smaller and smaller arteries (small artery = **arteriole**) in order to get to the level of the capillary which i) is the smallest blood vessel; ii) often forms branching networks called *capillary beds*; and iii) is the level at which the exchange of wastes and gases (i.e. O_2 and CO_2) occurs by diffusion. Next the newly deoxygenated blood enters very small veins (= **venules**) and then into larger and larger veins until the blood enters the venae cavae and then the right atrium. There are two venae cavae: one drains blood from the upper body while the other drains blood from the lower body (*superior* and *inferior* venae cavae, respectively). Coronary arteries branch off the aorta to supply the heart muscle.

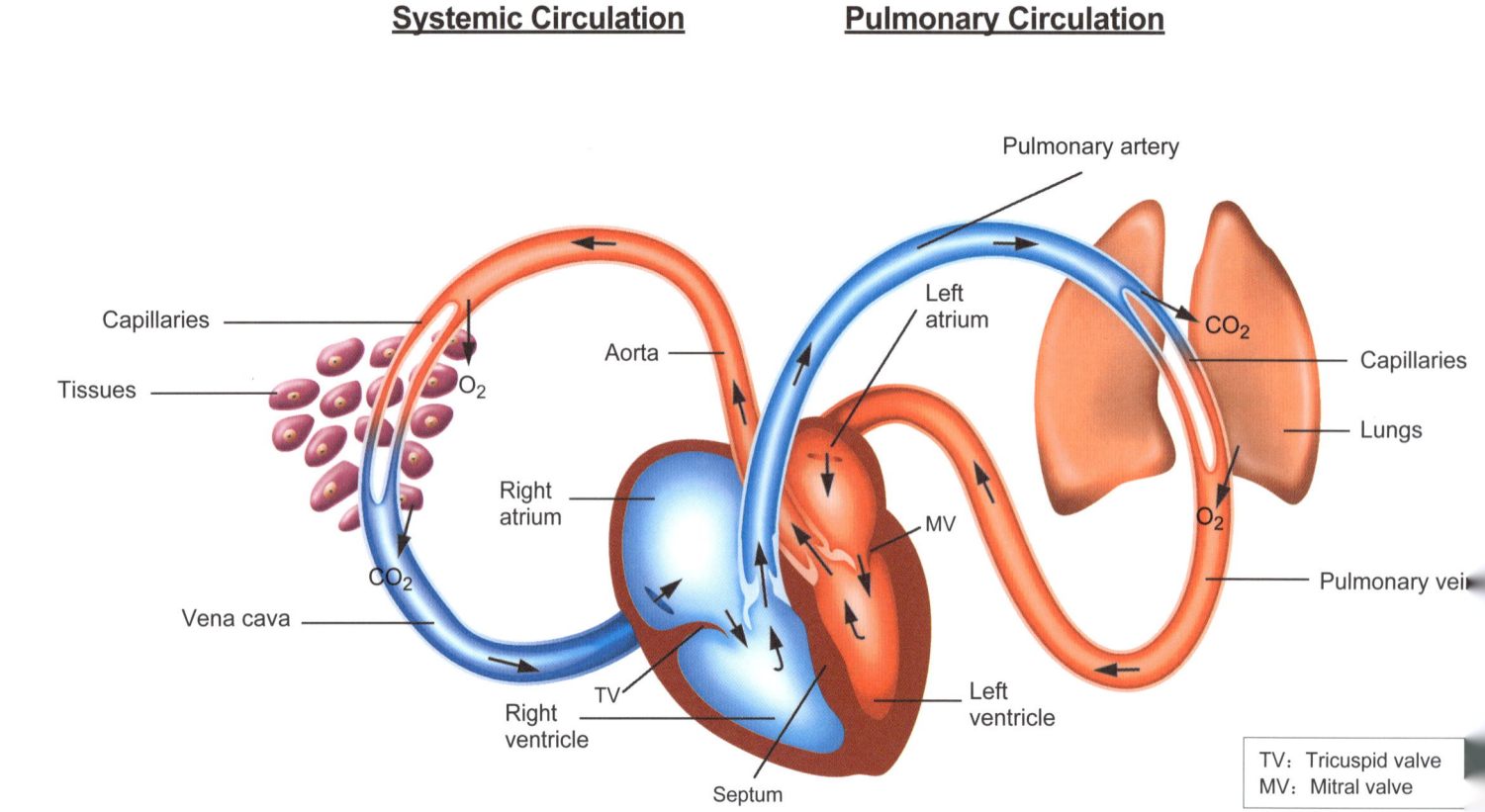

Figure IV.A.7.1: Schematic representation of the circulatory system.

7.4 Blood Pressure

Blood pressure is the force exerted by the blood against the inner walls of blood vessels (esp. arteries). Maximum arterial pressure is when the ventricles contract (= *systolic pressure*). Minimal pressure is when the ventricles relax (= *diastolic pressure*). Blood pressure is usually measured in the brachial artery in the arm. A pressure of 120/80 signifies a systolic pressure of 120 mmHg and a diastolic pressure of 80 mmHg. The *pulse pressure* is the difference (i.e. 40 mmHg).

Peripheral resistance is essentially the result of arterioles and capillaries which resist the flow of blood from arteries to veins (the narrower the vessel, the higher the resistance). An increase in peripheral resistance causes a rise in blood pressure.

BIOLOGY

7.5 Blood Composition

Blood contains *plasma* (55%) and *formed elements* (45%). Plasma is a straw colored liquid which is mostly composed of water (92%), electrolytes, and the following plasma proteins:

* **Albumin** which is important in maintaining the osmotic pressure and helps to transport many substances in the blood

* **Globulins** which include both transport proteins and the proteins which form antibodies

* **Fibrinogen** which polymerizes to form the insoluble protein *fibrin* which is essential for normal blood clotting. If you take away fibrinogen and some other clotting factors from plasma you will be left with a fluid called *serum*.

The formed elements of the blood originate from precursors in the bone marrow which produce the following for the circulatory system: 99% red blood cells (= *erythrocytes*), then there are platelets (= *thrombocytes*), and white blood cells (= *leukocytes*). **Red blood cells** are biconcave cells without nuclei whose primary function is the transport of O_2 and CO_2.

Platelets are cytoplasmic fragments of large bone marrow cells (*megakaryocytes*) which are involved in blood clotting by adhering to the collagen of injured vessels, releasing mediators which cause blood vessels to constrict (= *vasoconstriction*), etc.

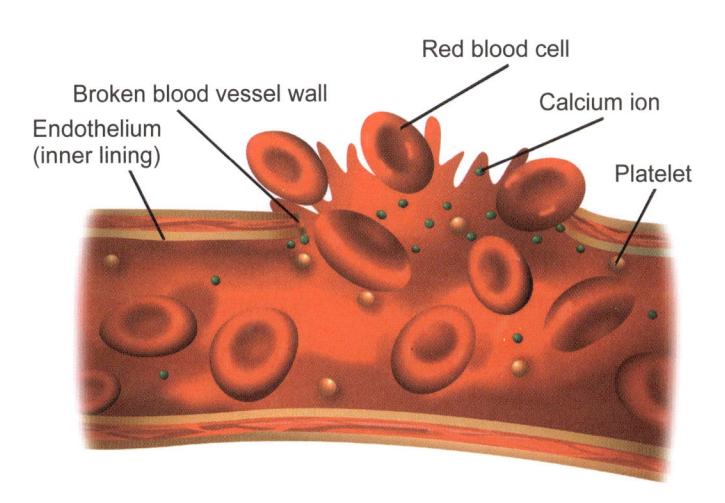

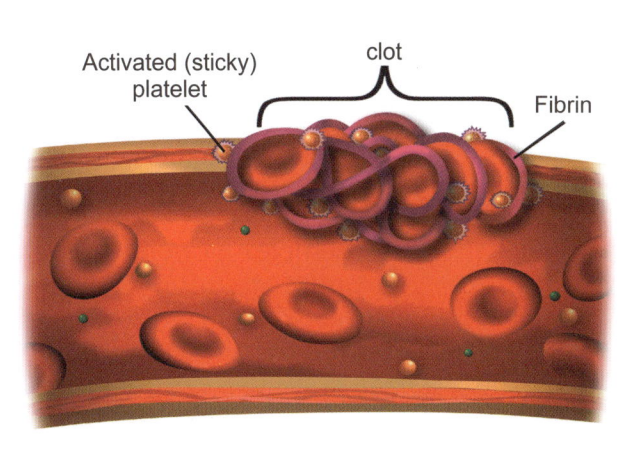

Figure IV.A.7.1.1: Schematic representation of blood clotting.

Calcium ions (Ca²⁺) are important in blood clotting because they help in signaling platelets to aggregate.

White blood cells help in the defense against infection; they are divided into *granulocytes* and *agranulocytes* depending on whether or not the cell does or does not contain granules, respectively.

Granulocytes (= *polymorphonuclear leukocytes*) are divided into: i) neutrophils which are the first white blood cells to respond to injury, they destroy microorganisms (i.e. bacteria, viruses) by phagocytosis and are the main cellular constituent of pus; ii) eosinophils which, like neutrophils, are phagocytic and have a variety of inflammatory and immune responses; iii) basophils which can release both anticoagulants (heparin) and substances important in hypersensitivity reactions (histamine).

Agranulocytes (= *mononuclear leukocytes*) are divided into: i) lymphocytes which are vital to the immune system (*see Immune System*, chapter 8); and monocytes (often called *phagocytes* or *macrophages* when they are outside of the circulatory system) which can phagocytose large particles. {See BIO 15.2 *for ABO Blood Types*}

The hematocrit measures how much space (volume) in the blood is occupied by red blood cells. Normal hematocrit in adults is about 45%.

7.5.1 Hemoglobin

Each red blood cell carries hundreds of molecules of a substance which is responsible for their red color: **hemoglobin**. Hemoglobin (Hb) is a complex of *heme*, which contains iron, and *globin*, which is a protein. In the lungs, oxygen concentration or *partial pressure* is high, thus O_2 dissolves in the blood; oxygen can then quickly combine with the iron in Hb forming bright red *oxyhemoglobin*. The binding of oxygen to hemoglobin is cooperative. In other words, each oxygen that binds to Hb facilitates the binding of the next

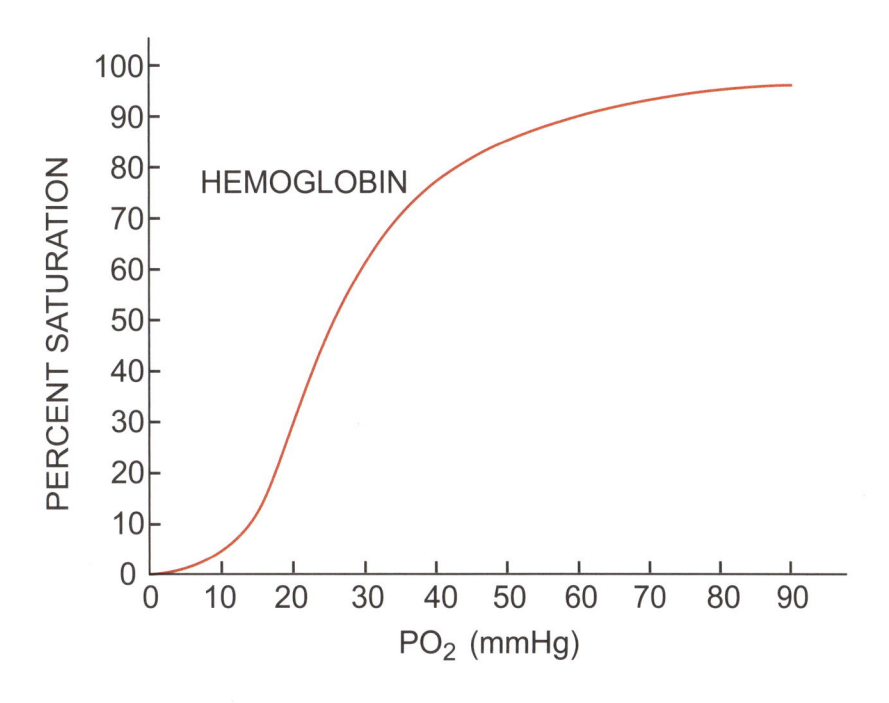

Figure IV.A.7.2: Oxygen dissociation curve: percent O₂ saturation versus O₂ partial pressure.

oxygen. Consequently, the dissociation curve for oxyhemoglobin is sigmoidal.

Examine Figure IV.A.7.2 carefully. Notice that P_{50}, which is the partial pressure of oxygen (PO_2) when the per cent saturation is 50, is approximately 27 mmHg. The curve can: (i) <u>shift to the left</u> which means that for a given PO_2 in the tissue capillary there is *decreased* unloading (release) of oxygen; or (ii) <u>shift to the right</u> which means that for a given PO_2 in the tissue capillary there is increased unloading of oxygen. The latter occurs when the tissue (i.e. muscle) is very active and thus requires more oxygen. Thus a rightward shift occurs when the muscle is hot (↑ temperature), acid (↓ pH due to lactic acid, *see* BIO 4.4 and 4.5), hypercarbic (↑CO_2 means ↓ pH, *see* BIO 4.4 and 12.4.1), or contains high levels of organic phosphates (esp. 2,3 DPG in red blood cells).

In the body tissues where the partial pressure of O_2 is low and CO_2 is high, O_2 is released and CO_2 combines with the protein component of Hb forming the darker colored *carbaminohemoglobin* (also called: deoxyhemoglobin). The red color of muscle is due to a different form of hemoglobin concentrated in muscle called *myoglobin*.

7.5.2 Capillaries: A Closer Look

Capillary fluid movement can occur as a result of two processes: diffusion (dominant role) and filtration (secondary role but critical for the proper function of organs, especially the kidney; BIO 10.3). Osmotic pressure (CHM 5.1.3) due to proteins in blood plasma is sometimes called colloid osmotic pressure or oncotic pressure. The Starling equation is an equation that describes the role of hydrostatic and oncotic forces (= Starling forces) in the movement of fluid across capillary membranes as a result of filtration.

When blood enters the arteriole end of a capillary, it is still under pressure produced by the contraction of the ventricle. As a result of this pressure, a substantial amount of water (hydrostatic) and some plasma proteins filter through the walls of the capillaries into the tissue space. This fluid, called interstitial fluid (BIO 7.6), is simply blood plasma minus most of the proteins.

Interstitial fluid bathes the cells in the tissue space and substances in it can enter the cells by diffusion (mostly) or active transport. Substances, like carbon dioxide, can diffuse out of cells and into the interstitial fluid.

Near the venous end of a capillary, the blood pressure is greatly reduced. Here

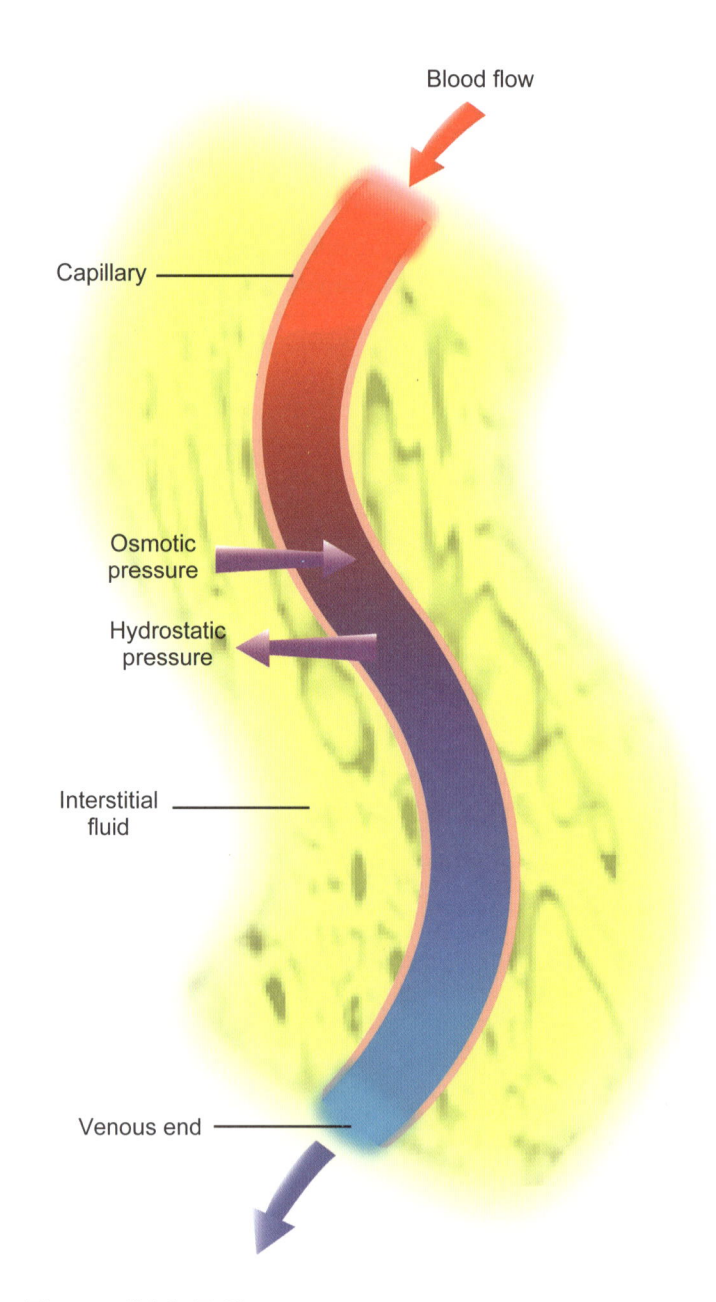

Figure IV.A.7.2b: Circulation at the level of the capillary. The exchange of water, oxygen, carbon dioxide, and many other nutrient and waste chemical substances between blood and surrounding tissues occurs at the level of the capillary.

another force comes into play. Although the composition of interstitial fluid is similar to that of blood plasma, it contains a smaller concentration of proteins than plasma and thus a somewhat greater concentration of water. This difference sets up an osmotic pressure. Although the osmotic pressure is small, it is greater than the blood pressure at the venous end of the capillary. Thus the fluid reenters the capillary here.

To summarize: when the blood pressure is greater than the osmotic pressure, filtration of interstitial fluid occurs; when the blood pressure is less than the osmotic pressure, reabsorption of interstitial fluid occurs.

7.6 The Lymphatic System

Body fluids can exist in blood vessels (intravascular), in cells (intracellular) or in a *3rd space* which is intercellular (between cells) or extracellular (outside cells). Such fluids are called <u>interstitial fluids</u>. The **lymphatic system** is a network of vessels which can circulate fluid from the 3rd space to the cardiovascular system.

Aided by osmotic pressure, interstitial fluids enter the lymphatic system via small closed-ended tubes called *lymphatic capillaries* (in the small intestine they are called *lacteals*). Once the fluid enters it is called **lymph**. The lymph continues to flow into larger and larger vessels propelled by muscular contraction (esp. skeletal) and one-way valves. Then the lymph will usually pass through *lymph nodes* and then into a large vessel (esp. *the thoracic duct*) which drains into one of the large veins which eventually leads to the right atrium.

Lymph functions in important ways. Most protein molecules which leak out of blood capillaries are returned to the bloodstream by lymph. Also, microorganisms which invade tissue fluids are carried to lymph nodes by lymph. Lymph nodes contain *lymph*ocytes and macrophages which are components of the immune system.

GOLD NOTES

THE IMMUNE SYSTEM

Chapter 8

Memorize

Roles in immunity: T-lymphocytes; B-lymphocytes
Tissues in the immune system including bone marrow
Spleen, thymus, lymph nodes

Understand

* Concepts of antigen, antibody, interaction
* Structure of antibody molecule
* Mechanism of stimulation by antigen

Not Required*

* Advanced level college info
* The 5 antibody isotypes
* Life cycle of pathogens
* Anatomy of lymph nodes
* Class switching

GAMSAT-Prep.com

Introduction

The immune system protects against disease. Many processes are used in order to identify and kill various microbes (see Microbiology, Chapter 2, for examples) as well as tumor cells (more detail when you get into medical school!). There are 2 acquired responses of the immune system: cell-mediated and humoral.

Additional Resources

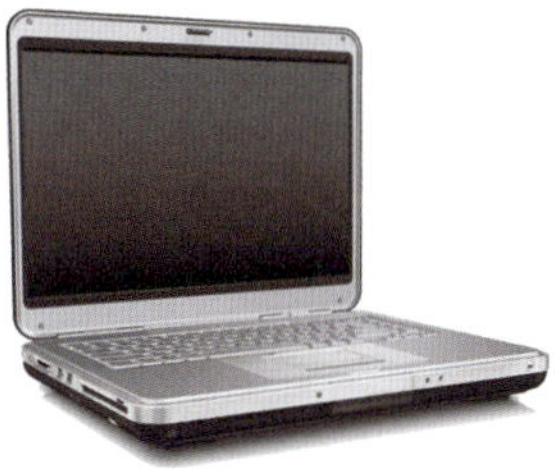

Free Online Q&A + Forum

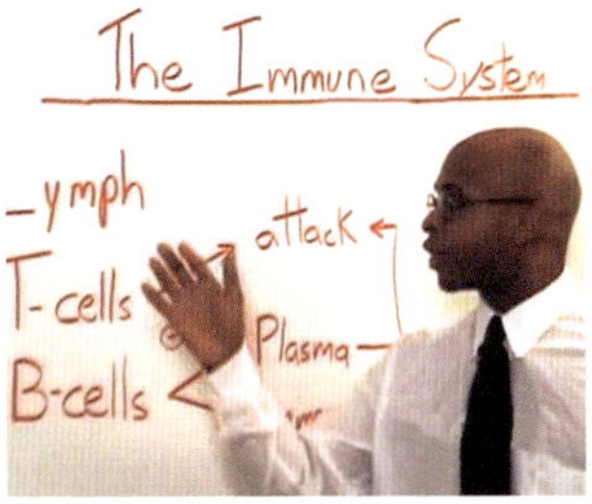

Video: Online or DVD 3

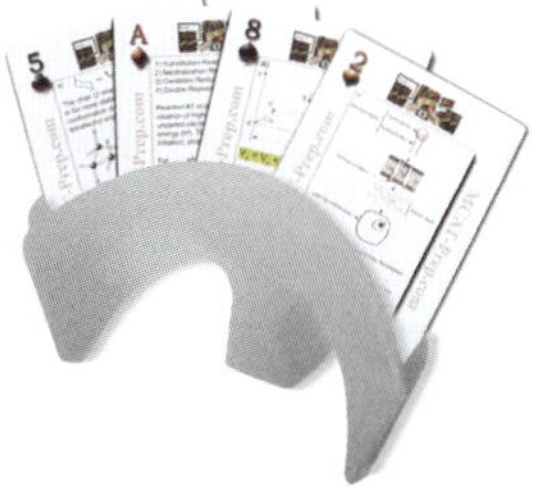

Flashcards

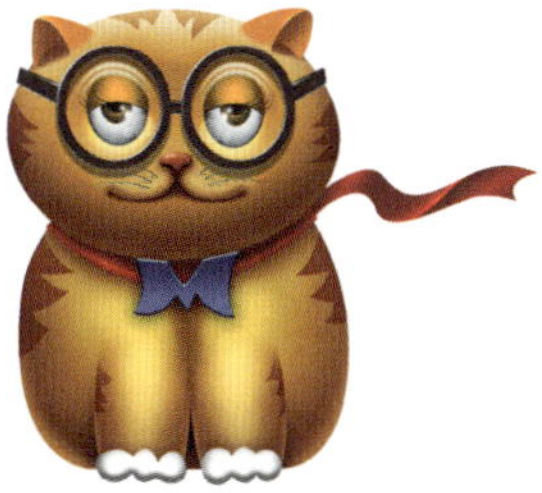

Special Guest

* The real GAMSAT may have advanced level information presented (ie. in a passage) but previous knowledge of said information is not required to answer the questions that would follow. Practice ACER and GS practice GAMSATs can help you clarify this point.

8.1 Overview

The immune system is composed of various cells and organs which defend the body against pathogens, toxins or any other foreign agents. Substances (usu. proteins) on the foreign agent causing an immune response are called **antigens**. There are two acquired responses to an antigen: the **cell-mediated response** where T-lymphocytes are the dominant force and the **humoral response** where B-lymphocytes are the dominant force.

8.2 Cells of the Immune System

B-lymphocytes originate in the bone marrow. Though T-lymphocytes also originate in the bone marrow, they go on to mature in the thymus gland. T-lymphocytes learn with the help of macrophages to recognize and attack only *foreign* substances (i.e. antigens) in a direct cell to cell manner (= *cell-mediated* or *cellular immunity*). Some T-cells (T_4, T_H or T *h*elper) mediate the cellular response by secreting substances to activate macrophages, other T-cells and even B-cells. {T_H-cells are specifically targeted and killed by the HIV virus in AIDS patients}

B-lymphocytes act indirectly against the foreign agent by producing and secreting antigen-specific proteins called **antibodies**, which are sometimes called immunoglobulins (= *humoral immunity*). Antibodies are "designer" proteins which can specifically attack the antigen for which it was designed. The antibodies along with other proteins (i.e. *complement proteins*) can attack the antigen-bearing particle in many ways:

* **Lysis** by digesting the plasma membrane of the foreign cell

* **Opsonization** which is the altering of cell membranes so the foreign particle is more susceptible to phagocytosis by neutrophils and macrophages

* **Agglutination** which is the clumping of antigen-bearing cells

* **Chemotaxis** which is the attracting of other cells (i.e. phagocytes) to the area

* **Inflammation** which includes migration of cells, release of fluids and dilatation of blood vessels.

The activated antibody secreting B-lymphocyte is called a *plasma cell*. After the first or *primary* response to an antigen, both T- and B-cells produce *memory cells* which will make the next or *secondary* response much faster. {Note: though lymphocytes are vital to the immune system, it is the neutrophil which responds to injury first; BIO 7.5}

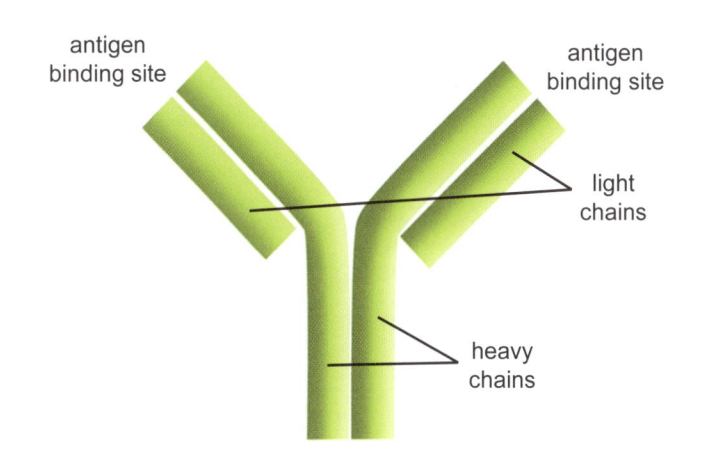

Figure IV.A.8.1: Schematic representation of an antibody.

8.3 Tissues of the Immune System

The important tissues of the immune system are the bone marrow, and the lymphatic organs which include the thymus, the lymph nodes and the spleen. The roles of the bone marrow and the thymus have already been discussed. It is of value to add that the thymus secretes a hormone (= *thymosin*) which appears to help stimulate the activity of T-lymphocytes.

Lymph nodes are often the size of a pea and are found in groups or chains along the paths of the larger lymphatic vessels. Their functions can be broken down into two general categories: i) a non-specific filtration of bacteria and other particles from the lymph using the phagocytic activity of macrophages; ii) the storage and proliferation of T-cells, B-cells and antibody production.

GAMSAT-Prep.com
THE GOLD STANDARD

The **spleen** is the largest lymphatic organ and is situated in the upper left part of the abdominal cavity. Within its lobules it has tissue called red and white pulp. In the white pulp there are white blood cells which help to filter: i) damaged red blood cells; ii) cellular debris, and iii) foreign particles from the blood. The spleen is sometimes considered a blood storage organ (the red pulp has a high concentration of red blood cells).

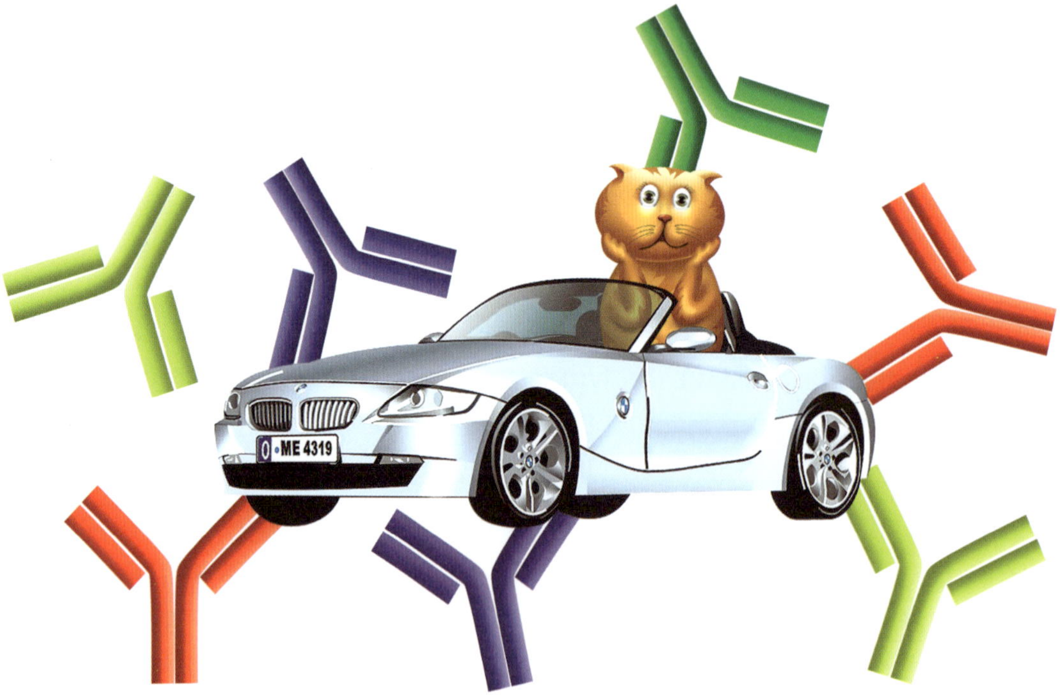

Autoimmunity!

Figure IV.A.8.1: Actually "autoimmunity" refers to a disease process where the immune system attacks one's own cells and tissues as opposed to one's own car.

BIO-94   THE IMMUNE SYSTEM

GOLD NOTES

GOLD NOTES

THE DIGESTIVE SYSTEM
Chapter 9

Memorize
* Saliva as lubrication and enzyme source
* Stomach low pH, gastric juice, mucal protection against self-destruction

Understand
* Basic function of the upper GI and lower GI tracts
* Bile: storage in gallbladder, function
* Pancreas: production of enzymes; transport of enzymes to small intestine
* Small intestine: production of enzymes, site of digestion, neutralize stomach acid
* Peristalsis; structure and function of villi

Not Required*
* Advanced level college info

GAMSAT-Prep.com

Introduction

The digestive system is involved in the mechanical and chemical break down of food into smaller components with the aim of absorption into, for example, blood or lymph. Thus digestion is a form of catabolism.

Additional Resources

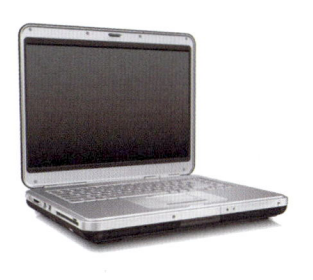

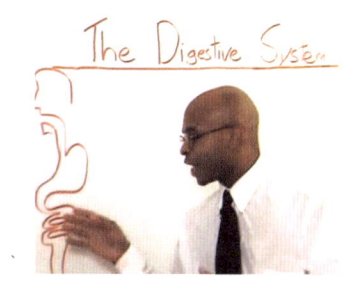

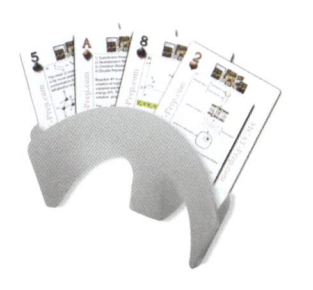

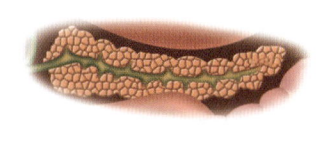

Free Online Q&A + Forum   Video: Online or DVD 3   Flashcards   Special Guest

THE BIOLOGICAL SCIENCES   BIO-97

* The real GAMSAT may have advanced level information presented (ie. in a passage) but previous knowledge of said information is not required to answer the questions that would follow. Practice ACER and GS practice GAMSATs can help you clarify this point.

9.1 Overview

The digestive or *gastrointestinal* (= GI) system is principally concerned with the intake and reduction of food into subunits for absorption. These events occur in five main phases which are located in specific parts of the GI system: i) **ingestion** which is the taking of food or liquid into the mouth; ii) **fragmentation** which is when larger pieces of food are *mechanically* broken down; iii) **digestion** where macromolecules are *chemically* broken down into subunits which can be absorbed; iv) **absorption** through cell membranes; and v) **elimination** of the waste products.

The GI tract or *alimentary canal* is a muscular tract about 9 meters long covered by a layer of mucosa which has definable characteristics in each area along the tract. The GI tract includes the oral cavity (mouth), pharynx, esophagus, stomach, small intestine, large intestine, and anus. The GI system includes the accessory organs which release secretions into the tract: the salivary glands, gallbladder, liver, and pancreas (*see Figure IV.A.9.1*).

9.2 The Oral Cavity and Esophagus

Ingestion, fragmentation and digestion begin in the oral cavity. Children have twenty teeth (= *deciduous*) and adults have thirty-two (= *permanent*). From front to back, each quadrant (= quarter) of the mouth contains: two incisors for cutting, one cuspid (= *canine*) for tearing, two bicuspids (= *premolars*) for crushing, and three molars for grinding. Chewing fragments the food as three pairs of salivary glands (*parotid, sublingual,* and *submaxillary*) secrete their products - esp. salivary amylase and mucous. Amylase is an enzyme which splits starch and glycogen into disaccharide subunits. The mucous helps to bind food particles together and lubricate it as it is swallowed. Swallowing (= *deglutition*) occurs by the action of the tongue and pharyngeal muscles which role the bolus of food into the esophagus. The epiglottis is a small flap of tissue which covers the opening to the airway (= *glottis*) while swallowing. Gravity and peristalsis help bring the food through the esophagus to the stomach.

Peristalsis, which is largely the result of two muscle layers in the GI tract (i.e. the inner circular and outer longitudinal layers), is the sequential wave-like muscular contractions which propel food along the tract. The rate, strength and velocity of muscular contractions

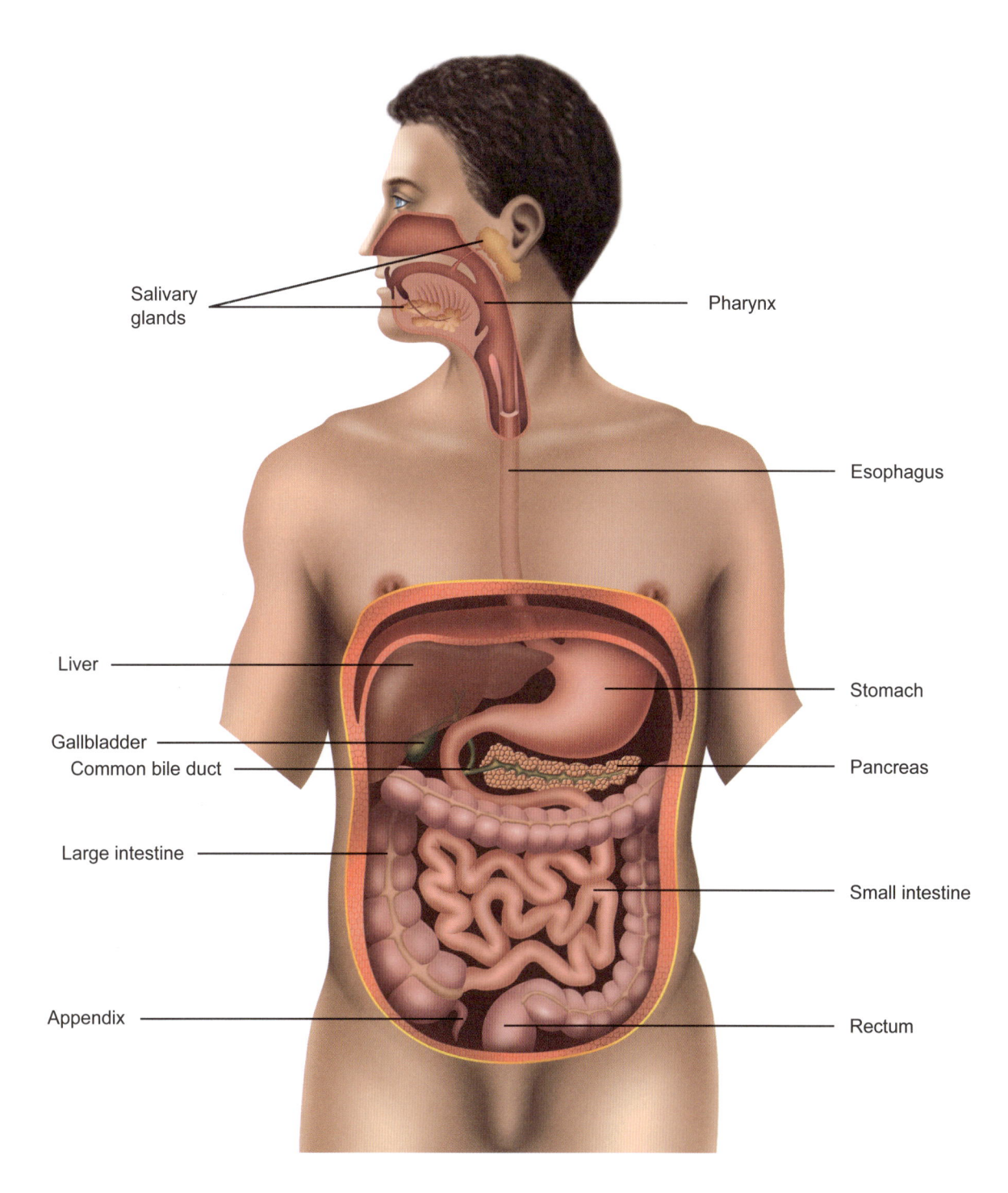

Figure IV.A.9.1: Schematic drawing of the major components of the digestive system.

are modulated by the ANS. Parasympathetic impulses tend to activate the GI system while sympathetic impulses tend to do the opposite.

9.3 The Stomach

The stomach continues in fragmenting the food with its strong muscular activity and it more completely aids in digestion due to the secretion of gastric juice. Goblet cells of the G.I. tract protect the lumen from the acidic gastric juice by secreting mucous. Both the hormone *gastrin*, which is produced in the stomach, and parasympathetic impulses can increase the production of gastric juice. The important components of gastric juice are: i) HCl which keeps the pH low (approx. = 2) to kill microorganisms, to aid in hydrolysis, and to provide the environment for ii) *pepsinogen* which is an inactive enzyme (= *zymogen*) which is converted to its active form *pepsin* in the presence of a low pH. Pepsin digests proteins.

The preceding events turns food into a semi-digested fluid called chyme. Chyme is squirted through a muscular sphincter in the stomach, the *pylorus*, into the first part of the small intestine, the *duodenum*. Many secretions are produced by exocrine glands in the liver and pancreas and enter the duodenum via the *common bile duct*. Exocrine secretions eventually exit the body through ducts which includes any gland or cell which secretes its product to the skin or into the intestine. For example, *goblet cells*, which are found in the stomach and throughout the intestine, are exocrine secretory cells which produce mucus which lines the epithelium of the gastrointestinal tract.

9.4 The Exocrine Roles of the Liver and Pancreas

9.4.1 The Liver

The liver occupies the upper right part of the abdominal cavity. It has many roles including: the conversion of glucose to glycogen; the synthesis of glucose from non-carbohydrates; the production of plasma proteins; the destruction of red blood cells; the deamination of amino acids and the formation of urea; the storage of iron and certain vitamins; the alteration of toxic substances (*detoxification*); and its exocrine role - the production of **bile** by liver cells (= *hepatocytes*).

Bile is a yellowish-green fluid mainly composed of water, cholesterol, pigments (from the destruction of red blood cells) and salts. It is the **bile salts** which have a digestive function by the emulsification of fats. Emulsification is the dissolving of fat globules into tiny droplets called *micelles* which have hydrophobic interiors and hydrophilic exteriors (cf. Plasma Membrane, BIO 1.1). Emulsification also helps in the absorption of the fat-soluble vitamins A, D, E, and K.

Thus bile is produced by the liver, stored and concentrated in a small muscular sac, the **gallbladder**, and then secreted into the duodenum via the common bile duct.

9.4.2 The Pancreas

The pancreas is close to the duodenum and extends behind the stomach. The pancreas has both endocrine (*see Endocrine Systems*; BIO 6.3.4) and exocrine functions. It secretes pancreatic juice into the pancreatic duct which joins the common bile duct. Pancreatic juice is secreted both due to parasympathetic and hormonal stimuli. The hormones *secretin* and *CCK* are produced and released by the duodenum in response to the presence of chyme. They make the pancreas secrete alkaline bicarbonate ions (to neutralize the acidic chyme) and digestive enzymes, respectively. The **digestive enzymes** can break down molecules of carbohydrates (*pancreatic amylase*), fat (*pancreatic lipase*), nucleic acids (*nucleases*), and proteins in a very specific manner (*trypsin, chymotrypsin, carboxypeptidase*).

9.5 The Intestines

The **small intestine** is divided into the duodenum, the jejunum, and the ileum, in that order. It is this part of the GI system that completes the digestion of chyme, absorbs the nutrients (i.e. monosaccharides, amino acids, nucleic acids, etc.), and passes the rest onto the large intestine. Peristalsis is the primary mode of transport.

Absorption is aided by the great surface area involved including the finger-like projections **villi** (which contain blood capillaries and lacteals) and **microvilli** (*see the Generalized Eukaryotic Cell,* BIO 1.1F and 1.2). They both project into the passageway or lumen of the small intestines. The lacteals absorb most fat products into the lymphatic system while the blood capillaries absorb the rest taking these nutrients to the liver for processing via a special vein - the *hepatic portal vein* [A portal vein carries blood from one capillary bed to another]. Goblet cells secrete a copious amount of mucus in order to lubricate the passage of material through the intestine and to protect the epithelium from abrasive chemicals (i.e. acids, enzymes, etc.).

The **large intestine** is divided into: the cecum which connects to the ileum and projects a closed-ended tube - the *appendix*; the colon which is subdivided into ascending, transverse, descending, and sigmoid portions; the rectum which can store feces; and the anal canal which can expel feces (*defecation*) through the anus with the relaxation of the anal sphincter and the increase in abdominal pressure. The large intestine has little or no digestive functions. It absorbs water and electrolytes from the residual chyme and it forms feces. Feces is mostly water, undigested material, bacteria, mucous, bile pigments (responsible for the characteristic color) and bacteria (= gut flora = 60% of the dry weight of feces). The average human body consists of about 10 trillion (10,000,000,000,000) cells but about ten times that number of bacteria are in the lower GI tract (mostly colon).

Essentially, it is a mutualistic, symbiotic relationship (BIO 2.2). Though people can survive with no bacterial flora, these microorganisms perform a host of useful functions, such as fermenting unused energy substrates, training the immune system, preventing growth of harmful species, producing vitamins for the host (i.e. vitamin K), etc. and bile pigments.

BIOLOGY

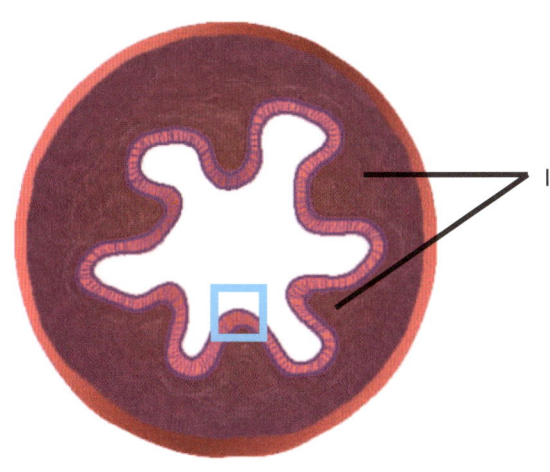

Intestinal folds (plicae circulares)

Cross-section of the small intestine.

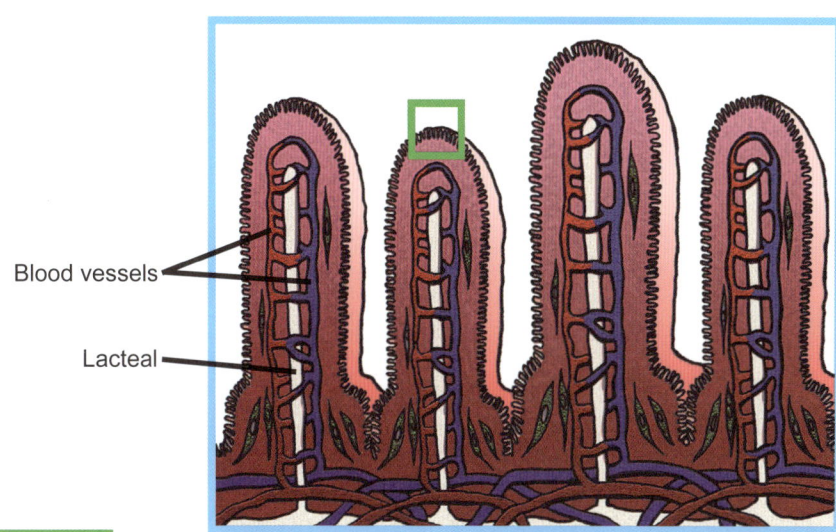

Blood vessels

Lacteal

4 intestinal villi.

Microvilli

Columnar cells (i.e. intestinal cells arranged in columns) with microvilli facing the lumen (brush border).

Figure IV.A.9.2: Levels of organization of the small intestine.

GOLD NOTES

THE EXCRETORY SYSTEM
Chapter 10

Memorize

Kidney structure: cortex, medulla
Nephron structure: glomerulus, Bowman's capsule, proximal tubule, etc.
Loop of Henle, distal tubule, collecting duct
Storage and elimination: ureter, bladder, urethra

Understand

* Roles of the excretory system in homeostasis
* Blood pressure, osmoregulation, acid-base balance, N waste removal
* Formation of urine: glomerular filtration, secretion and reabsorption of solutes
* Concentration of urine; counter-current multiplier mechanism

Not Required*

*Advanced level college info

GAMSAT-Prep.com

Introduction

The excretory system excretes waste. The focus of this chapter is to examine the kidney's role in excretion. This includes eliminating nitrogen waste products of metabolism such as urea.

Additional Resources

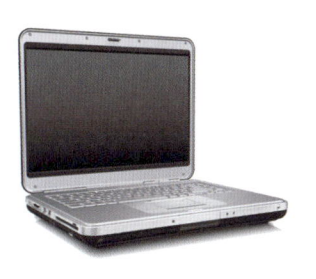

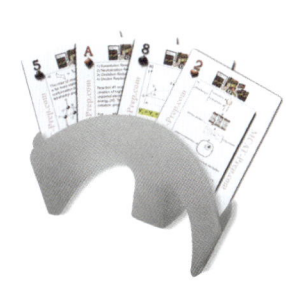

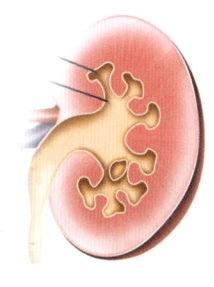

Free Online Q&A + Forum

Video: Online or DVD 4

Flashcards

Special Guest

THE BIOLOGICAL SCIENCES   BIO-105

* The real GAMSAT may have advanced level information presented (ie. in a passage) but previous knowledge of said information is not required to answer the questions that would follow. Practice ACER and GS practice GAMSATs can help you clarify this point.

10.1 Overview

Excretion is the elimination of substances (usu. wastes) from the body. It begins at the level of the cell. Broken down red blood cells are excreted as bile pigments into the GI tract; CO_2, an end product of cellular aerobic respiration, is blown away in the lungs; urea and ammonia (NH_3), breakdown products of amino acid metabolism, creatinine, a product of muscle metabolism, and H_2O, a breakdown product of aerobic metabolism, are eliminated by the urinary system. In fact, the urinary system eliminates such a great quantity of waste it is often called the excretory system.

The composition of body fluids remains within a fairly narrow range. The urinary system is the dominant organ system involved in electrolyte and water homeostasis (*osmoregulation*). It is also responsible for the excretion of toxic nitrogenous compounds (i.e. urea, uric acid, creatinine) and many drugs into the urine. The urine is produced in the kidneys (mostly by the filtration of blood) and is transported, with the help of peristaltic waves, down the tubular ureters to the muscular sack which can store urine, the bladder. Through the process of urination (= *micturition*), urine is expelled from the bladder to the outside via a tubular urethra.

The amount of volume within blood vessels (= *intravascular* or blood volume) and blood pressure are proportional to the rate the kidneys filter blood. Hormones act on the kidney to affect urine formation (*see Endocrine Systems,* BIO 6.3).

10.2 Kidney Structure

The kidney resembles a bean with a concave border (= *the hilum*) where the ureter, nerves, and vessels (blood and lymph) attach. The upper end of the ureter expands into the *renal pelvis* which can be divided into two or three *major calyces*. Each major calyx can be divided into *minor calyces*. The kidney can be grossly divided into an outer granular-looking **cortex** and an inner dark striated **medulla**.

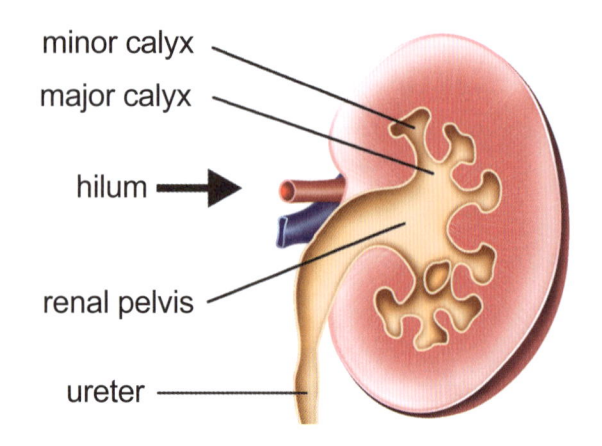

Figure IV.A.10.1: Kidney structure.

The kidney is a *filtration-reabsorption-secretion* (excretion) organ. These events are clearly demonstrated at the level of the nephron.

10.3 The Nephron

The nephron is the functional unit of the kidney and consists of the **renal corpuscle** and the **renal tubule**. A renal corpuscle is responsible for the filtration of blood and is composed of a tangled ball of blood capillaries (= *the glomerulus*) and a sac-like structure which surrounds the glomerulus (= *Bowman's capsule*). *Afferent* and *efferent* arterioles lead towards and away from the glomerulus, respectively. The renal tubule is divided into *proximal* and *distal convoluted tubules* with a *loop of Henle* in between. The tube ends in a *collecting duct*.

Blood plasma is **filtered** by the glomerulus through three layers before entering Bowman's capsule. The first layer is formed by the *endothelial cells* of the capillary; the second layer is the *glomerular basement membrane*; and the third layer is formed by the negatively charged cells (= *podocytes*) in Bowman's capsule which help repel proteins (most proteins are negatively charged). The rate of filtration is proportional to the *hydrostatic* (or blood) pressure and osmotic pressure (BIO 7.5.2).

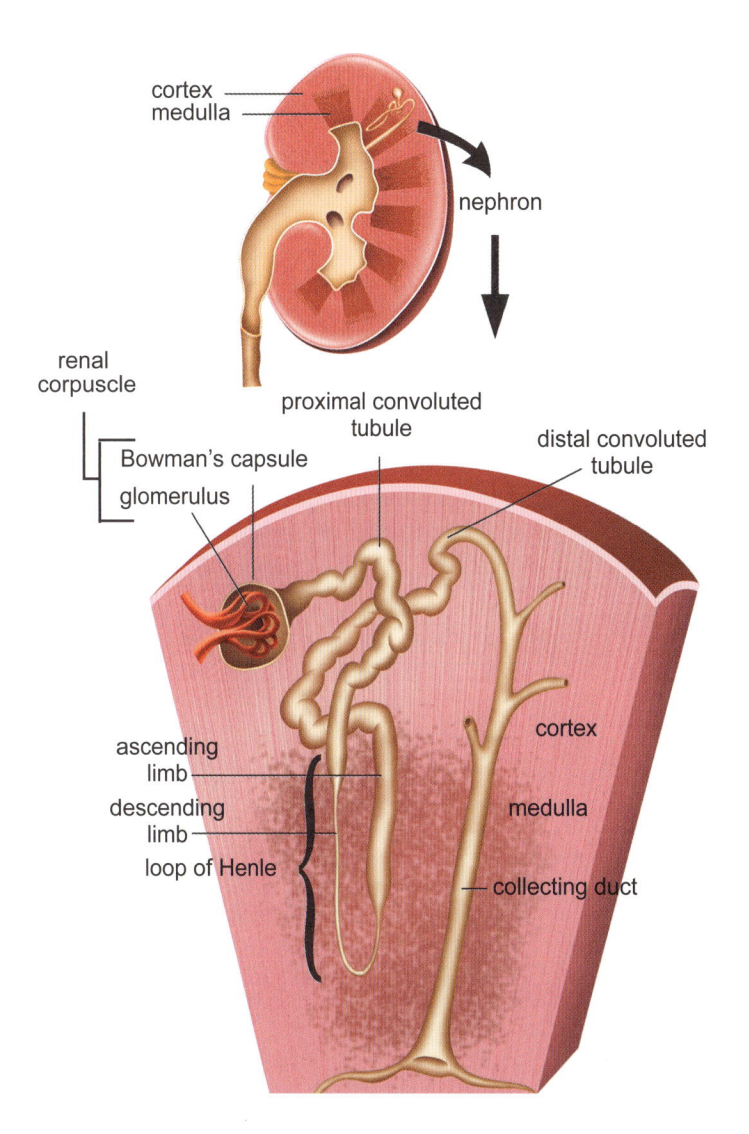

Figure IV.A.10.2: The kidney and its functional unit, the nephron.

GAMSAT-Prep.com
THE GOLD STANDARD

FRESH AIR INTAKE

EXHAUST FUMES

COLD

0° ← 50°

100° ← 150° — Insulator

200° ← 250° — Conductor ("Permeable" to heat)

300° ← 350°

temperature

HOT

Furnace

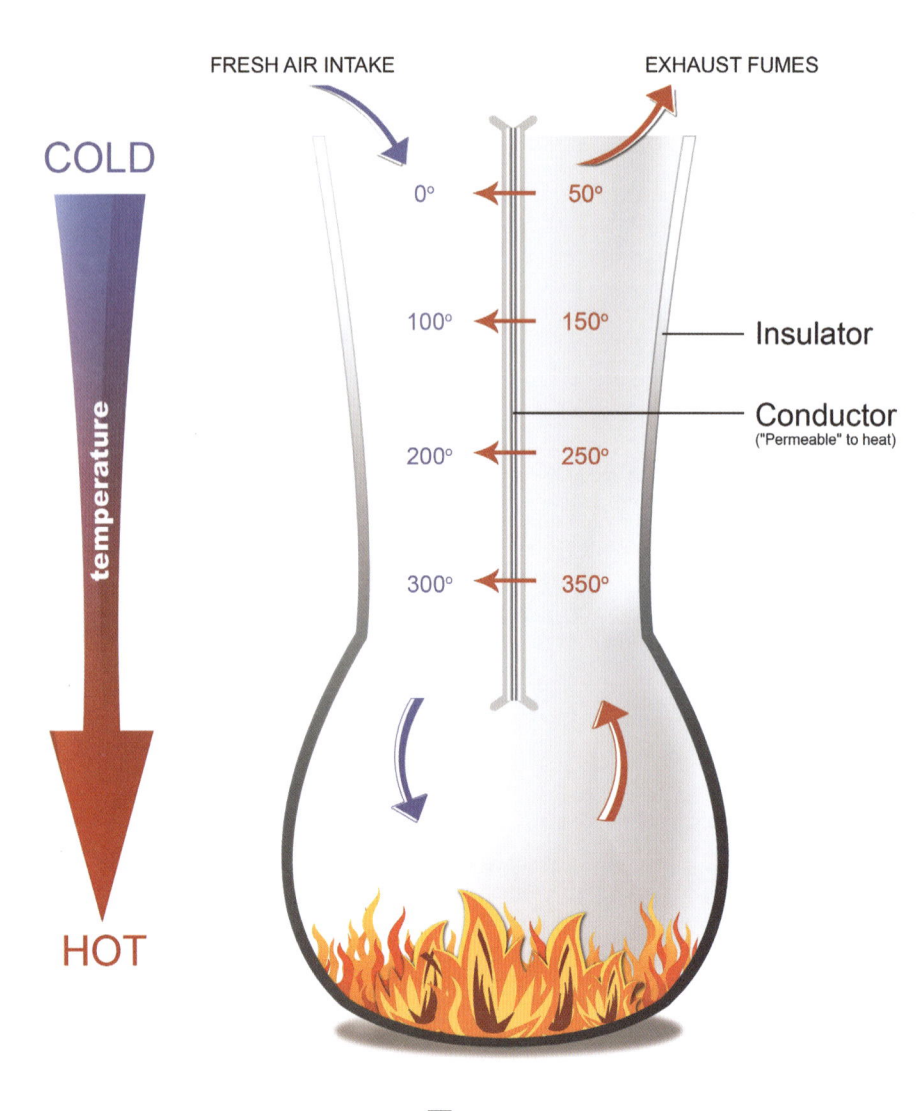

The countercurrent principle depends on a parallel flow arrangement moving in 2 different directions (countercurrent) in close proximity to each other. Our example is that of the air intake and exhaust pipe in this simplified schematic of a furnace.

Heat is transferred from the exhaust fumes to the incoming air.

The small horizontal temperature gradient of only 50° is multiplied longitudinally to a gradient of 300°. This conserves heat that would otherwise be lost.

Figure IV.A.10.3: The countercurrent principle (= counter-current mechanism) using a simplified furnace as an example.

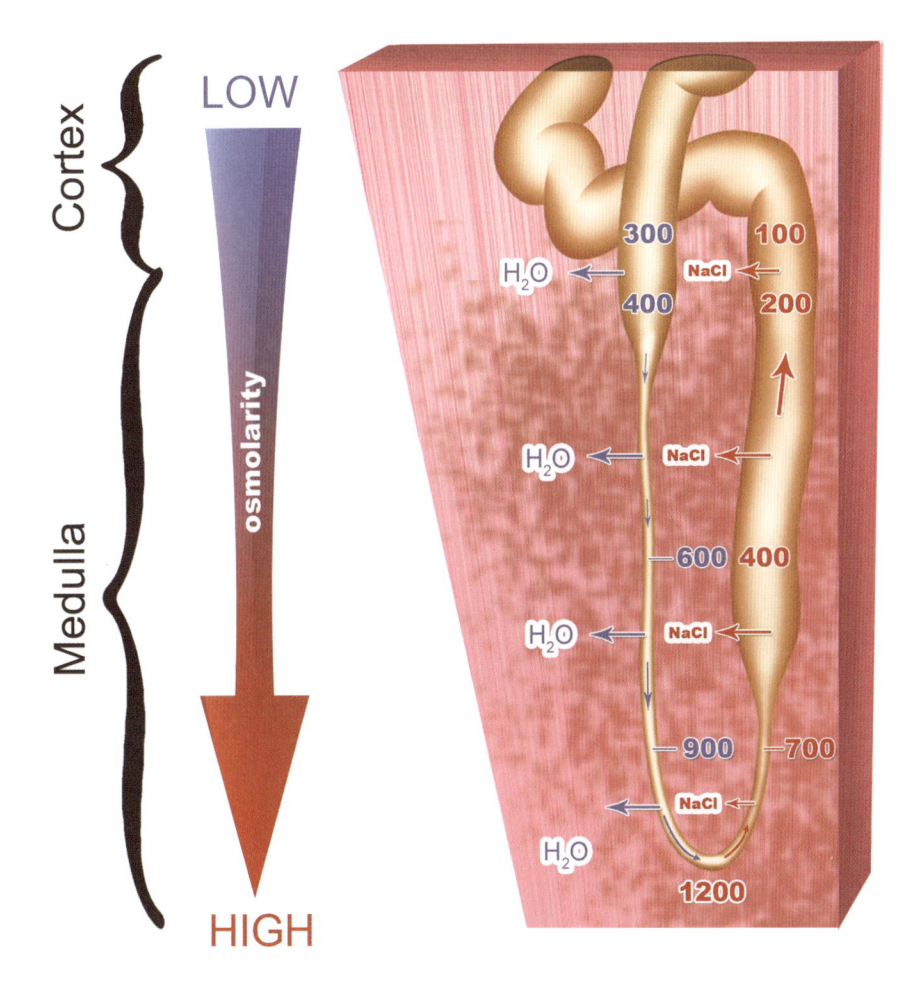

The descending limb of the loop of Henle is highly permeable to water and relatively impermeable to NaCl. The ascending limb is impermeable to water but relatively (through active transport) permeable to NaCl.

Due to the increased osmolarity of the interstitial fluid, water moves out of the descending limb into the interstitial fluid by osmosis. Volume of the filtrate decreases as water leaves. Osmotic concentration of the filtrate increases (1200) as it rounds the hairpin turn of the loop of Henle.

Some of the NaCl leaving the ascending limb moves by diffusion into the descending limb from the interstitial fluid thus increasing the solute concentration in the descending limb. Also, new NaCl in the filtrate continuously enters the tubule inflow to be transported out of the ascending limb into the interstitial fluid. Thus this recycling multiplies NaCl concentration.

Loop of Henle

Figure IV.A.10.4: The countercurrent principle (= counter-current mechanism) in the loop of Henle.

10.3 The Nephron (cont'd)

The <u>filtrate</u>, which is similar to plasma but with minimal proteins, now passes into the proximal convoluted tubule (PCT). It is here that the body actively **reabsorbs** compounds that it needs (i.e. proteins, amino acids, and especially glucose); and over 75% of all ions and water are reabsorbed by *obligate* (= required) reabsorption from the PCT. To increase the surface area for absorption, the cells of the PCT have a lot of microvilli (= *brush border*; cf. BIO 1.2). Some substances like H^+, urea and penicillin are **secreted** into the PCT.

From the PCT the filtrate goes through the descending and ascending limbs of the loop of Henle which extend into the renal medulla. The purpose of the loop of Henle is to concentrate the filtrate by the transport of ions (Na^+ and Cl^-) into the medulla which produces an osmotic gradient (= *a counter-current mechanism*). As a consequence of this system, the medulla of the kidney becomes concentrated with ions and tends to "pull" water out of the renal tubule by osmosis.

The filtrate now passes on to the distal convoluted tubule (DCT) which reabsorbs ions actively and water passively <u>and</u> secretes various ions (i.e. H^+). Hormones can modulate the reabsorption of substances from the DCT (= *facultative* reabsorption). Aldosterone acts at the DCT to absorb Na^+ which is coupled to the secretion of K^+ and the passive retention of H_2O.

Finally the filtrate, now called urine, passes into the collecting duct which drains into larger and larger ducts which lead to renal papillae, calyces, the renal pelvis, and then the ureter. ADH concentrates urine by increasing the permeability of the DCT and the collecting ducts allowing the medulla to draw water out by osmosis. Water returns to the circulation via a system of vessels called the *vasa recta*.

Renin is a hormone (BIO 6.3.5) which is secreted by cells that are "near the glomerulus" (= *juxtaglomerular* cells). At the beginning of the DCT is a region of modified tubular cells which can influence the secretion of renin (= *macula densa*). The juxtaglomerular cells and the macula densa are collectively known as the juxtaglomerular apparatus.

GOLD NOTES

GOLD NOTES

THE MUSCULOSKELETAL SYSTEM
Chapter 11

Memorize
ucture of three basic muscle types: striated, ooth, cardiac
untary/involuntary muscles; sympathetic/ asympathetic innervation

Understand
* Muscle system, important functions
* Support, mobility, peripheral circulatory assistance, thermoregulation (shivering reflex)
* Control: motor neurons, neuromuscular junctions, motor end plates
* Skeletal system: structural rigidity/support, calcium storage, physical protection
* Skeletal structure: specialization of bone types, basic joint, endo/exoskeleton

Not Required*
* Advanced level college info

GAMSAT-Prep.com

Introduction

The musculoskeletal system (= locomotor system) permits the movement of organisms with the use of muscle and bone. Other uses include providing form and stability for the organism; protection of vital organs (i.e. skull, rib cage); storage for calcium and phosphorous as well as containing a critical component to the production of blood cells (skeletal system).

Additional Resources

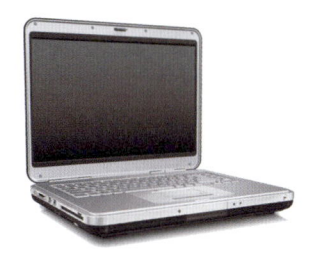

Free Online Q&A + Forum

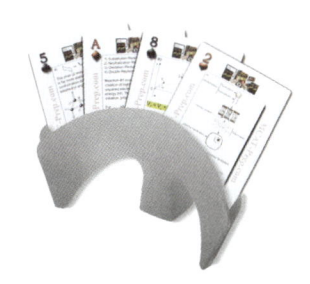

Flashcards

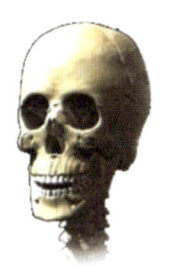

Special Guest

THE BIOLOGICAL SCIENCES   BIO-113

* The real GAMSAT may have advanced level information presented (ie. in a passage) but previous knowledge of said information is not required to answer the questions that would follow. Practice ACER and GS practice GAMSATs can help you clarify this point.

11.1 Overview

The musculoskeletal system supports, protects and enables body parts to move. Muscles convert chemical energy (i.e. ATP, creatine phosphate) into mechanical energy (→ contraction). Thus body heat is produced, body fluids are moved (i.e. lymph), and body parts can move in accordance with lever systems of muscle and bone.

11.2 Muscle

There are many general features of muscle. A latent period is the lag between the stimulation of a muscle and its response. A twitch is a single contraction which lasts for a fraction of a second. Muscles can either *contract* or *relax* but they can not actively expand. Tetany is a sustained contraction (a summation of multiple contractions) that lacks even partial relaxation. Muscle tone (*tonus*) occurs because even when a muscle appears to be at rest, some degree of sustained contraction is occurring.

The cellular characteristics of muscle have already been described (*see Contractile Cells and Tissues,* BIO 5.2). We will now examine the gross features of the three basic muscle types.

Cardiac muscle forms the walls of the heart and is responsible for the pumping action. Its contractions are continuous and are initiated by inherent mechanisms and modulated by the autonomic nervous system. Its activity is decreased by the parasympathetic nervous system and increased by the sympathetic nervous system. The sinoatrial node (SA node) or *pacemaker* contains specialized cells in the right atrium which initiate the contraction of the heart.

Smooth Muscle has two forms. One type occurs as separate fibers and can contract in response to motor nerve stimuli. These are found in the iris (*pupillary dilation or constriction*) and the walls of blood vessels (*vasodilation or constriction*). The second and more dominant form occurs as sheets of muscle fibers and is sometimes called *visceral muscle*. It forms the walls of many hollow visceral organs like the stomach, intestines, uterus, and the urinary bladder. Like cardiac muscle, its contractions are inherent, involuntary, and rhythmic. Visceral muscle is responsible for peristalsis. Its contractility is usually slow and can be modulated by the autonomic nervous system, hormones, and local metabolites. The activity of visceral muscle is increased by the parasympathetic nervous system and decreased by the sympathetic nervous system.

Skeletal muscle is responsible for voluntary movements. This includes the skeleton and organs such as the tongue and the globe of the eye. Its cells can form a syncytium which is a mass of cells which merge and can function together. Thus skeletal muscle can contract and relax relatively rapidly (*see the Reflex Arc*, BIO 6.1.3). Control of skeletal muscle originates in the cerebral cortex. Most skeletal muscles act across joints. Each muscle has a movable end (= *the insertion*) and an immovable end (= *the origin*). When a muscle contracts its insertion is moved towards its origin. When the angle of the joint decreases it is called flexion, when it increases it is called extension. Abduction is movement away from the midline of the body and adduction is movement toward the midline. {Adduction is addicted to the middle (= midline)}

Muscles which assist each other are synergistic (for example: while the deltoid muscle abducts the arm, other muscles hold the shoulder steady). Muscles that can move a joint in opposite directions are antagonistic (for example: at the elbow the biceps can flex while the triceps can extend).

Skeletal muscle is innervated by the somatic nervous system. Motor (*efferent*) neurons carry nerve impulses from the CNS to synapse with muscle fibers at the *neuromuscular junction*. The terminal end of the motor neuron (motor end plate) can secrete acetylcholine which can depolarize the muscle fiber. One motor neuron can depolarize many muscle fibers (= a *motor unit*).

The autonomic nervous system can supply skeletal muscle with more oxygenated blood in emergencies (sympathetic response) or redirect the blood to the viscera during relaxed states (parasympathetic response).

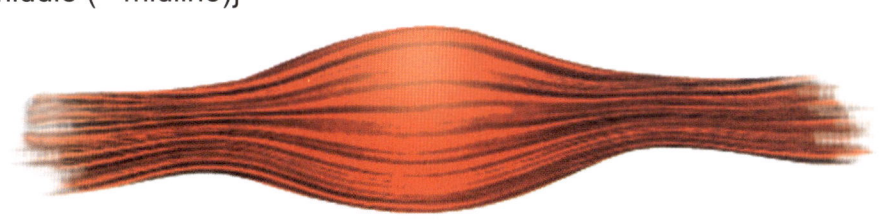

Skeletal muscle

11.3 The Skeletal System

The microscopic features of bone and cartilage have already been described (*see Connective Cells and Tissues*, BIO 5.4.3/4). We will now examine the relevant gross features of the skeletal system.

The bones of the skeleton have many functions: i) acting like levers that aid in **body movement**; ii) the **storage** of inorganic salts like calcium and phosphorus (and to a lesser extent sodium and magnesium); iii) the production of blood cells (= **hematopoiesis**) in the metabolically active red marrow of the spongy parts of many bones. Bone also has a yellow marrow which contains fat storage cells.

11.3.1 Bone Structure and Development

Bone structure can be classified as follows: i) long bones which have a long longitudinal axis and expanded ends, like arm and leg bones; ii) short bones which are shaped like long bones but are smaller and have less prominent ends; iii) flat bones which have broad surfaces like the skull, ribs, and the scapula; iv) irregular bones like the vertebrae and many facial bones.

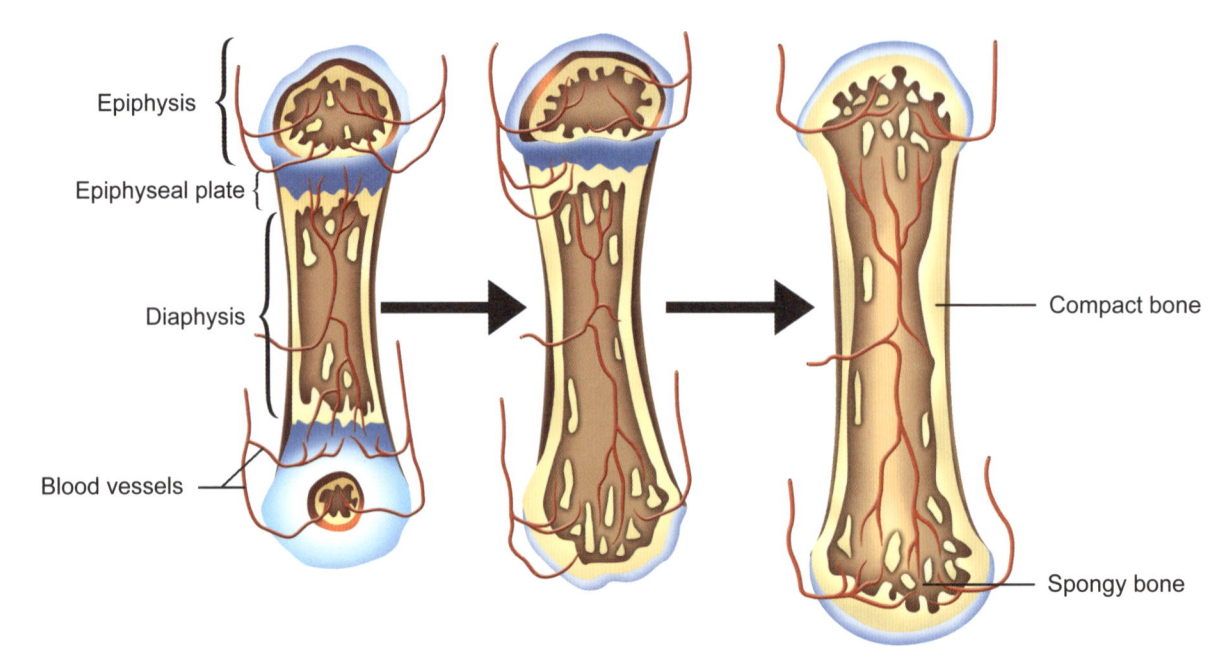

Figure IV.A.11.1: Bone structure and development.

The rounded expanded end of a long bone is called the *epiphysis* which contains spongy bone. The epiphysis is covered by fibrous tissue (*the periosteum*) and it forms a joint with another bone. Spongy bone contains bony plates called *trabeculae*. The shaft of the bone which connects the expanded ends is called the *diaphysis*. It is predominately composed of compact bone. This kind of bone is very strong and resistant to bending. Animals that fly have less dense, more light bones (spongy bone) in order to facilitate flying. Animals that swim do not need to have as strong bones as land animals as the buoyant force of the water takes away from the everyday stress on the bones. In the adult, yellow marrow is likely to be found in the diaphysis while red marrow is likely to be found in the epiphysis.

Bone growth occurs in two ways: i) the bone first appears as layers of membranous connective tissue and is thus called membranous bone; ii) cartilage appears first and is replaced by bone which is then called cartilaginous or endochondral bone. In children one can detect an **epiphyseal growth plate** on X-ray. This plate is a disk of cartilage between the epiphysis and diaphysis where bone is being actively deposited (= *ossification*).

11.3.2 Joint Structure

Articulations or joints are junctions between bones. They can be **immovable** like the dense connective tissue sutures which hold the flat bones of the skull together; **partly movable** like the hyaline and fibrocartilage joints on disks of the vertebrae; or **freely movable** like the synovial joints which are the most prominent joints in the skeletal system. Synovial joints contain a joint capsule composed of outer ligaments and an inner layer (= *the synovial membrane*) which secretes a lubricant (= *synovial fluid*).

Freely movable joints can be of many types. For example, ball and socket joints have a wide range of motion, like the shoulder and hip joints. On the other hand, hinge joints allow motion in only one plane like a hinged door (i.e. the knee, elbow, and interphalangeal joints).

11.3.3 Cartilage

The microscopic aspects of cartilage have already been discussed (*see Dense Connective Tissue,* BIO 5.4.2/3). Opposing and mobile surfaces of bone are covered by various forms of cartilage. As already mentioned, joints with hyaline or fibrocartilage allow little movement.

Ligaments attach bone to bone. They are formed by dense bands of fibrous connective tissue which reinforce the joint capsule and help to maintain bones in the proper anatomical arrangement.

Tendons connect muscle to bone. They are formed by the densest kind of fibrous connective tissue. Tendons allow muscular forces to be exerted even when the body (*or belly*) of the muscle is at some distance from the action.

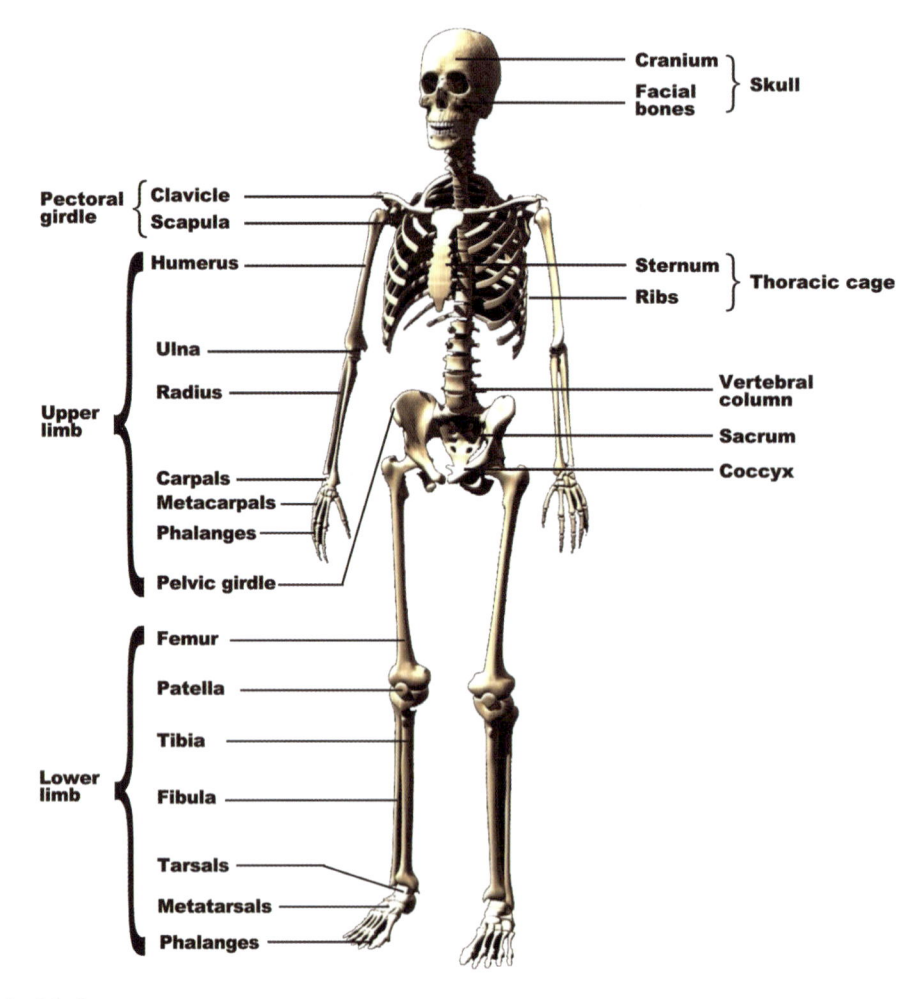

Figure IV.A.11.2: Skeletal structure. Note: in brackets some common relations - scapula (shoulder blade), clavicle (collarbone), carpals (wrist), metacarpals (palm), phalanges (fingers), tibia (shin), patella (kneecap), tarsals (ankle), metatarsals (foot), phalanges (toes), vertebral column (backbone).

GOLD NOTES

GOLD NOTES

THE RESPIRATORY SYSTEM
Chapter 12

Memorize	Understand	Not Required*
* Basic anatomy and order	* Basic functions: gas exchange, thermoregulation * Protection against disease, particulate matter * Breathing mechanisms: diaphragm, rib cage, differential pressure * Resiliency and surface tension effects	* Advanced level college info

GAMSAT-Prep.com

Introduction

The respiratory system permits the exchange of gases with the organism's environment. This critical process occurs in the microscopic space between alveoli and capillaries. It is here where molecules of oxygen and carbon dioxide passively diffuse between the gaseous external environment and the blood.

Additional Resources

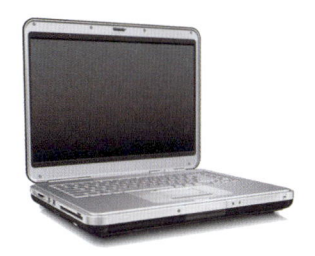

Free Online Q&A + Forum   Flashcards   Special Guest

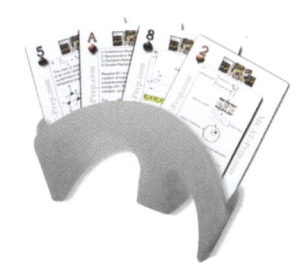

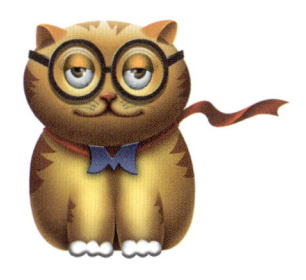

THE BIOLOGICAL SCIENCES   BIO-121

* The real GAMSAT may have advanced level information presented (ie. in a passage) but previous knowledge of said information is not required to answer the questions that would follow. Practice ACER and GS practice GAMSATs can help you clarify this point.

12.1 Overview

There are two forms of respiration: <u>cellular respiration</u> which refers to the oxidation of organic molecules (*see* BIO 4.4 - 4.10) and <u>mechanical respiration</u> where the gases related to cellular respiration are exchanged between the atmosphere and the circulatory system (O_2 in and CO_2 out).

The respiratory system, which is concerned with mechanical respiration, has the following principal functions:

* providing a <u>conducting system</u> for the exchange of gases
* the <u>filtration</u> of incoming particles
* to help control the <u>water content and temperature</u> (= *thermoregulation*) of the incoming air
* to assist in <u>speech production</u>, the <u>sense of smell</u>, and the <u>regulation of pH</u>.

12.2 The Upper Respiratory Tract

The <u>respiratory system</u> can be divided into an *upper* and *lower respiratory tract* which are separated by the pharynx. The **upper respiratory tract** is composed of <u>the nose</u>, <u>the nasal cavity</u>, <u>the sinuses</u>, and <u>the nasopharynx</u>. The nose (*nares*) has receptors for the sense of smell. It is guarded by hair to entrap coarse particles. The nasal cavity, the hollow space behind the nose, contains a ciliated mucous membrane (= a form of *respiratory epithelium*) to entrap smaller particles and prevent infection (this arrangement is common throughout the respiratory tract; for cilia *see the Generalized Eukaryotic Cell*, BIO 1.2). The nasal cavity adjusts the humidity and temperature of incoming air. The nasopharynx helps to equilibrate pressure between the environment and the middle ear via the eustachian tube.

12.3 The Lower Respiratory Tract

The **lower respiratory tract** is composed of <u>the larynx</u> which contains the vocal cords, <u>the trachea</u> which divides into left and right <u>main bronchi</u> which continue to divide into smaller airways (→ 2° bronchi → 3° bronchi → bronchioles → terminal bronchioles → respiratory bronchioles → alveolar ducts → alveolar sacs) until the level of <u>the alveolus</u>.

BIOLOGY

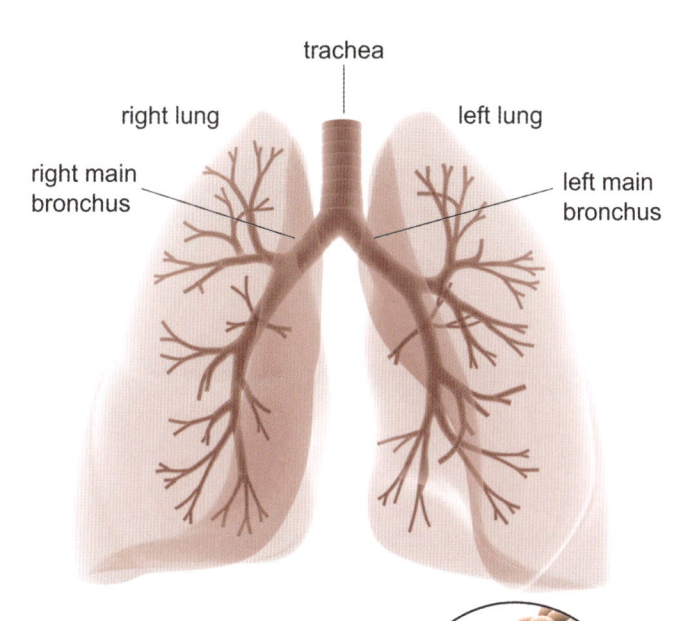

Figure IV.A.12.1: Illustration representing the lower respiratory tract including the dividing bronchial tree and grape-shaped alveoli with blood supply. Note that "right" refers to the patient's perspective which means the left side from your perspective.

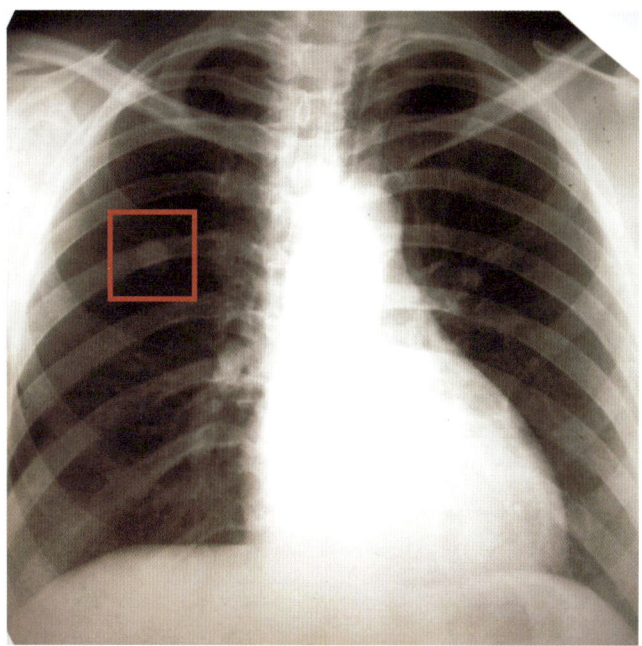

Figure IV.A.12.2: Chest x-ray of an adult male smoker. Notice the coin-shaped shadow in the right lung which presented with coughing blood. Further tests confirmed the presence of a right lung cancer. Cancer-causing chemicals (carcinogens) can irritate any of the cells lining the lower respiratory tract.

It is in these microscopic air sacs called *alveoli* that O_2 diffuses through the alveolar walls and enters the blood in nearby capillaries (where the concentration or *partial pressure* of O_2 is lowest and CO_2 is highest) and CO_2 diffuses from the blood through the walls to enter the alveoli (where the partial pressure of CO_2 is lowest and O_2 is highest). *Alveolar macrophages* are phagocytes which help to engulf particles which reach the alveolus. A *surfactant* is secreted into alveoli by special lung cells (*pneumocytes type II*). The surfactant reduces surface tension and prevents the fragile alveoli from collapsing.

Sneezing and coughing, which are reflexes mediated by the medulla, can expel particles from the upper and lower respiratory tract, respectively.

The **lungs** are separated into left and right and are enclosed by the diaphragm and the thoracic cage. It is covered by a membrane (= *pleura*) which secretes a lubricant to reduce friction while breathing. The lungs contain the air passages, nerves, alveoli, blood and lymphatic vessels of the lower respiratory tract.

THE BIOLOGICAL SCIENCES   BIO-123

12.4 Breathing: Structures and Mechanisms

Inspiration is <u>active</u> and occurs according to the following main events: i) nerve impulses from the <u>phrenic nerve</u> cause the muscular <u>diaphragm</u> to contract; as the dome shaped diaphragm moves downward, the thoracic cavity increases; ii) simultaneously, the intercostal (= *between ribs*) muscles and/or certain neck muscles may contract further increasing the thoracic cavity (the muscles mentioned here are called *accessory respiratory muscles* and under normal circumstances the action of the diaphragm is much more important); iii) as the size of the thoracic cavity increases, its <u>internal pressure</u> decreases leaving it relatively negative; iv) the relatively positive <u>atmospheric pressure</u> forces air into the respiratory tract thus inflating the lungs.

Expiration is <u>passive</u> and occurs according to the following main events: i) the diaphragm and the accessory respiratory muscles relax; ii) the elastic tissues of the lung, thoracic cage, and abdominal organs suddenly recoil; iii) this recoil increases the pressure within the lungs (making the pressure relatively positive) thus forcing air out of the lungs and passageways.

12.4.1 Control of Breathing

Though voluntary breathing is possible (!), normally breathing is involuntary, rhythmic, and controlled by the *respiratory center* in the medulla of the brain stem. <u>Low</u> blood O_2 but more importantly <u>high</u> blood CO_2 or <u>low</u> pH increase the breathing rate. The latter two events are interrelated since CO_2 can be picked up by hemoglobin forming carbamino-hemoglobin (about 20%, BIO 7.5.1), but it can also be <u>converted into carbonic acid</u> by dissolving in blood plasma (about 5%) or by conversion in red blood cells by the enzyme *carbonic anhydrase* (about 75%). The reaction is summarized as follows:

$$CO_2 + H_2O \leftrightarrow \underset{\text{carbonic acid}}{H_2CO_3} \leftrightarrow \underset{\text{bicarbonate}}{HCO_3^-} + H^+$$

According to Henry's Law, the concentration of a gas dissolved in solution is directly proportional to its partial pressure. From the preceding you can see why the respiratory system, through the regulation of the partial pressure of CO_2 in blood, also helps in maintaining pH homeostasis.

GOLD NOTES

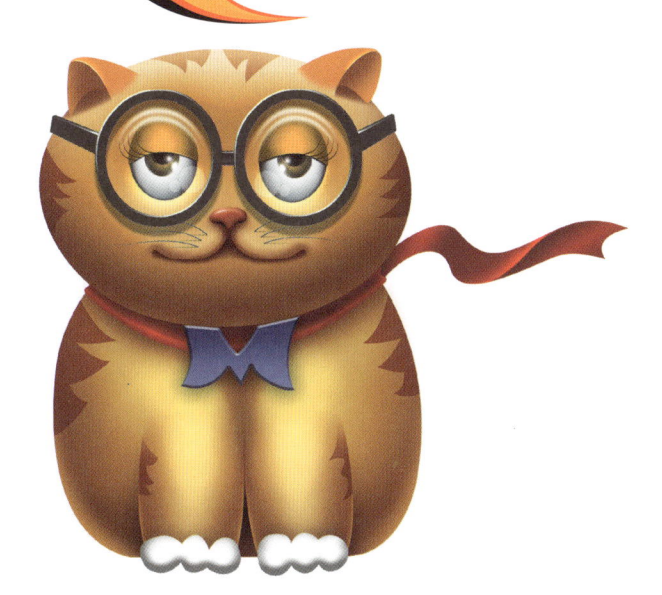

GOLD NOTES

THE SKIN AS AN ORGAN SYSTEM
Chapter 13

Memorize
* Structure and function of skin, layer differentiation
* Sweat glands, location in dermis

Understand
* Skin system: homeostasis and osmoregulation
* Functions in thermoregulation: hair, erectile musculature, fat layer for insulation
* Vasoconstriction and vasodilation in surface capillaries
* Physical protection: nails, calluses, hair; protection against abrasion, disease organisms
* Relative impermeability to water

Not Required*
* Advanced level college info

GAMSAT-Prep.com

Introduction

Skin is composed of layers of epithelial tissues which protect underlying muscle, bone, ligaments and internal organs. Thus skin has many roles including protecting the body from microbes, insulation, temperature regulation, sensation and synthesis of vitamin D.

Additional Resources

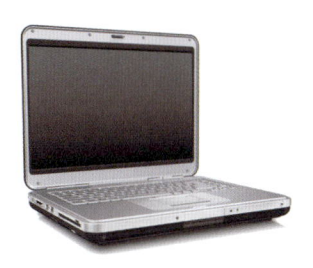

Free Online Q&A + Forum   Flashcards   Special Guest

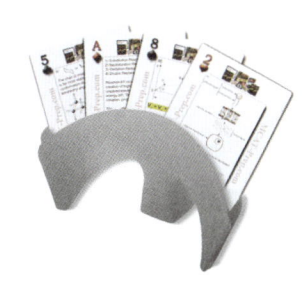

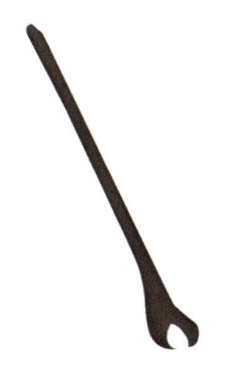

THE BIOLOGICAL SCIENCES   BIO-127

* The real GAMSAT may have advanced level information presented (ie. in a passage) but previous knowledge of said information is not required to answer the questions that would follow. Practice ACER and GS practice GAMSATs can help you clarify this point.

13.1 Overview

The skin, or *integument*, is the body's largest organ. The following represents its major functions:

* **Physical protection**: The skin protects against the onslaught of the environment including uv light, chemical, thermal or even mechanical agents. It also serves as a barrier to the invasion of microorganisms.

* **Sensation**: The skin, being the body's largest sensory organ, contains a wide range of sensory receptors including those for pain, temperature, light touch, and pressure.

* **Metabolism**: Vitamin D synthesis can occur in the epidermis of skin (*see Endocrine Systems*, BIO 6.3). Also, energy is stored as fat in subcutaneous adipose tissue.

* **Thermoregulation and osmoregulation**: Skin is vital for the homeostatic mechanism of thermoregulation and to a lesser degree osmoregulation. Hair (*piloerection*, which can trap a layer of warm air against the skin's surface) and especially subcutaneous fat (*adipose tissue*) insulate the body against heat loss. Shivering, which allows muscle to generate heat, and decreasing blood flow to the skin (= *vasoconstriction*) are important in emergencies. On the other hand, heat and water loss can be increased by increasing blood flow to the multitude of blood vessels (= *vasodilation*) in the dermis (cooling by radiation), the production of sweat, and the evaporation of sweat due to the heat at the surface of the skin; thus the skin cools. {Remember: the **hypothalamus** also regulates body temperature (*see The Nervous System*, BIO 6.1); it is like a thermostat which uses other organs as tools to maintain our body temperatures at about 37 °C (98.6 °F)}.

13.2 The Structure of Skin

Skin is divided into three layers: i) the outer **epidermis** which contains a stratified squamous epithelium; ii) the inner **dermis** which contains vessels, nerves, muscle, and connective tissues; iii) the innermost **subcutaneous layer** which contains adipose and a loose connective tissue; this layer binds to any underlying organs.

The epidermis is divided into several different layers or *strata*. The deepest layer, *stratum basale*, contains actively dividing cells which are nourished by the vessels in the dermis. As these cells continue to divide, older epidermal cells are pushed towards the surface of the skin - *away from the nutrient providing dermal layer*; thus in time they die. Simultaneously, these cells are actively producing strands of a tough, fibrous, waterproof protein called keratin. This process is called *keratinization*. The two preceding events lead to the formation of an outermost layer (= the *stratum corneum*) of keratin-filled dead cells which are devoid of organelles and can be easily shed (= *desquamation*).

Melanin is a dark pigment produced by cells (= *melanocytes*) whose cell bodies are usually found in the stratum basale. Melanin absorbs light thus protects against uv light induced cell damage (i.e. sunburns, skin cancer). Individuals have about the same number of melanocytes - regardless of race. Melanin production depends on genetic factors (i.e. race) and it can be stimulated by exposure to sunlight (i.e. tanning).

The dermis contains the blood vessels which nourish the various cells in the skin. It also contains motor and many sensory nerve fibers.

13.3 Skin Appendages

The **appendages** of the skin include hair, sebaceous glands and sweat glands. Hair is a modified keratinized structure produced by a cylindrical downgrowth of epithelium (= *hair follicle*). The follicle extends into the dermis (sometimes the subcutaneous tissue as well). When the bundle of smooth muscle which is attached to the connective tissue of the follicle contracts (= *piloerection*), 'goose bumps' are produced.

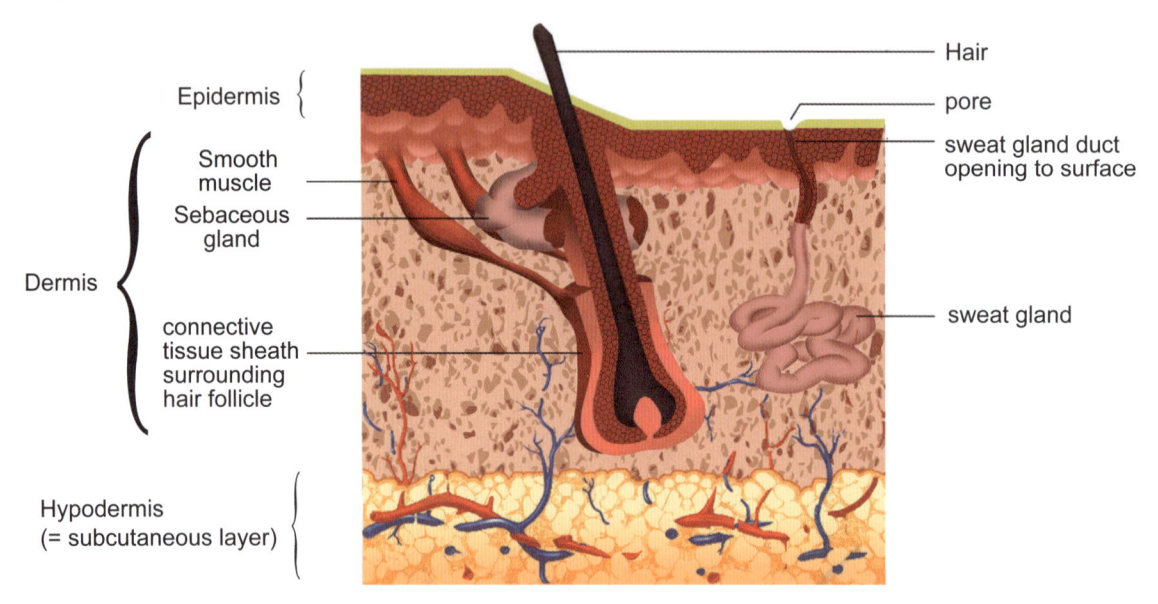

Figure IV.A.13.1: Skin structure with appendages.

13.3.1 Nails, Calluses

Nails are flat, translucent, keratinized coverings near the tip of fingers and toes. They are useful for scratching and fine manipulation (including picking up dimes!).

A callus is a toughened, thickened area of skin. It is usually created in response to repeated friction or pressure thus they are normally found on the hands or feet.

GOLD NOTES

REPRODUCTION AND DEVELOPMENT
Chapter 14

Memorize
Male and female reproductive structures, functions
Ovum, sperm: differences in formation, relative contribution to next generation
Reproductive sequence: fertilization; implantation; development
Major structures arising out of primary germ layers

Understand
* Gametogenesis by meiosis
* Formation of primary germ layers: endoderm, mesoderm, ectoderm
* Embryogenesis: stages of early development: order and general features of each
* Cell specialization, communication in development, gene regulation in development
* Programmed cell death; basic: the menstrual cycle

Not Required*
* Advanced level college info

GAMSAT-Prep.com

Introduction

Reproduction refers to the process by which new organisms are produced. The process of development follows as the single celled zygote grows into a fully formed adult. These two processes are fundamental to life as we know it.

Additional Resources

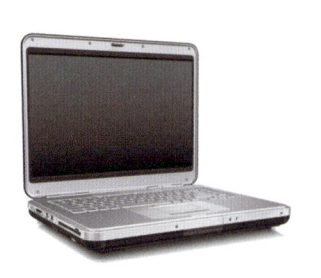

Free Online Q&A + Forum   Video: Online or DVD 3, 4   Flashcards   Special Guest

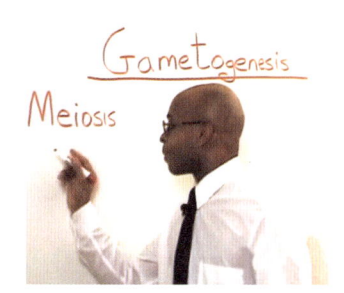

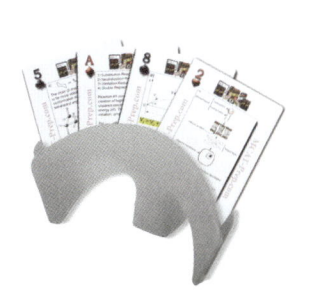

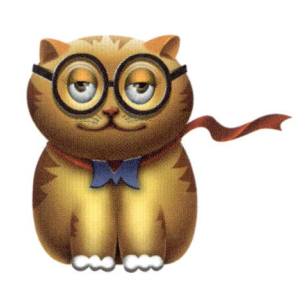

THE BIOLOGICAL SCIENCES   BIO-133

* The real GAMSAT may have advanced level information presented (ie. in a passage) but previous knowledge of said information is not required for the questions that would follow. Practice ACER and GS practice GAMSATs can help you clarify this point.

14.1 Organs of the Reproductive System

The female gonads are the two ovaries which lie in the pelvic cavity. Opening around the ovaries and connecting to the uterus are the Fallopian tubes (= *oviducts*) which conduct the egg (= *ovum*) from the ovary to the uterus. The uterus is a muscular organ. Part of the uterus (= the cervix) protrudes into the vagina or *birth canal*. The vagina leads to the external genitalia. The vulva includes the openings of the vagina, various glands, and folds of skin which are large (= labia majora) and small (= labia minora). The clitoris is found between the labia minora at the anterior end of the vulva. Like the glans penis, it is very sensitive as it is richly innervated.

The male gonads are the two testicles (= *testes*) which are suspended by spermatic cords in a sac-like scrotum outside the body cavity (this is because the optimal temperature for spermatogenesis is less than body temperature). Sperm (= *spermatozoa*) are produced in the seminiferous tubules in the testes and then continue along a system of ducts including: the epididymis where sperm complete their maturation and are collected and stored; the vas deferens which leads to the ejaculatory duct which in turn leads to the penile urethra which conducts to the exterior. The accessory organs include the seminal vesicles, the bulbourethral and prostate glands. They are exocrine glands whose secretions contribute greatly to the volume of the *ejaculate* (= semen = seminal fluid). The penis is composed of a body or shaft, which contains an erectile tissue which can be engorged by blood; a penile urethra which can conduct either urine or sperm; and a very sensitive head or glans penis which may be covered by foreskin (= *prepuce*, which is removed by circumcision).

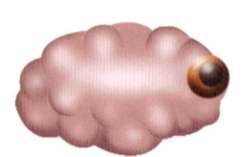

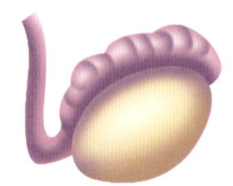

Figure IV.A.14.0: An ovulating ovary and a testicle with spermatic cord.

14.2 Gametogenesis

Gametogenesis refers to the production of gametes (eggs and sperm) which occurs by meiosis (*see Mitosis, BIO 1.3, for comparison*). Meiosis involves two successive divisions which can produce four cells from one parent cell. The first division, the reduction division, reduces the number of chromosomes from 2N (= *diploid*) to N (= *hap-*

loid) where N = 23 for humans. This reduction division occurs as follows: i) in **prophase I** the chromosomes appear (= *condense*), the nuclear membrane and nucleoli disappear, the spindle fibers become organized, homologous chromosomes pair[1] (= *synapsis*) and exchange genetic information by crossing over at particular sites (= *chiasmata formation*); ii) in **metaphase I** the synaptic pairs of chromosomes line up midway between the poles of the developing spindle (= *the equatorial plate*). Thus each pair consists of 2 chromosomes (= 4 chromatids), each attached to a spindle fiber; iii) in **anaphase I** the homologous chromosomes migrate to opposite poles of the spindle. Consequently, the centromeres do *not* divide; iv) in **telophase I** the parent cell divides into two daughter cells (= *cytokinesis*), the nuclear membranes and nucleoli reappear, and the spindle fibers are no longer visible.

The first meiotic division is followed by a short interphase I and then the second meiotic division which proceeds essentially the same as mitosis. Thus prophase II, metaphase II, anaphase II, and telophase II proceed like the corresponding mitotic phases.

Gametogenesis in males (= *spermatogenesis*) proceeds as follows: before the age of sexual maturity only a small number of primordial germ cells (= *spermatogonia*) are present in the testes. After sexual maturation these cells prolifically multiply throughout a male's life. In the seminiferous tubules, the spermatogonia (2N) differentiate by mitosis into primary spermatocytes (2N) which undergo meiotic divisions producing secondary spermatocytes (1N) followed by spermatids (1N). Each primary spermatocyte results in the production of **four** spermatids which are transformed into **four** motile sperm by *spermiogenesis*.

Sperm can be divided into: i) a *head* which is oval and contains the nucleus with its 23 chromosomes {since the nucleus carries either an X or Y sex chromosome, sperm determine the sex of the offspring}. The head is partly surrounded by the *acrosome* which contains enzymes (esp. *hyaluronidase*) which help the sperm penetrate the egg; ii) the *body* of the sperm contains a central core surrounded by a large number of mitochondria for power; and iii) the *tail* constitutes a flagellum which is critical for the cell's locomotion. Also in the seminiferous tubules are Sertoli cells which support and nourish developing sperm and Leydig cells which produce and secrete testosterone. While LH stimulates the latter, FSH stimulates primary spermatocytes to undergo meiosis. {Remember:

---

[1] synapsing homologous chromosomes are often called *tetrads* or *bivalents*.

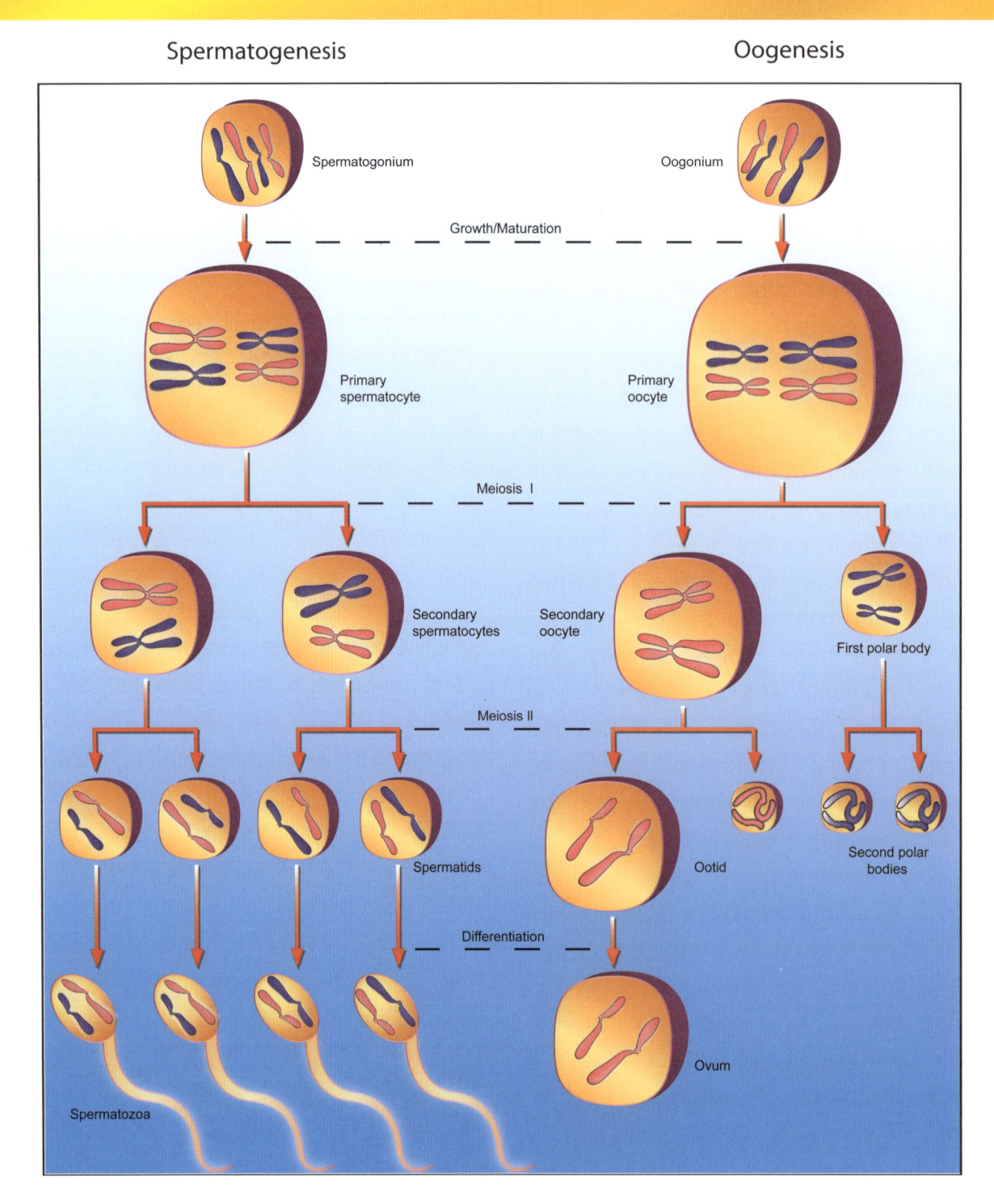

Figure IV.A.14.0a: Gametogenesis.

LH = Leydig, FSH = spermatogenesis}

Gametogenesis in females (= *oogenesis*) proceeds as follows: in fetal development, groups of cells (= *ovarian* or *primordial follicles*) develop from the germinal epithelium of the ovary. Oogonia (2N) produce primary oocytes (2N) which are surrounded by epithelia (= *follicular cells*) in the primordial follicle. The oocytes remain arrested in prophase I of meiosis until ovulation which occurs between the ages of about 13 (sexual maturity) and 50 (menopause). Thus, unlike males, all female germ cells are present at birth. Some follicles degenerate and are called *atretic*. During puberty, when the ovarian cycle begins, up to 20 primordial follicles may begin to differentiate to Graafian follicles. During this development meiosis continues as the primary oocyte (2N) produces a secondary oocyte (1N) by a reduction division. The latter is surrounded by (from the inside out): a thick, tough membrane (= *the zona pellucida*), follicular cells (= *the corona radiata*), and estrogen-secreting *thecal* cells.

Of the twenty or so maturing follicles, all will degenerate (= *atresia*) except one which is expelled from the ovary in the process called ovulation. This ovum, along with its zona pellucida and corona radiata, migrate to and through the Fallopian tubes where a sperm may penetrate the ovum (= *fertilization*). If fertilization occurs then the second meiotic division proceeds; if fertilization does not occur, then the ovum degenerates. Unlike in males, each primary germ cell (oocyte) produces one gamete and not four. This is a consequence of the production of *polar bodies* which are degenerated nuclear material. Up to three polar bodies can be formed: one from the division of the primary oocyte, one from the division of the secondary oocyte, and sometimes the first polar body divides.

14.3 The Menstrual Cycle

The "period" or menstrual cycle occurs in about 28 days and can be divided as follows: i) **Menses**: the first five days of the cycle are notable for the menstrual blood flow. This occurs as a result of an estrogen and progesterone withdrawal which leads to vasoconstriction in the uterus causing the uterine lining (= *endometrium*) to disintegrate and slough away; ii) **Follicular** (ovary) or **Proliferative Phase** (uterus): FSH stimulates the maturation of the follicle which in turn produces and secretes estrogen. Estrogen causes the uterine lining to thicken (= proliferate); iii) **Ovulation**: a very high concentration of estrogen is followed by an LH surge at about day 14 (midcycle) which stimulates ovulation; iv) **Luteal** (ovary) or **Secretory Phase** (uterus): the follicular cells degenerate into the corpus luteum which secretes estrogen *and* progesterone. Progesterone is responsible for a transient body temperature rise immediately after ovulation and it stimulates the uterine lining to become more vascular and glandular. Estrogen continues to stimulate uterine wall development and, along with progesterone, inhibits the secretion of LH and FSH (= negative feedback).

If the ovum is fertilized, the implanted embryo would produce the hormone *human chorionic gonadotropin* (= hCG) which would stimulate the corpus luteum to continue the secretion of estrogen and progesterone {hCG is the basis for most pregnancy tests}. If there is no fertilization, the corpus luteum degenerates causing a withdrawal of estrogen and progesterone thus the cycle continues [*see* i) *above*].

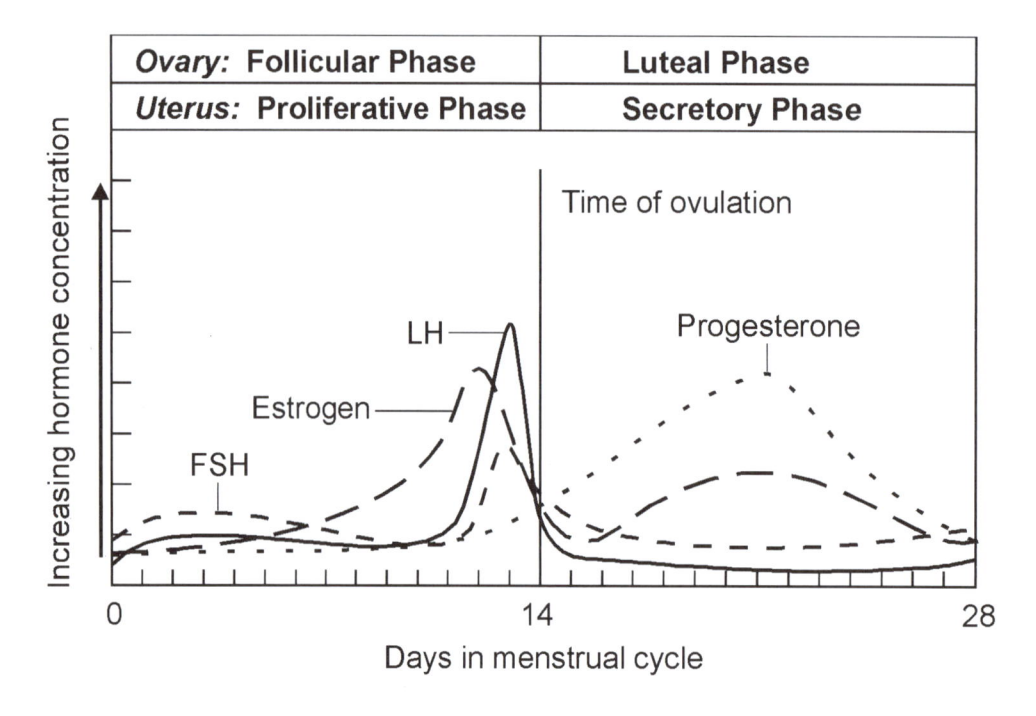

Figure IV.A.14.1: Changing hormone concentration during the menstrual cycle.

14.4 The Reproductive Sequence

During sexual stimulation parasympathetic impulses in the male lead to the dilatation of penile arteries combined with restricted flow in the veins resulting in the engorgement of the penis with blood (= *an erection*). In the female, the preceding occurs in a similar manner to the clitoris, along with the expansion and increase in secretions in the vagina. Intercourse or copulation may lead to orgasm which includes many responses from the sympathetic nervous system. In the male, the ejaculation of semen accompanies orgasm. In the female, orgasm is accompanied by many reflexes including an increase in muscular activity of the uterus and the Fallopian tubes. The latter may help in the transport of the already motile sperm to reach the tubes where the egg might be.

14.5 Embryogenesis

The formation of the embryo or *embryogenesis* occurs in a number of steps within two weeks of fertilization. Many parts of the developing embryo take shape during this period (= *morphogenesis*).

Fertilization is a sequence of events which include: the sperm penetrating the corona radiata and the zona pellucidum due to the release of lytic enzymes from the acrosome; the fusion of the plasma membranes of the sperm and egg; the egg, which is really a secondary oocyte, becomes a mature ovum by completing the second meiotic division; the nuclei of the ovum and sperm are now called *pronuclei*; the male and female pronuclei fuse forming a zygote (2N). Fertilization, which normally occurs in the Fallopian tubes, is completed within 24 hours of ovulation.

Cleavage consists of rapid, repeated mitotic divisions beginning with the zygote. Because the resultant daughter cells or blastomeres are still contained within the zona pellucidum, the cytoplasmic mass remains constant. Thus the increasing number of cells requires that each daughter cell be smaller than its parent cell. A morula is a solid ball of about 16 blastomeres which enters the uterus.

Blastulation is the process by which the morula develops a fluid filled cavity (= *blastocoel*) thus converting it to a blastocyst (= *blastula*). Since the zona pellucidum degenerates at this point, the blastocyst is free to implant in the uterine lining or endometrium. The blastocyst contains some centrally located cells (= *the inner cell mass*) which develops into the embryo.

Gastrulation is the process by which the blastula invaginates, and the inner cell mass is converted into a three layered (= *trilaminar*) disk. The trilaminar disk includes the **three primary germ layers**: an outer ectoderm, a middle mesoderm, and an inner endoderm. The ectoderm will develop into the epidermis and the nervous system; the mesoderm will become muscle, connective tissue (incl. blood, bone), and circulatory, reproductive and excretory organs; the endoderm will become the epithelial linings of the respiratory tract, and digestive tract, including the glands of the accessory organs (i.e. the liver and pancreas). During this stage the embryo may be called a gastrula.

Neurulation is the process by which the neural plate and neural folds form and close to produce the neural tube. The neural plate is formed by the thickening of ectoderm which is induced by the developing *notochord*. The notochord is a cellular rod that defines the axis of the embryo and provides some rigidity. Days later, the neural plate invaginates along its central axis producing a central neural groove with neural folds on each side. The neural folds come together and fuse thus converting the neural plate into a neural tube which separates from the surface ectoderm. Special cells on the crest of the neural folds (= *neural crest cells*) migrate to either side of the developing neural tube to a region called the neural crest.

As a consequence, we are left with **three** regions: the surface ectoderm which will become the epidermis; the neural tube which will become the central nervous system (CNS); and the neural crest which will become cranial and spinal ganglia and nerves and the medulla of the adrenal gland. During this stage the embryo may be called a *neurula*.

14.5.1 Mechanisms of Development

Though this is a subject which is still poorly understood, it seems clear that morphogenesis relies on the coordinated interaction of genetic and environmental factors. When the zygote passes through its first few divisions, the blastomeres remain indeterminate or uncommitted to a specific fate. As development proceeds the cells become increasingly committed to a specific outcome (i.e. neural tube cells → CNS). This is called **determination**.

In order for a cell to specialize it must differentiate into a committed or determined cell. Since essentially all cells in a person's body have the same amount of genetic information, differentiation relies on the *difference* in the way these genes are *activated*. For example, though brain cells (neurons) have the same genes as osteoblasts, neurons do not activate such genes (otherwise we would have bone forming in our brains!). The general mechanism by which cells differentiate is called **induction**.

Induction can occur by many means. If two cells divide unevenly, the cell with more cytoplasm might have the necessary amount of a substance which could *induce* its chromosomes to activate cell-specific genes. Furthermore, sometimes a cell, through contact (i.e. *contact inhibition*) or the release of a chemical mediator, can influence the development of nearby cells (*recall that the notochord induces the development of the neural plate*). The physical environment (pH, temperature, etc.) may also influence the development of certain cells. Irrespective of what form of induction is used, the signal must be translated into an intracellular message which influences the genetic activity of the responding cells.

Programmed cell-death (PCD = apoptosis) is death of a cell in any form, which is controlled by an intracellular program. PCD is carried out in a regulated process directed by DNA which normally confers advantage during an organism's life-cycle. PCD serves fundamental functions during tissue development. For example, the development of the spaces between your fingers requires cells to undergo PCD.

Thus cells specialize and develop into organ systems (morphogenesis). The embryo develops from the second to the ninth week, followed by the fetus which develops from the ninth week to birth (*parturition*).

14.6 The Placenta

The **placenta** is a complex vascular structure formed by part of the maternal endometrium (= *the decidua basalis*) and cells of embryonic origin (= *the chorion*). The placenta begins to form when the blastocyst implants in the endometrium. A cell layer from the embryo invades the endometrium with fingerlike bumps (= *chorionic villi*) which project into intervillous spaces which contain maternal blood. Maternal spiral arteries enter the intervillous spaces allowing blood to circulate.

The placenta has three main functions: i) the **transfer** of substances necessary for the development of the embryo or fetus from the mother (O_2, H_2O, carbohydrates, amino acids, certain antibodies, vitamins, etc.) and the **transfer** of wastes from the embryo or fetus to the mother (CO_2, urea, uric acid, etc.); ii) the placenta can synthesize substances (i.e. glycogen, fatty acids) to use as an energy source for itself and the embryo or fetus; iii) the placenta produces and secretes a number of hormones including hCG, estrogen and progesterone.

14.7 Fetal Circulation

Consider the following: the fetus has lungs but does not breathe O_2. In fact, the placenta is, metaphorically, the "fetal lung." Oxygenated blood from the placenta carried via umbilical veins is largely directed to the inferior vena cava by the ductus venosus. Most of this oxygenated blood is diverted from pulmonary circulation to the left atrium via a hole in the atrial septum: the patent foramen ovale (for adult circulation and anatomy, see chapter 7).

Deoxygenated blood from the superior vena cava enters the right heart then pulmonary artery as in an adult. However, resistance in the collapsed lung is high. Thus pulmonary artery pressure is higher than it is in the aorta. Consequently, most of the blood bypasses the lung via the ductus arteriosus to the aorta. Blood from the aorta now enters systemic circulation. Umbilical arteries divert some aortal blood to the placenta for oxygenation. In normal infants, the foramen ovale and the ductus arteriosus both fuse shut. {Consider what would happen if they remained open}

14.8 Fetal Sexual Development

The normal sexual development of the fetus depends on the genotype (XX female, XY male), the morphology of the internal organs and gonads, and the phenotype or external genitalia. Later, these many factors combine to influence the individual's self-perception along with the development of secondary sexual characteristics (i.e. breast development in females, hair growth and lower pitched voice in males).

Every fetus, regardless of genotype, has the capacity to become a normally formed individual of either sex. Development naturally proceeds towards "female" unless there is a Y chromosome factor present. Thus the XX genotype leads to the maturation of the Müllerian ducts into the uterus, fallopian tubes, and part of the vagina. The primitive gonad will develop into a testis only if the Y chromosome is present and encodes the appropriate factor and eventually the secretion of testosterone. Thus the XY genotype leads to the involution of the Müllerian ducts and the maturation of the Wolffian ducts into the vas deferens, seminiferous tubules and prostate.

> Reproductive biology is the only science where multiplication and division mean the same thing.

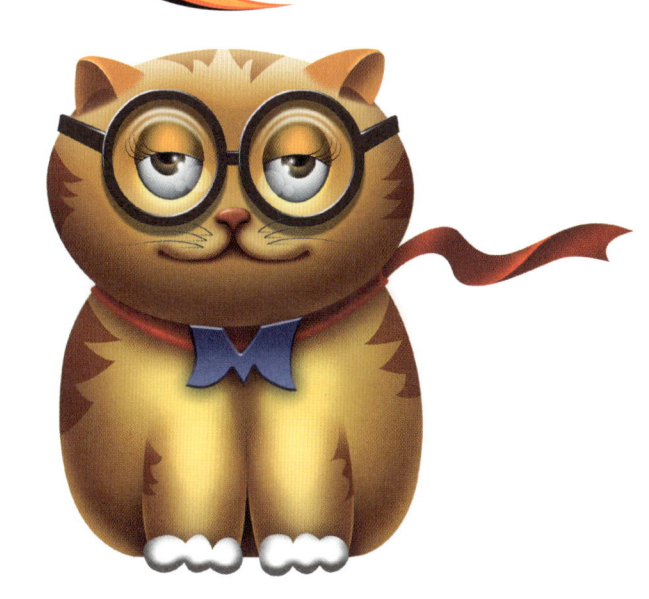

GOLD NOTES

GENETICS

Chapter 15

Memorize	Understand	Not Required*
Define: phenotype, genotype, gene, locus, allele: single and multiple Homo/heterozygosity, wild type, recessiveness, complete/co-dominance Incomplete dominance, gene pool Sex-linked characteristics, sex determination Types of mutations: random, translation error, transcription error, base subs., etc.	*Importance of meiosis; compare/contrast with mitosis *Segregation of genes, assortment, linkage, recombination *Single/double crossovers; relationship of mutagens to carcinogens *Hardy-Weinberg Principle, inborn errors of metabolism *Test cross: back cross, concepts of parental, F1 and F2 generations	* Advanced level college info

GAMSAT-Prep.com

Introduction

Genetics is the study of heredity and variation in organisms. The observations of Gregor Mendel in the mid-nineteenth century gave birth to the science which would reveal the physical basis for his conclusions, DNA, about 100 years later.

Additional Resources

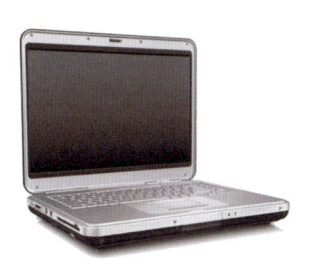

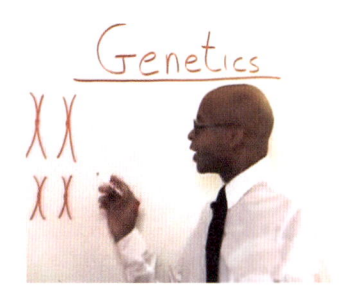

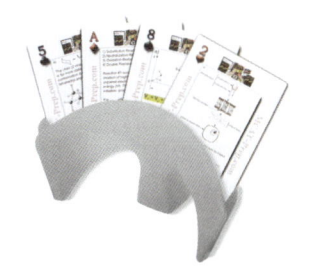

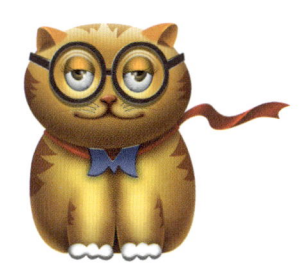

Free Online Q&A + Forum | Video: Online or DVD 4 | Flashcards | Special Guest

THE BIOLOGICAL SCIENCES   BIO-145

* The real GAMSAT may have advanced level information presented (ie. in a passage) but previous knowledge of said information is not required to answer the questions that would follow. Practice ACER and GS practice GAMSATs can help you clarify this point.

15.1 Background Information

Genetics is a branch of biology which deals with the principles and mechanics of heredity; in other words, the *means* by which *traits* are passed from parents to offspring. To begin, we will first examine some relevant definitions - a few of which we have already discussed.

Chromosomes are a complex of DNA and proteins (incl. histones). A gene is that sequence of DNA that codes for a protein or polypeptide. A locus is the *position* of the gene on the DNA molecule. Recall that humans inherit 46 chromosomes - 23 from maternal origin and 23 from paternal origin (BIO 14.2). A given chromosome from maternal origin has a counterpart from paternal origin which codes for the same products. This is called a **homologous pair** of chromosomes. Any homologous pair of chromosomes have a pair of genes which codes for the same product (i.e. hair color). Such pairs of genes are called **alleles**. Thus for one gene product, a nucleus contains one allele from maternal origin and one allele from paternal origin. If both alleles are identical (i.e. they code for the same hair color), then the individual is called **homozygous** for that trait. If the two alleles differ (i.e. one codes for dark hair while the other codes for light hair), then the individual is called **heterozygous** for that trait.

The set of genes possessed by a particular organism is its genotype. The appearance or phenotype of an individual is expressed as a consequence of the genotype and the environment. Consider a heterozygote that expressed one gene (dark hair) but not the other (light hair). The expressed gene would be called dominant while its allele is recessive. The individual would have dark hair as their phenotype, yet their genotype would be heterozygous for that trait.

It is common to symbolize dominant genes with capital letters (A) and recessive genes with small letters (a). From the preceding paragraphs, we can conclude that with two alleles, three genotypes are possible: homozygous dominant (AA), heterozygous (Aa), and homozygous recessive (aa). Note that this only results in two phenotypes since both AA and Aa express the dominant gene, while only aa expresses the recessive gene.

Each individual carries **two** alleles while populations may have many or **multiple alleles**. Sometimes these genes are not strictly dominant or recessive. There may be degrees of blending (= *incomplete dominance*) or sometimes two alleles may be equally dominant (= *codominance*). ABO blood types are an important example of multiple alleles with codominance.

15.2 ABO Blood Types

Red blood cells can have various antigens or *agglutinogens* on their plasma membranes which aid in blood typing. The important two are antigens A and B. If the red blood cells have only antigen A, the blood type is A; if they have only antigen B, then the blood type is B; if they have both antigens, the blood type is AB; if neither antigen is present, the blood type is O. There are three allelic genes in the population (I^A, I^B, i^O). Two are codominant (I^A, I^B) and one is recessive (i^O). Thus in a given population, there are six possible genotypes which result in four possible phenotypes:

Genotype	Phenotype
$I^A I^A$, $I^A i^O$	blood type A
$I^B I^B$, $I^B i^O$	blood type B
$I^A I^B$	blood type AB
$i^O i^O$	blood type O

Blood typing is critical before doing a blood transfusion. This is because people with blood type A have anti-B antibodies, those with type B have anti-A, those with type AB have neither antibody, while type O has both anti-A and anti-B antibodies. If a person with type O blood is given types A, B, or AB, the clumping of the red blood cells will occur (= *agglutination*). Though type O can only receive from type O, it can give to the other blood types since its red blood cells have **no** antigens {type O = universal donor}. Type AB has neither antibody so it can receive blood from all blood types. The only other antigens which have some importance are the Rh factors which are coded by different genes at different loci from the A and B antigens. Rh factors are either there (Rh^+) or they are not there (Rh^-). 85% of the population are Rh^+. The problem occurs when a woman is Rh^- and has been exposed to Rh^+ blood and then forms anti-Rh^+ antibodies (note: unlike the previous case, exposure is necessary to produce these antibodies). If this woman is pregnant with an Rh^+ fetus her antibodies may cross the placenta and cause the fetus' red blood cells to agglutinate (*erythroblastosis fetalis*). This condition is fatal if left untreated.

15.3 Mendelian Genetics

Recall that in gametogenesis homologous chromosomes separate during the first meiotic division. Thus alleles that code for the same trait are segregated: this is **Mendel's First Law of Segregation. Mendel's Second Law of Independent Assortment** states that different chromosomes (*or factors which carry different traits*) separate independently of each other. For example, consider a primary spermatocyte (2N) undergoing its first meiotic division. It is <u>not</u> the case that all 23 chromosomes of paternal origin will end up in one secondary spermatocyte while the other 23 chromosomes of maternal origin ends up in the other. Rather, each chromosome in a homologous pair separates *independently* of any other chromosome in other homologous pairs.

However, it has been noted experimentally that sometimes traits on the same chromosome assort independently! This non-Mendelian concept is a result of *crossing over* (recall that this is when homologous chromosomes exchange parts, BIO 14.2). In fact, it has been shown that two traits located far apart on a chromosome are more likely to cross over and thus assort independently, as compared to two traits that are close. The propensity for some traits to refrain from assorting independently is called <u>linkage</u>. Double crossovers occur when two crossovers happen in a chromosomal region being studied.

Another exception to Mendel's laws involves **sex linkage**. Mendel's laws would predict that the results of a genetic cross should be the same regardless of which parent introduces the allele. However, it can be shown that some traits follow the inheritance of the sex chromosomes. Humans have one pair of sex chromosomes (XX = female, XY = male), and the remaining 22 pairs of homologous chromosomes are called **autosomes**. Since females have <u>two</u> X chromosomes and a male only has <u>one</u>, a *single* recessive allele on an X chromosome could be expressed in a male! {the preceding occurs only when the Y chromosome has no homologous counterpart to the X chromosome - which is commonly the case} In fact, a typical pattern of sex linkage is when a mother passes her phenotype to **all** her sons but **none** of her daughters. Her daughters become *carriers* for the recessive allele. Certain forms of <u>hemophilia</u>, <u>colorblindness</u>, and one kind of <u>muscular dystrophy</u> are well-known recessive sex-linked traits.{*in what was once known as* <u>Lyon's Hypothesis</u>, *it has been shown that every female has a condensed, inactivated X chromosome in her body or* <u>somatic</u> *cells called a* <u>Barr body</u>}

Let us examine the predictions of Mendel's First Law. Consider two parents, one homozygous dominant (AA) and the other homozygous recessive (aa). Each parent can only form one type of gamete with respect to that trait (*either* A *or* a, *respectively*). The next generation (*called* first filial *or* **F₁**) must then be uniformly heterozygotes or *hybrids* (Aa). Now the F_1 hybrids can produce gametes that can be either A half the time or a half the time. With this information we can predict the outcome in the next generation (F_2) using a Punnett square:

	1/2 A	1/2 a
1/2 A	1/4 AA	1/4 Aa
1/2 a	1/4 Aa	1/4 aa

Here is an example as to how you derive the information within the square: when you cross A with A you get AA (i.e. 1/2 A × 1/2 A = 1/4 AA). Thus by doing a simple *mono*hybrid cross (Aa × Aa) with random mating, the Punnett square indicates that in the F_2 generation, 1/4 of the population would be AA, 1/2 would be Aa (1/4 + 1/4), and 1/4 would be aa. In other words the *genotypic* ratio of homozygous dominant to heterozygous to homozygous recessive is 1:2:1. However, since AA and Aa demonstrate the same *phenotype* (i.e. dominant) the ratio of dominant to recessive is 3:1.

Now we will consider the predictions of Mendel's Second Law. To examine independent assortment, we will have to consider a case with two traits (usu. on different chromosomes) or a *di*hybrid cross. Imagine a parent which is homozygous dominant for two traits (AABB) while the other is homozygous recessive (aabb). Each parent can only form one type of gamete with respect to those traits (*either* AB *or* ab, *respectively*). The F_1 generation will be uniform for the dominant trait (i.e. *the* genotypes *would all be* AaBb). In the gametes of the F_1 generation, the alleles will assort independently. Consequently, an equal amount of all the possible gametes will form: 1/4 AB, 1/4 Ab, 1/4 aB, and 1/4 ab. With this information we can predict the outcome in the F_2 generation using the Punnett square:

	1/4 AB	1/4 Ab	1/4 aB	1/4 ab
1/4 AB	1/16 AABB	1/16 AABb	1/16 AaBB	1/16 AaBb
1/4 Ab	1/16 AABb	1/16 AAbb	1/16 AaBb	1/16 Aabb
1/4 aB	1/16 AaBB	1/16 AaBb	1/16 aaBB	1/16 aaBb
1/4 ab	1/16 AaBb	1/16 Aabb	1/16 aaBb	1/16 aabb

Thus by doing a dihybrid cross with random mating, the Punnett square indicates that there are nine possible genotypes (*the frequency is given in brackets*): AABB (1), AABb (2), AaBb (4), AaBB (2), Aabb (2), aaBb (2), AAbb (1), aaBB (1), and aabb (1). Since A and B are dominant, there are only four phenotypic classes in the ratio 9:3:3:1 which are: the expression of <u>both</u> traits (AABB + AABb + AaBb + AaBB = 9), the expression of only the <u>first</u> trait (AAbb + Aabb = 3), the expression of only the <u>second</u> trait (aaBB + aaBb = 3), and the expression of <u>neither</u> trait (aabb = 1). Now we know, for example, that 9/16 represents that fraction of the population which will have the phenotype of both dominant traits.

15.3.1 A Word about Probability

If you were to flip a quarter, the probability of getting "heads" is 50% (p = 0.5). If you flipped the quarter ten times and each time it came up heads, the probability of getting heads on the next trial is still 50%. After all, previous trials have no effect on the next trial.

Since chance events, such as fertilization of a particular kind of egg by a particular kind of sperm, occur independently, the genotype of one child has no effect on the genotypes of other children produced by a set of parents. Thus in the previous example of the dihybrid cross, the chance of producing the genotype AaBb is 4/16 (25%) irrespective of the genotypes which have already been produced.

BIO-150 GENETICS

BIOLOGY

15.4 The Hardy-Weinberg Law

The Hardy-Weinberg Law deals with population genetics. A **population** includes all the members of a species which occupy a more or less well defined geographical area and have demonstrated the ability to reproduce from generation to generation. A **gene pool** is the sum of all the genes in a population. A central component to evolution is the changing of alleles in a gene pool from one generation to the next. The Hardy-Weinberg Law or *equilibrium* predicts the outcome of a randomly mating population of sexually reproducing diploid organisms who are not undergoing evolution.

For the Hardy-Weinberg Law to be applied, the idealized population must meet the following conditions: i) **random mating**: the members of the population must have no mating preferences; ii) **no mutations**: there must be no errors in replication nor similar event resulting in a change in the genome; iii) **isolation**: there must be no exchange of genes between the population being considered and any other population; iv) **large population**: since the law is based on statistical probabilities, to avoid sampling errors, the population cannot be small; v) **no selection pressures**: there must be no reproductive advantage of one allele over the other.

To illustrate a use of the law, consider an idealized population that abides by the preceding conditions and have a gene locus occupied by either A or a. Let p = the frequency of allele A in the population and let q = the frequency of allele a. Since they are the only alleles, p + q = 1. Squaring both sides we get:

$$(p + q)^2 = (1)^2$$
$$\text{OR}$$
$$p^2 + 2pq + q^2 = 1$$

The preceding equation (= *the Hardy-Weinberg equation*) can be used to calculate genotype frequencies once the allelic frequencies are given. This can be summarized by the following:

	pA	qa
pA	p^2AA	pqAa
qa	pqAa	q^2aa

The Punnett square illustrates the expected frequencies of the three genotypes in the next generation: AA = p^2, Aa = 2pq, and aa = q^2.

THE BIOLOGICAL SCIENCES

For example, let us calculate the percentage of heterozygous individuals in a population where the recessive allele q has a frequency of 0.2. Since p + q = 1, then p = 0.8. Using the Hardy-Weinberg equation and squaring p and q we get:

$$0.64 + 2pq + 0.04 = 1$$
$$2pq = 1 - 0.68 = 0.32$$

Thus the percentage of heterozygous (2pq) individuals is 32%.

A practical application of the Hardy-Weinberg equation is the prediction of how many people in a generation are carriers for a particular recessive allele. The values would have to be recalculated for every generation since humans do not abide by all the conditions of the Hardy-Weinberg Law (i.e. *humans continually evolve*).

15.4.1 Back Cross, Test Cross

A back cross is the cross of an individual (F_1) with one of its parents (P) or an organism with the same genotype as a parent. Back crosses can be used to help identify the genotypes of the individual in a specific type of back cross called a test cross. A test cross is a cross between an organism whose genotype for a certain trait is unknown and an organism that is homozygous recessive for that trait so the unknown genotype can be determined from that of the offspring. For example, for P: AA x aa and F1: Aa, we get:

Backcross #1: Aa x AA
Progeny #1: 1/2 Aa and 1/2 AA

Backcross #2: Aa x aa
Progeny #2: 1/2 Aa and 1/2 aa

15.5 Genetic Variability

Meiosis and mutations are sources of genetic variability. During the first division of meiosis, crossing over occurs which leads to a **recombination** of parental genes in a new way. Thus recombination can result in alleles of linked traits separating into different gametes. However, the closer two traits are on a chromosome, the more likely they will be linked and thus remain together, and vice versa.

Further recombination occurs during the random fusion of gametes during fertilization. Consequently, taking Mendel's two laws and recombination together, we can predict that parents can give their offspring combinations of alleles which the parents never had. This leads to **genetic variability**.

Mutations are rare, inheritable, random changes in the genetic material (DNA) of a cell. Mutations are much more likely to be either neutral (esp. *silent mutations*) or negative (i.e. cancer) than positive for an organism's survival. Nonetheless, such a change in the genome increases genetic variability. Only mutations of gametes, and not somatic cells, are passed on to offspring.

The following are some forms of mutations:

* **Point mutation** is a change affecting a single base pair in a gene

* **Deletion** is the removal of a sequence of DNA, the regions on either side being joined together

* **Inversion** is the reversal of a segment of DNA

* **Translocation** is when one chromosome breaks and attaches to another

* **Duplication** is when a sequence of DNA is repeated.

* **Frame shift mutations** occur when bases are added or deleted in numbers other than multiples of three. Such deletions or additions cause the rest of the sequence to be shifted such that each triplet reading frame is altered.

A mutagen is any substance or agent that can cause a mutation. A mutagen is not the same as a carcinogen. Carcinogens are agents that cause cancer. While many mutagens are carcinogens as well, many others are not. The Ames test is a widely used test to screen chemicals used in foods or medications for mutagenic potential.

Mutations can produce many types of genetic diseases including inborn errors of metabolism. These disorders in normal metabolism are usually due to defects of a single gene that codes for one enzyme.

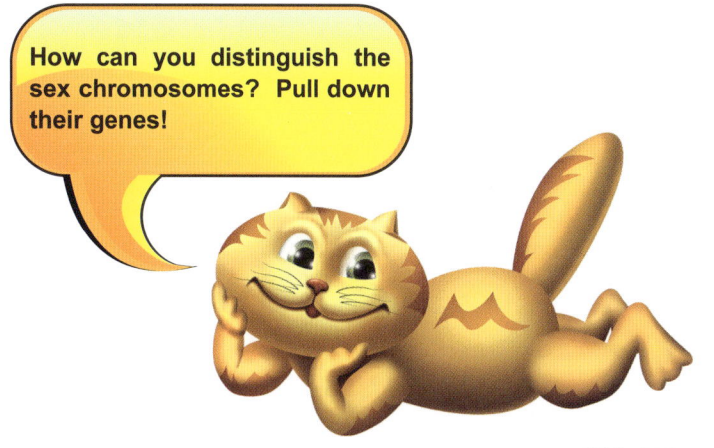

How can you distinguish the sex chromosomes? Pull down their genes!

GOLD NOTES

EVOLUTION

Chapter 16

Memorize	Understand	Not Required*
* Define: species, genetic drift * Basics: chordates, vertebrates	* Natural selection, speciation * Genetic drift * Basics: origin of life * Basics: comparative anatomy	* Advanced level college info

GAMSAT-Prep.com

Introduction

Evolution is, quite simply, the change in the inherited traits of a population of organisms from one generation to another. This change over time can be traced to 3 main processes: variation, reproduction and selection. The major mechanisms that drive evolution are natural selection and genetic drift.

Additional Resources

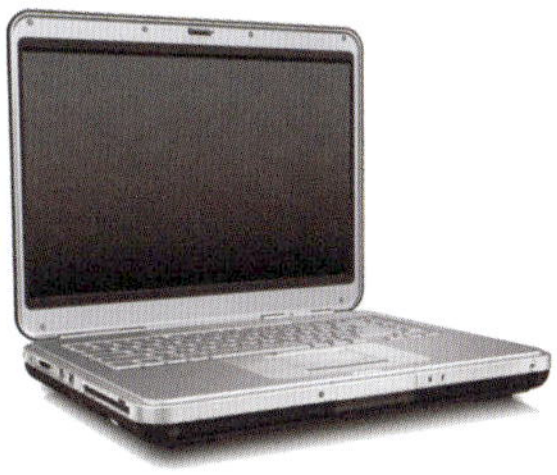

Free Online Q&A + Forum

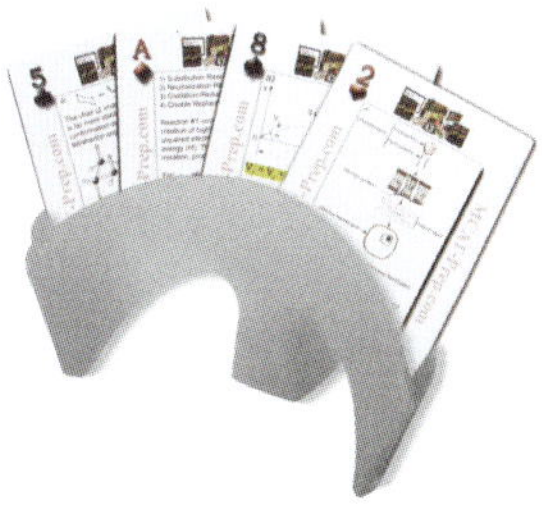

Flashcards

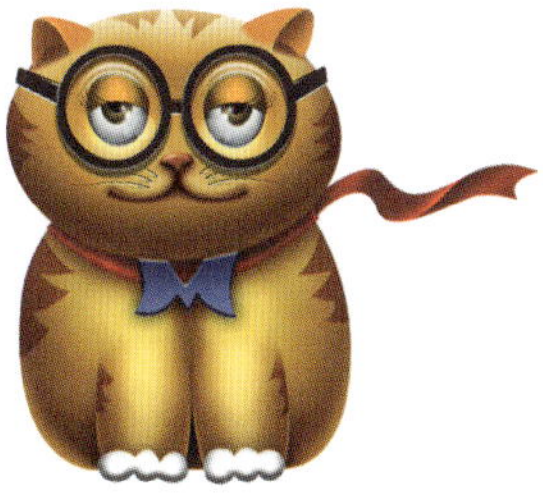

Special Guest

THE BIOLOGICAL SCIENCES BIO-155

* The real GAMSAT may have advanced level information presented (ie. in a passage) but previous knowledge of said information is not required to answer the questions that would follow. Practice ACER and GS practice GAMSATs can help you clarify this point.

GAMSAT-Prep.com
THE GOLD STANDARD

16.1 Overview

Evolution is the change in frequency of one or more alleles in a population's gene pool from one generation to the next. The evidence for evolution lies in the fossil record, biogeography, embryology, comparative anatomy, and experiments from artificial selection. The most important mechanism of evolution is the **selection** of certain phenotypes provided by the **genetic variability** of a population.

16.2 Natural Selection

Natural selection is the non-random differential survival and reproduction from one generation to the next. Natural selection contains the following premises: i) genetic and phenotypic variability exist in populations; ii) more individuals are produced than live to grow up and reproduce; iii) individuals with some genes are more likely to survive (*greater fitness*) than those with other genes.

It is not necessarily true that natural selection leads to the "survival of the fittest"; rather it is the genes, and not necessarily the individual, which are likely to survive.

Evolution goes against the foundations of the Hardy-Weinberg Law. For example, natural selection leads to non-random mating due to phenotypic differences. Evolution occurs when those phenotypic changes depend on an underlying genotype; thus non-random mating can lead to changes in allelic frequencies. Consider an example: if female peacocks decide to only mate with a male with long feathers, then there will be a selection pressure against any male with a genotype which is expressed as short feathers. Because of this differential reproduction, the alleles which are expressed as short feathers will be eliminated from the population. Thus this population evolves.

The two common forms of natural selection are: i) **stabilizing selection** in which average phenotypes have a selective advantage over extremes (*phenotypes have a 'bell curve' distribution*); ii) **directional selection** when one extreme has a selective advantage over the average phenotype (*thus the curve can become squewed to the left or right*). A derivative of directional selection is disruptive selection where both extremes are selected over the average phenotype; this would produce a split down the middle of the 'bell curve' such that two new and separate 'bell curves' would result. For example, if a bird only ate medium sized seeds and left the large and small ones alone, two new populations or groups of seeds would have a reproductive advantage. Thus by selecting against one group of seeds, two new groups of seeds with, possibly, different allelic frequencies for seed size will result. This is an example of *group selection* causing *disruptive selection*.

16.3 Species and Speciation

Species can be defined as the members of populations that interbreed or can interbreed under natural conditions. There are great variations within species. A **cline** is a gradient of variation in a species across a geographical area. **Speciation** is the evolution of new species by the isolation of gene pools of related populations. The isolation of gene pools is typically geographic. An ocean, a glacier, a river or any other physical barrier can isolate a population and prevent it from mating with other populations of the same species. The two populations may begin to differ because their mutations may be different, or, there may be different selection pressures from the two different environments, or, genetic drift may play a role.

Genetic drift is the random change in frequencies of alleles or genotypes in a population (recall that this is antagonistic to the Hardy-Weinberg Law). Genetic drift normally occurs when a small population is isolated from a large population. Since the allelic frequencies in the small population may be different from the large population (*sampling error*), the two populations may evolve in different directions.

Populations or species can be sympatric (= live together), or allopatric (= live apart). Mechanisms involved in allopatric speciation are represented in the two preceding paragraphs. The following represents some isolating mechanisms that prevent sympatric populations of different species from breeding together: i) habitat differences; ii) different breeding times or seasons; iii) mechanical differences (i.e. different anatomy of the genitalia); iv) behavioral specificity (i.e. different courtship behavior); v) gametic isolation (= fertilization cannot occur); vi) hybrid inviability (i.e. the hybrid zygote dies before reaching the age of sexual maturity); vii) hybrid sterility; viii) hybrid breakdown: the hybrid offspring is fertile but produces a next generation (F_2) which is infertile or inviable.

16.4 Origin of Life

Evidence suggests that the primitive earth had a reducing atmosphere with gases such as H_2 and the reduced compounds H_2O (vapor), $NH_{3(g)}$ (ammonia) and $CH_{4(g)}$ (methane). Such an atmosphere has been shown (i.e. Miller, Fox) to be conducive to the formation and stabilization of organic compounds. Such compounds can sometimes polymerize (*possibly due to autocatalysis*) and evolve into living systems with metabolism, reproduction, digestion, excretion, etc...

Critical in the early history of the earth was the evolution of: photosynthesis which releases O_2 and thus converted the atmosphere into an oxidizing one; respiration, which could use the O_2 to efficiently produce ATP; and the development of membrane bound organelles (*a subset of prokaryotes which evolved into eukaryotes*) which allowed eukaryotes to develop meiosis, sexual reproduction, and fertilization.

It is important to recognize that throughout the evolution of the earth, organisms and the environment have and will continue to shape each other.

16.5 Comparative Anatomy

Anatomical features of organisms can be compared in order to derive information about their evolutionary histories. Structures which originate from the same part of the embryo are called homologous. **Homologous** structures may have different functions in different species. **Analogous** structures have similar functions but arise from different embryological structures. **Vestigial** structures represent further evidence for evolution since they are organs which are useless in their present owners, but are homologous with organs which are important in other species.

Taxonomy is the branch of biology which deals with the classification of organisms. Humans are classified as follows:

Kingdom	Animalia
Phylum (= Division)	Chordata
Class	Mammalia
Order	Primates
Family	Hominidae
Genus	*Homo*
Species	*Homo sapiens*

{Mnemonic for remembering the taxonomic categories: King Philip came over for great soup}

BIOLOGY

The subphyla Vertebrata and Invertebrata are subdivisions of the phylum Chordata. Acorn worms, tunicates, sea squirts and amphioxus are invertebrates. Humans, birds, frogs, fish, and crocodiles are vertebrates. We will examine features of both the chordates and the vertebrates.

Chordates have the following characteristics at some stage of their development: i) a notochord; ii) pharyngeal gill slits which lead from the pharynx to the exterior; iii) a hollow dorsal nerve cord. Other features which are less defining but are nonetheless present in chordates are: i) a more or less segmented anatomy; ii) an internal skeleton (= *endoskeleton*); iii) a tail at some point in their development.

Vertebrates have all the characteristics of chordates. In addition, vertebrates have: i) a vertebral column; ii) well developed sensory and nervous systems; iii) a ventral heart with a closed vascular system; iv) some sort of a liver, endocrine organs, and kidneys; and v) cephalization which is the concentration of sense organs and nerves to the front end of the body producing an obvious head.

Why did the dinosaur cross the road? Because chickens hadn't evolved yet.

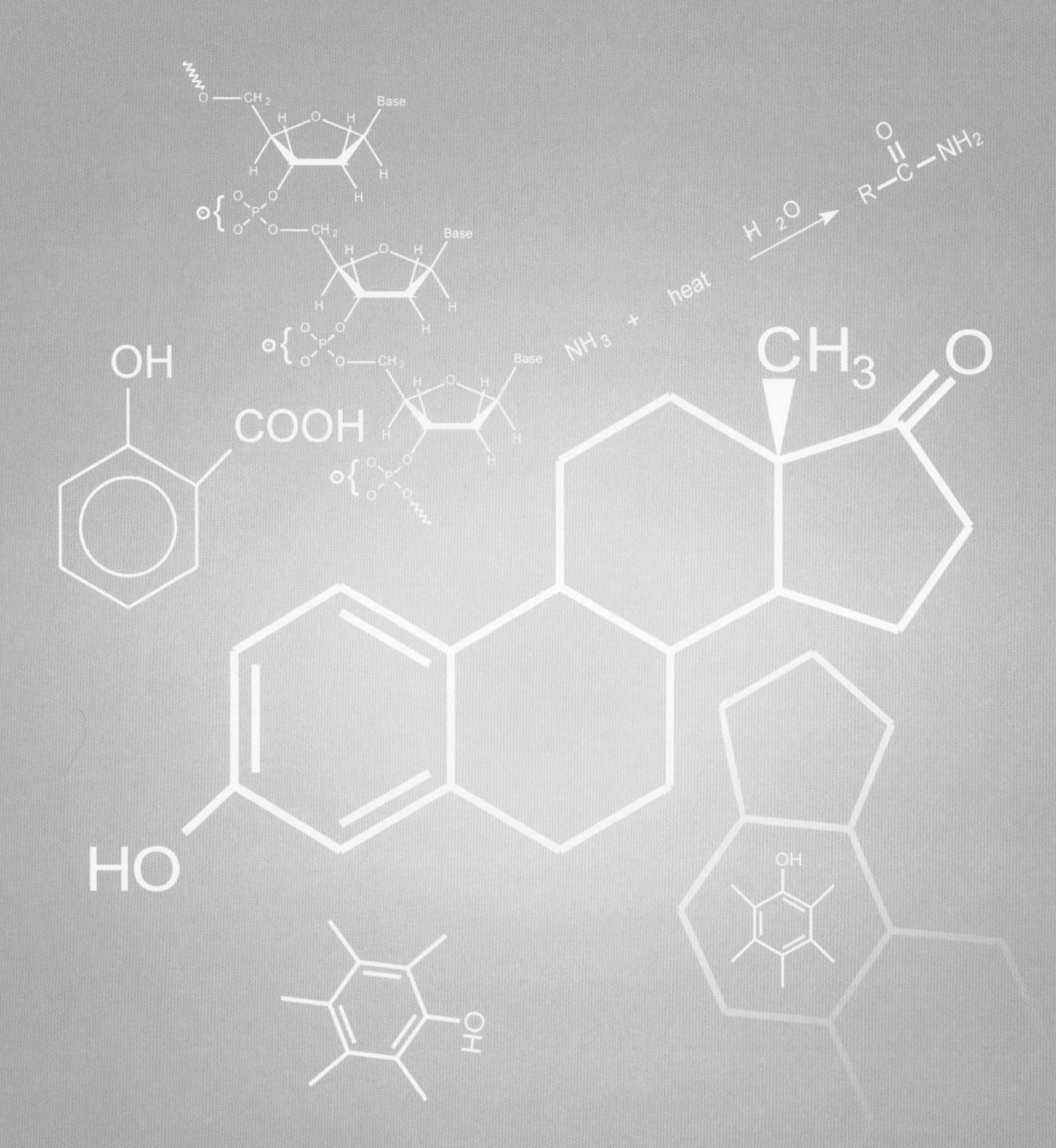

GAMSAT-Prep.com
ORGANIC CHEMISTRY
PART IV.B: BIOLOGICAL SCIENCES

IMPORTANT: Before doing your science survey for the GAMSAT, be sure you have read the Preface, Introduction and Part II, Chapter 2. The beginning of each science chapter provides guidelines as to what you should Memorize, Understand and what is Not Required. These are guides to get you a top score without getting lost in the details. Our guides have been determined from an analysis of all ACER materials plus student surveys. Additionally, the original owner of this book gets a full year access to many online features described in the Preface and Introduction including an online Forum where each chapter can be discussed.

MOLECULAR STRUCTURE OF ORGANIC COMPOUNDS
Chapter 1

Memorize
* Hybrid orbitals and geometries
* Periodic table trends
* Define: Lewis, dipole moments
* Ground rules for reaction mechanisms

Understand
* Delocalized electrons and resonance
* Multiple bonds, length, energies
* Basic stereochemistry
* Principles for reaction mechanisms

Not Required *
* Advanced level college info
* Hybrids involving d, f, etc.

GAMSAT-Prep.com

Introduction

Organic chemistry is the study of the structure, properties, composition, reactions, and preparation (i.e. synthesis) of chemical compounds containing carbon. Such compounds may contain hydrogen, nitrogen, oxygen, the halogens as well as phosphorus, silicon and sulfur. If you master the basic rules in this chapter, you will be able to conquer GAMSAT mechanisms with little or no further memorization.

Additional Resources

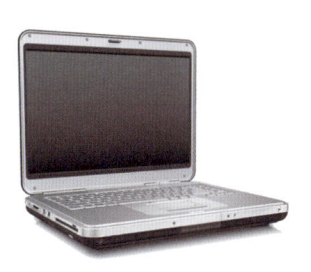

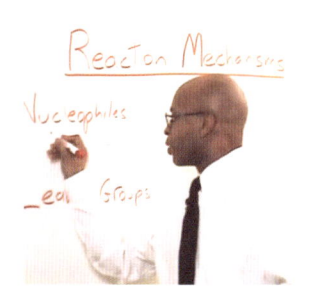

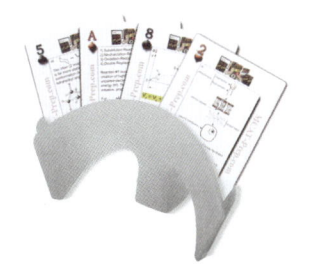

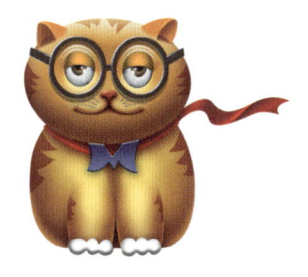

Free Online Q&A + Forum   Video   Flashcards   Special guest

THE BIOLOGICAL SCIENCES   ORG-03

* The real GAMSAT may have advanced level information presented (ie. in a passage) but previous knowledge of said information is not required to answer the questions that would follow. Practice ACER and GS practice GAMSATs can help you clarify this point.

1.1 Overview: The Atoms of Organic Chemistry

Organic chemistry may be defined as the chemistry of the compounds of carbon. Organic chemistry is very important, as living systems are composed mainly of water and organic compounds. Other important organic molecules form essential components of fuels, plastics and other petroleum derivatives.

Carbon (C), hydrogen (H), oxygen (O), nitrogen (N) and the halides (i.e. fluorine – F, chlorine – Cl, bromine – Br, etc.) are the most common atoms found in organic compounds. The atoms in most organic compounds are held together by covalent bonds (*the sharing of an electron pair between two atoms*). Some ionic bonding (*the transfer of electrons from one atom to another*) does exist. Common to both types of chemical bonds is the fact that the atoms bond such that they can achieve the electron configuration of the nearest noble gas, usually eight electrons. This is known as the *octet rule*.

A **carbon** atom has one s and three p orbitals in its outermost shell, allowing it to form 4 single bonds. As well, a carbon atom may be involved in a double bond, where two electron pairs are shared, or a triple bond, where three electron pairs are shared. An **oxygen** atom may form 2 single bonds, or one double bond. It has 2 unshared (lone) electron pairs. A **hydrogen** atom will form only one single bond. A **nitrogen** atom may form 3 single bonds. As well, it is capable of double and triple bonds. It has one unshared electron pair. The **halides** are all able to form only one (single) bond. Halides all have three unshared electron pairs.

Throughout the following chapters we will be examining the structural formulas of molecules involving H, C, N, O, halides and phosphorus (P). However it should be noted that less common atoms often have similar structural formulas within molecules as compared to common atoms. For example, silicon (Si) is found in the same group as carbon in the periodic table; thus they have similar properties. In fact, Si can also form 4 single bonds leading to a tetrahedral structure (i.e. SiH_4, SiO_4). Likewise sulfur (S) is found in the same group as oxygen. Though it can be found as a solid (S_8), it still has many properties similar to those of oxygen. For example, like O in H_2O, sulfur can form a bent, polar molecule which can hydrogen bond (H_2S). We will later see that sulfur is an important component in the amino acid cysteine. {*To learn more about molecular structure, hybrid orbitals, polarity and bonding, review General Chemistry chapters 2 and 3*}

HONC!!!
H requires 1 more electron in its outer shell to become stable
O requires 2
N requires 3
C requires 4

ORGANIC CHEMISTRY

1.2 Hybrid Orbitals

In organic molecules, the orbitals of the atoms are combined to form **hybrid orbitals**, consisting of a mixture of the s and p orbitals. In a carbon atom, if the one s and three p orbitals are mixed, the result is four hybrid sp^3 orbitals. Three hybridized sp^2 orbitals result from the mixing of one s and two p orbitals, and two hybridized sp orbitals result from the mixing of one s and one p. The geometry of the hybridized orbitals is shown in Figure IV.B.1.1.

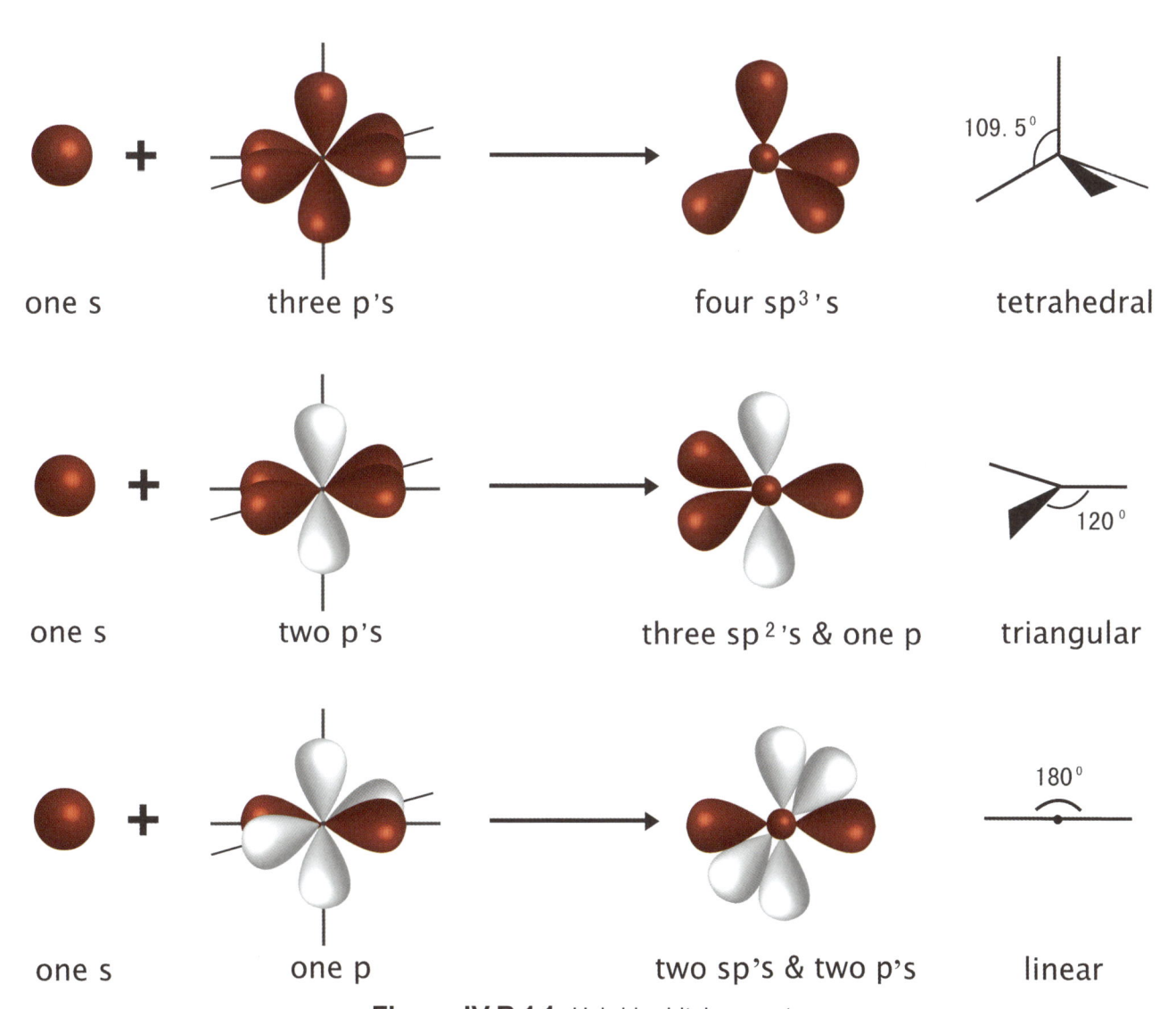

Figure IV.B.1.1: Hybrid orbital geometry

THE BIOLOGICAL SCIENCES ORG-05

1.3 Bonding

Sigma (or single) bonds are those in which the electron density is between the nuclei. They are symmetric about the axis, can freely rotate, and are formed when orbitals (regular or hybridized) overlap directly. They are characterized by the fact that they are circular when a cross section is taken and the bond is viewed along the bond axis. The electron density in pi bonds overlaps both above and below the plane of the atoms. A single bond is a sigma bond; a double bond is one sigma and one pi bond; a triple bond is one sigma (σ) and two pi (π) bonds.

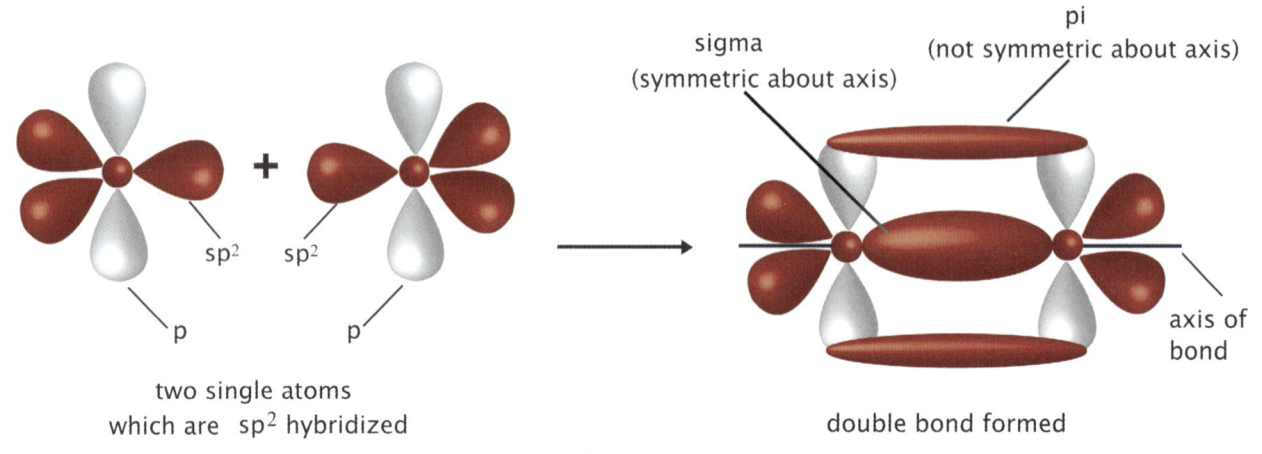

Figure IV.B.1.2: Sigma and pi bonds. The sp^2 hybrids overlap between the nuclei to form a σ bond; the p orbitals overlap above and below the axis between the nuclei to form a π bond.

1.3.1 The Effects of Multiple Bonds

The pi bonds in doubly and triply bonded molecules create a barrier to free rotation about the axis of the bond. Thus multiple bonds create molecules which are much more rigid than a molecule with only a single bond which can freely rotate about its axis.

As a rule, the length of a bond decreases with multiple bonds. For example, the carbon-carbon triple bond is shorter than the carbon-carbon double bond which is shorter than the carbon-carbon single bond.

Bond strength and thus the amount of energy required to break a bond (= *BE, the bond dissociation energy*) varies with the number of bonds. One σ bond has a BE ≈ 110 kcal/mole and one π bond has a BE ≈ 60 kcal/mole. Thus a single bond (one σ) has a BE ≈ 110 kcal/mole while a double bond (one σ + one π) has a BE ≈ 170 kcal/mole. Hence multiple bonds have greater bond strength than single bonds.

ORGANIC CHEMISTRY

1.4 Delocalized Electrons and Resonance

Delocalization of charges in the pi bonds is possible when there are hybridized orbitals in adjacent atoms. This delocalization may be represented in two different ways, the molecular orbital (MO) approach or the resonance (*valence bond*) approach. The differences are found in Figure IV.B.1.3.

The MO approach takes a linear combination of atomic orbitals to form molecular orbitals, in which electrons form the bonds. These molecular orbitals cover the whole molecule, and thus the delocalization of electrons is depicted. In the resonance approach, there is a linear combination of different structures with localized pi bonds and electrons, which together depict the true molecule, or **resonance hybrid**. There is no single structure that represents the molecule.

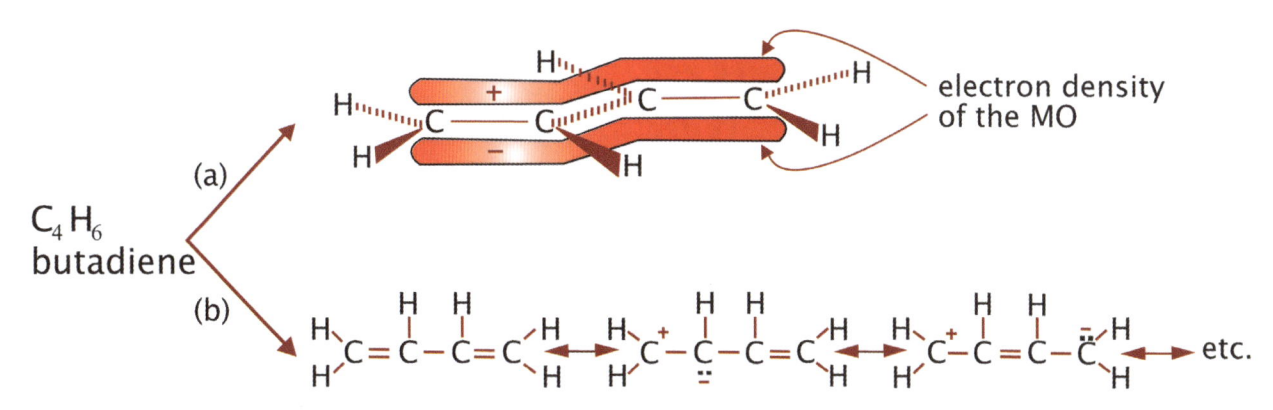

Figure IV.B.1.3: A comparison of MO and resonance approaches. (a) The electron density of the MO covers the entire molecule such that π bonds and p orbitals are not distinguishable. (b) No singular resonance structure accurately portrays butadiene; rather, the true molecule is a composite of all of its resonance structures.

1.5 Lewis Structures, Charge Separation and Dipole Moments

The outer shell (or **valence**) electrons are those that form chemical bonds. **Lewis dot structures** are a method of showing the valence electrons and how they form bonds. These electrons, along with the octet rule (*which states that a maximum of eight electrons are allowed in the outermost shell of an atom*) holds only for the elements in the second row of the periodic table (C,N,O,F). The elements of the third row (Si, P, S, Cl) use d orbitals, and thus can have more than eight electrons in their outer shell.

Let us use CO_2 as an example. Carbon has four valence electrons and oxygen has six. By covalently bonding, electrons are shared and the octet rule is followed,

·C· + 2 :Ö: ⟶

:Ö::C::Ö: or :Ö=C=Ö:

Carbon and oxygen can form resonance structures in the molecule CO_3^{-2}. The −2 denotes two extra electrons to place in the molecule. Once again the octet rule is followed,

In the final structure, each element counts one half of the electrons in a bond as its own, and any unpaired electrons are counted as its own. The sum of these two quantities should equal the number of valence electrons that were originally around the atom.

If the chemical bond is made up of atoms of different electronegativity, there is a **charge separation:**

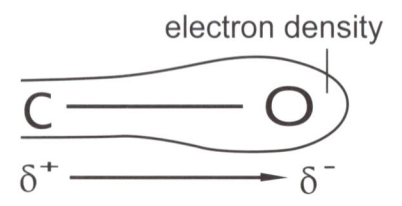

electron density

C————O

δ^+ ⟶ δ^-

There is a slight pulling of electron density by the more electronegative atom (oxygen in the preceding example) from the less electronegative atom (carbon in the preceding example). This results in the C–O bond having **partial ionic character** (i.e. *a polar bond; see CHM 3.3*). The charge separation also causes an electrical dipole to be set up in the direction of the arrow. A dipole has a positive end (carbon) and a negative end (oxygen). A dipole will line up in an electric field.

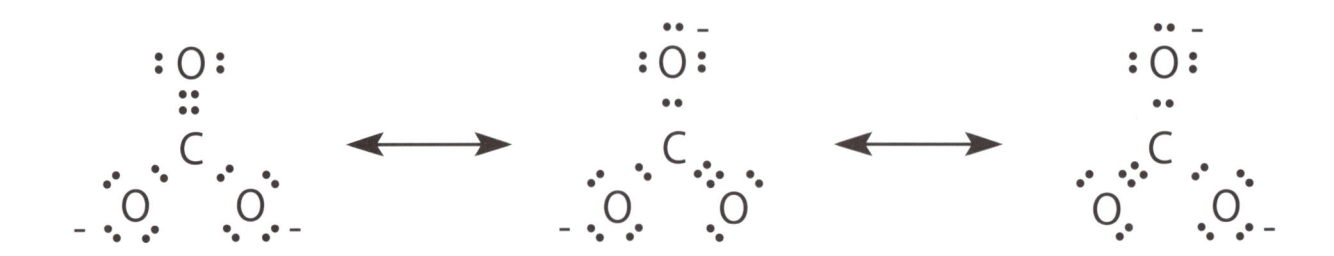

ORG-08   MOLECULAR STRUCTURE OF ORGANIC COMPOUNDS

The most electronegative elements (in order, with electronegativities in brackets) are fluorine (4.0), oxygen (3.5), nitrogen (3.0), and chlorine (3.0) [To examine trends, see the periodic table in CHM 2.3]. These elements will often be paired with hydrogen (2.1) and carbon (2.5), resulting in bonds with partial ionic character. The **dipole moment** is a measure of the charge separation and thus, the electronegativities of the elements that make up the bond; the larger the dipole moment, the larger the charge separation.

No dipole moment is found in molecules with no charge separation between atoms (i.e. Cl_2, Br_2), or, when the charge separation is symmetric resulting in a cancellation of bond polarity like vector addition in physics (i.e. CH_4, CO_2).

A molecule where the charge separation between atoms is not symmetric will have a non-zero dipole moment (i.e. CH_3F, H_2O, NH_3 - see ORG 11.1.2).

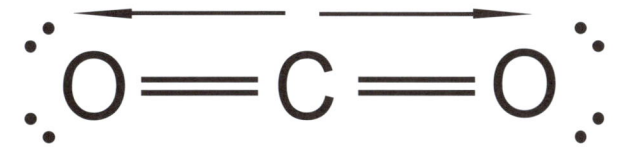

Figure IV.B.1.4: CO_2 - polar bonds but overall it is a non-polar molecule; therefore, CO_2 has a zero dipole moment.

1.5.1 Strength of Polar vs. Non-Polar Bonds

Non-polar bonds are generally stronger than polar covalent and ionic bonds, with ionic bonds being the weakest. However, in compounds with ionic bonding, there is generally a large number of bonds between molecules and this makes the compound as a whole very strong. For instance, although the ionic bonds in one compound are weaker than the non-polar covalent bonds in another compound, the ionic compound's melting point will be higher than the melting point of the covalent compound. Polar covalent bonds have a partially ionic character, and thus the bond strength is usually intermediate between that of ionic and that of non-polar covalent bonds. The strength of bonds generally decreases with increasing ionic character.

1.6 Ground Rules

Opposites attract. Like charges repel. Such simple statements are fundamental in solving over 90% of mechanisms in organic chemistry. Once you are comfortable with the basics - electronegativity, polarity and resonance - you will not need to memorize the grand majority of outcomes of given reactions. You will be capable of quickly deducing the answer even when new scenarios are presented.

A substance which has a formal positive charge (+) or a partial positive charge ("delta+" or δ^+) is attracted to a substance with a formal negative charge (-) or a partial negative charge (δ^-). In general, a substance with a formal charge would have a greater force of attraction than one with a partial charge when faced with an oppositely charged species. There is an important exception: spectator ions. Ions formed by elements in the first two groups of the periodic table (i.e. Na^+, K^+, Ca^{++}) do not actively engage in reactions in organic chemistry. They simply watch the reaction occur then at the very end they associate with the negatively charged product.

In most carbon-based compounds the carbon atom is bonded to a more electronegative atom. For example, in a carbon-oxygen bond the oxygen is δ^- resulting in a δ^+ carbon (see ORG 1.5). Because opposites attract, a δ^- carbon (which is unusual) could create a carbon-carbon bond with a δ^+ carbon (which is common). There are two important categories of compounds which can create a carbon-carbon bond; a) alkyl lithiums (RLi) and b) Grignard reagents (RMgBr), because they each have a δ^- carbon. Note that the carbon is δ^- since lithium is to the left of carbon on the periodic table (for electronegativity trends see CHM 2.3).

For nucleophiles, the general trend is that the stronger the nucleophile, the stronger the base it is. For example:

$$RO^- > HO^- \gg RCOO^- > ROH > H_2O$$

For information on the quality of leaving groups, see ORG 6.2.4.

ORGANIC CHEMISTRY

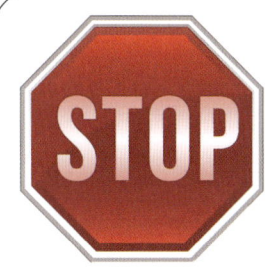

Reminder: Chapter review questions are available online for the original owner of this textbook. Doing practice questions will help clarify concepts and ensure that you study in a targeted way. First, register at gamsat-prep.com, then login and click on GAMSAT Textbook Owners in the right column so you can use your Online Access Card to have access to the Lessons section.

No science background? Consider watching the relevant videos at gamsat-prep.com and you have support at gamsat-prep.com/forum. Don't forget to check the Index at the beginning of this book to see which chapters are HIGH, MEDIUM and LOW relative importance for the GAMSAT.

Your online access continues for one full year from your online registration.

GOLD NOTES

STEREOCHEMISTRY

Chapter 2

Memorize
* Categories of stereoisomers
* Define enantiomers, diastereomers
* Define ligand, chiral, racemic mixture

Understand
* Basic stereochemistry
* Identify meso compounds
* Assign R/S/E/Z
* Fischer projections

Not Required*
* Advanced level college info
* Memorize specific rotation equation

GAMSAT-Prep.com

Introduction

Stereochemistry is the study of the relative spatial (3-D) arrangement of atoms within molecules. An important branch of stereochemistry, and most relevant to the new GAMSAT, is the study of chiral molecules.

More than 1/3 of organic chemistry questions from ACER practice materials test content presented in this chapter. Of course, this does not guarantee the balance of questions on your upcoming exam but it underlines the relative importance of this chapter. Normally, but not always, ACER will reiterate - in the exam's stimulus material - the rules for assigning R/S/E/Z configuration ("stimulus material" refers to the passage, article, graphs, tables or diagrams that precede multiple-choice questions).

Additional Resources

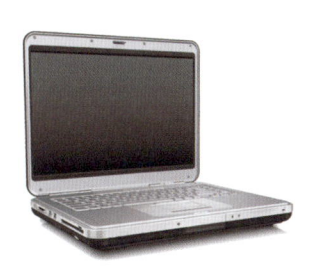

Free Online Q&A + Forum   Video: DVD Disc 1   Flashcards   Special Guest

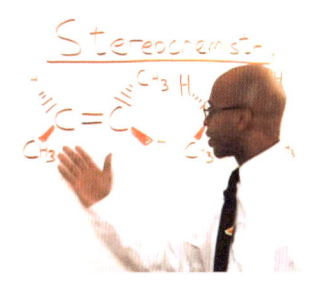

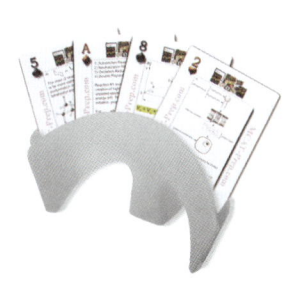

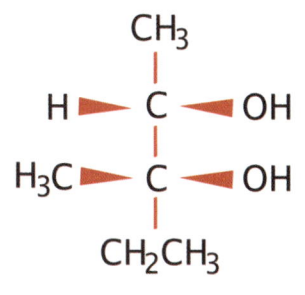

THE BIOLOGICAL SCIENCES ORG-13

* The real GAMSAT may have advanced level information presented (ie. in a passage) but previous knowledge of said information is not required to answer the questions that would follow. Practice ACER and GS practice GAMSATs can help you clarify this point.

2.1 Isomers

Stereochemistry is the study of the arrangement of atoms in a molecule, in three dimensions. Two *different molecules* with the same number and type of atoms (= *the same molecular formula*) are called isomers. There are several different types of isomers:

Structural isomers have different atoms and/or bonding patterns in relation to each other:

$$H_3C-\underset{\underset{H}{|}}{\overset{\overset{CH_3}{|}}{C}}-CH_2CH_2CH_3$$

and

$$H_3C-\underset{\underset{CH_3}{\underset{|}{CH_2}}}{\overset{\overset{H}{|}}{C}}-CH_2CH_3$$

Conformational isomers are isomers which differ only by the rotation about single bonds. As a result, substituents (= *ligands* = *attached atoms or groups*) can be maximally close (*eclipsed conformation*), maximally apart (*anti or staggered conformation*) or anywhere in between (i.e. *gauche conformation*). Though all conformations occur at room temperature, anti is most stable since it minimizes electron shell repulsion.

Geometric isomers occur because carbons that are in a ring or double bond structure are *unable* to freely rotate. Geometric isomers occur only as alkenes and cyclic compounds. This results in *cis* and *trans* compounds. When the substituents (i.e. Br) are on the same side of the ring or double bond, it is designated cis. When they are on opposite sides, it is designated trans. The trans isomer is more stable since the substituents are further apart, thus electron shell repulsion is minimized.

$$\underset{Br}{\overset{H}{\diagdown}}C=C\underset{Br}{\overset{H}{\diagup}}$$

cis-dibromoethene

and

$$\underset{Br}{\overset{H}{\diagdown}}C=C\underset{H}{\overset{Br}{\diagup}}$$

trans-dibromoethene

In general, structural and geometric isomers have different reactivity, spectra and physical properties (i.e. boiling points, melting points, etc.).

Stereoisomers are different compounds with the same structure, differing only in the spatial orientation of the atoms (= *configuration*). Stereoisomers may be further divided into enantiomers and diastereomers.

A stereocenter (= stereogenic center) is an atom bearing attachments such that interchanging any two groups produces a stereoisomer. If a molecule has n stereocenters, then it can have up to 2^n different non-superimposable (non-superposable) structures (= enantiomers).

ORGANIC CHEMISTRY

2.2 Enantiomers and Diastereomers

<u>Enantiomers</u> come in pairs. They are two non-superimposable molecules, which are mirror images of each other. In order to have an enantiomer, a molecule must be chiral. Chiral molecules contain at least one chiral carbon which is a carbon atom that has four different substituents attached. For the purposes of the GAMSAT, the concepts of a chiral carbon, asymmetric carbon and stereocenter are interchangeable.

Enantiomers have the same chemical and physical properties. The only difference is with their interactions with other chiral molecules, and their rotation of plane polarized light.

Conversely, <u>diastereomers</u> are any pair of stereoisomers that are not enantiomers. Diastereomers are both chemically and physically different from each other.

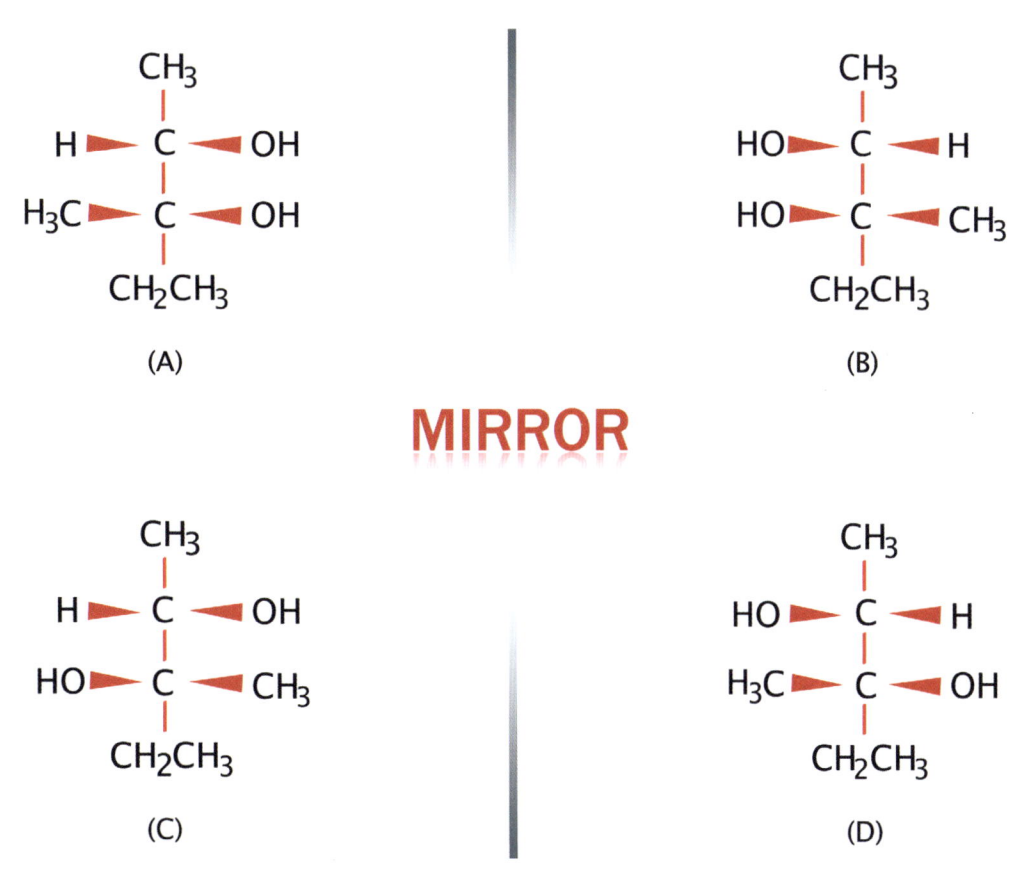

Figure IV.B.2.1: Enantiomers and diastereomers. The enantiomers are A & B, C & D. The diastereomers are A & C, A & D, B & D, B & C. Thus there are 2 pairs of enantiomers. This is consistent with the 2^n equation since each of the structures above have exactly 2 chiral carbons (stereocenters) and thus $2^2 = 4$ enantiomers.

THE BIOLOGICAL SCIENCES ORG-15

2.3 Absolute and Relative Configuration

Absolute configuration uses the R, S system of naming compounds (*nomenclature;* ORG 2.3.1) and relative configuration uses the D, L system (ORG 2.3.2).

Before 1951, the absolute three dimensional arrangement or configuration of chiral molecules was not known. Instead chiral molecules were compared to an arbitrary standard (*glyceraldehyde*). Thus the *relative* configuration could be determined. Once the actual spatial arrangements of groups in molecules were finally determined, the *absolute* configuration could be known.

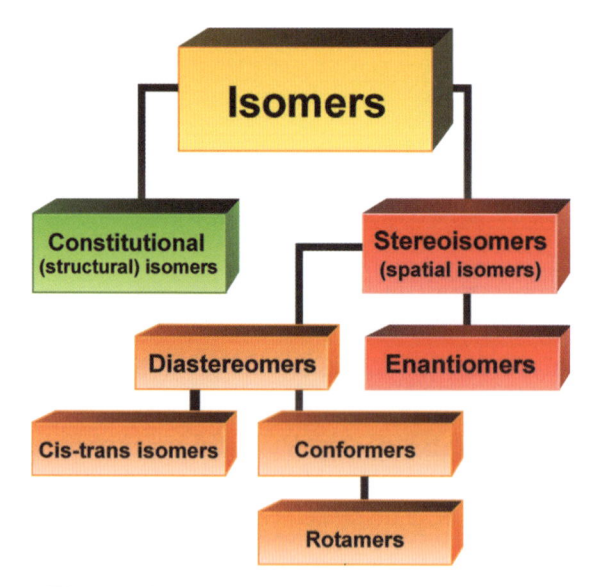

Figure IV.B.2.1.1: Categories of isomers

2.3.1 The R, S System and Fischer Projections

One consequence of the existence of enantiomers, is a special system of nomenclature: the R, S system. This system provides information about the absolute configuration of a molecule. This is done by assigning a stereochemical configuration at each asymmetric (*chiral*) carbon in the molecule by using the following steps:

1. Identify an asymmetric carbon, and the four attached groups.

2. Assign priorities to the four groups, using the following rules:
   i. Atoms of higher atomic number have higher priority.
   ii. An isotope of higher atomic mass receives higher priority.
   iii. The higher priority is assigned to the group with the atom of higher atomic number or mass at the first point of difference.
   iv. If the difference between the two groups is due to the number of otherwise identical atoms, the higher priority is assigned to the group with the greater number of atoms of higher atomic number or mass.
   v. To assign priority of double and triple bonded groups, these atoms are replicated:

ORG-16   STEREOCHEMISTRY

−CH=CH is taken as
```
    −CH−CH
     |  |
     C  C
```

−CH≡CH is taken as
```
     C  C
     |  |
    −C−−CH
     |  |
     C  C
```

3. View the molecule along the bond from the asymmetric carbon to the group of lowest priority (i.e. the asymmetric carbon is near, and the low priority group is far away).

4. Consider the clockwise or counterclockwise order of the priorities of the remaining groups. If they increase in a clockwise direction, the asymmetric carbon is said to have the R configuration. If they decrease in a clockwise direction, the asymmetric carbon is said to have the S configuration.

A stereoisomer is named by indicating the configurations of each of the asymmetric carbons.

A Fischer projection is a 2-D way of looking at 3-D structures. All horizontal bonds project toward the viewer, while vertical bonds project away from the viewer. In organic chemistry, Fischer projections are used mostly for carbohydrates (see ORG 12.3.1, 12.3.2). To determine if 2 Fischer projections are superimposable, you can: (1) rotate one projection 180° or (2) keep one substituent in a fixed position and then you can rotate the other 3 groups either clockwise or counterclockwise. Using either technique preserves the 3-D configuration of the molecule.

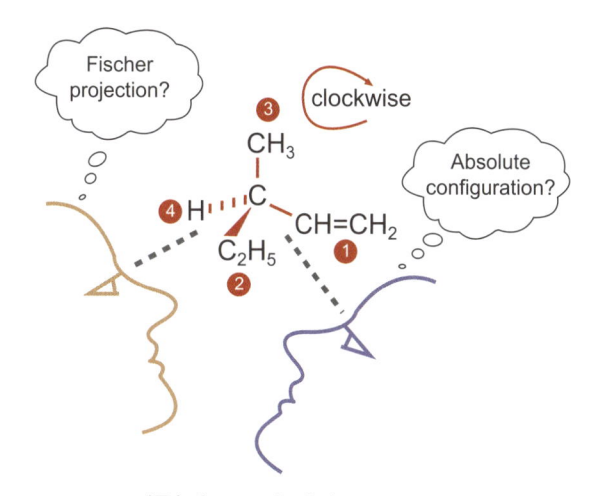

(R)-3-methyl-1-pentene

Figure IV.B.2.2(a): Assigning Absolute Configuration. In organic chemistry, the directions of the bonds are symbolized as follows: a broken line extends away from the viewer (i.e. INTO the page), a solid triangle projects towards the viewer, and a straight line extends in the plane of the paper. According to rule #3, we must imagine that the lowest priority group (H) points away from the viewer.

Fischer Projection

Figure IV.B.2.2(b): Creating the Fischer projection of (R)-3-methyl-1-pentene. Notice that the perspective of the viewer in the image is the identical perspective of the viewer on the left of Figure IV.B.2.2(a). In either case, a perspective is chosen so that the horizontal groups project towards the viewer.

2.3.2 Optical Isomers and the D, L System

Optical isomers are enantiomers and thus are stereoisomers that differ by different spatial orientations about a chiral carbon atom. Light is an electromagnetic wave that contains oscillating fields. In ordinary light, the electric field oscillates in all directions. However, it is possible to obtain light with an electric field that oscillates in only one plane. This type of light is known as **plane polarized light**. When plane polarized light is passed through a sample of a chiral substance, it will emerge vibrating in a different plane than it started. Optical isomers differ only in this rotation. If the light is rotated in a clockwise direction, the compound is dextrorotary, and is designated by a D or (+). If the light is rotated in a counterclockwise direction, the compound is levrorotary, and is designated by an L or (−). All L compounds have the same relative configuration as L-glyceraldehyde.

A racemic mixture will show no rotation of plane polarized light. This is a consequence of the fact that a racemate is a mixture with equal amounts of the D and L forms of a substance.

Specific rotation (α) is an inherent physical property of a molecule. It is defined as follows:

$$\alpha = \frac{\text{Observed rotation in degrees}}{(\text{tube length in dm})(\text{concentration in g/ml})}$$

The observed rotation is the rotation of the light passed through the substance. The tube length is the length of the tube that contains the sample in question. The specific rotation is dependent on the solvent used, the temperature of the sample, and the wavelength of the light.

It should be noted that there is no clear correlation between the absolute configuration (i.e. R, S) and the direction of rotation of plane polarized light.

MIRROR

Figure IV.B.2.3: Optical isomers and their Fischer projections. To prove to yourself that the 2 molecules are non-superimposable mirror images (enantiomers), review the rules for Fischer projections (ORG 2.3.1) and compare.

2.3.3 Meso Compounds

Tartaric acid (= 2,3-dihydroxybutanedioic acid which, in the chapters to come, is a compound that you will be able to name systematically = IUPAC) has two chiral centers that have the same four substituents and are equivalent. As a result, two of the four possible stereoisomers of this compound are identical due to a plane of symmetry. Thus there are only three stereoisomeric tartaric acids. Two of these stereoisomers are enantiomers and the third is an achiral diastereomer, called a meso compound. Meso compounds are achiral (optically inactive) diastereomers of chiral stereoisomers.

In a meso compound, an internal plane of symmetry exists by drawing a line that will cut the molecule in half. For example, notice that in meso-tartaric acid, you can draw a line perpendicular to the vertical carbon chain creating 2 symmetric halves {**MeSo** = **M**irror of **S**ymmetry}.

2.3.4 E, Z Designation

The E, Z notation is the IUPAC preferred method for designating the stereochemistry of double bonds. ORG 2.1 reviewed how to use cis/trans. The E, Z notation is quite similar but more precise.

To begin with, each substituent at the double bond is assigned a priority (see 2.3.1 for rules). If the two groups of higher priority are on opposite sides of the double bond, the bond is assigned the configuration E, (from *entgegen*, the German word for "opposite"). If the two groups of higher priority are on the same side of the double bond, the bond is assigned the configuration Z, (from *zusammen,* the German word for "together"). {Generally speaking, learning German is NOT required for the GAMSAT!}

GOLD NOTES

ALKANES

Chapter 3

Memorize
* IUPAC nomenclature
* Physical properties

Understand
* Trends based on length, branching
* Ring strain, ESR
* Complete combustion
* Free Radicals

Not Required*
* Advanced level college info
* Technical categorization of "cyclic alkanes"

GAMSAT-Prep.com

Introduction

Alkanes (a.k.a. paraffins) are compounds that consist only of the elements carbon (C) and hydrogen (H) (i.e. hydrocarbons). In addition, C and H are linked together exclusively by single bonds (i.e. they are saturated compounds). Methane is the simplest possible alkane while saturated oils and fats are much larger.

Additional Resources

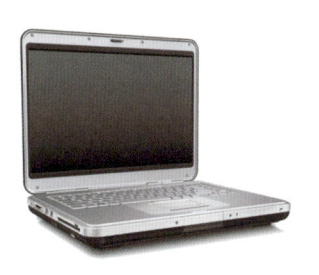

Free Online Q&A + Forum   Video: DVD Discs 1,3   Flashcards   Special Guest

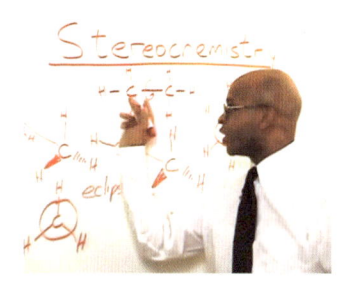

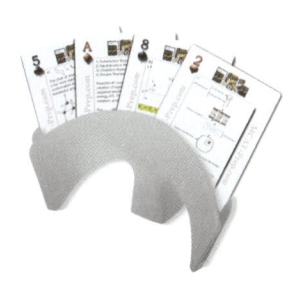

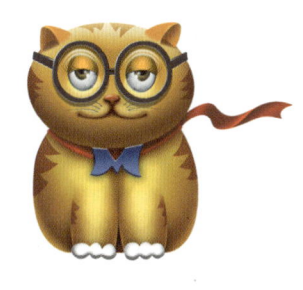

THE BIOLOGICAL SCIENCES   ORG-21

* The real GAMSAT may have advanced level information presented (ie. in a passage) but previous knowledge of said information is not required to answer the questions that would follow. Practice ACER and GS practice GAMSATs can help you clarify this point.

3.1 Description and Nomenclature

Alkanes are hydrocarbon molecules containing only sp³ hybridized carbon atoms (single bonds). They may be unbranched, branched or cyclic. Their general formula is C_nH_{2n+2} for a straight chain molecule; 2 hydrogen (H) atoms are subtracted for each ring. They contain no functional groups and are fully saturated molecules (= *no double or triple bonds*). As a result, they are chemically unreactive except when exposed to heat or light.

Systematic naming of compounds (= *nomenclature*) has evolved from the International Union of Pure and Applied Chemistry (IUPAC). **The nomenclature of alkanes is the basis of that for many other organic molecules.** The root of the compound is named according to the number of carbons in the longest carbon chain:

C_1 = meth C_5 = pent C_8 = oct
C_2 = eth C_6 = hex C_9 = non
C_3 = prop C_7 = hept C_{10} = dec
C_4 = but

When naming these as fragments, (alkyl fragments: *the alkane minus one H atom*, symbol: R), the suffix '–yl' is used. If naming the alkane, the suffix '-ane' is used. Some prefixes result from the fact that a carbon with *one* R group attached is a *primary* (normal or n –) carbon, *two* R groups is *secondary* (sec) and with *three* R groups it is a *tertiary* (tert or t –) carbon. Some alkyl groups have special names:

C—C—C—   n-propyl (= propyl)

C—C—C—C—   n-butyl (= butyl)

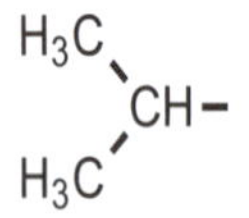

isopropyl
(= 2-propyl or propan-2-yl)

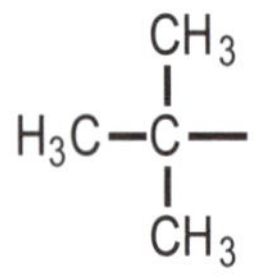

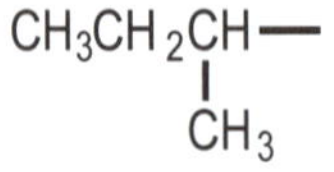

sec-butyl
(= 1-methylpropyl)

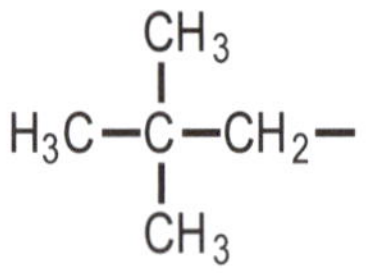

tert-butyl
(= 1,1-dimethylethyl)

neopentyl
(= dimethylpropyl)

Cyclic alkanes are named in the same way (according to the number of carbons), but the prefix 'cyclo' is added. The shorthand for organic compounds is a geometric figure where each corner represents a carbon; hydrogens need not be written, though it should be remembered that the number of hydrogens would exist such that the number of bonds at each carbon is four.

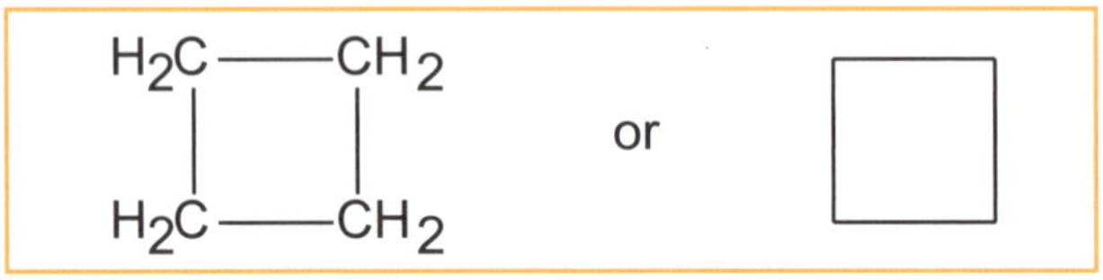

cyclobutane

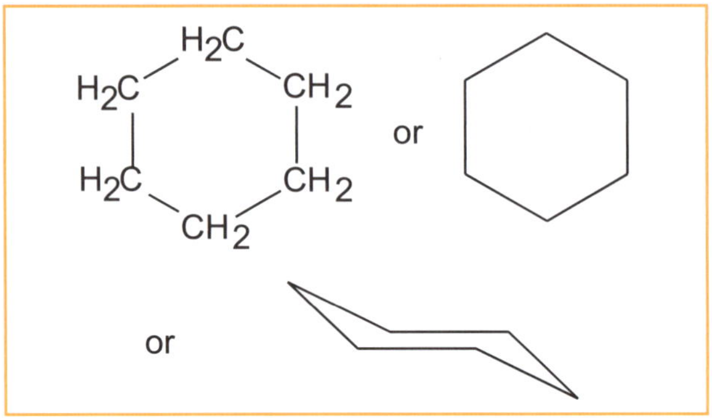

cyclohexane

ORGANIC CHEMISTRY

The nomenclature for <u>branched-chain alkanes</u> begins by determining the longest <u>straight chain</u> (i.e. *the highest number of carbons attached in a row*). The groups attached to the straight or *main* chain are numbered so as to achieve the lowest set of numbers. Groups are cited in alphabetical order. If a group appears more than once, the prefixes di-(2), tri-(3), tetra-(4) are used. If two chains of equal length compete for selection as the main chain, choose the chain with the most substituents. For example:

4,6-Diethyl-2,5,5,6,7-pentamethyl octane (7 substituents) or 3,5-Diethyl-2,3,4,4,7-pentamethyl octane (a bit better for keeners! i.e. not GAMSAT level) NOT 2,5,5,6-Tetramethyl-4-ethyl-6-isopropyl octane (6 substituents)

3.1.1 Physical Properties of Alkanes

At room temperature and one atmosphere of pressure straight chain alkanes with 1 to 4 carbons are gases (i.e. CH_4 – methane, CH_3CH_3 – ethane, etc.), 5 to 17 carbons are liquids, and more than 17 carbons are solid. Boiling points of straight chain alkanes (= *aliphatic*) show a regular increase with increasing number of carbons. This is because they are nonpolar molecules, and have weak intermolecular forces. Branching of alkanes leads to a dramatic decrease in the boiling point. As a rule, as the number of carbons increase the melting points also increase.

Alkanes are soluble in nonpolar solvents (i.e. benzene, CCl_4 – carbon tetrachloride, etc.), and not in aqueous solvents (= *hydrophobic*). They are insoluble in water because of their low polarity and their inability to hydrogen bond. Alkanes are the least dense of all classes of organic compounds (<< ρ_{water}, 1 g/ml). Thus petroleum, a mixture of hydrocarbons rich in alkanes, floats on water.

3.2 Important Reactions of Alkanes

3.2.1 Combustion

Combustion may be either complete or incomplete. In complete combustion, the hydrocarbon is converted to carbon dioxide (CO_2) and water (H_2O). If there is insufficient oxygen for complete combustion, the reaction gives other products, such as carbon monoxide (CO) and soot (molecular C). This strongly exothermic reaction may be summarized:

$$C_nH_{2n+2} + \text{excess } O_2 \rightarrow nCO_2 + (n+1)H_2O.$$

3.2.2 Radical Substitution Reactions

Radical substitution reactions with halogens may be summarized:

$$RH + X_2 + \text{uv light}(hf) \text{ or heat} \rightarrow RX + HX$$

The halogen X_2, may be F_2, Cl_2, or Br_2. I_2 does not react. The mechanism of *halogenation* may be explained and summarized by example:

i. Initiation: This step involves the formation of *free radicals* (highly reactive substances which contain an unpaired electron, which is symbolized by a single dot):

$$Cl:Cl + \text{uv light or heat} \rightarrow 2Cl\cdot$$

ii. Propagation: In this step, the chlorine free radical begins a series of reactions that form new free radicals:

$$CH_4 + Cl\cdot \rightarrow \cdot CH_3 + HCl$$
$$\cdot CH_3 + Cl_2 \rightarrow CH_3Cl + Cl\cdot$$

iii. Termination: These reactions end the radical propagation steps. Termination reactions destroy the free radicals (coupling).

$$Cl\cdot + \cdot CH_3 \rightarrow CH_3Cl$$
$$\cdot CH_3 + \cdot CH_3 \rightarrow CH_3CH_3$$
$$Cl\cdot + Cl\cdot \rightarrow Cl_2$$

Radical substitution reactions can also occur with halide acids (i.e. HCl, HBr) and peroxides (i.e. HOOH – hydrogen peroxide). Chain propagation (step ii) can destroy many organic compounds fairly quick. This step can be inhibited by using a resonance stabilized free radical to "mop up" (*termination*) other destructive free radicals in the medium. For example, BHT is a resonance stabilized free radical added to packaging of many breakfast cereals in order to inhibit free radical destruction of the cereal (= *spoiling*).

The stability of a free radical depends on the ability of the compound to stabilize the unpaired electron. This is analogous to stabilizing a positively charged carbon (= *carbocation*). Thus, in both cases, a tertiary compound is more stable than secondary which, in turn, is more stable than a primary compound.

3.3 Ring Strain in Cyclic Alkanes

Cyclic alkanes are strained compounds. This **ring strain** results from the bending of the bond angles in greater amounts than normal. This strain causes cyclic compounds of 3 and 4 carbons to be unstable, and thus not often found in nature. The usual angle between bonds in an sp³ hybridized carbon is 109.5° (= *the normal tetrahedral angle*).

The expected angles in some cyclic compounds can be determined geometrically: 60° in cyclopropane; 90° in cyclobutane and 108° in cyclopentane. Cyclohexane, in the chair conformation, has normal bond angles of 109.5°. The closer the angle is to the normal tetrahedral angle of 109.5°, the more stable the compound. In fact, cyclohexane can be found in a chair or boat conformation or any conformation in between; however, at any given moment, 99% of the cyclohexane molecules would be found in the chair conformation because it is the most stable (lower energy).

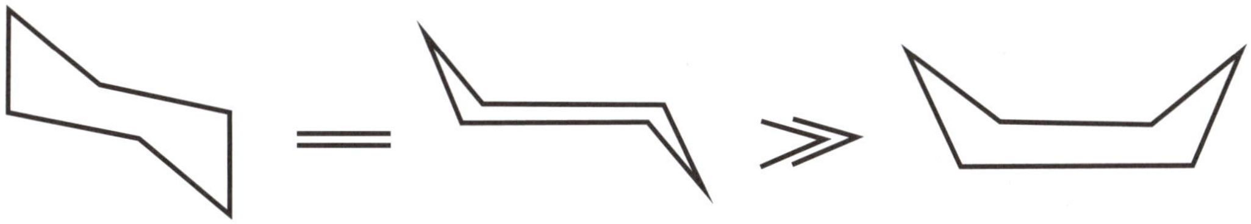

Figure IV.B.3.1: The chair and boat conformations of cyclohexane.

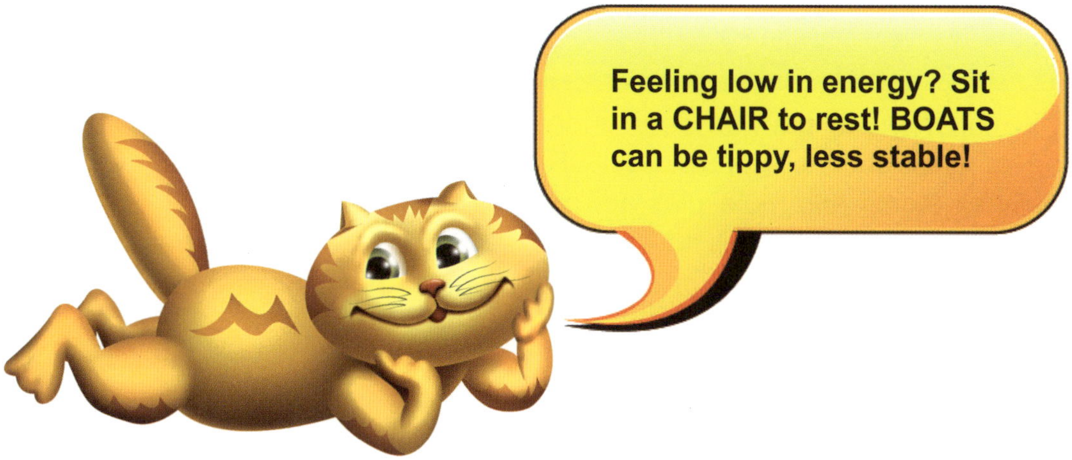

Feeling low in energy? Sit in a CHAIR to rest! BOATS can be tippy, less stable!

- axial hydrogen
- equatorial hydrogen
- carbon

Figure IV.B.3.2: The chair conformation of cyclohexane. The hydrogens which are generally in the same plane as the ring are equatorial. The hydrogens which are generally perpendicular to the ring are axial. The hydrogen atoms are maximally separated and staggered to minimize electron shell repulsion.

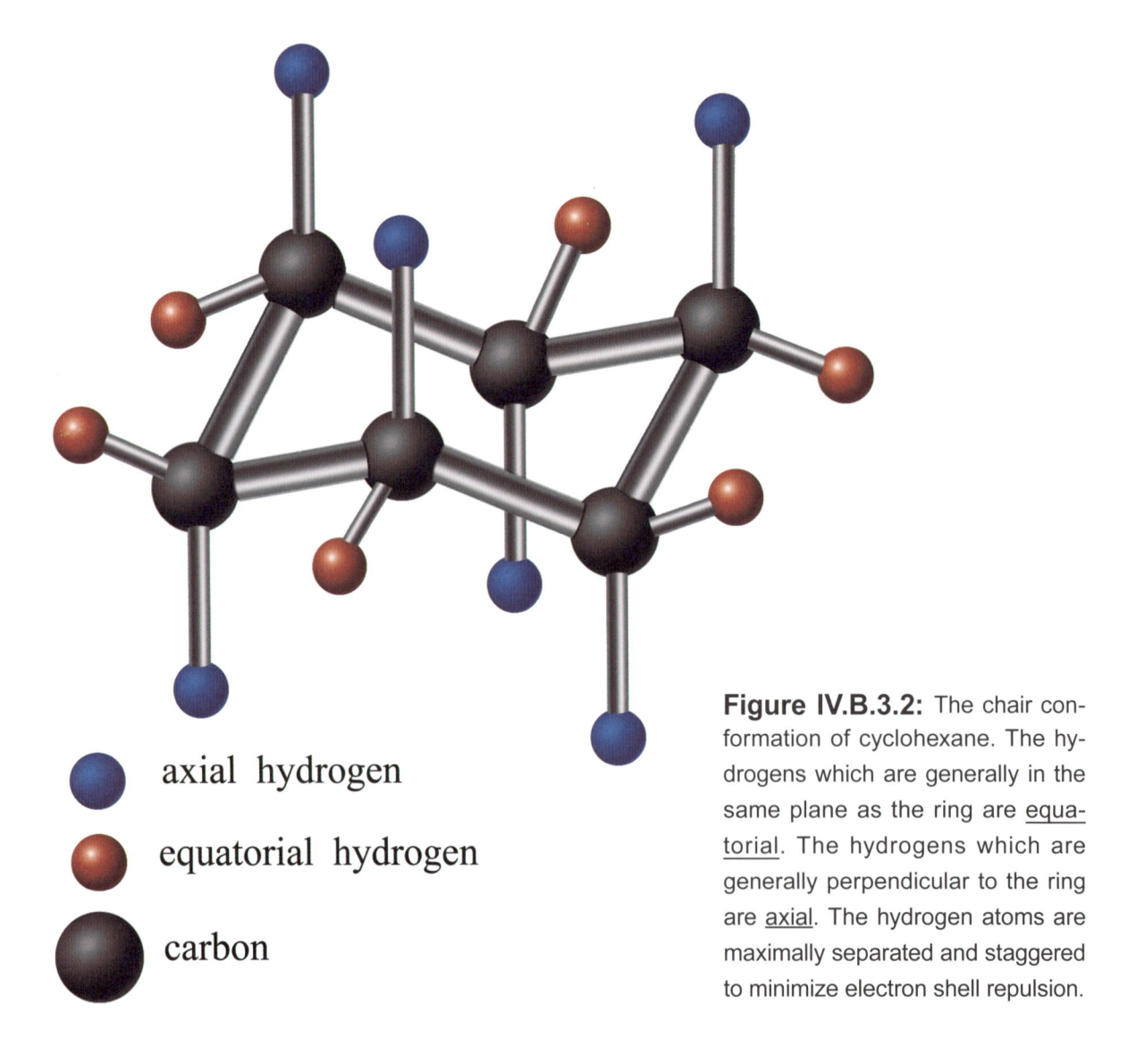

It is important to have a clear understanding of electron shell repulsion (ESR). Essentially all atoms and molecules are surrounded by an electron shell (CHM 2.1, ORG 1.2) which is more like a cloud of electrons. Because like charges repel, when there are options, atoms and molecules assume the conformation which minimizes ESR.

For example, when substituents are added to a cyclic compound (i.e. Fig. IV.B.3.2), the most stable position is equatorial (equivalent to the anti conformation, ORG 2.1) which minimizes ESR. This conformation is most pronounced when the substituent is bulky (i.e. isopropyl, t-butyl, phenyl, etc.). In other words, a large substituent takes up more space thus ESR has a more prominent effect.

ORGANIC CHEMISTRY

GOLD NOTES

ALKENES

Chapter 4

Memorize
* Basic nomenclature

Understand
* Electrophilic addition, hydrogenation, Markovnikoff's rule, oxidation

Not Required*
* Advanced level college info

GAMSAT-Prep.com

Introduction

An alkene (a.k.a. olefin) is an unsaturated chemical compound containing at least one carbon-to-carbon double bond.

Additional Resources

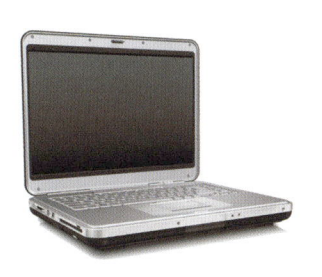

Free Online Q&A + Forum

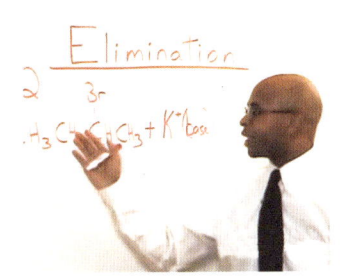

Video: DVD Discs 1,3,4

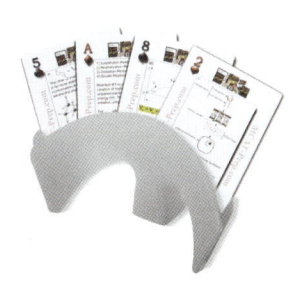

Flashcards

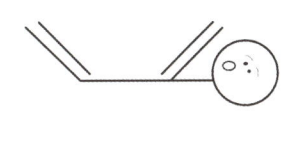

Special Guest

THE BIOLOGICAL SCIENCES ORG-29

* The real GAMSAT may have advanced level information presented (ie. in a passage) but previous knowledge of said information is not required to answer the questions that would follow. Practice ACER and GS practice GAMSATs can help you clarify this point.

4.1 Description and Nomenclature

Alkenes are unsaturated hydrocarbon molecules containing carbon-carbon double bonds. Their general formula is C_nH_{2n} for a straight chain molecule; 2 hydrogen (H) atoms are subtracted for each ring. The *functional group* in these molecules is the double bond which determines the chemical properties of alkenes. Double bonds are sp^2 hybridized (*see* ORG 1.2, 1.3). The nomenclature is the same as that for alkanes, except that i) the suffix 'ene' replaces 'ane' and ii) the double bond is (are) numbered in the molecule, trying to get the smallest number for the double bond(s). For cycloalkenes, the carbons of the double bond are given the 1– and 2– positions.

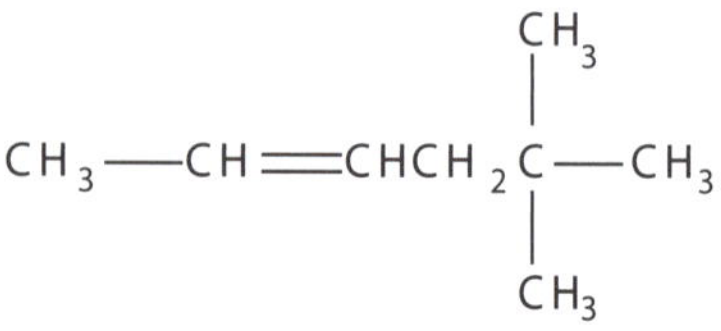

5,5-Dimethyl-2-hexene 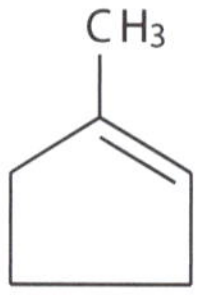   1-methylcyclopentene

Two frequently encountered groups are sometimes named as if they were substituents.

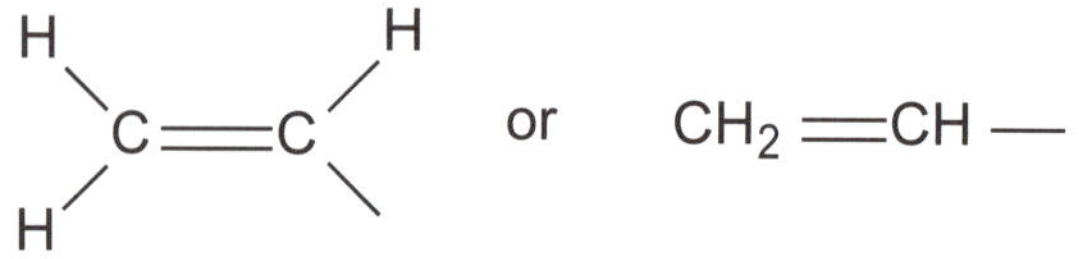

the vinyl group

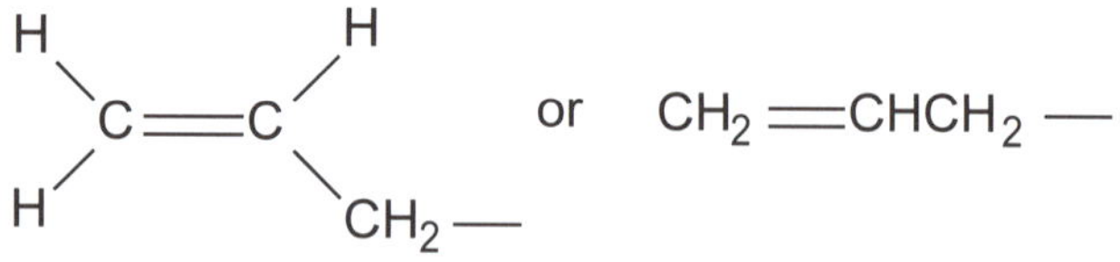

the allyl group

Alkenes have similar physical properties to alkanes. Trans compounds tend to have higher melting points (due to better symmetry), and lower boiling points (due to less polarity) than its corresponding cis isomer. Alkenes, however, due to the nature of the double bond may be polar:

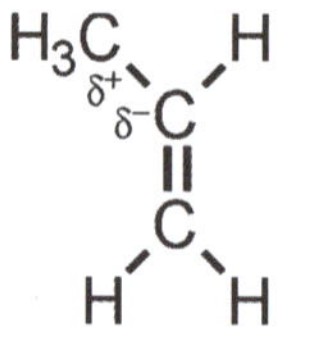

has a small dipole moment

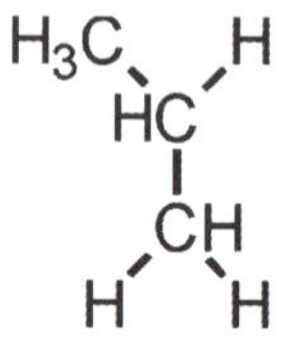

has no dipole moment

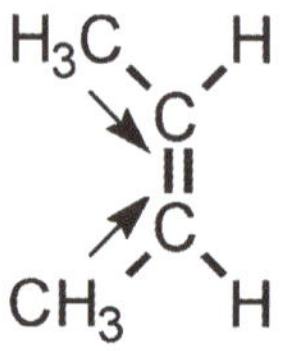

(cis) small dipole moment

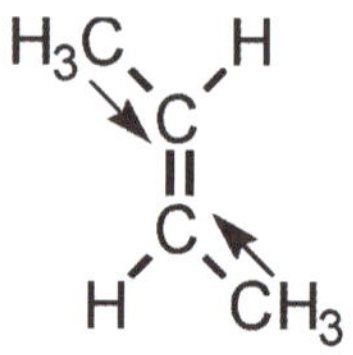

(trans) no dipole moment

ORG-30   ALKENES

ORGANIC CHEMISTRY

The greater the number of attached alkyl groups (i.e. *the more highly substituted the double bond*), the greater is the alkene's stability. The reason is that <u>alkyl</u> groups are somewhat electron donating, thus they stabilize the double bond.

An alkene with 2 double bonds is a diene, 3 is a triene. A diene with one single bond in between is a conjugated diene. Conjugated dienes are more stable than non-conjugated dienes primarily due to resonance stabilization (see the resonance stabilized conjugated molecule 1,3-butadiene in ORG 1.4).

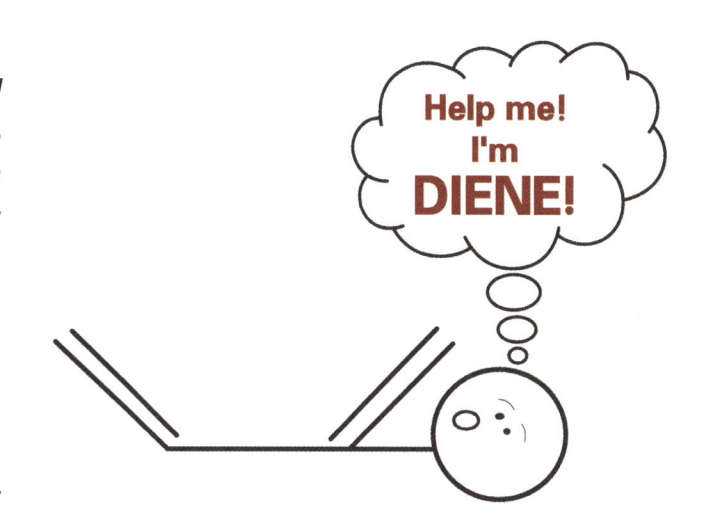

4.2 Important Chemical Reactions

4.2.1 Electrophilic Addition

The chemistry of alkenes may be understood in terms of their functional group, the double bond. When <u>electrophiles</u> (*substances which seek electrons*) add to alkenes, carbocations (= *carbonium ions*) are formed. An important electrophile is H^+ (i.e. in HBr, H_2O, etc.). A <u>nucleophile</u> is a molecule with a free pair of electrons, and sometimes a negative charge, that seeks out partially or completely positively charged species (i.e. a carbon nucleus). Some important nucleophiles are OH^- and CN^-.

E = electrophile   carbocation (intermediate)   Nu = nucleophile

Another important property of the double bond is its ability to stabilize carbocations, carbanions or radicals attached to adjacent carbons (*allylic carbons*). Note that all the following are resonance stabilized:

$$\text{C}=\text{C}-\overset{\oplus}{\text{C}} \longleftrightarrow \overset{\oplus}{\text{C}}-\text{C}=\text{C}$$

carbocation

$$\text{C}=\text{C}-\overset{\ominus}{\text{C}} \longleftrightarrow \overset{\ominus}{\text{C}}-\text{C}=\text{C}$$

carbanion

$$\text{C}=\text{C}-\overset{\cdot}{\text{C}} \longleftrightarrow \overset{\cdot}{\text{C}}-\text{C}=\text{C}$$

carbon radical

The stability of the intermediate carbocation depends on the groups attached to it, which can either stabilize or destabilize it. In general, groups which can share electrons by pi orbital overlap (resonance) stabilize the carbocation. As well, groups which place a partial or total positive charge adjacent to the carbocation withdraw electrons inductively, by sigma bonds, to destabilize it.

These points are useful in predicting which carbon will become the carbocation, and to which carbon the electrophile and nucleophile will bond. The intermediate carbocation formed must be the most stable. **Markovnikoff's rule** is a result of this, and it states: *the nucleophile will be bonded to the most substituted carbon* (fewest hydrogens attached) *in the product. Equivalently, the electrophile will be bonded to the least substituted carbon* (most hydrogens attached) *in the product*. An example of this is:

$$(H_3C)_2C=CH(H) + HBr \xrightarrow{H^+} (H_3C)_2\overset{+}{C}—CH_2(H) \xrightarrow{Br^-} (H_3C)_2C(Br)—CH(CH_3)(H)$$

① ②

H⁺ = electrophile
Br⁻ = nucleophile

① most substituted carbon
② least substituted carbon

① forms the most stable carbonium ion.

ORG-32 ALKENES

ORGANIC CHEMISTRY

The product, 2-bromo-2-methyl butane, is the more likely or major product (*the Markovnikoff product*). Had the H+ added to the most substituted carbon (which has a much lower probability of occurrence) the less likely or minor product would be formed (*the anti-Markovnikoff product*).

Markovnikoff's rule is true for the ionic conditions presented in the preceding reaction. However, for radical conditions the reverse occurs. Thus *anti-Markovnikoff* products are the major products under free radical conditions.

4.2.2 Oxidation

Alkenes can undergo a variety of reactions in which the carbon-carbon double bond is oxidized. Using potassium permanganate ($KMnO_4$) under mild conditions (*no heat*), or osmium tetroxide (OsO_4), a glycol (= *a dialcohol*) can be produced.

In the following chapters, you will learn how to derive systematic nomenclature (these are names of compounds based on rules as opposed to "common" names often based on tradition). IUPAC (official) nomenclature is usually systematic (i.e. ethane-1,2-diol) but sometimes it is not (i.e. acetic acid). Knowing both the common and the systematic names is the safest way to approach the GAMSAT though it is not necessary to memorize which is common, systematic or IUPAC. The first reaction that follows is the oxidation of ethene (= ethylene) under mild conditions and the second is the oxidation of 2-butene under abrasive conditions.

$$CH_2 = CH_2 + KMnO_4 \xrightarrow[OH^-]{Cold} \begin{array}{c} CH_2 - CH_2 \\ | \quad\quad\quad | \\ OH \quad\quad OH \end{array}$$

Ethylene glycol
(1,2-ethanediol or ethane-1,2-diol)

Using $KMnO_4$ under more abrasive conditions leads to an oxidative cleavage of the double bond:

$$CH_3CH = CHCH_3 \xrightarrow[heat]{KMnO_4, OH^-} 2CH_3C\begin{array}{c}=O \\ \diagdown O^- \end{array} \xrightarrow{H^+} 2CH_3C\begin{array}{c}=O \\ \diagdown OH \end{array}$$

Acetate ion
(ethanoate ion)

Acetic acid
(ethanoic acid)

Ozone (O₃) reacts vigorously with alkenes. The reaction (= *ozonolysis*) leads to an oxidative cleavage of the double bond which can produce a ketone and an aldehyde:

$$\underset{\text{2-Methyl-2-butene}}{CH_3\underset{\underset{CH_3}{|}}{C}=CHCH_3} \xrightarrow[\text{(2) Zn, H}_2\text{O}]{\text{(1) O}_3} \underset{\underset{\text{(propanone)}}{\text{Acetone}}}{CH_3\underset{\underset{CH_3}{|}}{C}=O} + \underset{\underset{\text{(ethanal)}}{\text{Acetaldehyde}}}{CH_3\overset{\overset{O}{\|}}{C}H}$$

4.2.3 Hydrogenation

Alkenes react with hydrogen in the presence of a variety of metal catalysts (i.e. Ni – nickel, Pd – palladium, Pt – platinum). The reaction that occurs is an *addition* reaction since one atom of hydrogen adds to each carbon of the double bond (= *hydrogenation*). Since there are two phases present in the process of hydrogenation (the hydrogen and the metal catalyst), the process is referred to as a heterogenous catalysis.

A carbon with multiple bonds is not bonded to the maximum number of atoms that potentially that carbon could possess. Thus it is *unsaturated*. Alkanes, which can be formed by hydrogenation, are *saturated* since each carbon is bonded to the maximum number of atoms it could possess (= *four*). Thus hydrogenation is sometimes called the process of saturation.

$$CH_3CH=CH_2 + H_2 \longrightarrow CH_3CH_2—CH_3$$

4.3 Alkynes

Alkynes are unsaturated hydrocarbon molecules containing carbon-carbon triple bonds. The nomenclature is the same as that for alkenes, except that the suffix 'yne' replaces 'ene'. Alkynes have similar physical properties and chemical reactions (i.e. electrophilic addition, oxidation) to alkenes. The current GAMSAT exam does not require any knowledge specific to alkyne chemistry.

ORGANIC CHEMISTRY

GOLD NOTES

AROMATICS

Chapter 5

Memorize
* Basic nomenclature

Understand
* Electrophilic aromatic substitution

Not Required*
* Advanced level college info
* Memorizing O-P or meta directors

GAMSAT-Prep.com

Introduction

Aromatics are cyclic compounds with unusual stability due to cyclic delocalization and resonance.

Additional Resources

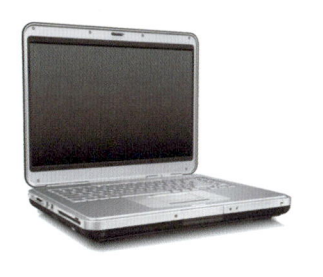

Free Online Q&A + Forum   Video: DVD Disc 4   Flashcards   Special Guest

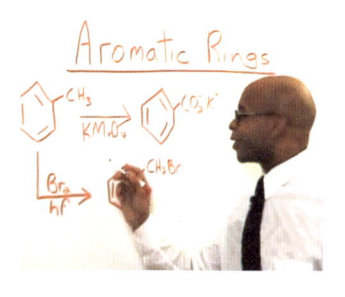

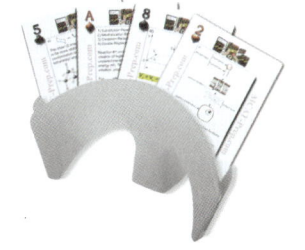

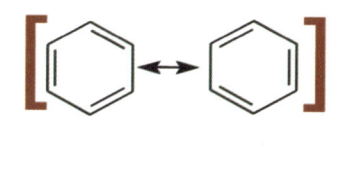

THE BIOLOGICAL SCIENCES ORG-37

* The real GAMSAT may have advanced level information presented (ie. in a passage) but previous knowledge of said information is not required to answer the questions that would follow. Practice ACER and GS practice GAMSATs can help you clarify this point.

5.1 Description and Nomenclature

Aromatic compounds are cyclic and have their π electrons delocalized over the entire ring and are thus stabilized by π-electron delocalization. Benzene is the simplest of all the aromatic hydrocarbons. The term *aromatic* has historical significance in that many well known fragrant compounds were found to be derivatives of benzene. Although at present, it is known that not all benzene derivatives have fragrance, the term remains in use today to describe benzene derivatives and related compounds.

Benzene is known to have only one type of carbon-carbon bond, with a bond length of ≈ 1.4 Å (angstroms, 10^{-10}m) somewhere between that of a single and double bond. The benzene molecule may thus be represented by two different resonance structures, showing it to be the average of the two:

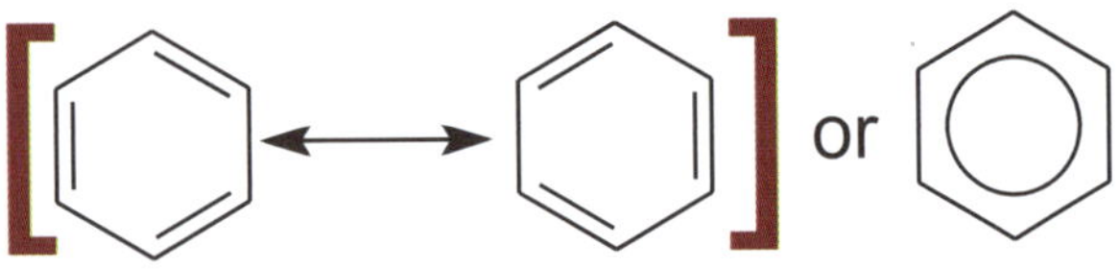

Many monosubstituted benzenes have common names by which they are known. Others are named by substituents attached to the aromatic ring. Some of these are:

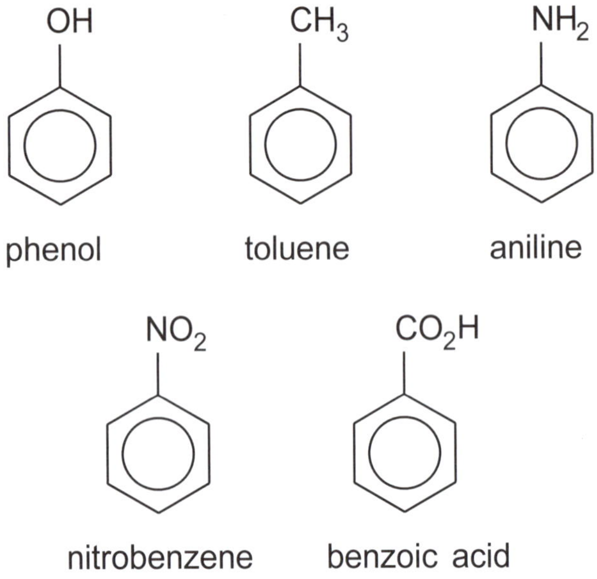

phenol   toluene   aniline

nitrobenzene   benzoic acid

Disubstituted benzenes are named as derivatives of their primary substituents. In this case, either the usual numbering or the ortho-meta-para system may be used. Ortho (*o*) substituents are at the 2nd position from the primary substituent; meta (*m*) substituents are at the 3rd position; para (*p*) substituents are at the 4th position. If there are more than two substituents on the aromatic ring, the numbering system is used. Some examples are:

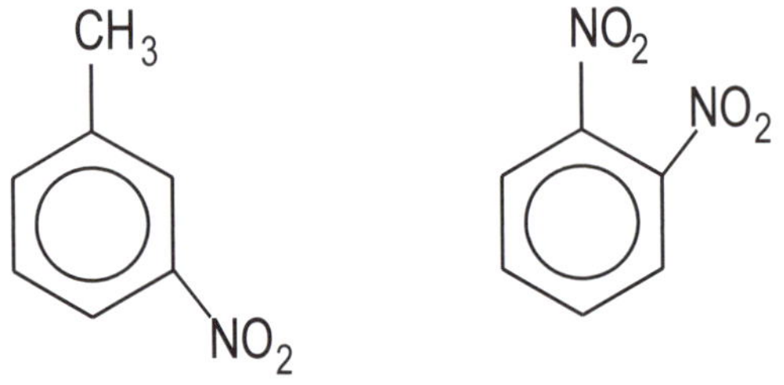

m - Nitrotoluene   o - Dinitrobenzene

ORGANIC CHEMISTRY

o - Methylaniline
o - Aminotoluene

3 - nitro - 4 - hydroxybenzoic acid

When benzene is a substituent, it is called a *phenyl or aryl group*. The shorthand for phenyl is Ph. Toluene without a hydrogen on the methyl substituent is called a *benzyl group*.

5.2 Electrophilic Aromatic Substitution

One important reaction of aromatic compounds is known as electrophilic aromatic substitution, which occurs with electrophilic reagents. The reaction is similar to a S_N1 mechanism in that an addition leads to a rearrangement which produces a substitution. However, in this case it is the electrophile (*not a nucleophile*) which substitutes for an atom in the original molecule. The reaction may be summarized:

Note that the intermediate positive charge is stabilized by resonance.

It is important to understand that the electrophile used in electrophilic aromatic substitution must always be a powerful electrophile. After all, the resonance stabilized aromatic ring is resistant to many types of routine chemical reactions (i.e. oxidation with $KMnO_4$ – ORG 4.2.2, electrophilic addition with acid - ORG 4.2.1, and hydrogenation - ORG 4.2.3). Remembering that Br, a halide, is already very electronegative (CHM

2.3), Br⁺ is an example of a powerful electrophile. In a reaction called bromination, Br₂/FeBr₃ is used to generate the Br⁺ species which adds to the aromatic ring. Similar reactions are performed to "juice up" other potential substituents (i.e. alkyl, acyl, iodine, etc.) to become powerful electrophiles to add to the aromatic ring.

When groups are attached to the aromatic ring, the intermediate charge delocalization is affected. There are two classes of substituents: ortho-para (o–p) directors and meta directors. As implied, these groups indicate where most of the electrophile will end up in the reaction.

5.2.1 O-P Directors

If a substituted benzene reacts more rapidly than a benzene alone, the substituent group is said to be an <u>activating group</u>. Activating groups can *donate* electrons to the ring. Thus the ring is more attractive to an electrophile. All activating groups are o/p directors. Some examples are $-OH, -NH_2, -OR, -NR_2$, and alkyl groups.

Note that the partial electron density (δ^-) is at the ortho and para positions, so the electrophile favors attack at these positions. Good stabilization results with a substituent at the ortho or para positions:

ORG-40   AROMATICS

When there is a substituent at the meta position, the –OH can no longer help to delocalize the positive charge, so the o-p positions are favored over the meta:

Note that even though the substituents are o-p directors, probability suggests that there will still be a small percentage of the electrophile that will add at the meta position.

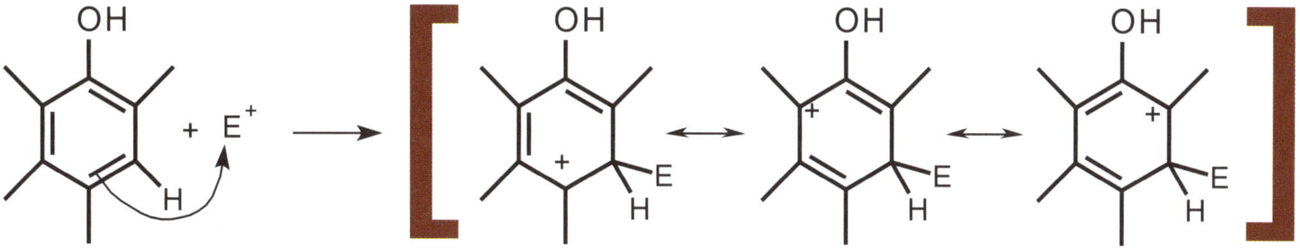

5.2.2 Meta Directors

If a substituted benzene reacts more slowly than the benzene alone, the substituent group is said to be a <u>deactivating group</u>. Deactivating groups can *withdraw* electrons from the ring. Thus the ring is less attractive to an electrophile. All deactivating groups are meta directors, with the exception of the weakly deactivating halides which are o–p directors.

Some examples of meta directors are $-NO_2$, $-SO_2$, $-CN$.

Without any substituents, the partial positive charge density (δ^+) will be at the o–p positions. Thus the electrophile avoids the positive charge and favors attack at the meta position:

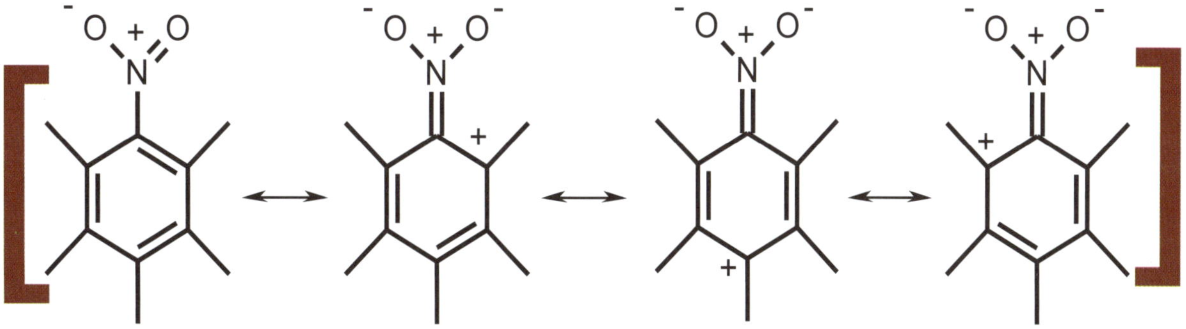

THE BIOLOGICAL SCIENCES   ORG-41

With a substituent at the meta position:

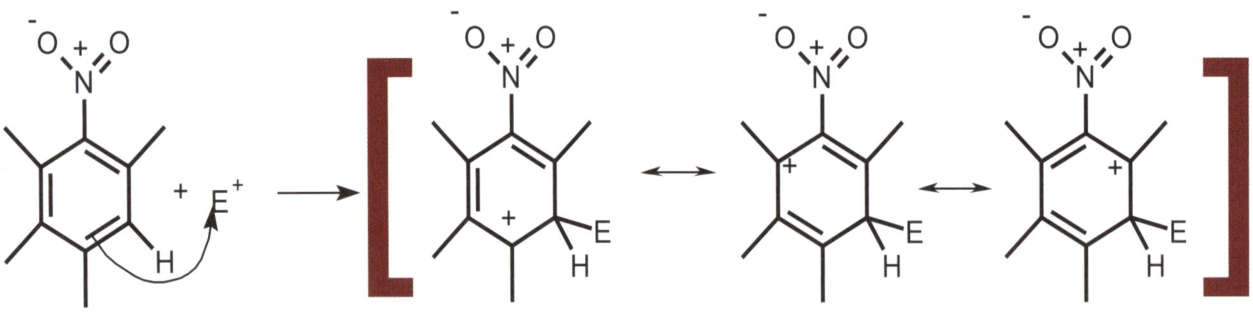

Note that even though the substituents are meta directors, probability suggests that there will still be a smaller percentage of the electrophile that will add at the o–p positions.

If you are seeking another way to learn, consider logging into your gamsat-prep.com account and clicking on Videos to choose the Aromatic Chemistry videos.

ORGANIC CHEMISTRY

GOLD NOTES

ALCOHOLS

Chapter 6

Memorize

* IUPAC nomenclature
* Physical properties
* Products of oxidation
* Define: steric hindrance

Understand

* Trends based on length, branching
* Effect of hydrogen bonds
* Mechanisms of reactions
* Nucleophilic substitution

Not Required*

* Advanced level college info

GAMSAT-Prep.com

Introduction

An alcohol is any organic compound in which a hydroxyl group (-OH) is bound to a carbon atom of an alkyl or substituted alkyl group.

Additional Resources

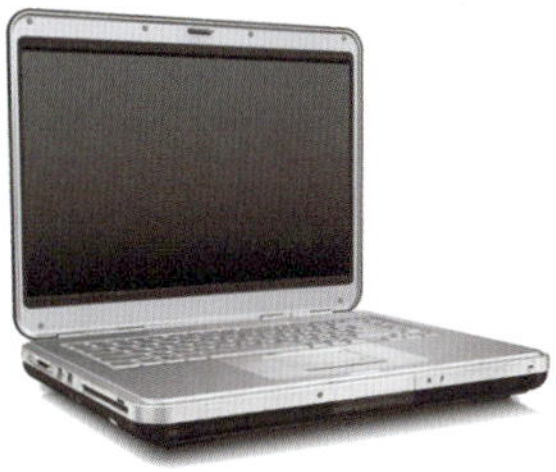

Free Online Q&A + Forum

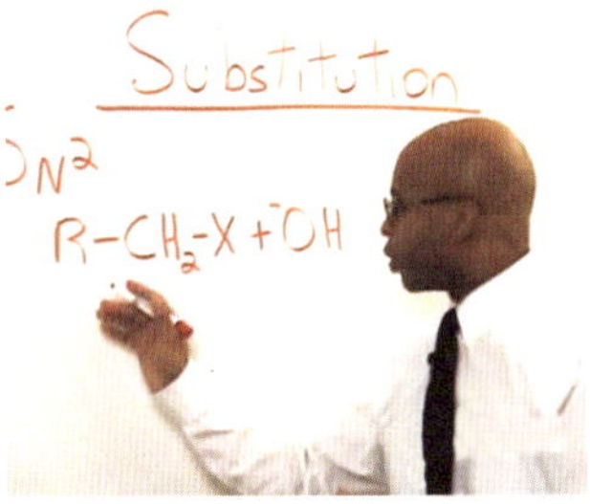

Video: DVD Discs 2,3,4

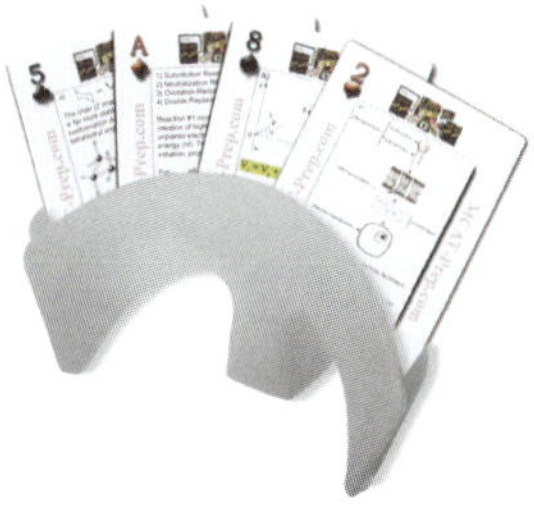

Flashcards

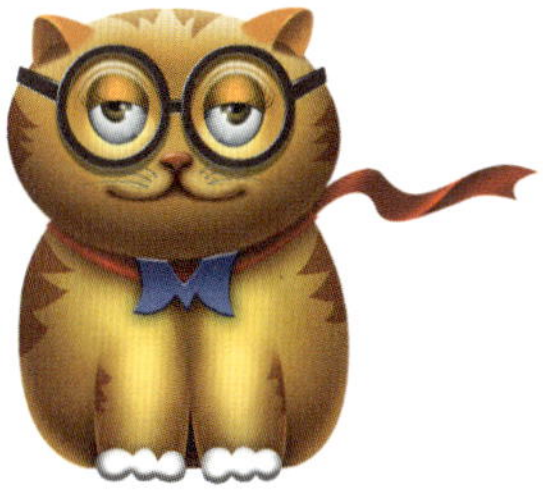

Special Guest

THE BIOLOGICAL SCIENCES ORG-45

* The real GAMSAT may have advanced level information presented (ie. in a passage) but previous knowledge of said information is not required to answer the questions that would follow. Practice ACER and GS practice GAMSATs can help you clarify this point.

6.1 Description and Nomenclature

The systematic naming of alcohols is accomplished by replacing the –e of the corresponding alkane with –ol. As with alkanes, special names are used for branched groups:

$$CH_3-CH(OH)-CH_3$$
IUPAC: 2-propanol
- Isopropanol
- Isopropyl alcohol

$$CH_3-C(OH)(CH_3)-CH_3$$
IUPAC: 2-methylpropan-2-ol
- 2-methyl-2-propanol
- tert-butanol

The alcohols are always numbered to give the carbon with the attached hydroxy (–OH) group the lowest number:

$$CH_3CH_2CH_2CH(OH)CH_2CH_3$$
3-hexanol NOT 4-hexanol

$$CH_3CH_2CH_2CH(CH_3)CH_2CH(OH)CH_2CH(CH_3)$$
2,6-dimethyl-4-nonanol

The shorthand for methanol is MeOH, and the shorthand for ethanol is EtOH. Alcohols are weak acids ($K_a \approx 10^{-18}$), being weaker acids than water. Their conjugate bases are called alkoxides, very little of which will be present in solution:

$$C_2H_5OH + OH^- \rightleftharpoons C_2H_5O^- + H_2O$$
ethanol ethoxide

The acidity of an alcohol decreases with increasing number of attached carbons. Thus CH_3OH is more acidic than CH_3CH_2OH; and CH_3CH_2OH (a primary alcohol) is more acidic than $(CH_3)_2CHOH$ (a secondary alcohol), which is, in turn, more acidic than $(CH_3)_3COH$ (a tertiary alcohol).

Alcohols have higher boiling points and a greater solubility than comparable alkanes, alkenes, aldehydes, ketones and alkyl halides. This greater solubility is due to the greater polarity and hydrogen bonding of the alcohol. In alcohols, hydrogen bonding is a weak association of the –OH proton of one molecule, with the oxygen of another. To form the hydrogen bond, both a donor, and an acceptor are required:

donor → O—H----O ← acceptor
       | |
      CH₃ δ+ δ- CH₃

Sometimes an atom may act as both a donor and acceptor of hydrogen bonds. One example of this is the oxygen atom in an alcohol:

hydrogen bonds

As the length of the carbon chain (= R) of the alcohol molecule increases, the non-polar chain becomes more meaningful, and the alcohol becomes less water soluble. The hydroxyl group of a primary alcohol is able to form hydrogen bonds with molecules such

… as water more easily than the hydroxyl group of a tertiary alcohol. The hydroxyl group of a tertiary alcohol is crowded by the surrounding methyl groups and thus its ability to participate in hydrogen bonds is lessened. As well, in solution, primary alcohols are more acidic than secondary alcohols, and secondary alcohols are more acidic than tertiary alcohols. In the gas phase, however, the order of acidity is reversed.

6.2 Important Reactions of Alcohols

6.2.1 Dehydration

Dehydration (= *loss of water*) reactions of alcohols produce alkenes. The general dehydration reaction is shown in Figure IV.B.6.1.

$$\text{alcohol} \xrightarrow[-H_2O]{+H^+} \text{carbocation} \xrightarrow{-H^+} \text{alkene}$$

Consumption of alcohol may make you think you are whispering when you are not!

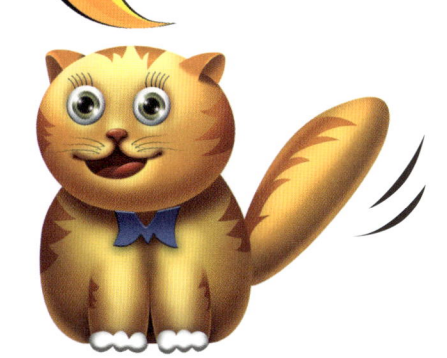

For the preceding reaction to occur, the temperature must be between 300 and 400 degrees Celsius, and the vapors must be passed over a metal oxide catalyst. Alternatively, strong, hot acids, such as H_2SO_4 or H_3PO_4 at 100 to 200 degrees Celsius may be used.

The reactivity depends upon the type of alcohol. A tertiary alcohol is more reactive than a secondary alcohol which is, in turn, more reactive than a primary alcohol. The faster reactions have the most stable carbocation intermediates. The alkene that is formed is the most stable one. A phenyl group will take preference over one or two alkyl groups, otherwise the most substituted double bond is the most stable (= *major product*) and the least substituted is less stable (= *minor product*).

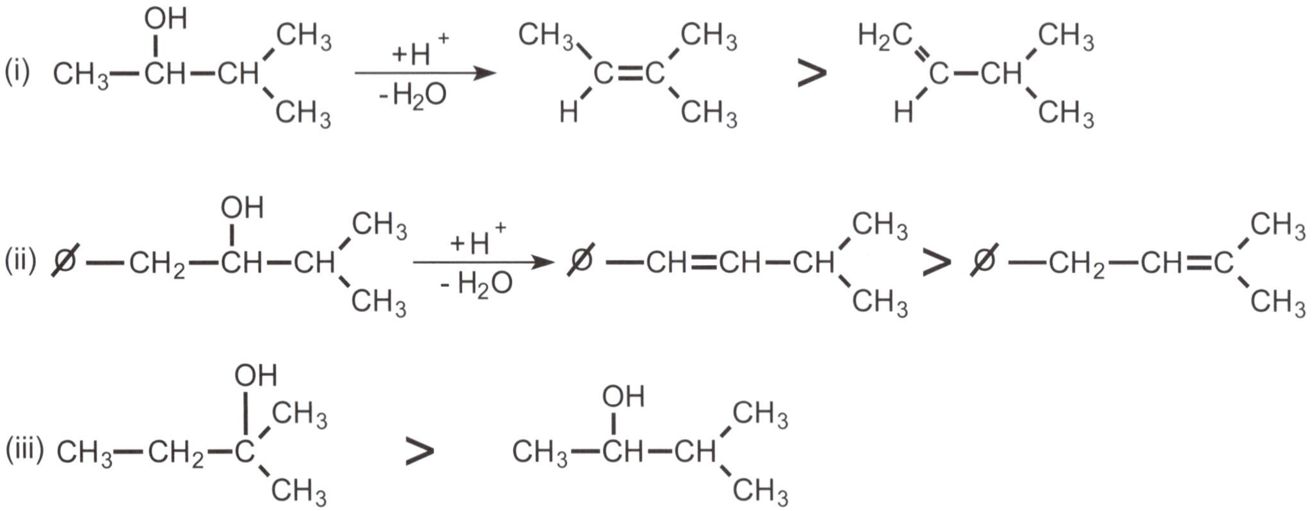

Figure IV.B.6.2: Dehydration of substituted alcohols. Major and minor products, respectively, are represented in reactions (i) and (ii). An example of a reactant with a greater reaction rate due to more substituents as an intermediate is represented by (iii). ϕ = a phenyl group.

6.2.2 Oxidation-Reduction

In organic chemistry, oxidation (O) is the increasing of oxygen or decreasing of hydrogen content, and reduction (H) is the opposite. Primary alcohols are converted to aldehydes using the mild oxidizing agents CrO_3 or $K_2Cr_2O_7/H_2SO_4$ or by using the powerful oxidizing agent, $KMnO_4$, under mild conditions (i.e. room temperature, neutral pH). Primary alcohols can produce carboxylic acids in the presence of $KMnO_4$ under abrasive conditions (i.e. increased temperature, presence of OH^-). Secondary alcohols are converted to ketones by any of the preceding oxidizing agents. It is *very* difficult to oxidize a tertiary alcohol.

ORGANIC CHEMISTRY

Under acidic conditions, tertiary alcohols are unaffected; they may be oxidized under acidic conditions by dehydration and *then* oxidizing the double bond of the resultant alkene. Classic reducing agents (H) include LiAlH$_4$ (strong), H$_2$/metals (strong) and NaBH$_4$ (mild).

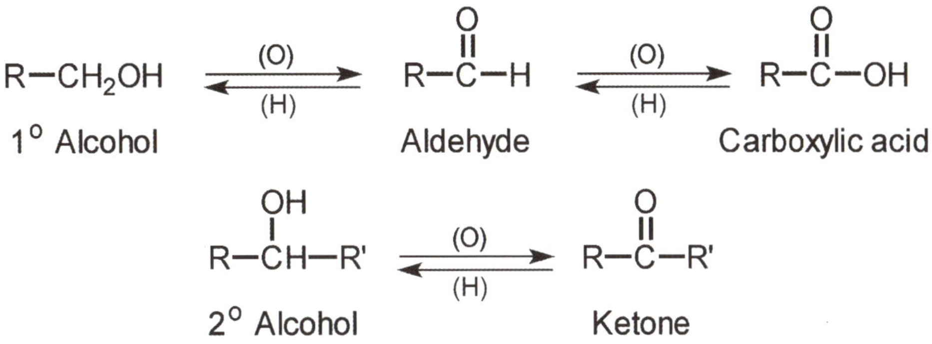

$$R-CH_2OH \xrightleftharpoons[(H)]{(O)} R-\overset{\overset{O}{\|}}{C}-H \xrightleftharpoons[(H)]{(O)} R-\overset{\overset{O}{\|}}{C}-OH$$

1° Alcohol — Aldehyde — Carboxylic acid

$$R-\overset{\overset{OH}{|}}{C}H-R' \xrightleftharpoons[(H)]{(O)} R-\overset{\overset{O}{\|}}{C}-R'$$

2° Alcohol — Ketone

Figure IV.B.6.3: Oxidation-Reduction. In organic chemistry, traditionally the symbols R and R' denote an attached hydrogen, or a hydrocarbon side chain of any length (which are consistent with the reactions above), but sometimes these symbols refer to any group of atoms.

6.2.3 Substitution

In a substitution reaction one atom or group is *substituted* or replaced by another atom or group. For an alcohol, the –OH group is replaced (*substituted*) by a halide (usually chlorine or bromine). A variety of reagents may be used, such as HCl, HBr or PCl$_3$. There are two different types of substitution reactions, S$_N$1 and S$_N$2.

In the S$_N$1 (*1st order or monomolecular nucleophilic substitution*) reaction, the transition state involves a carbocation, the formation of which is the rate-determining step. Alcohol substitutions that proceed by this mechanism are those involving benzyl groups, allyl groups, tertiary and secondary alcohols. The mechanism of this reaction is:

(i) R–L → R$^+$ + L$^-$
(ii) Nu$^-$ + R$^+$ → Nu–R

The important features of this reaction are:

- The reaction is first order (this means that the rate of the reaction depends only on the concentration of one compound); the rate depends on [R–L], where R represents an alkyl group, and L represents a substituent or ligand.

- There is a racemization of configuration, when a chiral molecule is involved.

- A stable carbonium ion should be formed; thus in terms of reaction rate, benzyl groups = allyl groups > tertiary alcohols > secondary alcohols >> primary alcohols.

- The stability of alkyl groups is as follows: primary alkyl groups < secondary alkyl groups < tertiary alkyl groups.

The mechanism of the S_N2 (*2nd order or bimolecular nucleophilic substitution*) reaction is:

$Nu^- + R{-}L \rightarrow [Nu\text{----}R\text{----}L]^- \rightarrow Nu{-}R + L^-$

There are several important points to know about this reaction:

- The reaction rate is second order overall (the rate depends on the concentration of two compounds); first order with respect to [R-L] and first order with respect to the concentration of the nucleophile [Nu^-].

- Note that the nucleophile adds to the alkyl group by *backside displacement* (i.e. Nu must add to the *opposite* site to the ligand). Thus optically active alcohols react to give an inversion of configuration, forming the opposite enantiomer.

- Large or bulky groups near or at the reacting site may hinder or retard a reaction. This is called *steric hindrance*. Size or steric factors are important since they affect S_N2 reaction rates; in terms of reaction rates, CH_3^- > primary alcohols > secondary alcohols >> tertiary alcohols.

The substitution reactions for methanol (CH_3OH) and other primary alcohols are by the S_N2 reaction mechanism.

6.2.4 Elimination

Elimination reactions occur when an atom or a group of atoms is removed (*eliminated*) from adjacent carbons leaving a multiple bond:

$$\begin{array}{c} -\underset{Y}{\overset{|}{C}}-\underset{Z}{\overset{|}{C}}- \end{array} \xrightarrow[(-YZ)]{\text{elimination}} \begin{array}{c} \diagdown \\ C=C \\ \diagup \end{array}$$

There are two different types of elimination reactions, E1 and E2. In the E1 (Elimination, 1st order) reaction, the rate of reaction depends on the concentration of one compound. E1 often occurs as minor products alongside S_N2 reactions. E1 can occur as major products in alkyl halides or, as in the following example, to an alcohol:

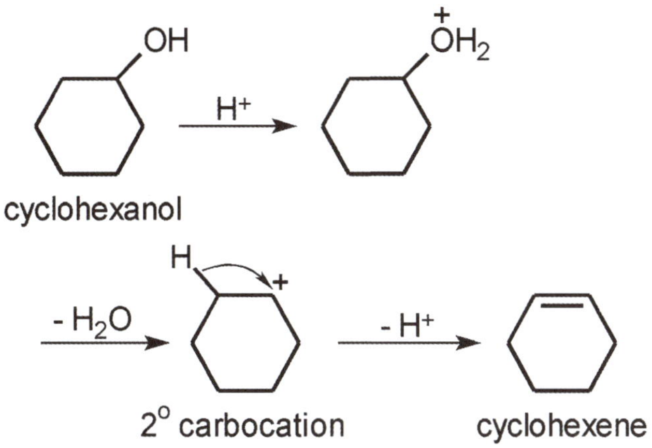

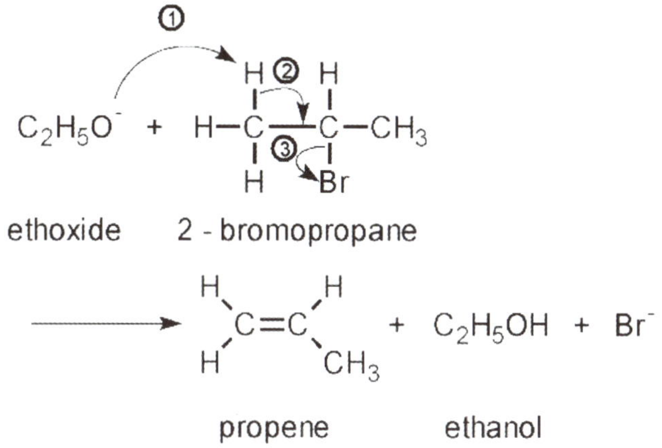

ORGANIC CHEMISTRY

In the E2 (Elimination, 2nd order) reaction the rate of reaction depends on the concentration of two compounds. E2 reactions require strong bases like KOH or the salt of an alcohol (i.e. *sodium alkoxide*). An alkoxide can be synthesized from an alcohol using either Na(s) or NaH (*sodium hydride*) as reducing agents. The hydride ion H⁻ is a powerful base:

$$R-OH + NaH \longrightarrow R-O^- Na^+ \text{ (sodium alkoxide)} + H_2$$

Now the alkoxide can be used as a proton acceptor in an E2 reaction involving an alkyl halide:

In the preceding reaction, the first step (1) involves the base (ethoxide) removing (*elimination*) a proton, thus carbon has a negative charge (*primary* carbanion, <u>very</u> *unstable*). The electron pair is quickly attracted to the δ⁺ neighboring carbon (2) forming a double bond (note that the carbon was δ⁺ because it was attached to the electronegative atom Br, *see* ORG 1.5). Simultaneously, Br (*a halide, which are good leaving groups*) is bumped (3) from the carbon as carbon can have only four bonds. {Notice that in organic chemistry the curved arrows always follow the movement of electrons}

The determination of the quality of a leaving group is quite simple: <u>good leaving groups</u> have *strong* conjugate acids. As examples, H_2O is a good leaving group because H_3O^+ is a strong acid, likewise for Br^-/HBr, Cl^-/HCl, HSO_4^-/H_2SO_4, etc.

GOLD NOTES

ALDEHYDES AND KETONES

Chapter 7

Memorize
* IUPAC nomenclature
* Redox reactions

Understand
* Effect of hydrogen bonds
* Mechanisms of reactions
* Acidity of the alpha H
* Resonance, polarity
* Grignards, organometallic reagents

Not Required*
* Advanced level college info
* The Wittig reaction

GAMSAT-Prep.com

Introduction

An aldehyde contains a terminal carbonyl group. The functional group is a carbon atom bonded to a hydrogen atom and double-bonded to an oxygen atom (O=CH-) and is called the aldehyde group. A ketone contains a carbonyl group (C=O) bonded to two other carbon atoms: R(CO)R'.

Additional Resources

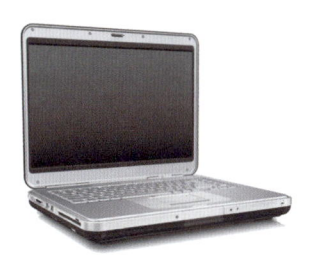

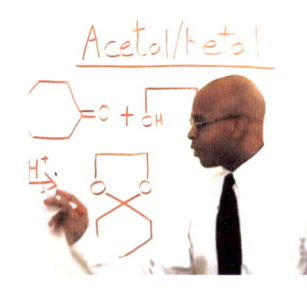

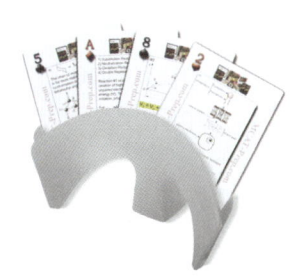

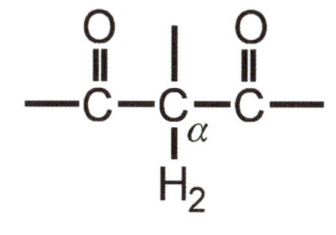

Free Online Q&A + Forum   Video: DVD Discs 1, 2, 3, 4   Flashcards   Special Guest

THE BIOLOGICAL SCIENCES ORG-53

* The real GAMSAT may have advanced level information presented (ie. in a passage) but previous knowledge of said information is not required to answer the questions that would follow. Practice ACER and GS practice GAMSATs can help you clarify this point.

7.1 Description and Nomenclature

Aldehydes and ketones are two types of molecules, both containing the carbonyl group, C=O, which is the basis for their chemistry.

The general structure of aldehydes and ketones is:

$$\underset{\text{Aldehyde}}{R-\overset{\overset{\displaystyle O}{\|}}{C}-H} \qquad \underset{\text{Ketone}}{R-\overset{\overset{\displaystyle O}{\|}}{C}-R'}$$

Aldehydes have at least one hydrogen bonded to the carbonyl carbon, as well as a second hydrogen (= *formaldehyde*) or either an alkyl or an aryl group (= *benzene minus one hydrogen*). Ketones have two alkyl or aryl groups bound to the carbonyl carbon (i.e. the carbon forming the double bond with oxygen).

Systematic naming of these compounds is done by replacing the '–e' of the corresponding alkane with '–al' for aldehydes, and '-one' for ketones. For ketones the chain is numbered as to give the lowest possible number to the carbonyl carbon. Common names are given in brackets:

$$\underset{\substack{\text{Ethanal}\\ \text{(acetaldehyde)}}}{CH_3\overset{\overset{\displaystyle O}{\|}}{C}-H} \qquad \underset{\substack{\text{Propanone}\\ \text{(acetone)}}}{CH_3\overset{\overset{\displaystyle O}{\|}}{C}CH_3}$$

$$\underset{\substack{\text{2-Pentanone}\\ \text{(methyl propyl ketone)}}}{CH_3\overset{\overset{\displaystyle O}{\|}}{C}CH_2CH_2CH_3}$$

The important features of the carbonyl group are:

- Resonance: There are two resonance forms of the carbonyl group:

$$R-\overset{\overset{\displaystyle \delta^-\,O}{\|}}{\underset{\delta^+}{C}}-R' \longleftrightarrow R-\overset{\overset{\displaystyle {}^-O}{|}}{\underset{+}{C}}-R'$$

- Polarity: Reactions about this group may be either nucleophilic, or electrophilic. Since opposite charges attract, nucleophiles (Nu⁻) attack the δ⁺ carbon, and electrophiles (E⁺) attack the δ⁻ oxygen. In both of these types of reactions, the character of the double bond is altered:

$$R-\overset{\overset{\displaystyle O\delta^-}{\|}}{\underset{\delta^+}{C}}-R \xrightarrow{E^+} \text{Electrophilic}$$

$$\left[R-\overset{\overset{\displaystyle {}^+O\!\!-\!\!E}{\|}}{C}-R \longleftrightarrow R-\overset{\overset{\displaystyle O\!\!-\!\!E}{|}}{\underset{+}{C}}-R \right]$$

$$\underset{Nu^-}{R}-\overset{\overset{\displaystyle O\delta^-}{\|}}{\underset{\delta^+}{C}}-R \xrightarrow{\text{Nucleophilic}} R-\overset{\overset{\displaystyle O^-}{|}}{\underset{Nu}{C}}-R$$

ORGANIC CHEMISTRY

- **Acidity of the α-hydrogen**: The α-hydrogen is the hydrogen attached to the carbon next to the carbonyl group (the α-carbon). The β-carbon is the carbon adjacent to the α-carbon. The α-hydrogen may be removed by a base. The acidity of this hydrogen is increased if it is between 2 carbonyl groups:

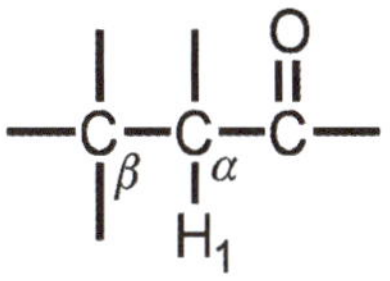

  $H_2 > H_1$ in acidity

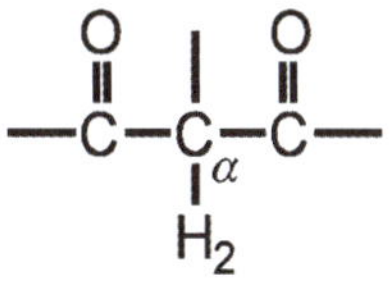

  This acidity is a result of the resonance stabilization of the α-carbanion formed. This stabilization will also permit addition at the β-carbon in α-β unsaturated carbonyls (*those with double or triple bonds*):

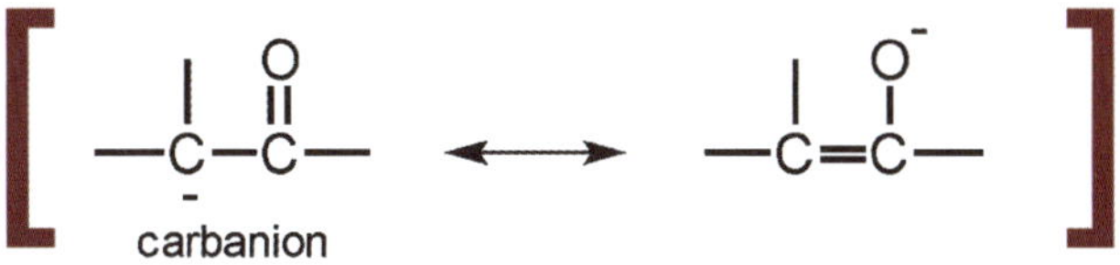

  carbanion
  resonance stabilization

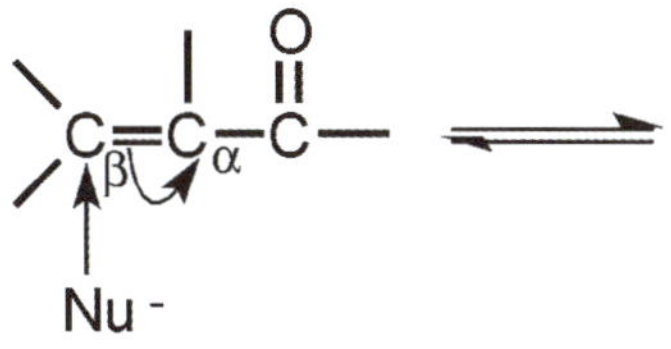

  α, β unsaturated carbonyl

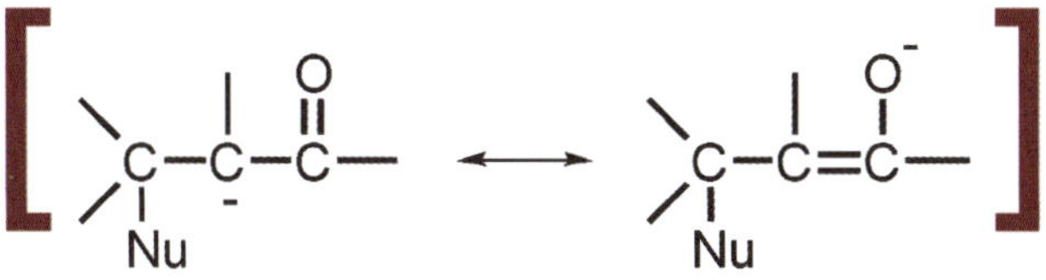

- **Keto-enol tautomerization**: The carbonyl exists in equilibrium with the enol form of the molecule. Although the carbonyl is usually the predominant one, if the enol double bond can be conjugated with other double bonds, it becomes stable (conjugated double bonds are those which are separated by a single bond):

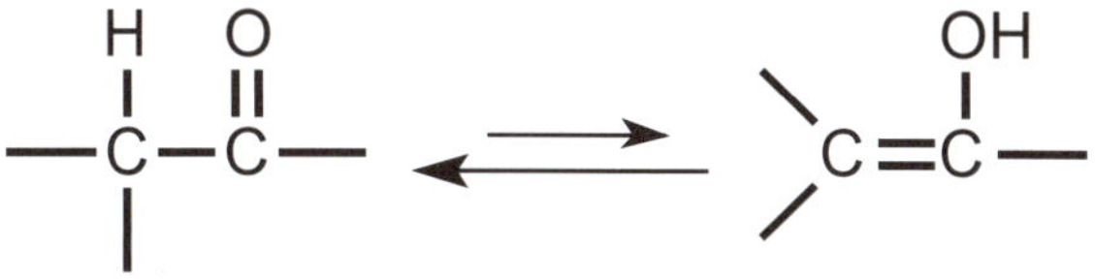

  carbonyl   enol

- **Hydrogen bonds**: The O of the carbonyl forms hydrogen bonds with the hydrogens attached to other electronegative atoms, such as O's or N's:

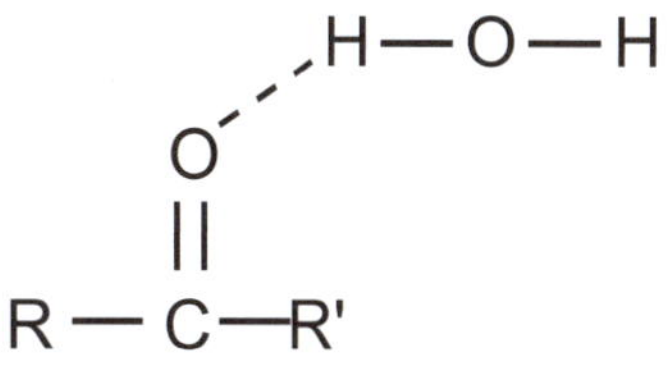

  or

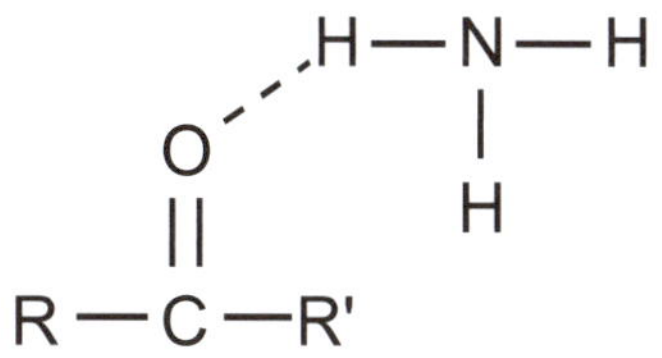

THE BIOLOGICAL SCIENCES ORG-55

7.2 Important Reactions of Aldehydes & Ketones

7.2.1 Overview

Since the carbonyl group is the functional group of aldehydes and ketones, groups adjacent to the carbonyl group affect the rate of reaction for the molecule. For example, an electron withdrawing ligand adjacent to the carbonyl group will increase the partial positive charge on the carbon making the carbonyl group more attractive to a nucleophile. Conversely, an electron donating ligand would decrease the reactivity of the carbonyl group.

Generally, aldehydes oxidize easier, and undergo nucleophilic additions easier than ketones. This is a consequence of steric hindrance.

Aldehydes will be oxidized to carboxylic acids with the standard oxidizing agents. Ketones rarely oxidize. Carbonyls are also reduced using reducing agents (i.e. the hydrides $NaBH_4$ and $LiAlH_4$) forming alcohols (see ORG 6.2.2 for this very important redox - oxidation/reduction - series of reactions). Aldehydes can be made by reacting an acetal with aqueous acid or by reacting a primary alcohol with CrO_3/pyridine, or by reacting an acid chloride with H_2/Pd/C.

There are two classes of reactions that will be investigated: nucleophilic addition reactions at C=O bond, and reactions at adjacent positions.

7.2.2 Acetal (ketal) and Hemiacetal (hemiketal) Formation

Aldehydes and ketones will form hemiacetals and hemiketals, respectively, when dissolved in an excess of a primary alcohol. In addition, if this mixture contains a trace of an acid catalyst, the hemiacetal (hemiketal) will react further to form acetals and ketals.

An acetal is a composite functional group in which two ether functions are joined to a carbon bearing a hydrogen and an alkyl group. A ketal is a composite functional group in which two ether functions are joined to a carbon bearing two alkyl groups.

This reaction may be summarised:

$$R-\underset{\underset{O}{\parallel}}{C}-R' + R''OH \underset{-H^+}{\overset{+H^+}{\rightleftharpoons}}$$

aldehyde (R' = H)   excess
or ketone (R' = alkyl)   alcohol

$$R-\underset{\underset{OR''}{|}}{\overset{\overset{OH}{|}}{C}}-R' \underset{+H_2O}{\overset{+H^+/-H_2O}{\rightleftharpoons}} R-\underset{\underset{OR''}{|}}{\overset{\overset{OR''}{|}}{C}}-R'$$

hemiacetal   acetal
or   or
hemiketal   ketal

The first step in the preceding reaction is that the most charged species (+, the hydrogen) attracts electrons from the δ- oxygen, leaving a carbocation intermediate. The second step involves the δ- oxygen from the alcohol *quickly* attracted to the current most charged species (+, carbon). A proton is lost which regenerates the catalyst, and produces the hemiacetal or hemiketal. Now the proton may attract electrons from –OH forming H₂O, a good leaving group. Again the δ- oxygen on the alcohol is attracted to the positive carbocation. And again the alcohol releases its proton, regenerating the catalyst, producing an acetal or ketal.

7.2.3 Imine and Enamine Formation

Imines and enamines are formed when aldehydes and ketones are allowed to react with amines.

When an aldehyde or ketone reacts with a primary amine, an imine (or Schiff base) is formed. A primary amine is a nitrogen compound with the general formula R–NH₂, where R represents an alkyl or aryl group. In an imine the carbonyl group of the aldehyde or ketone is replaced with a C=N–R group.

When an aldehyde or ketone reacts with a secondary amine, an enamine is formed. A secondary amine is a nitrogen with the general formula R₂N–H, where R represents aryl or alkyl groups (these groups need not be identical).

Tertiary amines (of the general form R₃N) do not react with the aldehydes or ketones.

The reaction may be summarised:

7.2.4 Aldol Condensation

Aldol condensation is a base catalyzed reaction of aldehydes and ketones that have α-hydrogens. The intermediate, an aldol, is both an ald*ehyde* and a *alcoh*ol. The aldol undergoes a dehydration reaction producing a carbon-carbon bond in the condensation product, an *enal* (= alk*ene* + *al*dehyde).

The reaction may be summarised:

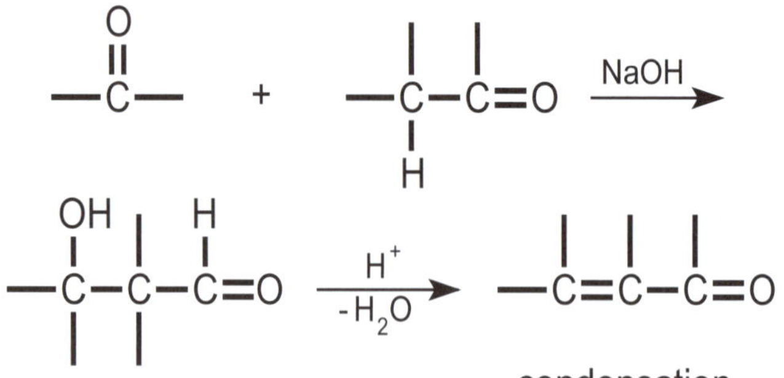

$$\underset{}{-\overset{O}{\underset{}{\overset{\|}{C}}}-} + -\overset{|}{\underset{H}{C}}-\overset{|}{C}=O \xrightarrow{NaOH}$$

$$-\overset{OH}{\underset{|}{C}}-\overset{H}{\underset{|}{C}}-\overset{|}{C}=O \xrightarrow[-H_2O]{H^+} -\overset{|}{C}=\overset{|}{C}-\overset{|}{C}=O$$

Aldol → condensation product

7.2.5 Conjugate Addition to α–β Unsaturated Carbonyls

α-β unsaturated carbonyls are unusually reactive with nucleophiles. This is best illustrated by example:

Examples of relevant nucleophiles includes CN^- from HCN, and R^- which can be generated by a Grignard Reagent (= RMgX) or as an alkyl lithium (= RLi).

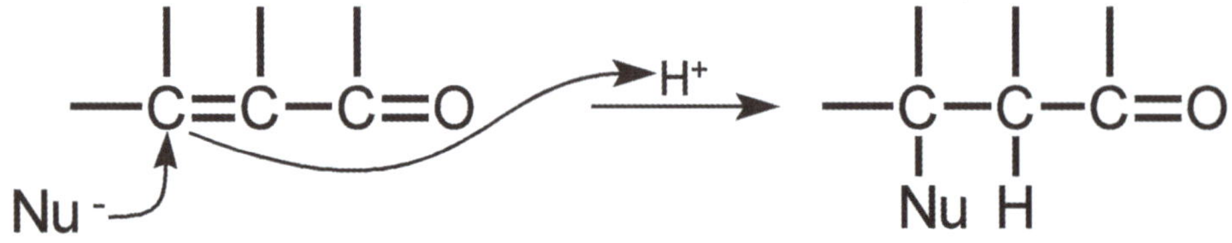

$$-\overset{|}{C}=\overset{|}{C}-\overset{|}{C}=O \xrightarrow{H^+} -\overset{|}{\underset{Nu}{C}}-\overset{|}{\underset{H}{C}}-\overset{|}{C}=O$$

Nu⁻

For Oxidation-Reduction reactions for aldehydes and ketones, see ORG 6.2.2.

ORGANIC CHEMISTRY

GOLD NOTES

CARBOXYLIC ACIDS

Chapter 8

Memorize
* IUPAC nomenclature
* Redox reactions

Understand
* Hydrogen bonding
* Mechanisms of reactions
* Relative acid strength
* Resonance, inductive effects
* Grignards, organometallic reagents

Not Required*
* Advanced level college info
* Nitrile reaction mechanisms

GAMSAT-Prep.com

Introduction

Carboxylic acids are organic acids with a carboxyl group, which has the formula -C(=O)OH, usually written -COOH or -CO$_2$H. Carboxylic acids are Brønsted-Lowry acids (proton donors) that are actually, in the grand scheme of chemistry, weak acids. Salts and anions of carboxylic acids are called carboxylates.

Additional Resources

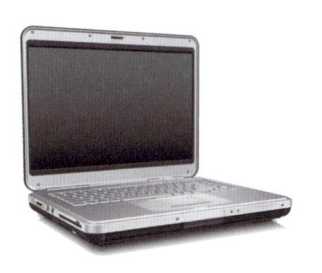

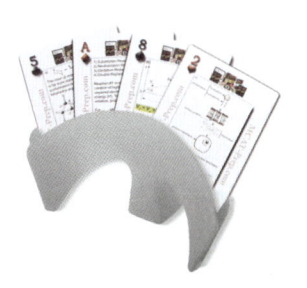

Free Online Q&A + Forum   Video: DVD Discs 2, 3   Flashcards   Special Guest

THE BIOLOGICAL SCIENCES   ORG-61

* The real GAMSAT may have advanced level information presented (ie. in a passage) but previous knowledge of said information is not required to answer the questions that would follow. Practice ACER and GS practice GAMSATs can help you clarify this point.

8.1 Description and Nomenclature

Carboxylic acids are molecules containing the *carboxylic group* (carbonyl + hydroxyl), which is the basis of their chemistry. The general structure of a carboxylic acid is:

$$R-\overset{\overset{O}{\|}}{C}-OH$$

Systematic naming of these compounds is done by replacing the '–e' of the corresponding alkane with '–oic acid'. The molecule is numbered such that the carbonyl carbon is carbon number one. Many carboxylic acids have common names by which they are usually known (systematic names in italics):

$$H-\overset{\overset{O}{\|}}{C}-OH \quad CH_3-\overset{\overset{O}{\|}}{C}-OH \quad HO-\overset{\overset{O}{\|}}{C}-OH$$

formic acid   acetic acid   carbonic acid
methanoic acid   *ethanoic acid*   *hydroxymethanoic acid*

$$HO-\overset{\overset{O}{\|}}{C}-CH_2CH_2-\overset{\overset{O}{\|}}{C}-OH$$

succinic acid
butanedioic acid

benzoic acid
same: *benzoic acid*

Low molecular weight carboxylic acids are liquids with strong odours and high boiling points. The high boiling point is due to the polarity and the hydrogen bonding capability of the molecule. Because of this hydrogen bonding, these molecules are water soluble. As well, carboxylic acids are soluble in dilute bases (NaOH or NaHCO$_3$), because of their acid properties. The carboxyl group is the basis of carboxylic acid chemistry, and there are four important features to remember. Looking at a general carboxylic acid:

- The hydrogen (H) is weakly acidic. This is due to its attachment to the oxygen atom, and because the carboxylate anion is resonance stabilized:

$$R-\overset{\overset{O}{\|}}{C}-OH \rightleftharpoons H^+ +$$

$$\left[R-\overset{\overset{O}{\|}}{C}-O^- \leftrightarrow R-\overset{\overset{O^-}{|}}{C}=O \right]$$

resonance forms

- The carboxyl carbon is very susceptible to nucleophilic attack. This is due to the attached oxygen atom, and the carbonyl oxygen, both atoms being electronegative:

$$R-\overset{\overset{\delta^- O}{\|}}{\underset{\delta^{++} \to \delta^-}{C}}-O-H$$

$$\underset{Nu^-}{R-\overset{\overset{O}{\|}}{C}-O-H} \longrightarrow R-\overset{\overset{O^-}{|}}{\underset{Nu}{C}}-O-H$$

- In basic conditions, the hydroxyl group, as is, is a good leaving group. In acidic conditions, the protonated hydroxyl (i.e. water) is an excellent leaving group. This promotes nucleophilic substitution:

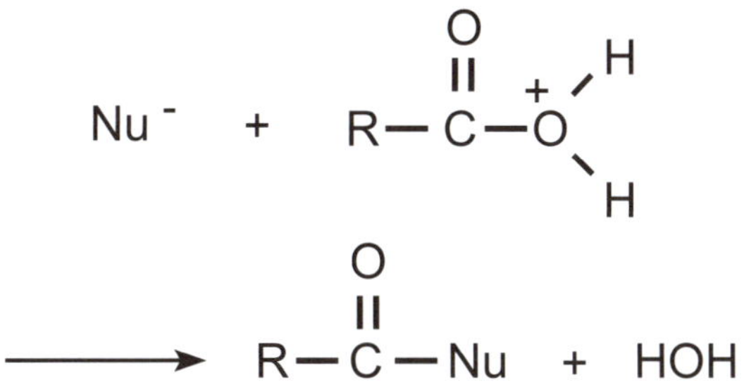

ORGANIC CHEMISTRY

$$Nu^- + R-\overset{\overset{O}{\|}}{C}-\overset{+}{O}\overset{H}{\underset{H}{\diagdown}} \longrightarrow R-\overset{\overset{O}{\|}}{C}-Nu + HOH$$

- Because of the carbonyl and hydroxyl moieties (i.e. parts), hydrogen bonding is possible both inter- and intramolecularly:

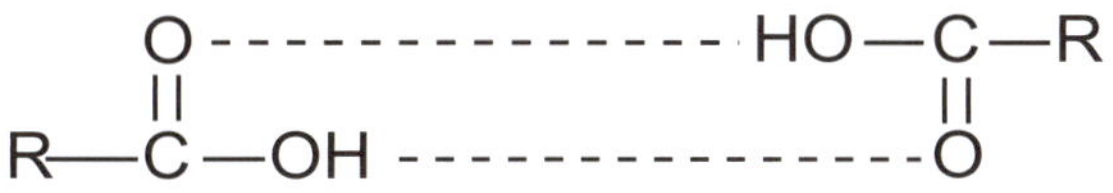

intermolecular (dimerization)

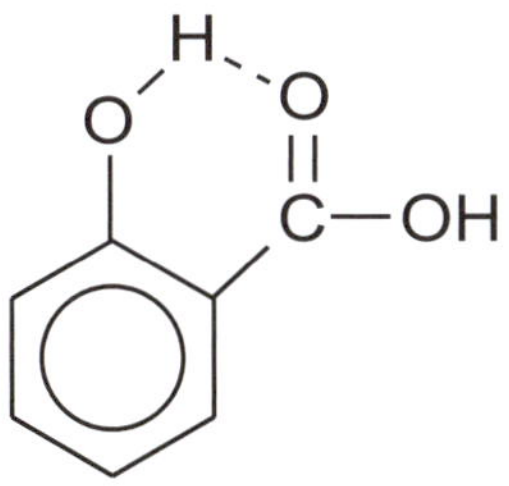

intramolecular

As implied by their name, carboxylic acids are acidic - the most common acid of all organic compounds. In fact, they are colloquially known as *organic acids*. Organic classes of molecules in order of increasing acid strength are:

alkanes < ammonia < alkynes < alcohols < water < carboxylic acids

Substituted phenols may be stronger acids than water.

The relative acid strength among carboxylic acids depends on the inductive effects of the attached groups, and their proximity to the carboxyl. For example:

$CH_3CH_2-C(Cl)_2-COOH$ *is a stronger acid than* $CH_3CH_2-CH(Cl)-COOH$.

The reason for this is that chlorine, which is electronegative, withdraws electron density and stabilizes the carboxylate anion. Proximity is important, as:

$CH_3CH_2-C(Cl)_2-COOH$ *is a stronger acid than* $CH_3-C(Cl)_2-CH_2COOH$.

8.1.1 Carboxylic Acid Formation

A carboxylic acid can be formed by reacting a Grignard reagent with carbon dioxide, or by reacting an aldehyde with $KMnO_4$ (*see* ORG 6.2.2). Carboxylic acids are also formed by reacting a nitrile (in which nitrogen shares a triple bond with a carbon) with aqueous acid.

8.2 Important Reactions of Carboxylic Acids

Carboxylic acids undergo nucleophilic substitution reactions with many different nucleophiles, under a variety of conditions:

$$Nu^- + R-\underset{\underset{O}{\|}}{C}-OH \longrightarrow R-\underset{\underset{O}{\|}}{C}-Nu + OH^-$$

If the nucleophile is –OR, the resulting compound is an ester. If it is –NH$_2$, the resulting compound is an amide. If it is Cl from SOCl$_2$, or PCl$_5$, the resulting compound is an acid chloride.

The typical esterification reaction may be summarized:

$$R'O^*H + R-\underset{\underset{O}{\|}}{C}-OH$$
alcohol   acid

$$\longrightarrow R-\underset{\underset{O}{\|}}{C}-O^*R' + H_2O$$
ester

Notice that an asterix* was added to the oxygen of the alcohol so that you can tell where that oxygen ended up in the product (i.e. the ester). In the lab, instead of an asterix (!), an isotope (CHM 1.3) of oxygen is used as a tracer or label.

The decarboxylation reaction involves the loss of the carboxyl group as CO$_2$:

$$HO-\underset{\underset{O}{\|}}{C}-\underset{\underset{R}{|}}{\overset{\overset{H}{|}}{C}}-\underset{\underset{O}{\|}}{C}-OH \xrightarrow[heat]{base} H-\underset{\underset{R}{|}}{\overset{\overset{H}{|}}{C}}-\underset{\underset{O}{\|}}{C}-OH + CO_2$$
β – diacid

$$R-\underset{\underset{O}{\|}}{C}-\underset{\underset{H}{|}}{\overset{\overset{H}{|}}{C}}-\underset{\underset{O}{\|}}{C}-OH \xrightarrow[heat]{base} R-\underset{\underset{O}{\|}}{C}-CH_3 + CO_2$$
β – keto acid

This reaction is not important for most ordinary carboxylic acids. There are certain types of carboxylic acids that decarboxylate easily, mainly:

- Those which have a keto group at the β position, known as β-keto acids.
- Malonic acids and its derivatives (i.e. β-diacids: those with two carboxyl groups, separated by one carbon).
- Carbonic acid and its derivatives.

Carboxylic acids are reduced to alcohols with lithium aluminum hydride, LiAlH$_4$, or H$_2$/metals (see ORG 6.2.2). Sodium borohydride, NaBH$_4$, being a milder reducing agent, only reduces aldehydes and ketones. Carboxylic acids may also be converted to esters or amides first, and then reduced:

$$LiAlH_4 + R-\underset{\underset{O}{\|}}{C}-OH$$

$$\longrightarrow R-CH_2-OH$$
alcohol

ORG-64   CARBOXYLIC ACIDS

ORGANIC CHEMISTRY

GOLD NOTES

CARBOXYLIC ACID DERIVATIVES
Chapter 9

Memorize
* IUPAC nomenclature

Understand
* Mechanisms of reactions
* Relative reactivity
* Steric, inductive effects

Not Required*
* Advanced level college info
* Nitrile reaction mechanisms

GAMSAT-Prep.com

Introduction

Carboxylic acid derivatives are a series of compounds that can be synthesized using carboxylic acid. For the GAMSAT, this includes acid chlorides, anhydrides, amides and esters.

Additional Resources

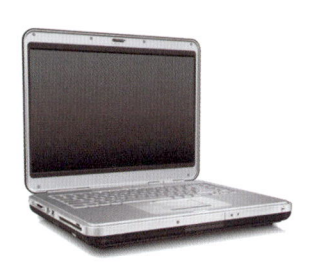

Free Online Q&A + Forum

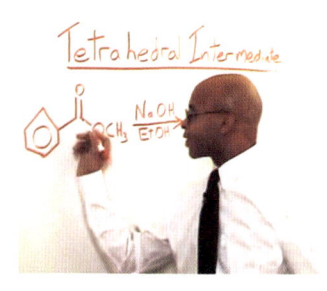

Video: DVD Disc 3

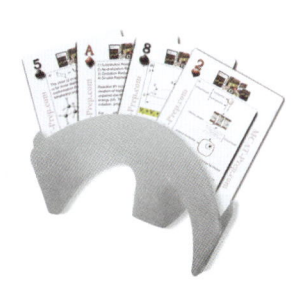

Flashcards

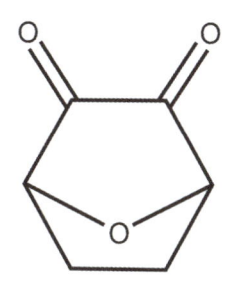

Special Guest

THE BIOLOGICAL SCIENCES ORG-67

* The real GAMSAT may have advanced level information presented (ie. in a passage) but previous knowledge of said information is not required to answer the questions that would follow. Practice ACER and GS practice GAMSATs can help you clarify this point.

9.1 Acid Halides

The general structure of an acid halide is:

$$R-\underset{\underset{O}{\|}}{C}-X \quad X = \text{Halide}$$

These are named by replacing the 'ic acid' of the parent carboxylic acid with the suffix 'yl halide.' For example:

$$CH_3CH_2CH_2-\underset{\underset{O}{\|}}{C}-Br \quad \text{Butanoyl bromide}$$

$$CH_3-\underset{\underset{O}{\|}}{C}-Cl \quad \text{Acetyl chloride (ethanoyl chloride)}$$

Acid chlorides are synthesized by reacting the parent carboxylic acid with PCl_5 or $SOCl_2$. Acid chlorides react with $NaBH_4$ to form alcohols. This can be done in one or two steps. In one step, the acid chloride reacts with $NaBH_4$ to immediately form an alcohol. In two steps, the acid chloride can react first with H_2/Pd/C to form a carboxylic acid; reaction of the carboxylic acid with $NaBH_4$ then produces an alcohol.

Acid halides can engage in nucleophilic reactions similar to carboxylic acids (*see* ORG 8.2); however, acid halides are more reactive (*see* ORG 9.6).

9.2 Acid Anhydrides

The general structure of an acid anhydride is:

$$R-\underset{\underset{O}{\|}}{C}-O-\underset{\underset{O}{\|}}{C}-R$$

These are named by replacing the 'acid' of the parent carboxylic acid with the word 'anhydride.' For example:

$$CH_3-\underset{\underset{O}{\|}}{C}-O-\underset{\underset{O}{\|}}{C}-CH_3$$
acetic anhydride
(ethanoic anhydride)

$$CH_3-\underset{\underset{O}{\|}}{C}-O-\underset{\underset{O}{\|}}{C}-H$$
acetic formic anhydride
(ethanoic methanoic anhydride)

Both acid chlorides and acid anhydrides have boiling points comparable to esters of similar molecular weight.

ORG-68 CARBOXYLIC ACID DERIVATIVES

9.3 Amides

The general structure of an amide is:

$$R-\underset{\underset{}{\overset{\overset{O}{\|}}{C}}}{}-NR'_2$$

These are named by replacing the '–ic (oic) acid' of the parent anhydride with the suffix '-amide.' If there are alkyl groups attached to the nitrogen, they are named as substituents, and designated by the letter N. For example:

$$CH_3-\overset{\overset{O}{\|}}{C}-N\underset{C_2H_5}{\overset{C_2H_5}{}} \quad \text{N,N-diethylacetamide}$$

$$CH_3CH_2-\overset{\overset{O}{\|}}{C}-NH_2 \quad \text{propanamide}$$

Unsubstituted and monosubstituted amides form very strong intermolecular hydrogen bonds, and as a result, they have very high boiling and melting points. The boiling points of disubstituted amides are similar to those of aldehydes and ketones. Amides are essentially neutral (no acidity, as compared to carboxylic acids, and no basicity, as compared to amines).

Amides may be prepared by reacting carboxylic acids (or other carboxylic acid derivatives) with ammonia:

$$R-\overset{\overset{O}{\|}}{C}-OH + NH_3 + \text{heat} \xrightarrow{-H_2O} R-\overset{\overset{O}{\|}}{C}-NH_2$$

As well, amides undergo nucleophilic substitution reactions at the carbonyl carbon:

$$R-\overset{\overset{O}{\|}}{C}-NH_2 + NuH \longrightarrow R-\overset{\overset{O}{\|}}{C}-Nu + NH_3$$

Amides can be hydrolyzed to yield the parent carboxylic acid and amine. This reaction may take place under acidic or basic conditions:

$$R-\overset{\overset{O}{\|}}{C}-NHR + H_2O \xrightarrow{H^+} R-\overset{\overset{O}{\|}}{C}-OH + RNH_2$$
amide → acid + amine

$$R-\overset{\overset{O}{\|}}{C}-NHR + H_2O \xrightarrow{OH^-}$$
amide

$$R-\overset{\overset{O}{\|}}{C}-O^- + RNH_2 \xrightarrow{H^+} R-\overset{\overset{O}{\|}}{C}-OH$$
carboxylate + amine → acid

Amides can also form amines by reacting with LiAlH$_4$.

9.4 Esters

The general structure of an ester is:

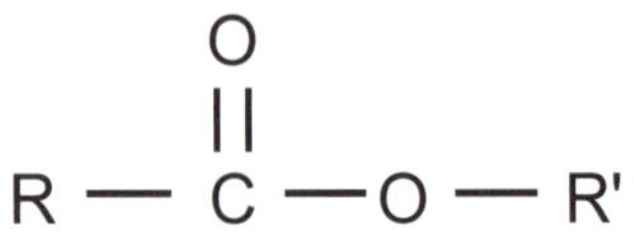

$$R-\underset{\underset{O}{\|}}{C}-O-R'$$

These are named by first citing the name of the alkyl group, followed by the parent acid, with the 'ic acid' replaced by 'ate.' For example:

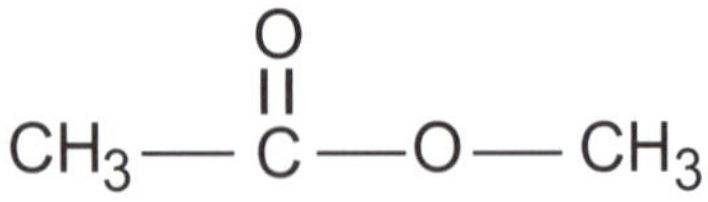

$$CH_3-\underset{\underset{O}{\|}}{C}-O-CH_3$$
methyl acetate
(methyl ethanoate)

The boiling points of esters are lower than those of comparable acids or alcohols, and similar to comparable aldehydes and ketones, because they are polar compounds, without hydrogens to form hydrogen bonds. Esters with longer side chains (R-groups) are more nonpolar than esters with shorter side chains (R-groups). Esters usually have pleasing, fruity odors.

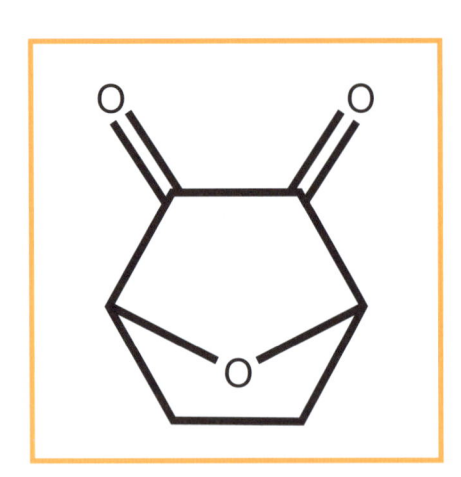

Esters may be synthesized by reacting carboxylic acids or their derivatives with alcohols under either basic or acidic conditions:

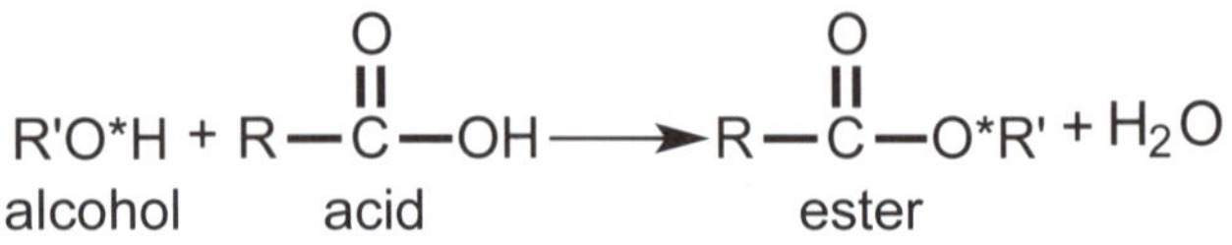

$$R'O^*H + R-\underset{\underset{O}{\|}}{C}-OH \longrightarrow R-\underset{\underset{O}{\|}}{C}-O^*R' + H_2O$$
alcohol   acid   ester

As well, esters undergo nucleophilic substitution reactions at the carbonyl carbon:

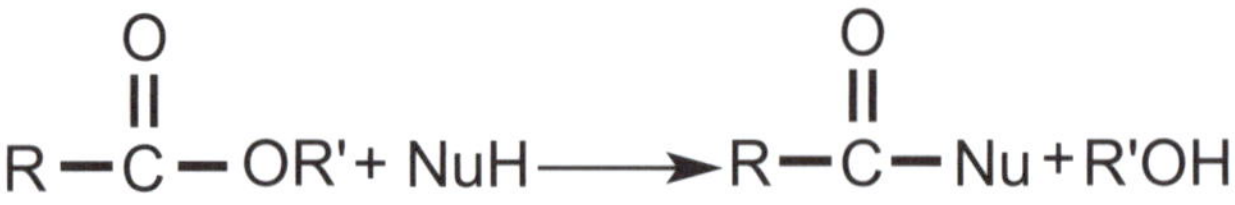

$$R-\underset{\underset{O}{\|}}{C}-OR' + NuH \longrightarrow R-\underset{\underset{O}{\|}}{C}-Nu + R'OH$$

Esters may also be hydrolyzed, to yield the parent carboxylic acid and alcohol. This reaction may take place under acidic or basic conditions.

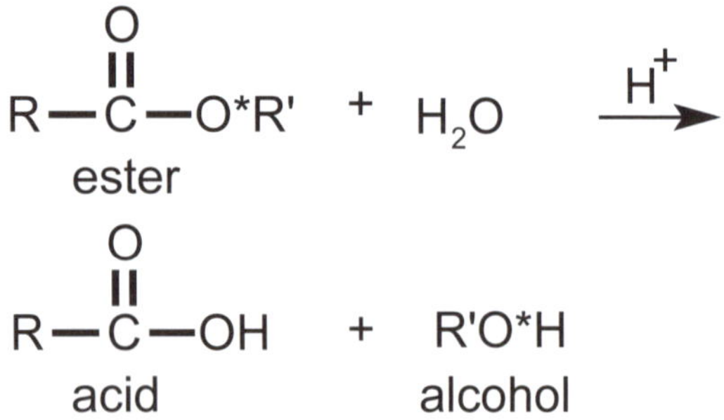

$$R-\underset{\underset{O}{\|}}{C}-O^*R' + H_2O \xrightarrow{H^+}$$
ester

$$R-\underset{\underset{O}{\|}}{C}-OH + R'O^*H$$
acid   alcohol

The Ester Bunny

NB: The Ester Bunny is NOT GAMSAT material. In fact for you super-keeners: is the Ester Bunny a real ester? Find out in our Forum!

ORG-70   CARBOXYLIC ACID DERIVATIVES

9.4.1 Fats, Glycerides and Saponification

A special class of esters is known as fats (i.e. mono-, di-, and triglycerides). These are biologically important molecules, and they are formed in the following reaction:

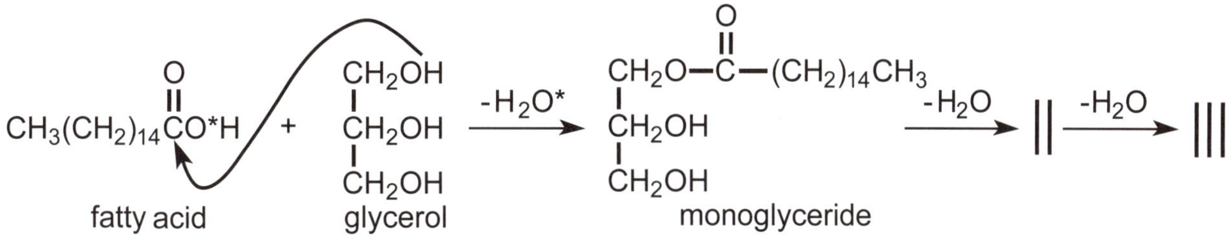

$$CH_3(CH_2)_{14}CO^*H \;+\; \begin{array}{c} CH_2OH \\ | \\ CH_2OH \\ | \\ CH_2OH \end{array} \xrightarrow{-H_2O^*} \begin{array}{c} CH_2O-\overset{O}{\underset{\|}{C}}-(CH_2)_{14}CH_3 \\ | \\ CH_2OH \\ | \\ CH_2OH \end{array} \xrightarrow{-H_2O} \;\|\| \xrightarrow{-H_2O} \;\|\|\|$$

fatty acid   glycerol   monoglyceride

Fatty acids (= *long chain carboxylic acids*) are formed through the condensation of C2 units derived from acetate, and may be added to the monoglyceride formed in the above reaction, forming diglycerides, and triglycerides. Fats may be hydrolyzed by a base to the components glycerol and the salt of the fatty acids. The salts of long chain carboxylic acids are called <u>soaps</u>. Thus this process is called *saponification*:

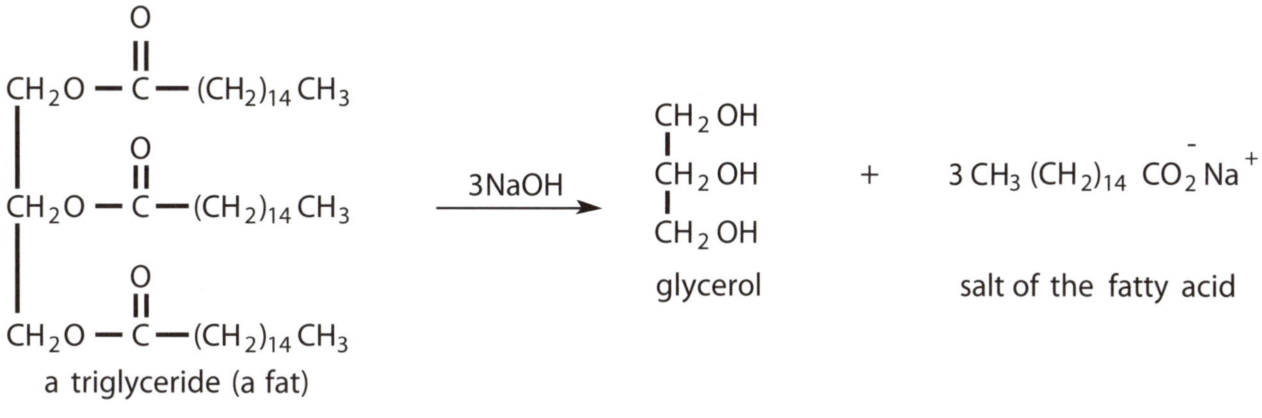

$$\begin{array}{c} CH_2O-\overset{O}{\underset{\|}{C}}-(CH_2)_{14}CH_3 \\ | \\ CH_2O-\overset{O}{\underset{\|}{C}}-(CH_2)_{14}CH_3 \\ | \\ CH_2O-\overset{O}{\underset{\|}{C}}-(CH_2)_{14}CH_3 \end{array} \xrightarrow{3NaOH} \begin{array}{c} CH_2OH \\ | \\ CH_2OH \\ | \\ CH_2OH \end{array} \;+\; 3\,CH_3(CH_2)_{14}CO_2^- Na^+$$

a triglyceride (a fat)   glycerol   salt of the fatty acid

9.5 β-Keto Acids

β-keto acids are carboxylic acids with a keto group (i.e. *ketone*) at the β position. Thus it is an acid with a carbonyl group one carbon removed from a carboxylic acid group.

Upon heating the carboxyl group can be readily removed as CO_2. This process is called *decarboxylation*. For example:

$$\text{R-CO-CH}_2\text{-COOH} \xrightarrow{\text{heat}} \text{RCOCH}_3 + CO_2$$

β – keto acid   →   ketone

9.6 Relative Reactivity of Carboxylic Acid Derivatives

In terms of nucleophilic substitution, generally, carboxylic acid derivatives are more reactive than comparable non-carboxylic acid derivatives. One important reason for the preceding is that the carbon in carboxylic acids is also attached to the electronegative oxygen atom of the carbonyl group; therefore, carbon is more δ+, thus being more attractive to a nucleophile. Hence an acid chloride (R-COCl) is more reactive than a comparable alkyl chloride (R-Cl); an ester (R-COOR') is more reactive than a comparable ether (R-OR'); and an amide (R-CONH$_2$) is more reactive than a comparable amine (R-NH$_2$).

Amongst carboxylic acid derivatives, the carbonyl reactivity in order from most to least reactive is:

acid chlorides > anhydrides >> esters > acids > amides > nitriles

The reasons for this may be attributed to resonance effects and inductive effects. The <u>resonance effect</u> is the ability of the substituent to stabilize the carbocation intermediate by delocalization of electrons. The <u>inductive effect</u> is the substituent group, by virtue of its electronegativity, to pull electrons away increasing the partial positivity of the carbonyl carbon.

Within each carboxylic acid derivative, <u>steric or bulk effects</u> also play an important role. The less the steric hindrance, the more access a nucleophile will have to attack the carbonyl carbon, and vice versa.

ORGANIC CHEMISTRY

GOLD NOTES

ETHERS AND PHENOLS

Chapter 10

Memorize	Understand	Not Required*
* Basic nomenclature	* Ether synthesis, electrophilic aromatic substitution	* Advanced level college info

GAMSAT-Prep.com

Introduction

Ethers are composed of an oxygen atom connected to two alkyl or aryl groups of the general formula R–O–R'. A classic example is the solvent and anesthetic diethyl ether, often just called "ether." Phenol is a toxic, white crystalline solid with a sweet tarry odor often referred to as a "hospital smell"! Its chemical formula is C_6H_5OH and its structure is that of a hydroxyl group (-OH) bonded to a phenyl ring thus it is an aromatic compound.

Additional Resources

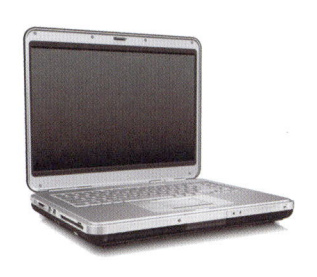

Free Online Q&A + Forum   Video: DVD Discs 1, 4   Flashcards   Special Guest

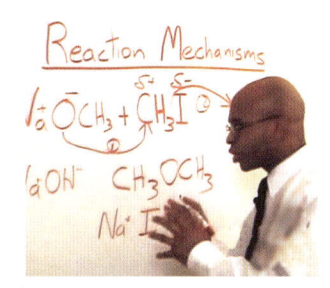

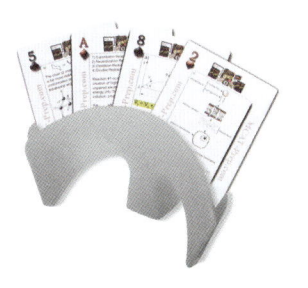

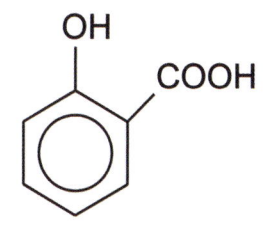

THE BIOLOGICAL SCIENCES   ORG-75

* The real GAMSAT may have advanced level information presented (ie. in a passage) but previous knowledge of said information is not required to answer the questions that would follow. Practice ACER and GS practice GAMSATs can help you clarify this point.

10.1 Description and Nomenclature of Ethers

The general structure of an ether is R-O-R', where the R's may be either aromatic or aliphatic (= *containing only carbon and hydrogen atoms*). In the common system of nomenclature, the two groups on either side of the oxygen are named, followed by the word ether:

$$CH_3-O-CH_3 \qquad CH_3-O-\underset{\underset{CH_3}{|}}{C}HCH_3$$
dimethyl ether　　　methyl isopropyl ether

In the systematic system of nomenclature, the alkoxy (RO-) groups are always named as substituents:

$$CH_3-O-CH_3 \qquad CH_3-O-\underset{\underset{CH_3}{|}}{C}HCH_3$$
methoxy methane　　　methoxy isopropane

The boiling points of ethers are comparable to that of other hydrocarbons. Ethers are more polar than other hydrocarbons, but are not capable of forming intermolecular hydrogen bonds (those between two ether molecules). Ethers are similar to alcohols in water solubility, as they can form intermolecular hydrogen bonds between the ether and the water molecules.

Ethers are <u>good solvents</u>, as the ether linkage is inert to many chemical reagents. Ethers are weak Lewis bases and can be protonated to form positively charged conjugate acids. In the presence of a high concentration of a strong acid (especially HI or HBr), the ether linkage will be cleaved, to form an alcohol and an alkyl halide:

$$CH_3-O-CH_3 + HI \longrightarrow$$
$$CH_3-OH + CH_3-I$$

Ether synthesis can proceed using alcohols or their derivatives. For example, the reverse of the preceding reaction would occur if $NaOCH_3$ (sodium methoxide) instead of $HOCH_3$ was in the reaction flask (the inorganic product would be $Na^+\ I^-$).

$$Na^+\ {}^-OCH_3 + {}^{\delta+}CH_3 - I^{\delta-} \longrightarrow$$
$$CH_3 - O - CH_3 + Na^+ I^-$$

ORGANIC CHEMISTRY

10.2 Phenols

A phenol is a molecule consisting of a hydroxyl (–OH) group attached to a benzene (aromatic) ring. The following are some phenols and derivatives which are important to biochemistry, medicine and nature:

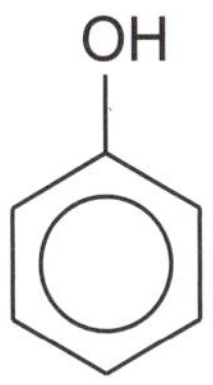

phenol

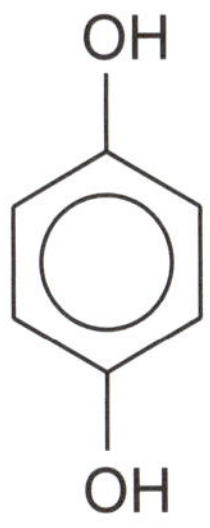

hydroquinone

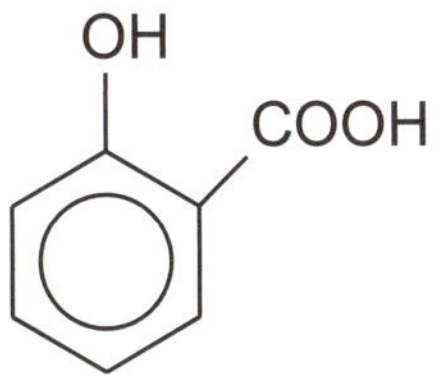

salicylic acid

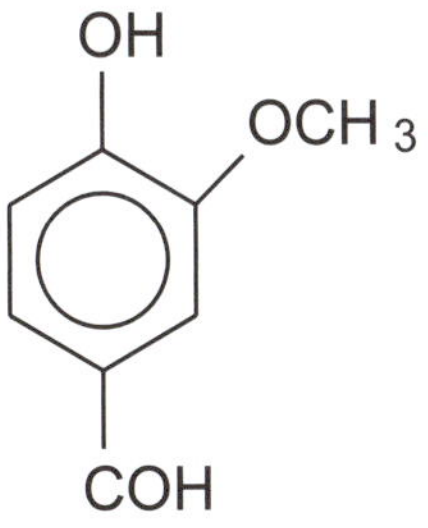

vanillin

Phenols are more acidic than their corresponding alcohols. This is due mainly to the electron withdrawing and resonance stabilization effects of the aromatic ring in the conjugate base anion (the phenoxide ion):

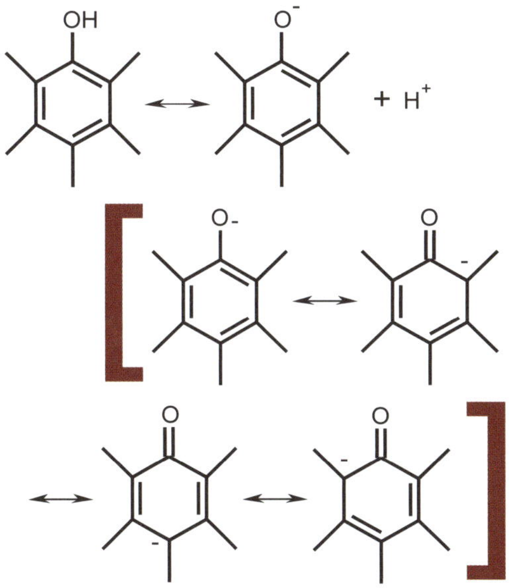

THE BIOLOGICAL SCIENCES ORG-77

Substituent groups on the ring affect the acidity of phenols by both inductive effects (as with alcohols) and resonance effects. The resonance structures show that electron stabilizing (*withdrawing* or *meta directing*) groups at the ortho or para positions should increase the acidity of the phenol. Examples of these groups include the nitro group ($-NO_2$), $-CN$, $-CO_2H$, and the weakly deactivating o-p directors - the halogens. Destabilizing groups, such as alkyl groups, or other ortho-para directors, will make the compound less acidic. Phenols are ortho-para directors.

Phenols can form hydrogen bonds, resulting in fairly high boiling points. Their solubility in water, however, is limited, because of the hydrophobic nature of the aromatic ring. Ortho phenols have lower boiling points than meta and para phenols, as they can form intramolecular hydrogen bonds. However, the para and even the ortho compounds can sometimes form intermolecular hydrogen bonds:

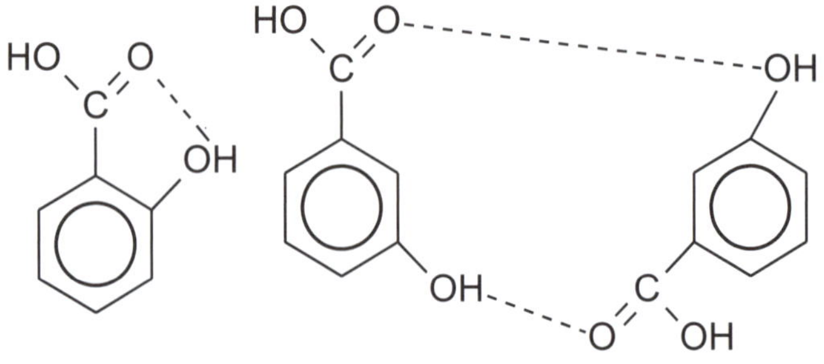

10.2.1 Electrophilic Aromatic Substitution for Phenols

Electrophilic aromatic substitution reactions of phenols may show some unusual effects, due to the hydroxyl group (*see* ORG 5.2.1). For example, phenols are fairly unreactive in the Friedel-Crafts acylation reaction (*a reaction in which an acyl group, R–C=O, is added to another molecule using $AlCl_3$ as a catalyst*), because the –OH group reacts with the catalyst.

The hydroxyl group is a powerful activating group and an ortho-para director in electrophilic substitutions. Thus phenols can brominate three times in bromine water as follows:

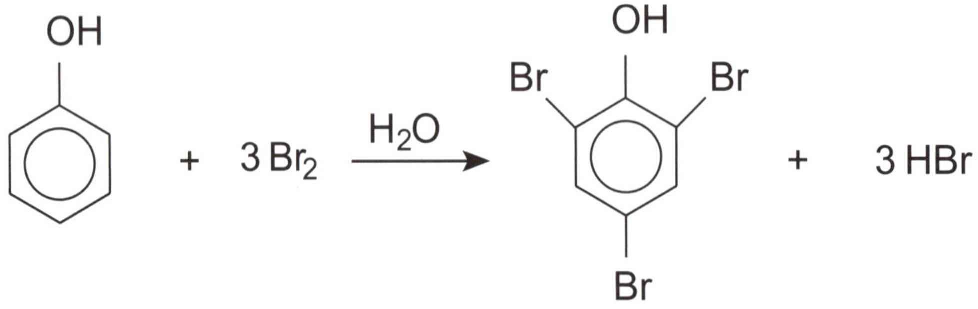

ORGANIC CHEMISTRY

GOLD NOTES

AMINES

Chapter 11

Memorize	Understand	Not Required*
* IUPAC nomenclature	* Effect of hydrogen bonds * Mechanisms of reactions * Trends in basicity * Resonance, delocalization of electrons	* Advanced level college info * Gabriel synthesis * Staudinger reduction

GAMSAT-Prep.com

Introduction

Amines are compounds and functional groups that contain a basic nitrogen atom with a lone pair. Amines are derivatives of ammonia (NH_3), where one or more hydrogen atoms are replaced by organic substituents such as alkyl and aryl groups.

Additional Resources

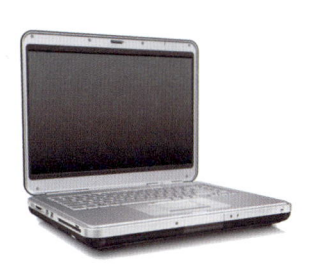

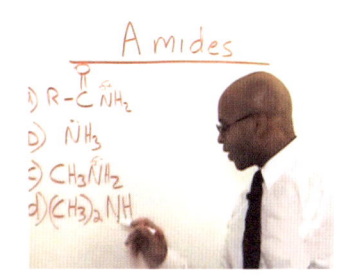

Free Online Q & A   Video: DVD Disc 3   Flashcards   Special Guest

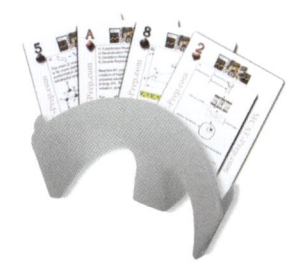

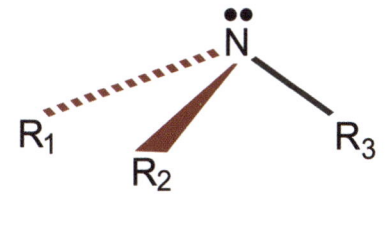

THE BIOLOGICAL SCIENCES   ORG-81

* The real GAMSAT may have advanced level information presented (ie. in a passage) but previous knowledge of said information is not required to answer the questions that would follow. Practice ACER and GS practice GAMSATs can help you clarify this point.

11.1 Description and Nomenclature

Organic compounds with a trivalent nitrogen atom bonded to one or more carbon atoms are called amines. These are organic derivatives of ammonia. They may be classified depending on the number of carbon atoms bonded to the nitrogen:

Primary Amine:	RNH_2
Secondary Amine:	R_2NH
Tertiary Amine:	R_3N
Quaternary Salt:	$R_4N^+ X^-$

In the common system of nomenclature, amines are named by adding the suffix '-amine' to the name of the alkyl group. In a secondary or tertiary amine, where there is more than one alkyl group, the groups are named as N-substituted derivatives of the larger group:

$$CH_3 - CH(CH_3) - N(CH_3) - CH_2 - CH_3$$

N,N - methyl ethyl isopropylamine

In the systematic system of nomenclature, amines are named analagous to alcohols, except the suffix '-amine' is used instead of the suffix '-ol'.

11.1.1 The Basicity of Amines

Along with the three attached groups, amines have an unbonded electron pair. Most of the chemistry of amines depends on this unbonded electron pair:

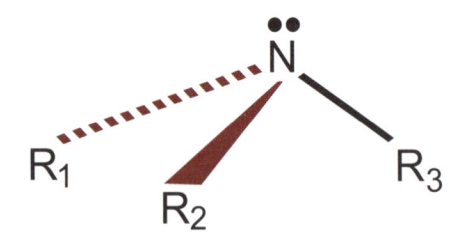

The electron pair is stabilized by the electron donating effects of alkyl groups. Thus the lone pair in tertiary amines is more stable than in secondary amines which, in turn, is more stable than in primary amines. As a result of this electron pair, amines are Lewis bases, and good nucleophiles. In aqueous solution, amines are weak bases, and can accept a proton:

$$R_3N + H_2O \longrightarrow R_3NH^+ + OH^-$$

The ammonium cation in the preceding reaction is stabilized, once again, by the electron donating effects of the alkyl groups. Conversely, should the nitrogen be adjacent to a carbocation, the lone pair can stabilize the carbocation by delocalizing the charge.

The relative basicity of amines is determined by the following:

- If the free amine is stabilized relative to the cation, the amine is less basic.
- If the cation is stabilized relative to the free amine, the amine is more stable, thus the stronger base.

Groups that withdraw electron density (such as halides or aromatics) decrease the availability of the unbonded electron pair. Electron releasing groups (such as alkyl groups) increase the availability of the unbonded electron pair. The base strength then increases in the following series (where Ø represents a phenyl group):

NO$_2$–Ø–NH$_2$ < Ø–NH$_2$ < Ø–CH$_2$–NH$_2$ < NH$_3$ < CH$_3$–NH$_2$ < (CH$_3$)$_2$–N–H < (CH$_3$)$_3$–N

Note that a substituent attached to an aromatic ring can greatly affect the basicity of the amine. For example, electron withdrawing groups (i.e. –NO$_2$) withdraw electrons from the ring which, in turn, withdraws the lone electron pair (*delocalization*) from nitrogen. Thus the lone pair is less available to bond witha proton; consequently, it is a weaker base. The opposite occurs with an electron donating group, making the amine, relatively, a better base.

11.1.2 More Properties of Amines

- The nitrogen atom can hydrogen bond (using its electron pair) to hydrogens attached to other N's or O's. It can also form hydrogen bonds from hydrogens attached to it with electron pairs of N, O, F or Cl:

Note that primary or secondary amines can hydrogen bond with each other, but tertiary amines cannot. This leads to boiling points which are higher than would be expected for compounds of similar molecular weight, like alkanes, but lower than similar alcohols or carboxylic acids. The hydrogen bonding also renders low weight amines soluble in water.

- A dipole moment is possible:

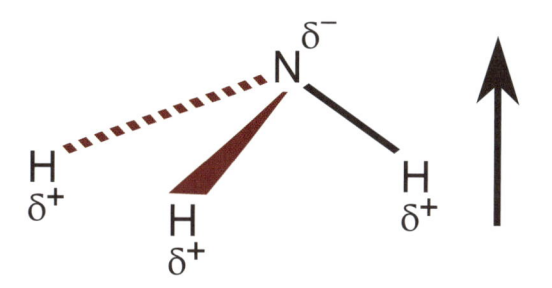

- The nitrogen in amines can contribute its lone pair electrons to activate a benzene ring. Thus amines are ortho-para directors.

- The solubility of quaternary salts decreases with increasing molecular weight. The quaternary structure has steric hindrance and the lone pair electrons on N is not available for H-bonding, thus their solubility is much less than other amines or even alkyl ammonium salts (i.e. R–NH$_3^+$X$^-$, R$_2$–NH$_2^+$X$^-$, R$_3$–NH$^+$X$^-$).

Quaternary ammonium salts can be synthesized from ammonium hydroxides which are very strong bases.

$$(CH_3)_4N^+OH^- + HCl \longrightarrow (CH_3)_4N^+Cl^- + H_2O$$
Quaternary hydroxide → Quaternary salt

11.2 Important Reactions of Amines

- <u>Amide formation</u> is an important reaction for protein synthesis. Primary and secondary amines will react with carboxylic acids and their derivatives to form *amides*:

$$R'NH_2 + R-\underset{\underset{O}{\|}}{C}-OH \longrightarrow R-\underset{\underset{O}{\|}}{C}-NHR' + H_2O$$

primary or secondary amine   acid   amide

Amides can engage in resonance such that the lone pair electrons on the nitrogen is delocalized. Thus amides are by far <u>less basic</u> than amines.

$$\left[R-\underset{\underset{O}{\|}}{C}-NR_2 \longleftrightarrow R-\underset{\underset{O^-}{|}}{C}=\overset{+}{N}R_2 \right]$$

As can be seen, the C–N bond has a partial double bond character. Thus there is restricted rotation about the C–N bond.

- <u>Alkylation</u> is another important reaction which involves amines with alkyl halides:

$$RCH_2Cl + R'NH_2 \longrightarrow RCH_2NHR' + HCl$$
1°, 2° or 3° amine

Both amide formation and alkylation make use of the nucleophilic character of the electrons on nitrogen.

ORG-84 AMINES

ORGANIC CHEMISTRY

GOLD NOTES

BIOLOGICAL MOLECULES

Chapter 12

Memorize	Understand	Not Required*
* Basic structures * Isoelectric point equation * Define: amphoteric, zwitterions	* Effect of H, S, hydrophobic bonds * Basic mechanisms of reactions * Effect of pH, isoelectric point * Protein structure * Different ways of drawing structures	* Advanced level college info * Memorizing all the names of amino acids * Detailed mech. specific to bio molecules

GAMSAT-Prep.com

Introduction

Biological molecules truly involve the chemistry of life. Such molecules include amino acids and proteins, carbohydrates (glucose, disaccharides, polysaccharides), lipids (triglycerides, steroids) and nucleic acids (DNA, RNA).

Additional Resources

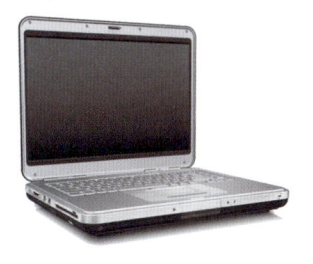

Free Online Q & A

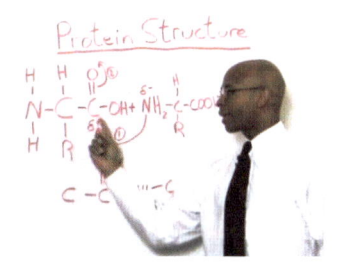

Video: DVD Disc 3

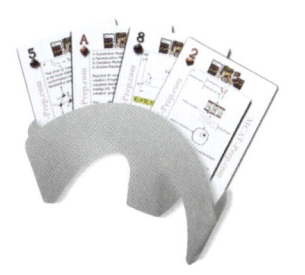

Flashcards

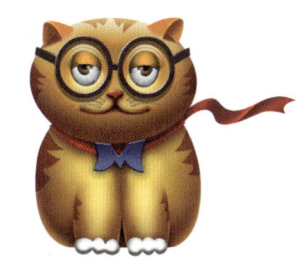

Special Guest

THE BIOLOGICAL SCIENCES ORG-87

* The real GAMSAT may have advanced level information presented (ie. in a passage) but previous knowledge of said information is not required to answer the questions that would follow. Practice ACER and GS practice GAMSATs can help you clarify this point.

12.1 Amino Acids

Amino acids are molecules that contain a side chain (R), a carboxylic acid, and an amino group at the α carbon. Thus the general structure of α-amino acids is:

L - amino acid   D - amino acid

Amino acids may be named systematically as substituted carboxylic acids, however, there are 20 important α-amino acids that are known by common names. These are naturally occurring and they form the building blocks of most proteins found in humans. The following are a few examples of α-amino acids:

Glycine   Alanine

Serine   Aspartic acid

Note that all amino acids have the same relative configuration, the L-configuration. However, the absolute configuration depends on the priority assigned to the side group (see ORG 2.3.1 for rules). In the preceding amino acids, the S-configuration prevails (except glycine which cannot be assigned any configuration since it is not chiral).

12.1.1 Hydrophilic vs. Hydrophobic

Different types of amino acids tend to be found in different areas of the proteins that they make up. Amino acids which are ionic and/or polar are hydrophilic, and tend to be found on the exterior of proteins (i.e. *exposed to water*). These include aspartic acid and its amide, glutamic acid and its amide, lysine, arginine and histidine. Certain other polar amino acids are found on either the interior or exterior of proteins. These include serine, threonine, and tyrosine. Hydrophobic amino acids which may be found on the interior of proteins include methionine, leucine, tryptophan, valine and phenylalanine. Hydrophobic molecules tend to cluster in aqueous solutions (= *hydrophobic bonding*). Alanine is a nonpolar amino acid which is unusual because it is less hydrophobic than most nonpolar amino acids. This is because its nonpolar side chain is very short.

ORG-88   BIOLOGICAL MOLECULES

Glycine is the smallest amino acid, and the only one that is not optically active. It is often found at the 'corners' of proteins.

Alanine is small and, although hydrophobic, is found on the surface of proteins.

12.1.2 Acidic vs. Basic

Amino acids have both an acid and basic components (= *amphoteric*). The amino acids with the R group containing an amino (–NH$_2$) group, are basic. The two basic amino acids are lysine and arginine. Amino acids with an R group containing a carboxyl (–COOH) group are acidic. The two acidic amino acids are aspartic acid and glutamic acid. One amino acid, histidine, may act as either an acid or a base, depending upon the pH of the resident solution. This makes histidine a very good physiologic buffer. The rest of the amino acids are considered to be neutral.

The basic –NH$_2$ group in the amino acid is present as an ammonium ion, –NH$_3^+$. The acidic carboxyl –COOH group is present as a carboxylate ion, –COO$^-$. As a result, amino acids are dipolar ions, or *zwitterions*. In an aqueous solution, there is an equilibrium present between the dipolar, the anionic, and the cationic forms of the amino acid:

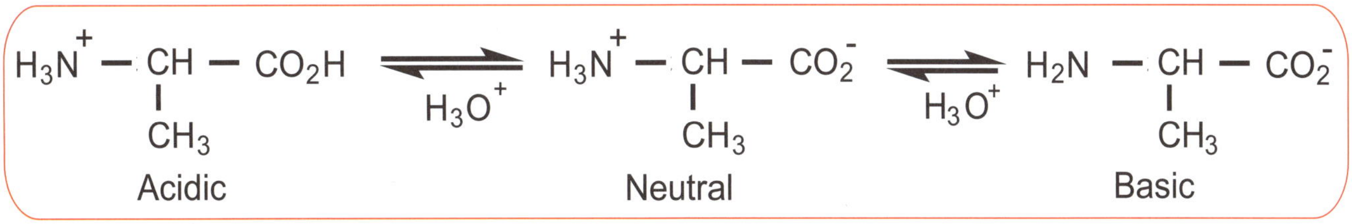

Therefore the charge on the amino acid will vary with the pH of the solution, and with the isoelectric point. This point is the pH where a given amino acid will be neutral (i.e. have no net charge). This isoelectric point is the average of the two pK$_a$ values of an amino acid (*depending on the dissociated group*):

$$\text{isoelectric point} = pI = (pK_{a1} + pK_{a2})/2$$

Above the isoelectric point (basic conditions), the amino acids will have a net negative charge. Below the isoelectric point (acidic conditions), the amino acids will have a net positive charge.

$$H_3N^+\!-\!CH(CH_3)\!-\!CO_2H \underset{H_3O^+}{\rightleftharpoons} H_3N^+\!-\!CH(CH_3)\!-\!CO_2^- \underset{H_3O^+}{\rightleftharpoons} H_2N\!-\!CH(CH_3)\!-\!CO_2^-$$

Acidic — Neutral — Basic

12.2 Proteins

12.2.1 General Principles

Proteins are long chain polypeptides which often form higher order structures. Polypeptides are polymers of 40 to 1000 α-amino acids joined together by amide (*peptide*) bonds. These peptide bonds are derived from the amino group of one amino acid, and the acid group of another. When a peptide bond is formed, a molecule of water is released (*condensation*). The bond can be broken by adding water (*hydrolysis*).

Since proteins are polymers of amino acids, they also have isoelectric points. Classification as to the acidity or basicity of a protein depends on the numbers of acidic and basic amino acids it contains. If there is an excess of acidic amino acids, the isoelectric point will be at a pH of less than 7. At pH = 7, these proteins will have a net negative charge. Similarly, those with an excess of basic amino acids will have an isoelectric point at a pH of greater than 7. Therefore, at pH = 7, these proteins will have a net positive charge.

12.2.2 Protein Structure

Protein structure may be divided into primary, secondary, tertiary and quaternary structures. The <u>primary structure</u> is the sequence of amino acids as determined by the DNA and the location of covalent bonds (*including disulfide bonds*). This structure determines the higher order structures.

The <u>secondary structure</u> is the orderly inter- or intramolecular *hydrogen bonding* of the protein chain. The resultant structure may be the more stable α-helix (e.g. keratin), or a β-pleated sheet (e.g. silk). Proline is an amino acid which cannot participate in the regular array of H-bonding in an α-helix. Proline disrupts the

ORG-90   BIOLOGICAL MOLECULES

α-helix, thus it is usually found at the beginning or end of a molecule (i.e. hemoglobin).

The tertiary structure is the further folding of the protein molecule onto itself, where many parts still remain α-helical. This structure is maintained by *noncovalent bonds* like hydrogen bonding, Van der Waals forces, hydrophobic bonding and electrostatic bonding. The resultant structure is a globular protein with a hydrophobic interior and hydrophilic exterior. Enzymes are classical examples of such a structure. In fact, enzyme activity often depends on tertiary structure.

The covalent bonding of cysteine (*disulfide bonds or bridge*) helps to stabilize the tertiary structure of proteins. Cysteine will form sulfur-sulfur covalent bonds with itself, producing *cystine*.

The quaternary structure is when there are two or more protein chains bonded together by noncovalent bonds. For example, hemoglobin consists of four polypeptide subunits (*globin*) held together by hydrophobic bonds forming a globular almost tetrahedryl arrangement.

$$2H_2N-CH(CH_2SH)-CO_2H \xrightarrow{-H_2} H_2N-CH(CH_2-S-S-CH_2)-CO_2H \cdots CH(NH_2)-CO_2H$$

cysteine → cystine

12.3 Carbohydrates

12.3.1 Description and Nomenclature

Carbohydrates are sugars and their derivatives. Formally they are 'carbon hydrates,' that is, they have the general formula $C_m(H_2O)_n$. Usually they are defined as polyhydroxy aldehydes and ketones, or substances that hydrolyze to yield polyhydroxy aldehydes and ketones. The basic units of carbohydrates are monosaccharides (sugars).

There are two ways to classify sugars. One way is to classify the molecule based on the type of carbonyl group it contains: one with an aldehyde carbonyl group is an *aldose*; one with a ketone carbonyl group is a *ketose*. The second method of classification depends on the number of carbons in the molecule: those with 6 carbons are *hexoses*, with 5 carbons are *pentoses*. Sugars may exist in either the ring form, as hemiacetals, or in the straight chain form, as polyhydroxy aldehydes. *Pyranoses* are 6 carbon sugars in the ring form; *furanoses* are 5 carbon sugars in the ring form.

In the ring form, there is the possibility of α or β *anomers*. Anomers occur when 2 cyclic forms of the molecule differ in conformation only at the hemiacetal carbon (carbon 1). Generally, pyranoses take the 'chair' conformation, as it is very stable, with all (usually) hydroxyl groups at the equatorial position. *Epimers* are 2 monosaccharides which differ in the conformation of one hydroxyl group.

To determine the number of possible optical isomers, one need only know the number of asymmetric carbons, normally 4 for hexoses and 3 for pentoses, designated as n. The number of optical isomers is then 2^n, where n is the number of asymmetric carbons (ORG 2.1).

Most but not all of the naturally occurring aldoses have the D-configuration. Thus they have the same *relative* configuration as D-glyceraldehyde. The configuration (D or L) is *only* assigned to the highest numbered chiral carbon. The *absolute* configuration can be determined for any chiral carbon. For example, using the rules from Section 2.3.1, it can be determined that the absolute configuration of D-glyceraldehyde is the R-configuration.

The names and structures of some common sugars are shown in Figure IV.B.12.1.

In the diagram that follows, you will notice a Fischer projection to the far left (*see* ORG 2.3.1). You will also find Fischer projections in the following pages since they are a common way to represent carbohydrates.

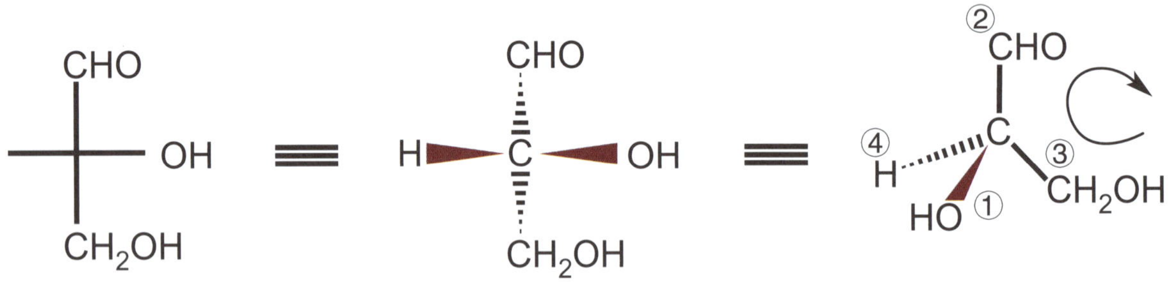

Fischer projection and 3-dimensional representation of D-glyceraldehyde, R-glyceraldehyde (*see* ORG 2.1, 2.2, 2.3 for rules).

ORGANIC CHEMISTRY

12.3.2 Important Reactions of Carbohydrates

A <u>disaccharide</u> is a molecule made up of two monosaccharides, joined by a *glycosidic bond* between the hemiacetal carbon of one molecule, and the hydroxyl group of another. The glycosidic bond forms an α-1,4-glycosidic linkage if the reactant is an α anomer. A β-1,4-glycosidic linkage is formed if the reactant is a β anomer. When the bond is formed, one molecule of water is released (condensation). In order to break the bond, water must be added (hydrolysis):

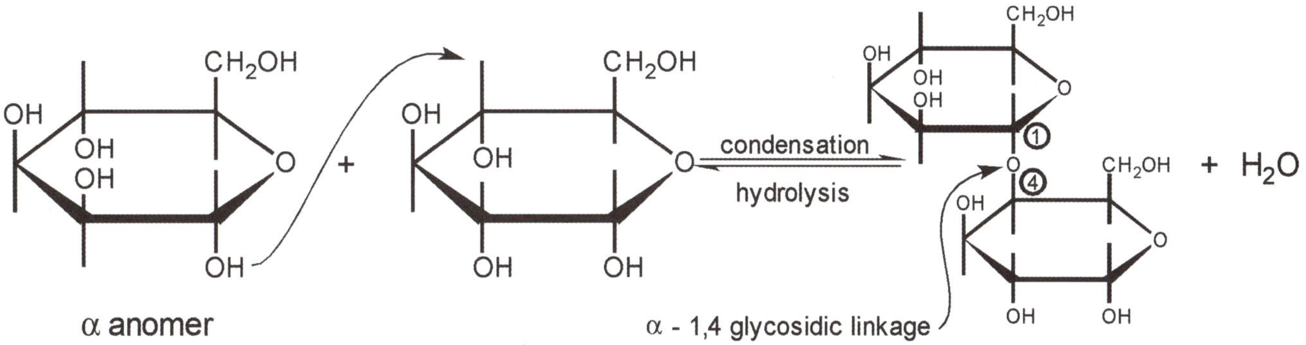

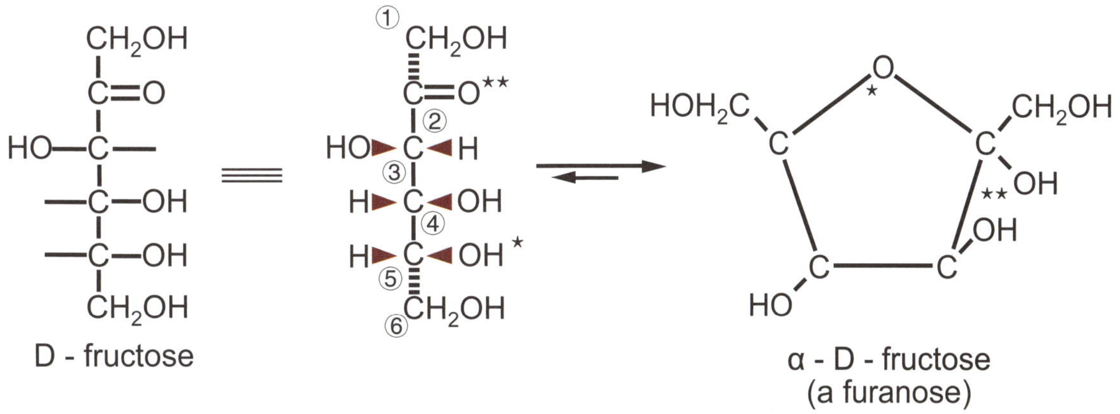

Figure IV.B.12.1 Part I: Names, structures and configurations of common sugars.

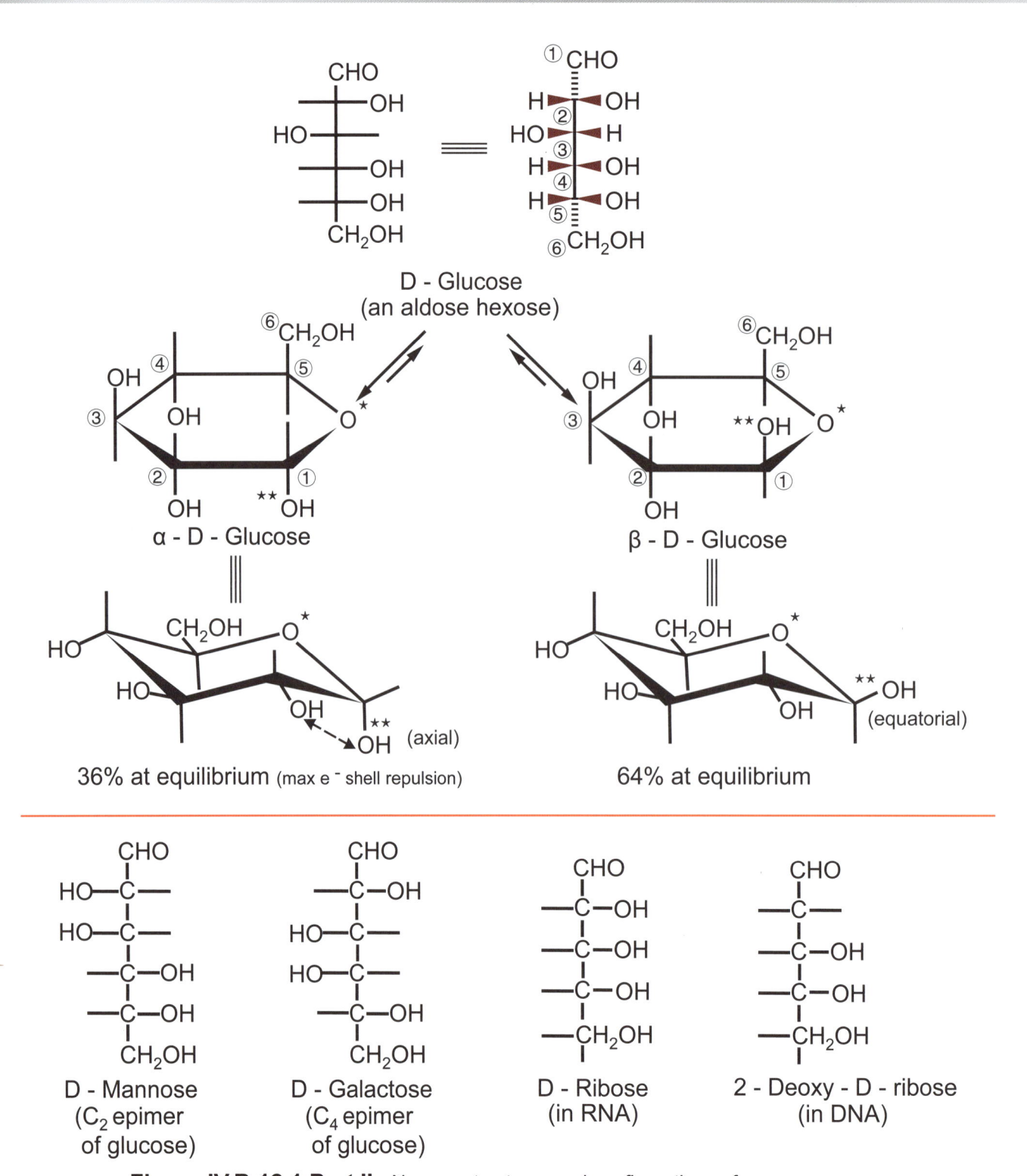

Figure IV.B.12.1 Part II: Names, structures and configurations of common sugars.

ORG-94 BIOLOGICAL MOLECULES

- Sucrose (common sugar) = glucose + fructose
- Lactose (milk sugar) = glucose + galactose
- Maltose (α-1,4 bond) = glucose + glucose
- Cellobiose (β-1,4 bond) = glucose + glucose

Sugars can undergo oxidation. When aldoses are treated with bromine water, the aldehyde is oxidized to a carboxylic acid group, resulting in a product known as an *aldonic acid*:

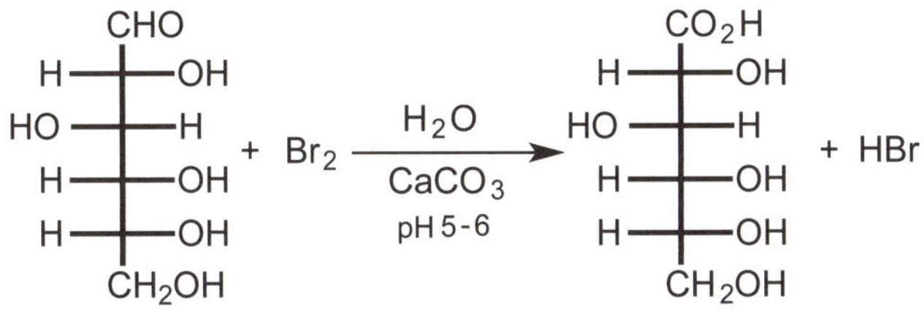

Aldoses treated with dilute nitric acid will have both the primary alcohol and aldehyde groups oxidize to carboxylic acid groups, resulting in a product known as an *aldaric acid*:

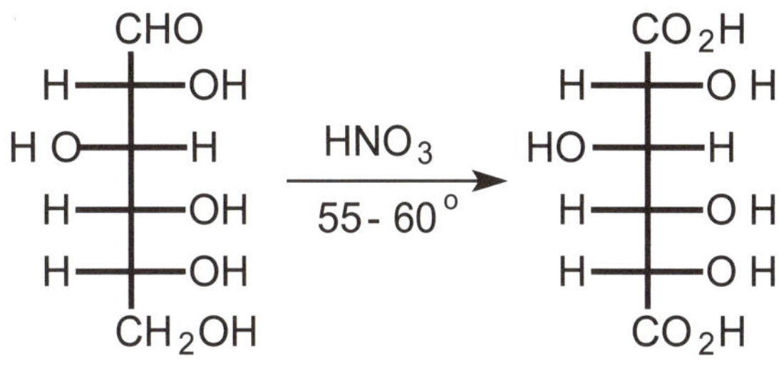

D-glucose (an aldose) + Br_2 $\xrightarrow{H_2O, CaCO_3, pH\ 5-6}$ D-Gluconic acid (an aldonic acid) + HBr

D-glucose (an aldose) $\xrightarrow{HNO_3, 55-60°}$ D-Glucaric acid (an aldaric acid)

12.3.3 Polysaccharides

Polymers of many monosaccharides are called <u>polysaccharides</u>. As in disaccharides, they are joined by glycosidic linkages. They may be straight chains, or branched chains. Some common polysaccharides are:

- Starch (plant energy storage)
- Cellulose (plant structural component)
- Glycocalyx (associated with the plasma membrane)
- Glycogen (animal energy storage in the form of glucose)
- Chitin (structural component found in shells or arthropods)

Carbohydrates are the most abundant organic constituents of plants. They are the source of chemical energy in living organisms, and, in plants, they are used in making the support structures.

12.4 Lipids

Lipids are a class of organic molecules containing many different types of substances, such as fatty acids, fats, waxes, triacyl glycerols, terpenes and steroids.

Triacyl glycerols are oils and fats of either animal or plant origin. In general, fats are solid at room temperature, and oils are liquid at room temperature. The general structure of a triacyl glycerol is:

$$\begin{array}{l} CH_2O-\overset{O}{\underset{\|}{C}}-R \\ CH_2O-\overset{O}{\underset{\|}{C}}-R' \\ CH_2O-\overset{O}{\underset{\|}{C}}-R'' \end{array}$$

The R groups may be the same or different, and are usually long chain alkyl groups. Upon hydrolysis of a triacyl glycerol, the products are three fatty acids and glycerol (see ORG 9.4.1). The fatty acids may be saturated (= no multiple bonds, i.e. *palmitic acid*) or unsaturated (= containing double or triple bonds, i.e. *oleic acid*). Unsaturated fatty acids are usually in the cis configuration. Saturated fatty acids have a higher melting point than unsaturated fatty acids. Some common fatty acids are:

$$CH_3(CH_2)_{14}COOH$$
palmitic acid

$$CH_3(CH_2)_{16}COOH$$
stearic acid

$$\underset{H}{\overset{CH_3(CH_2)_7}{\diagdown}}C=C\underset{H}{\overset{(CH_2)_7CO_2H}{\diagup}}$$
oleic acid

12.4.1 Steroids

Steroids are derivatives of the basic ring structure:

ORG-96 BIOLOGICAL MOLECULES

ORGANIC CHEMISTRY

The carbon atoms are numbered as shown. Many important substances are steroids, some examples include: cholesterol, D vitamins, bile acids, adrenocortical hormones, and male and female sex hormones.

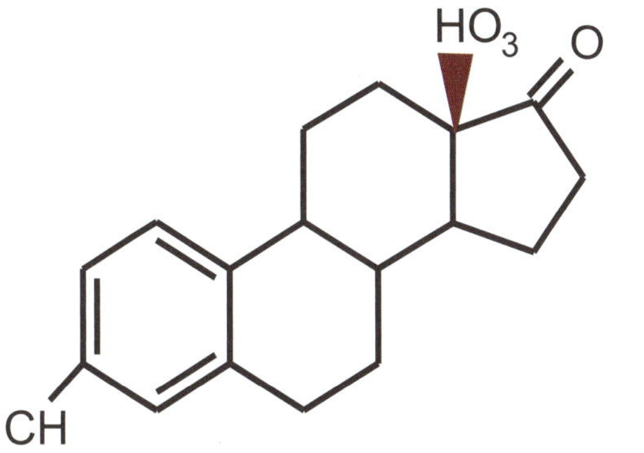

Estradiol
(an estrogen)

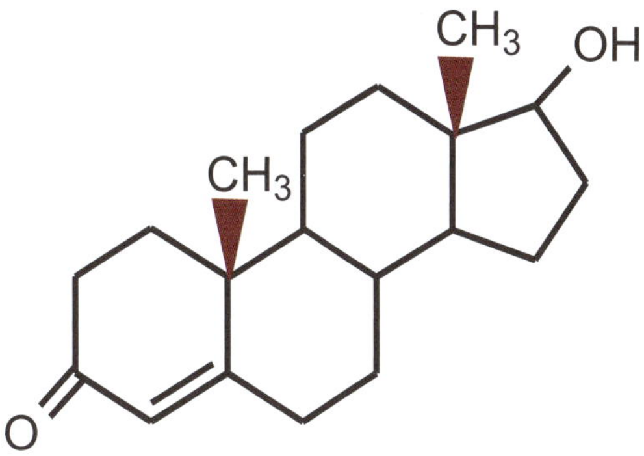

Testosterone
(an androgen)

Since such a significant portion of a steroid contains hydrocarbons, which are hydrophobic, steroids can dissolve through the hydrophobic interior of a cell's plasma membrane. Furthermore, steroid hormones contain polar side groups which allow the hormone to easily dissolve in water. Thus steroid hormones are well designed to be transported through the vascular space, to cross the plasma membranes of cells, and to have an effect either in the cell's cytosol or, as is usually the case, in the nucleus.

12.5 Phosphorous in Biological Molecules

Phosphorous is an essential component of various biological molecules including adenosine triphosphate (ATP), phospholipids in cell membranes, and the nucleic acids which form DNA. Phosphorus can also form phosphoric acid and several phosphate esters:

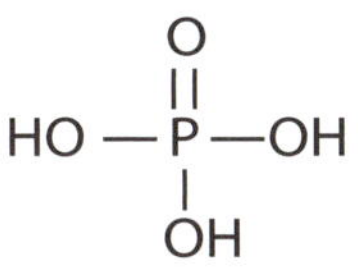

phosphoric acid

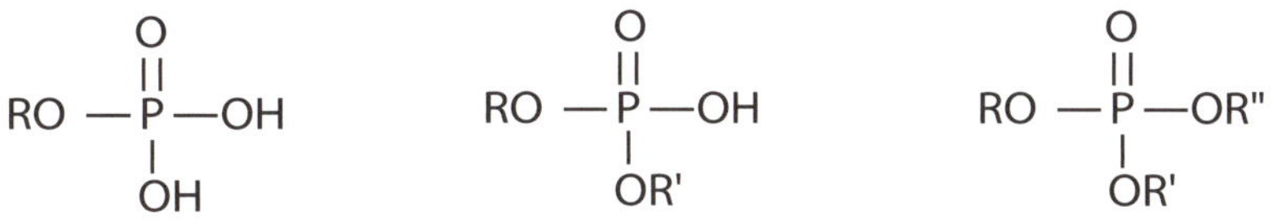

phosphate esters

THE BIOLOGICAL SCIENCES ORG-97

A phospholipid is produced from three ester linkages to glycerol. Phosphoric acid is ester linked to the terminal hydroxyl group and two fatty acids are ester linked to the two remaining hydroxyl groups of glycerol (*see Biology Section 1.1 for a schematic view of a phospholipid*).

In DNA the phosphate groups engage in two ester linkages creating phosphodiester bonds. It is the 5' phosphorylated position of one pentose ring which is linked to the 3' position of the next pentose ring (*see BIO 1.1.2*):

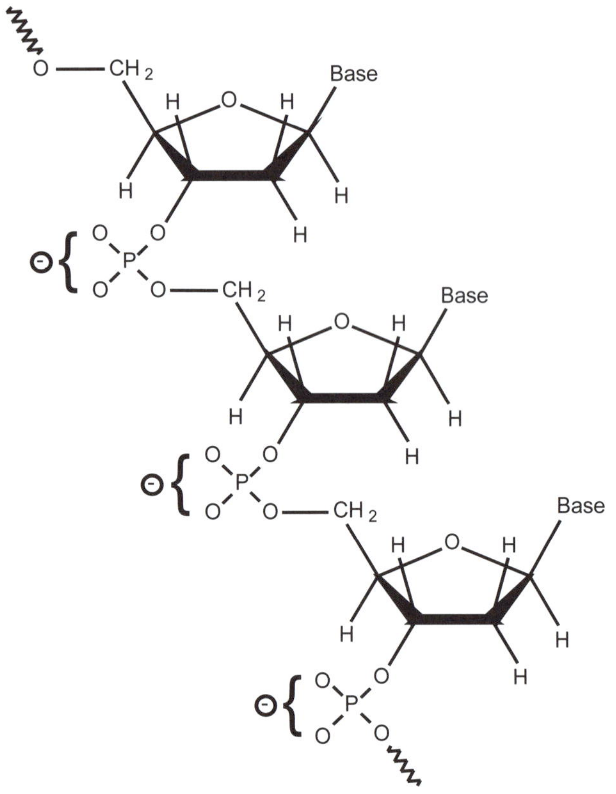

In Biology Chapter 4, the production of ATP was discussed. In each case the components ADP and P_i (= *inorganic phosphate*) combined using the energy generated from a coupled reaction to produce ATP. The linkage between the phosphate groups are via *anhydride bonds*:

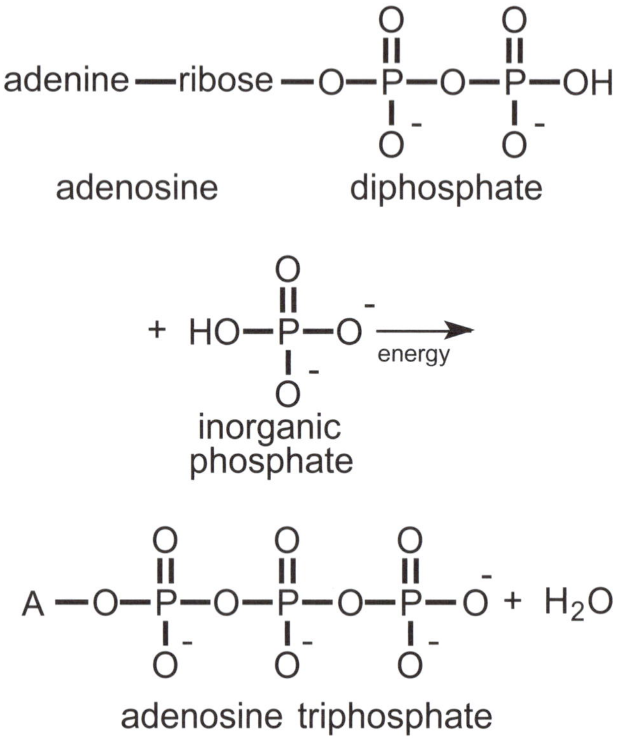

adenosine diphosphate

inorganic phosphate

adenosine triphosphate

ORG-98   BIOLOGICAL MOLECULES

ORGANIC CHEMISTRY

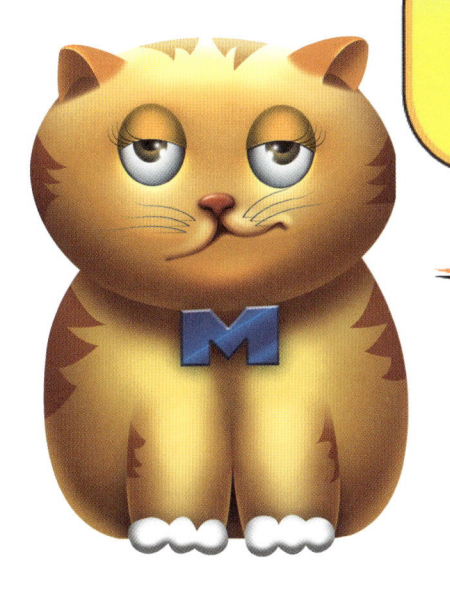

What does D.N.A. stand for? National Association of Dyslexics. Hmmm.

GOLD NOTES

SEPARATIONS AND PURIFICATIONS
Chapter 13

Memorize

* Definitions of the major techniques
* Interactions between organic molecules

Understand

* Different phases in the various techniques
* How to improve separation, purification
* How to avoid overheating (distillation)

Not Required*

* Advanced level college info
* Electrolysis, affinity purification
* Refining, smelting

GAMSAT-Prep.com

Introduction

Separation techniques are used to transform a mixture of substances into two or more distinct products. The separated products may be different in chemical properties or some physical property (i.e. size). Purification in organic chemistry is the physical separation of a chemical substance of interest from foreign or contaminating substances.

Additional Resources

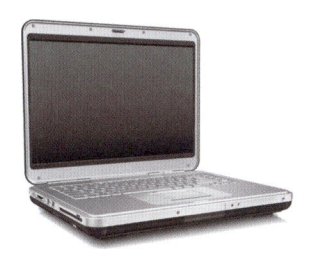

Free Online Q & A

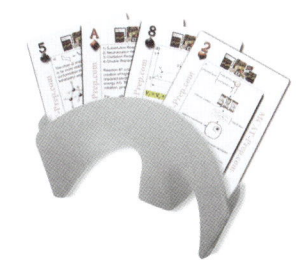

Flashcards

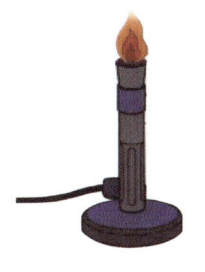

Special Guest

THE BIOLOGICAL SCIENCES   ORG-101

* The real GAMSAT may have advanced level information presented (ie. in a passage) but previous knowledge of said information is not required to answer the questions that would follow. Practice ACER and GS practice GAMSATs can help you clarify this point.

13.1 Extraction

Extraction is the process by which a solute is transferred (*extracted*) from one solvent and placed in another. This procedure is possible if the two solvents used cannot mix (= *immiscible*) and if the solute is more soluble in the solvent used for the extraction.

For example, consider the extraction of solute A which is dissolved in solvent X. We choose solvent Y for the extraction since solute A is highly soluble in it and because solvent Y is immiscible with solvent X. We now add solvent Y to the solution involving solute A and solvent X. The container is agitated. Solute A begins to dissolve in the solvent where it is most soluble, solvent Y. The container is left to stand, thus the two immiscible solvents separate. The phase containing solute A can now be removed.

In practice, solvent Y would be chosen such that it would be sufficiently easy to evaporate (= *volatile*) after the extraction so solute A can be easily recovered. Also, it is more efficient to perform several extractions using a small amount of solvent each time, rather than one extraction using a large amount of solvent.

13.2 Chromatography

Chromatography is the separation of a mixture of compounds by their distribution between two phases: one stationary and one moving. Molecules are separated based on differences in polarity and molecular weight.

13.2.1 Gas-Liquid Chromatography

In gas-liquid chromatography, the *stationary phase* is a liquid absorbed to an inert solid. The liquid can be polyethylene glycol, squalene, or others, depending on the polarity of the substances being separated.

The mobile phase is a gas (i.e. He, N_2) which is unreactive both to the stationary phase and to the substances being separated. The sample being analyzed can be injected in the direction of gas flow into one end of a column packed with the stationary phase. As the sample migrates through the column certain molecules will move faster than others. As mentioned the separation of the different types of molecules is dependent on size (*molecular weight*) and charge (*polarity*). Once the molecules reach the end of the column special detectors signal their arrival.

13.2.2 Thin-Layer Chromatography

Thin-layer chromatography is a solid-liquid technique, based on adsorptivity and solubility. The *stationary phase* is a type of finely divided polar material, usually silica gel or alumina, which is thinly coated onto a glass plate.

There are several types of interactions that may occur between the organic molecules in the sample and the silica gel, in order from weakest to strongest (see CHM 3.4, 4.2):

- Van der Waals force (nonpolar molecules)
- Dipole-dipole interaction (polar molecules)
- Hydrogen bonding (hydroxylic compounds)
- Coordination (Lewis bases)

Molecules with functional groups with the greatest polarity will bind more strongly to the stationary phase and thus will not rise as high on the glass plate.

Organic molecules will also interact with the *mobile phase* (= a solvent), or *eluent* used in the process. The more polar the solvent, the more easily it will dissolve polar molecules. The mobile phase usually contains organic solvents like ethanol, benzene, chloroform, acetone, etc.

As a result of the interactions of the organic molecules with the stationary and moving phases, for any adsorbed compound there is a dynamic distribution equilibrium between these phases. The different molecules will rise to different heights on the plate. Their presence can be detected using special stains (i.e. pH indicators, $KMnO_4$) or uv light (*if the compound can fluoresce*).

13.3 Distillation

Distillation is the process by which compounds are separated based on differences in boiling points. A classic example of simple distillation is the separation of salt from water. The solution is heated. Water will boil and vaporize at a far lower temperature than salt. Hence the water boils away leaving salt behind. Water vapor can now be condensed into pure liquid water (*distilled water*).

As long as one compound is more volatile, the distillation process is quite simple. If the difference between the two boiling points are low, it will be more difficult to separate the compounds by this method. Instead, fractional distillation can be used in which, for example, a column is filled with glass beads which is placed between the distillation flask and the condenser. The glass beads increase the surface area over which the less volatile compound can condense and drip back down to the distillation flask below. The more volatile compound boils away and condenses in the condenser. Thus the two compounds are separated.

The efficiency of the distillation process in producing a pure product is improved by repeating the distillation process, or, in the case of fractional distillation, increasing the length of the column and avoiding overheating. Overheating may destroy the pure compounds or increase the percent of impurities. Some of the methods which are used to prevent overheating include boiling slowly, the use of boiling chips (= *ebulliator*, which makes bubbles) and the use of a vacuum which decreases the vapor pressure and thus the boiling point (cf. CHM 4.3.2).

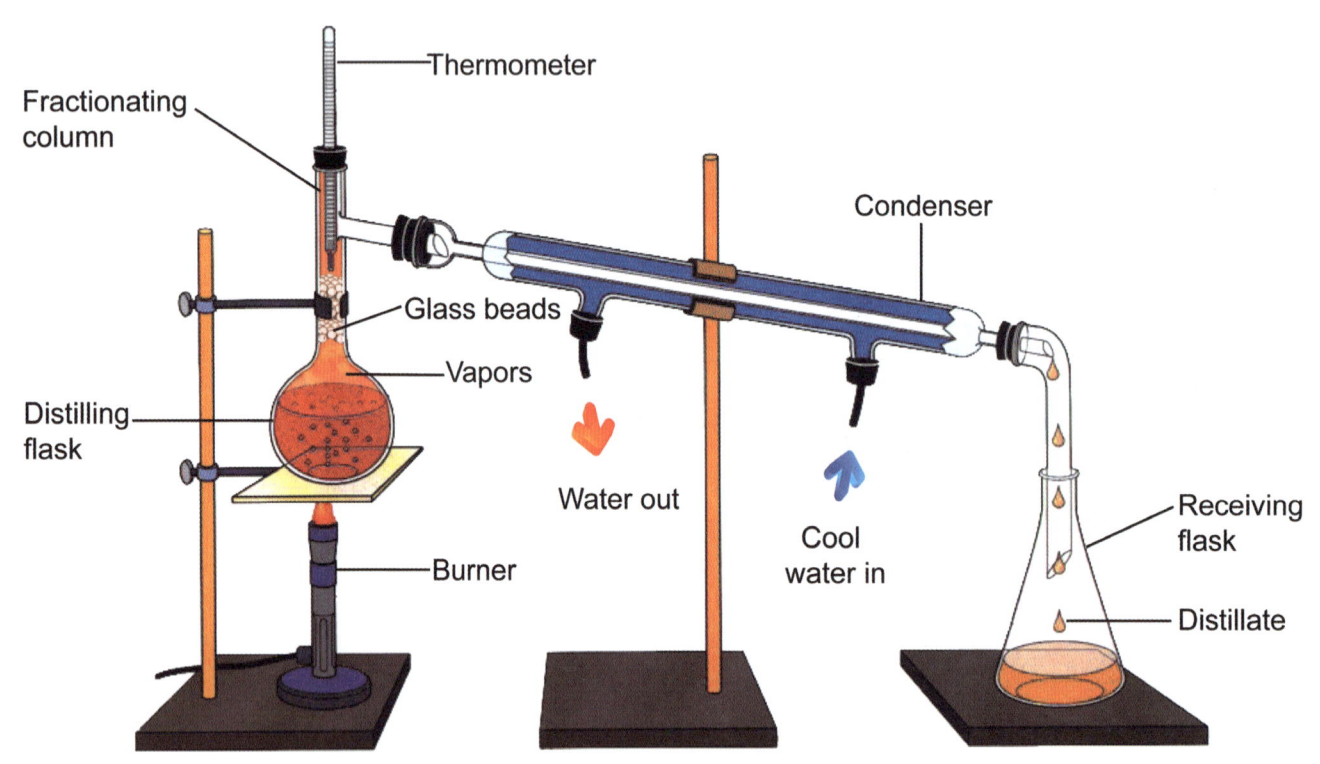

Figure IV.B.13.1: Standard distillation apparatus

13.4 Recrystallization

Recrystallization is a useful purification technique. A solid organic compound with some impurity is dissolved in a hot solvent, and then the solvent is slowly cooled to allow the pure compound to reform or *recrystallize*, while leaving the impurities behind in the solvent. This is possible because the impurities do not normally fit within the crystal structure of the compound.

In choosing a solvent, solubility data (e.g. K_{sp} at various temperatures, etc.) regarding both the compound to be purified and the impurities should be known. The data should be analyzed such that the solvent would:

- have the capability to dissolve alot of the compound (to be purified) at or near the boiling point of the solvent, while being able to dissolve little of the compound at room temperature. As well, the impurities should be soluble in the cold solvent.
- have a low boiling point, so as to be easily removed from the solid in a drying process.
- not react with the solid.

GOLD NOTES

SPECTROSCOPY

Chapter 14

Memorize	Understand	Not Required*
* Nothing	* Basic theory: IR spect., NMR * Very basic spectrum (graph) analysis	* Advanced level college info * mass spectrometry, x-ray, Raman * NMR other than proton NMR

GAMSAT-Prep.com

Introduction

Spectroscopy is the use of the absorption, emission, or scattering of electromagnetic radiation by matter to study the matter or to study physical processes. The matter can be atoms, molecules, atomic or molecular ions, or solids.

Additional Resources

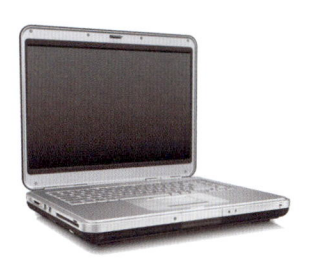

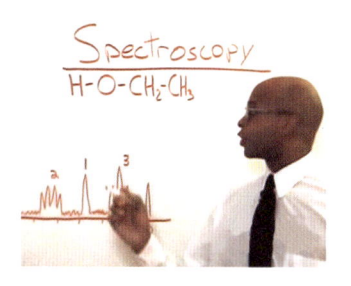

Free Online Q & A   Video: DVD Disc 4   Flashcards   Special Guest

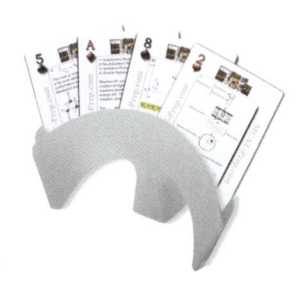

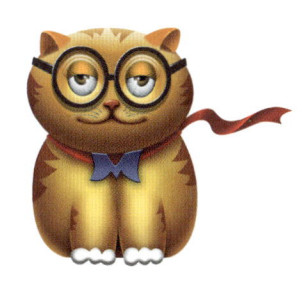

THE BIOLOGICAL SCIENCES   ORG-107

* The real GAMSAT may have advanced level information presented (ie. in a passage) but previous knowledge of said information is not required to answer the questions that would follow. Practice ACER and GS practice GAMSATs can help you clarify this point.

14.1 IR Spectroscopy

In an infrared spectrometer, a beam of infrared (IR) radiation is passed through a sample. The spectrometer will then analyze the amount of radiation transmitted (= % transmittance) through the sample as the incident radiation is varied. Ultimately, a plot results as a graph showing the transmittance or absorption (*the inverse of transmittance*) versus the frequency or wavelength of the incident radiation.

The location of an IR absorption band (*or peak*) can be specified in *frequency units* by its wave number, measured in cm^{-1}. As the wave number decreases, the wavelength increases, thus the energy decreases (recall from physics: $v = \lambda f$ and $E = hf$). A schematic representation of the IR spectrum of octane is:

Electromagnetic radiation consists of discrete units of energy called *quanta* or *photons*. All organic compounds are capable of absorbing many types of electromagnetic energy. The absorption of energy leads to an increase in the amplitude of intramolecular rotations and vibrations.

Intramolecular rotations are the rotations of a molecule about its center of gravity. The difference in rotational energy levels is inversely proportional to the moment of inertia of a molecule. Rotational energy is quantized and gives rise to absorption spectra in the microwave region of the electromagnetic spectrum.

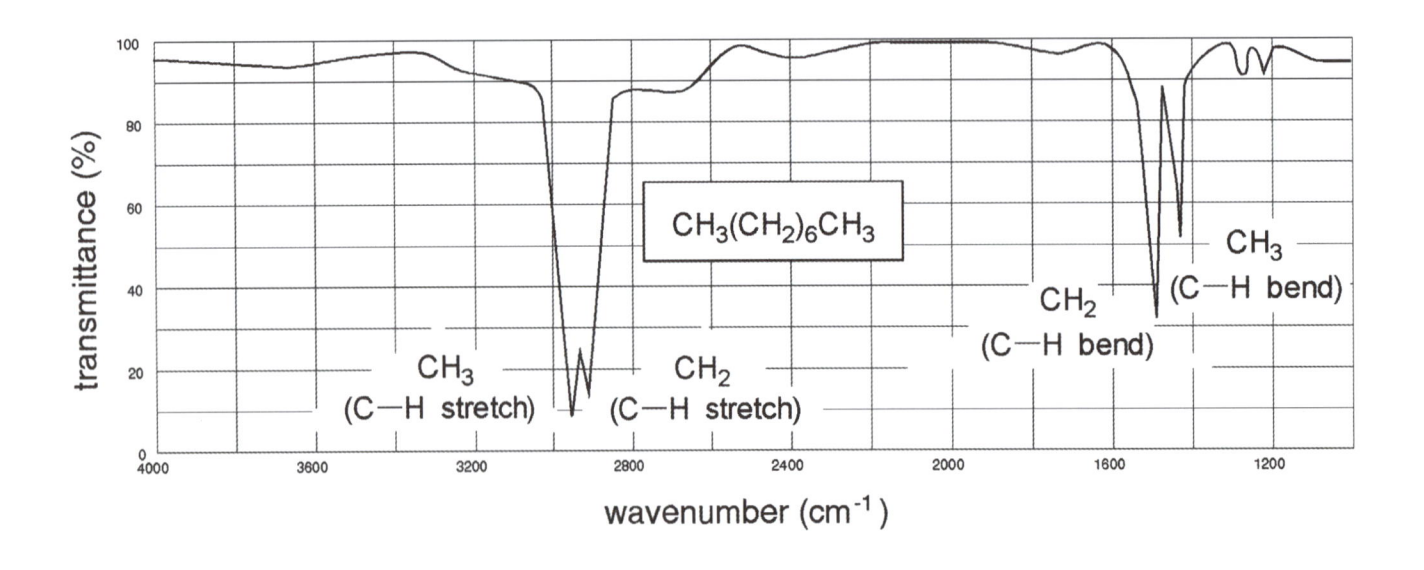

Intramolecular vibrations are the bending and stretching motions of bonds within a molecule. The relative spacing between vibrational energy levels increases with the increasing strength of an intramolecular bond. Vibrational energy is quantized and gives rise to absorption spectra in the infrared region of the electromagnetic spectrum.

Thus there are two types of bond vibration: stretching and bending. That is, after exposure to the IR radiation the bonds stretch and bend (*or contract*) to a greater degree once energy is absorbed. In general, bending vibrations will occur at lower frequencies (higher wavelengths) than stretching vibrations of the same groups. So, as seen in the sample spectra for octane, each group will have two characteristic peaks, one due to stretching, and one due to bending.

Different functional groups will have transmittances at characteristic wave numbers, which is why IR spectroscopy is useful.

Some examples (*approximate values*) of characteristic absorbances are:

Group	Frequency Range (cm^{-1})
Alkyl (C–H)	2850 – 2960
Alkene (C=C)	1620 – 1680
Alkyne (C≡C)	2100 – 2260
Alcohol (O–H)	3200 – 3650
Benzene (Ar–H)	3030
Carbonyl (C=O)	1630 – 1780
▶ Aldehyde	1680 – 1750
▶ Ketone	1735 – 1750
▶ Carboxylic Acid	1710 – 1780
▶ Amide	1630 – 1690
Amine (N–H)	3300 – 3500
Nitriles (C≡N)	2220 – 2260

By looking at the characteristic transmittances of a compound's spectrum, it is possible to identify the functional groups present in the molecule.

14.2 NMR Spectroscopy

Nuclear Magnetic Resonance (NMR) spectroscopy can be used to examine the environments of the hydrogen atoms in a molecule. In fact, using a (*proton*) NMR or ^{1}HNMR, one can determine both the number and types of hydrogens in a molecule. The basis of this stems from the magnetic properties of the hydrogen nucleus (proton). Similar to electrons, the hydrogen proton has a nuclear spin, able to take either of two values. These values are designated as +1/2 and –1/2. As a result of this spin, the nucleus will respond to a magnetic field by being oriented in the direction of the field. NMR spectrometers measure the absorption of energy by the hydrogen nuclei in an organic compound.

A schematic representation of an NMR spectrum, that of dimethoxymethane is shown:

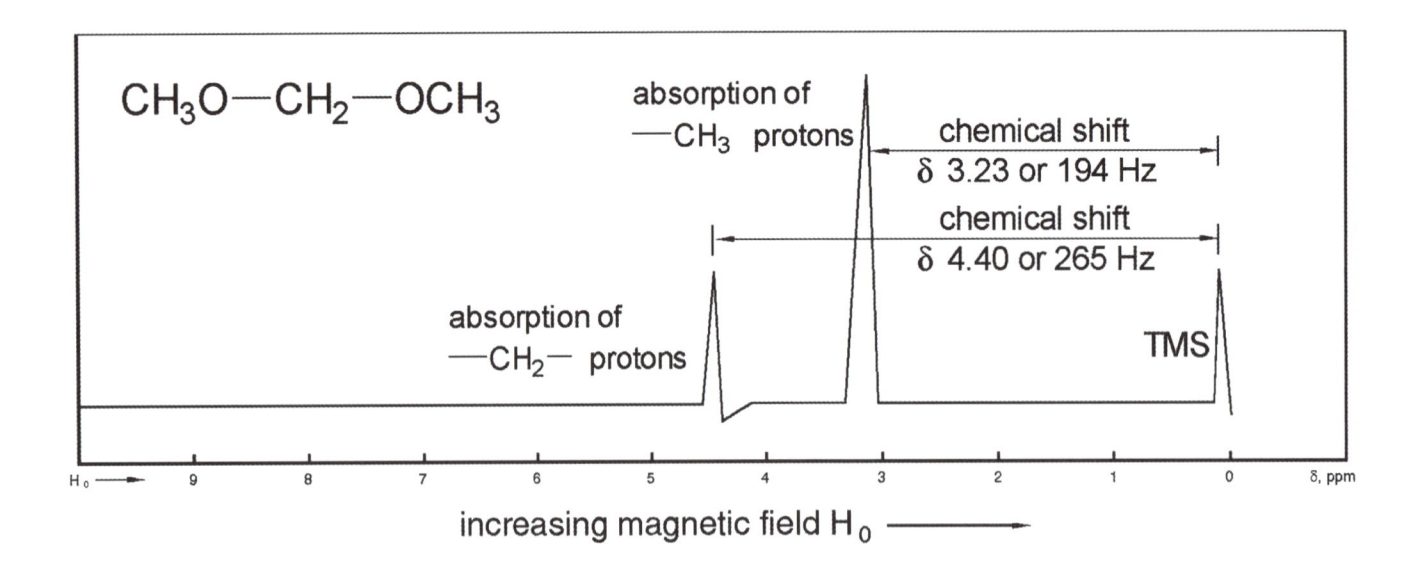

GAMSAT-Prep.com
THE GOLD STANDARD

[NMR spectrum of CH₃O—CH₂—OCH₃ showing absorption of —CH₃ protons (chemical shift δ 3.23 or 194 Hz), absorption of —CH₂— protons (chemical shift δ 4.40 or 265 Hz), and TMS peak. x-axis: δ, ppm from 9 to 0; increasing magnetic field H₀ →]

The small peak at the right is that of TMS, tetramethylsilane, shown here:

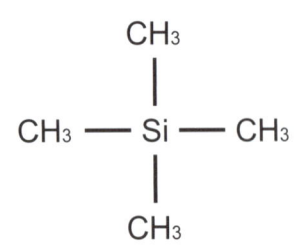

[Structure of TMS: Si bonded to four CH₃ groups]

This compound is added to the sample to be used as a reference, or standard. It is volatile, inert and absorbs at a higher field than most other organic chemicals.

The position of a peak relative to the standard is referred to as its *chemical shift*. Since NMR spectroscopy differentiates between types of protons, each type will have a different chemical shift, as shown. Protons in the same environment, like the three hydrogens in –CH₃, are called *equivalent protons*.

Dimethoxymethane is a symmetric molecule, thus the protons on either methyl group are equivalent. So, in the example above, the absorption of –CH₃ protons occurs at one peak (*a singlet*) 3.23 ppm downfield from TMS. In most organic molecules, the range of absorption will be in the 0–10 ppm (= *parts per million*) range.

The area under each peak is directly related to the number of protons contributing to it, and thus may be used to determine the relative number of protons in the molecule. Accurate measurements of the area under the two peaks above yield the ratio 1:3 which represents the relative number of hydrogens (i.e. 1:3 = 2:6).

Let us now examine a schematic representation of the NMR spectrum of ethyl bromide:

ORG-110   SPECTROSCOPY

ORGANIC CHEMISTRY

CH₃—CH₂—Br

absorption of —CH₂— protons
Rel. area = 2

absorption of —CH₃ protons
Rel. area = 3

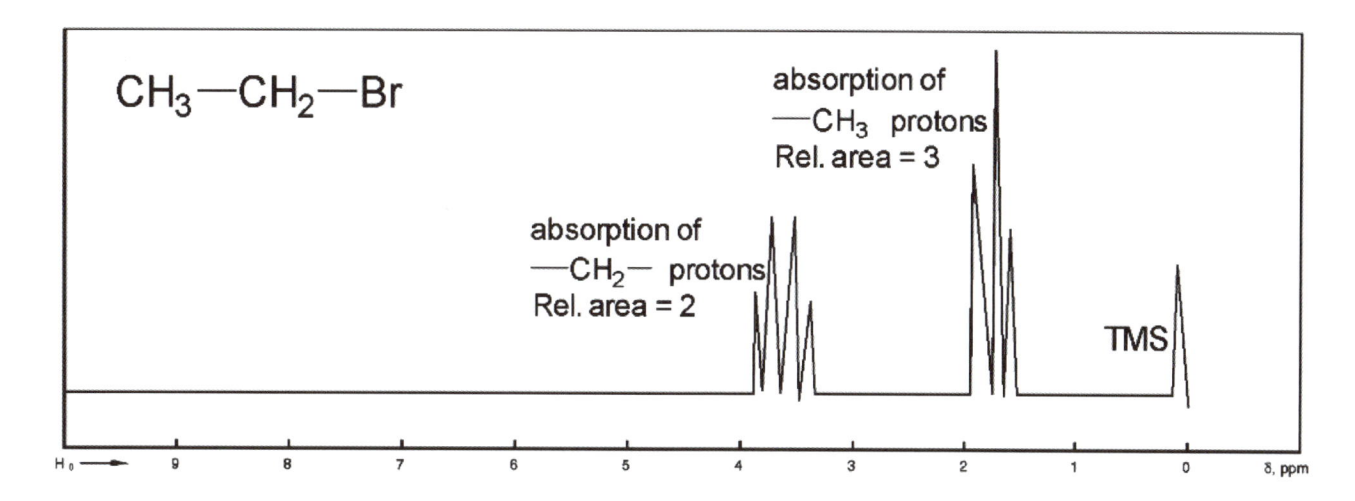

TMS

δ, ppm

It is obvious that something is different. Looking at the molecule, one can see that there are two different types of protons (*either far from Br or near to Br*). However, there are more than two signals in the spectrum. As such, the NMR signal for each group is said to be split. This type of splitting is called spin-spin splitting (= *spin-spin coupling*) and is caused by the presence of neighboring protons (*protons on an adjacent or vicinal carbon*) that are not equivalent to the proton in question.

The number of lines in the splitting pattern for a given set of equivalent protons depends on the number of adjacent protons according to the following rule: if there are n equivalent protons in adjacent positions, a proton NMR signal is split into n + 1 lines.

Therefore the NMR spectrum for ethyl bromide can be interpreted thus:

- There are two groups of lines (*two split peaks*), therefore there are two different environments for protons.

- The relative areas under each peak is 2:3, which represents the relative number of hydrogens in the molecule.

- There are 4 splits (*quartet*) in the peak which has relatively two hydrogens (–CH₂). Thus the number of adjacent hydrogens is n + 1 = 4; therefore, there are 3 hydrogens on the carbon adjacent to –CH₂.

- There are 3 splits (*triplet*) in the peak which has relatively three hydrogens (–CH₃). Thus the number of adjacent hydrogens is n + 1 = 3; therefore, there are 2 hydrogens on the carbon adjacent to –CH₃.

The relative areas under each peak may be expressed in three ways: (i) the information may simply be provided to you (*too easy!*); (ii) the integers may be written above the signals (=*integration integers*, i.e. 2,3 in the previous example); or (iii) a step-like *integration curve* above the signals where the relative height of each step equals the relative number of hydrogens.

THE BIOLOGICAL SCIENCES ORG-111

14.2.1 Deuterium Exchange

Deuterium, the hydrogen isotope ^{2}H or D, can be used to identify substances with readily exchangeable or acidic hydrogens. Rather than H$_2$O, D$_2$O is used to identify the chemical exchange:

$$ROH + DOD \rightleftharpoons ROD + HOD$$

The previous signal due to the acidic –O[H] would now disappear. However, if excess D$_2$O is used, a signal as a result of HOD may be observed.

Solvents may also be involved in exchange phenomena. The solvents carbon tetrachloride (CCl$_4$) and deuteriochloroform (CDCl$_3$) can also engage in exchange-induced decoupling of acidic hydrogens (usu. in alcohols).

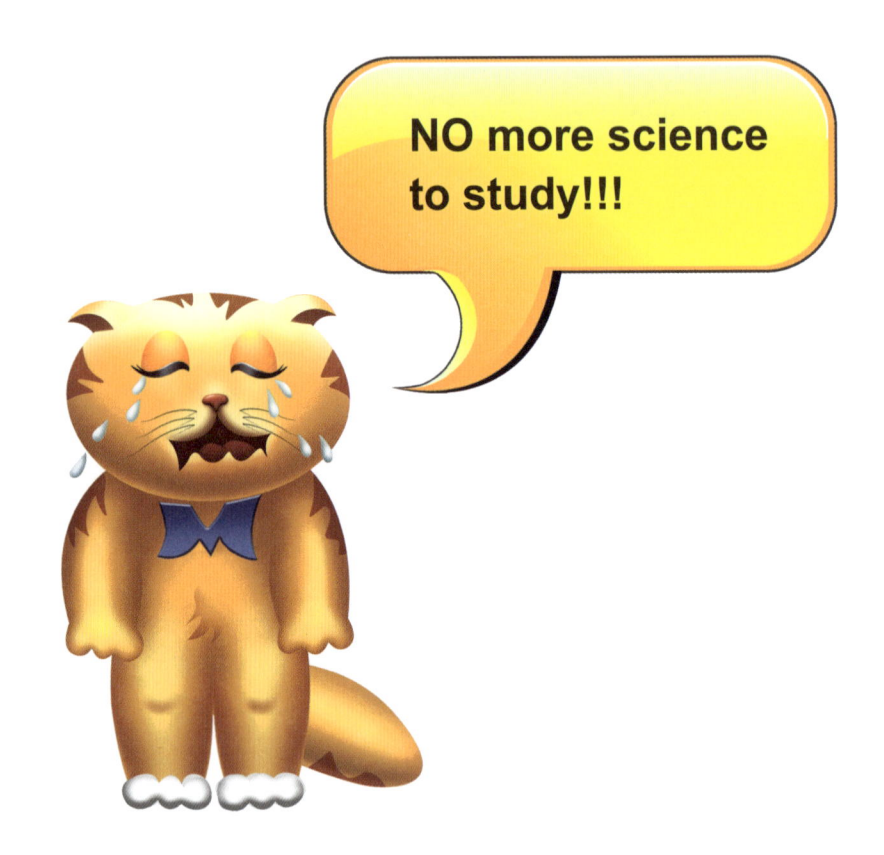

ORGANIC CHEMISTRY

CANDIDATE'S NAME _____ BOOKLET GS1-II

STUDENT ID _____

TEST GS-1

Section II: Written Communication

2 Writing Tasks (A and B); 60 Minutes (total)
Two 30 Minute Prompts, Timed Separately

INSTRUCTIONS: This test is designed to evaluate your writing skills. There are two writing assignments. You will have 30 minutes to complete each part. Your answers for Section II should be written in ANSWER DOCUMENT 2. Your response to Writing Task A must be written only on answer sheets marked "A," and your response to Writing Task B should be written only on answer sheets marked "B." The first 30 minutes may be used to respond to Task A only. The second 30 minutes may be used to respond to Task B only. If you finish writing before time is up, you may review your work ONLY on the response you have just completed.

Use your time in an efficient manner. Prior to writing your response, read the assignment carefully. The empty space on the page with the writing assignment may be used to make notes in planning your response. Scratch paper is not permitted. Corrections or additions can be made neatly between the lines but there should be no writing in the margins of the answer booklet. You are not expected to use each page of your answer document but do not skip lines. Use a black or blue pen to write your response. Illegible essays cannot be scored.

OPEN BOOKLET ONLY WHEN TIMER IS READY.

* GAMSAT is administered by ACER which is not associated with this product.
© RuveneCo Inc. All rights reserved. Reproduction without permission is illegal.

WRITING TASK A

Read the following statements and write a response to any one or more of the ideas presented.

Your essay will be evaluated on the value of your thoughts on the theme, logical organization of content and effective articulation of your key points.

* * * * * * * * *

Comment 1

    Whoever said the pen is mightier than the sword obviously never encountered automatic weapons.
Gen. Douglas MacArthur

* * * * *

Comment 2

    Political power grows out of the barrel of a gun.
Chairman Mao Zedong

* * * * *

Comment 3

    A man of courage never wants weapons.

* * * * *

Comment 4

    Before a standing army can rule, the people must be disarmed, as they are in almost every country in Europe.
Noah Webster

* * * * *

Comment 5

    You can get more with a kind word and a gun than you can with just a kind word.
Al Capone

WRITING TASK B

Read the following statements and write a response to any one or more of the ideas presented.

Your essay will be evaluated on the value of your thoughts on the theme, logical organization of content and effective articulation of your key points.

* * * * * * * * * *

Comment 1

Each friend represents a world in us, a world possibly not born until they arrive, and it is only by this meeting that a new world is born.

Anais Nin

* * * * *

Comment 2

A friend is one who walks in when the rest of the world walks out.

* * * * *

Comment 3

The best mirror is an old friend.

* * * * *

Comment 4

One friend in a lifetime is much; two are many; three are hardly possible. Friendship needs a certain parallelism of life, a community of thought, a rivalry of aim.

Henry Adams

* * * * *

Comment 5

Friendship is unnecessary, like philosophy, like art... It has no survival value; rather is one of those things that give value to survival.

C.S. Lewis

END OF WRITTEN COMMUNICATION.
DO NOT RETURN TO TASK A.

CANDIDATE'S NAME _____

STUDENT ID _____

BOOKLET GS1-III

TEST GS-1

Section III:
Reasoning in Biological and Physical Sciences

Questions 1-110
Time : 170 Minutes

INSTRUCTIONS: Of the 110 questions in this test, many are organized into groups preceded by a passage. After evaluating the passage, select the best answer to each question in the group. Some questions are independent of any descriptive passage or each other. Similarly, select the best answer to these questions. If you are unsure of an answer, eliminate the alternatives that you know to be incorrect and select an answer from the remaining alternatives. To indicate your selection, use a pencil to blacken the corresponding oval on Answer Document 1, GS-1. Rough work is to be done ONLY in the test booklet. No scrap paper is permitted. No calculator is permitted. No marks are deducted for wrong answers.

The Gold Standard GAMSAT* has been designed exclusively to test knowledge and thinking skills. The exam may contain hypothetical statements and/or express controversial ideas. Statements contained herein do not necessarily reflect the policy, position, or view of RuveneCo Inc.

OPEN BOOKLET ONLY WHEN TIMER IS READY.

Worked solutions are available to the original owner of this textbook at gamsat-prep.com.

* GAMSAT is administered by ACER which is not associated with this product.
© RuveneCo Inc. All rights reserved. Reproduction without permission is illegal.

UNIT 1

Questions 1–6

The sequence of events during synaptic transmission at the neuromuscular junction can be summarized as follows.

The depolarization produced by an action potential in the synaptic terminal opens voltage-dependent calcium channels in the terminal membrane. Calcium ions enter the terminal down their concentration and electrical gradients, inducing synaptic vesicles filled with acetylcholine (ACh) to fuse with the plasma membrane facing the muscle cell. The ACh is thereby dumped into the synaptic cleft, and some of it diffuses across the cleft to combine with specific receptors on ACh-activated channels. When ACh is bound, the channel opens and allows sodium and potassium ions to cross the membrane. This depolarizes the muscle membrane or *sarcolemma* and triggers an all-or-none action potential in the muscle cell. The action of ACh is terminated by the enzyme acetylcholinesterase, which splits ACh into acetate and choline.

In order to determine how, and under what conditions, ACh works, 2 experiments were done.

1. At the neuromuscular junction, the receptors on the ACh-activated channels are likely located:
   A   on the tubule of the T system.
   B   in the sarcolemma.
   C   on the muscle surface.
   D   in the synaptic cleft.

2. The depolarization across the muscle membrane triggers an all-or-none action potential in the muscle cell. This suggests that an increase in the amount of transmitter released at the neuromuscular junction would change:
   A   the amplitude of the action potential.
   B   the frequency of the nerve impulses.
   C   the direction of the action potential.
   D   the speed at which nerve impulses travel along the muscle cell.

3. A mutation in the gene which codes for acetylcholinesterase would inhibit all but which of the following processes?
   A   A hyperpolarization in the postsynaptic membrane
   B   A depolarization in the postsynaptic membrane
   C   The passage of a series of nerve impulses along the axon of the postsynaptic neuron
   D   The development of an inhibitory postsynaptic potential

Questions 4–6 refer to the following additional information:

Experiment 1

Determining the Effect of the Timing of Calcium Action on Transmitter Release

Calcium ions were removed from the bathing solution of a muscle cell so that release of ACh in response to nerve stimulation was virtually abolished. Calcium ions were then applied to the nerve terminal by ionophoreses, from a micropipette close to the terminal, just before the nerve was stimulated (N), without nerve stimulation, and just after the nerve was stimulated. The results obtained are shown in Fig. 1.

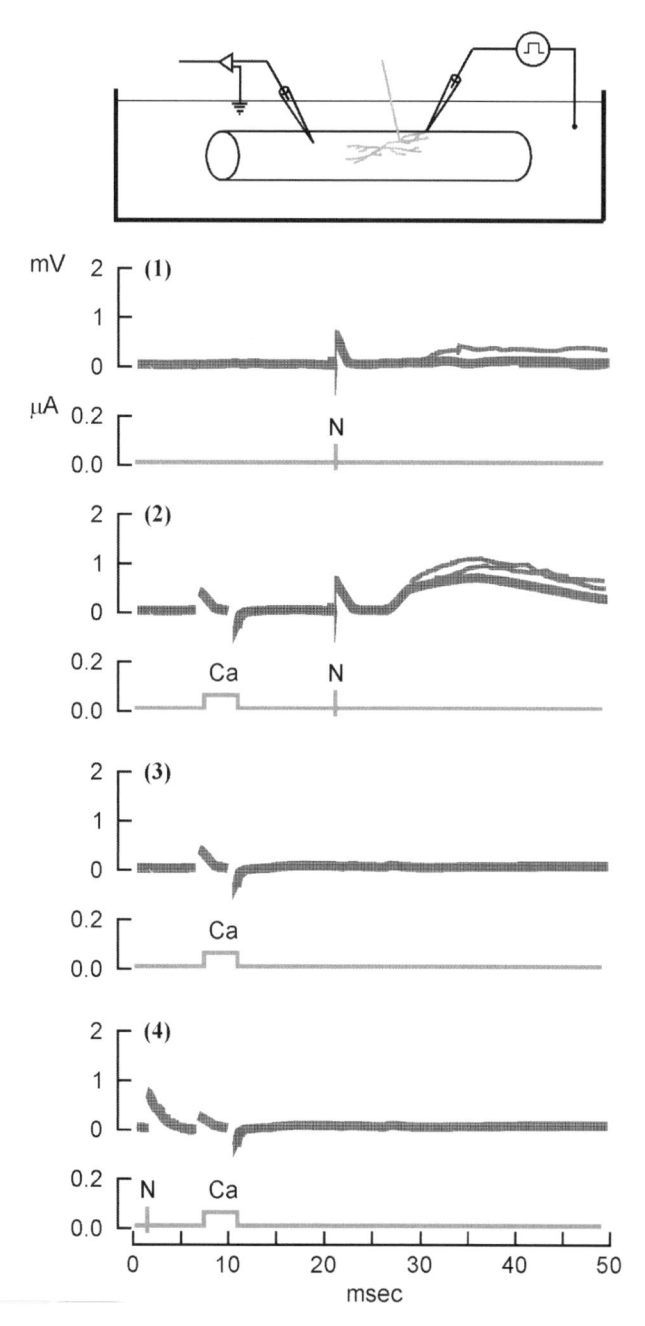

Figure 1

Experiment 2

Determining the Effect of ACh on Neuromuscular Transmission and its Subsequent Action on the Postsynaptic Membrane

Stimulating electrodes were placed on the nerve and a pair of recording electrodes was placed on the muscle. One of the electrodes was placed very close to the end plate region. First curare and then eserine were added to the solution bathing the muscle. The action potentials produced on stimulating the nerve were recorded. The results obtained are shown in Fig. 2.

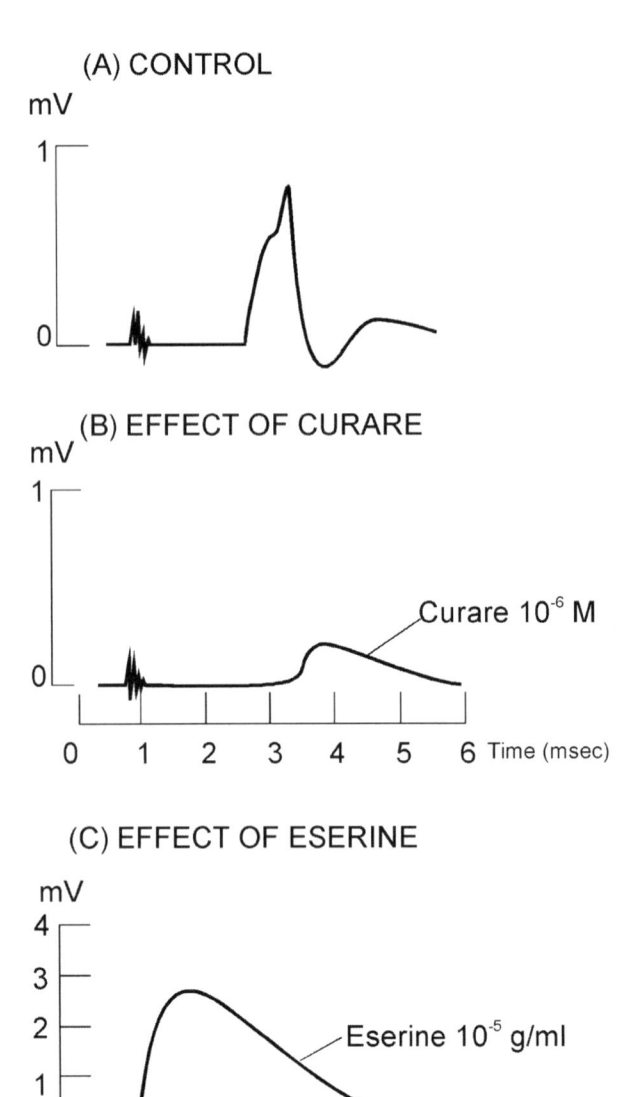

Figure 2

4. According to Fig. 1, which of the following conclusions was confirmed by the experiment?
   A For transmitter release to occur, calcium ions need only be present after the depolarization of the presynaptic membrane.
   B The presence of calcium ions is the only variable which affects transmitter release at the synapse.
   C For transmitter release to occur, calcium ions must be present before and after depolarization of the presynaptic membrane.
   D For transmitter release to occur, calcium ions must be present before depolarization of the presynaptic membrane.

5. According to Fig. 2, curare and eserine could act by, respectively:
   A blocking ion channels and binding to the receptors on ACh-activated channels.
   B blocking ion channels and preventing the hydrolysis of acetylcholinesterase.
   C initiating the entry of calcium ions into the synaptic knob and initiating the passage of a nerve impulse along the muscle cell.
   D binding to ACh receptor sites on the postsynaptic membrane and preventing the hydrolysis of acetylcholine.

6. According to Fig. 2, all of the following would be correct EXCEPT:
   A the post-stimulation peak in the eserine curve precedes the peak in the curare curve.
   B the curve for the control displays a shorter period of time with negative membrane potential compared to positive.
   C whether eserine or curare had been used in greater concentration cannot be determined from the information provided.
   D stimulating the nerves may create some artifact in the tracings.

UNIT 2

Questions 7–11

In the strictest sense, *crystal lattice* refers to an orderly arrangement of particles. Thus, any substance which solidifies forms its own crystal lattice, with orderly arrangements of atoms or molecules. Each atom, molecule or ion is said to occupy a lattice site as shown below in Figure 1.

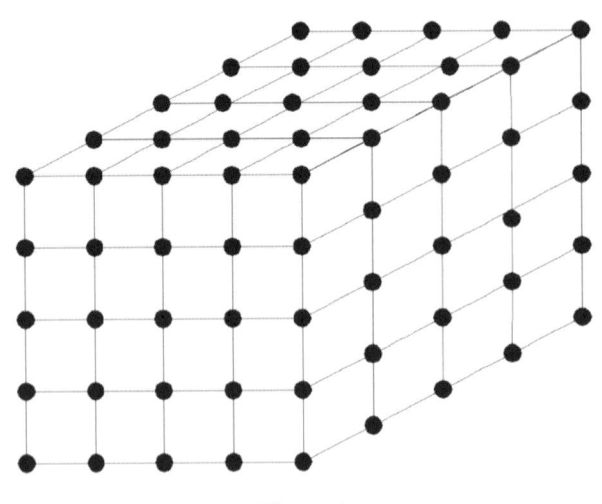

Figure 1

Usually, solidification or freezing occurs when the distance between individual particles is closer than in the liquid state. This leads to the mutual electrostatic attractive forces between the particles overcoming the mutual electrostatic forces of repulsion between the particles and the change from the liquid state to the solid state. In some substances, however, the distance over which the intermolecular forces act in the crystal lattice is greater than in the liquid state. This is due to certain intermolecular forces existing in the liquid state which become "fixed" in the lattice. An example of these types of bonds is the hydrogen bond. Thus, solid water (ice) floats on "liquid" water. The phenomenon gives rise to a phase diagram similar to that shown in Figure 2.

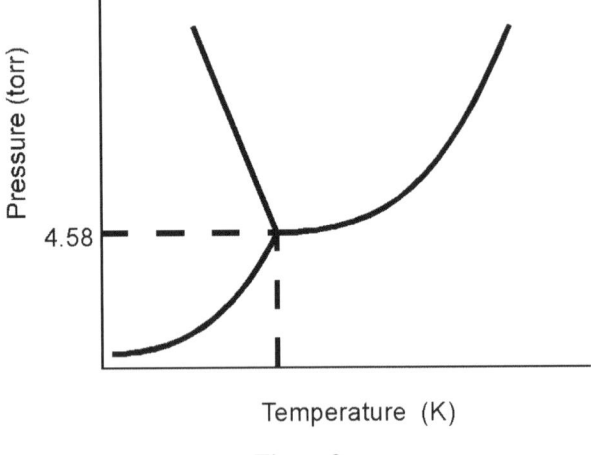

Figure 2

The freezing point of a solution can be depressed directly proportional to the molal concentration of the solute m (moles per kg of solvent). So mathematically,

$$\Delta T_f = K_f m$$

where ΔT_f = the decrease in the freezing point
and K_f = the freezing point depression constant.

7. Why does "solid" water (ice) float on "liquid" water?
   A   Because it is less dense.
   B   Because it occupies less volume.
   C   Because it exists at lower temperatures.
   D   Because it is a solid.

8. From Figure 2, what do you expect to happen to the melting point of solid water (ice) if an increased external pressure is applied to the system?
   A   The melting point would increase.
   B   The melting point would decrease.
   C   The melting point would remain at the same value.
   D   The direction of change in the value of the melting point depends on the magnitude of the applied pressure.

9. Which of the following molecules would yield a similar phase diagram to that of water?
   A CO_2
   B CH_4
   C NH_3
   D H_2

10. 50 grams of glucose ($C_6H_{12}O_6$) and 50 grams of sucrose ($C_{12}H_{22}O_{11}$) were each added to beakers of water (beaker 1 and beaker 2, respectively). Which of the following would be true?
    A   Boiling point elevation for beaker 1 would be greater than the boiling point elevation for beaker 2.
    B   Boiling point elevation for beaker 1 would be less than the boiling point elevation for beaker 2.
    C   The same degree of boiling point elevation will occur in both beakers.
    D   No boiling point elevation would be observed in either of the beakers.

11. The kelvin (symbol: K) is a unit of temperature and it is one of the seven SI base units. The kelvin and the degree Celsius are often used together, as they have the same interval, and 0 kelvin is –273.15 degrees Celsius. What would the freezing point in kelvin of a solution which is 0.5 molal in sucrose and 0.50 molal in acetic acid be?
    (K_f of water = 2.0 °C mol^{-1} and freezing point of water = 0 °C)
    A   –1.0 K
    B   –2.0 K
    C   272 K
    D   271 K

UNIT 3

Questions 12–16

The four forces that act on a plane are lift, weight, drag or air resistance, and thrust, the last of which is produced by the plane's engine.

Impact pressure produces 30% of the lift. It results from the fact that wings are given a *dihedral* angle where the distance from the tip of the wing to the ground is greater than that from the root of the wing to the ground.

The other 70% of lift can be accounted for by the Bernoulli effect. A cross-section of an airplane's wing reveals greater surface area above the wing compared to a flatter, lower surface. Thus air, moving in streamline flow, must move more rapidly over the top of the wing.

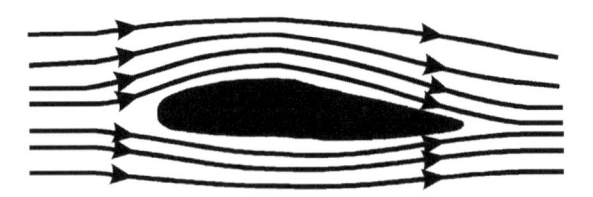

Bernoulli's equation, $P + 1/2\rho v^2 + \rho gh$ = constant, is often modified when discussing an airplane's wing. The "ρgh" component is usually left out since the difference in distance from the top of the wing to the ground compared to the bottom of the wing to the ground is usually negligible.

Note that:
- Streamline flow is governed by the continuity equation where $A_1v_1 = A_2v_2$
- For Bernoulli's and/or the continuity equation: P is pressure, ρ is density, v is velocity, g is gravity, h is the height and A is the cross-sectional area.

12. Newton's Third Law states that for every action there must be an equal and opposite reaction. This is applicable to lift and the dihedral angle because:
    - A the fast moving air above the wing increases the pressure.
    - B drag must be as low as possible to improve forward motion.
    - C there is a large pressure difference between the wings.
    - D the wing deflects the air downward and the air in turn deflects the wing upward.

13. Compared to the wing's upper surface, the air moving along the undersurface has:
    - A greater velocity, greater pressure.
    - B greater velocity, lower pressure.
    - C lower velocity, greater pressure.
    - D lower velocity, lower pressure.

14. An airplane is encircling an airport with DECREASING speed. When the airplane reaches point P, what is the general direction of its acceleration?

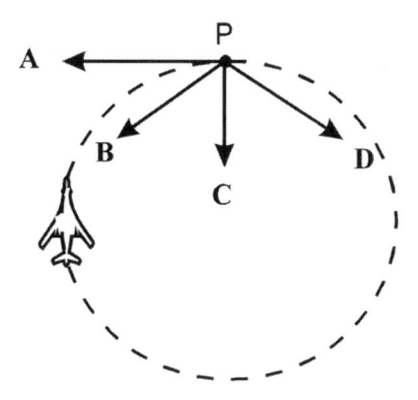

15. The following represents an incompressible fluid in laminar flow through pipes. Where is the pressure highest?

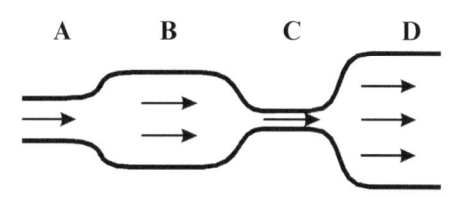

16. Flow is defined as volume per unit time. Concerning the preceding diagram, what can be determined regarding the flow?
    A   It is highest at C.
    B   It is highest at D.
    C   It cannot be determined.
    D   It is constant throughout.

UNIT 4

Question 17

Consider the following reduction potential table.

Electrochemical reaction	E° value (V)
$MnO_2 + 4H^+ + 2e^- \to Mn^{2+} + 2H_2O$	+1.23
$Fe^{3+} + e^- \to Fe^{2+}$	+0.771
$N_2 + 5H^+ + 4e^- \to N_2H_5^+$	−0.230
$Cr^{3+} + e^- \to Cr^{2+}$	−0.410

17. Given the data provided in the table, which of the following is the strongest reducing agent?
   A Cr^{3+}
   B Cr^{2+}
   C Mn^{2+}
   D MnO_2

UNIT 5

Question 18

18. The structure of β-D-glucose is shown below in two different projection systems. The circled hydroxyl group in Fig. 1 would be located at which position in the modified Fischer projection depicted in Fig. 2?

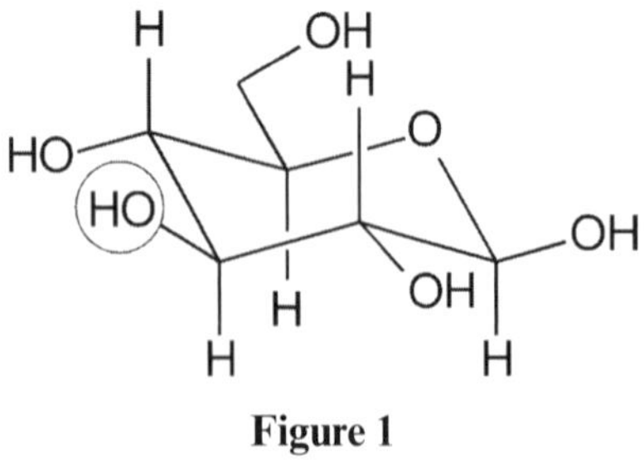

Figure 1

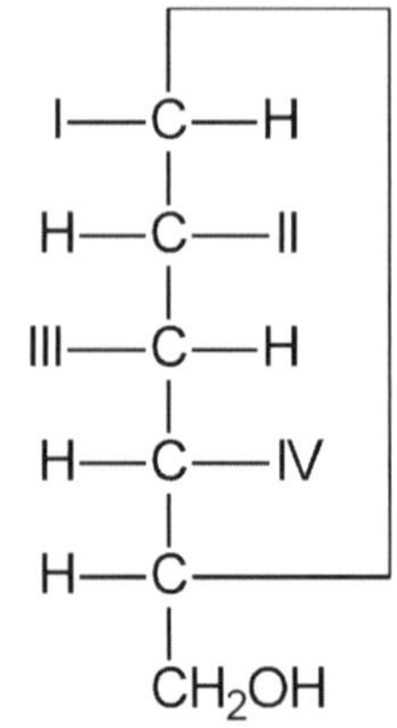

Figure 2

   A I
   B II
   C III
   D IV

UNIT 6

Questions 19–24

The essential stages in the manufacture of H_2SO_4 and H_2SO_3 involve the burning of sulfur or roasting of sulfide ores in air to produce SO_2. This is then mixed with air, purified and passed over a vanadium catalyst (either VO_3^- or V_2O_5) at 450 degrees Celsius. Thus the following reaction occurs.

$$2SO_2(g) + O_2(g) \rightleftharpoons 2SO_3(g) \quad \Delta H = -197 \text{ kJ mol}^{-1}$$

Reaction I

If the SO_2 is very carefully dissolved in water, sulfurous acid (H_2SO_3) is obtained. The first proton of this acid ionizes as if from a strong acid while the second ionizes as if from a weak acid.

$$H_2SO_3 + H_2O \rightarrow H_3O^+ + HSO_3^-$$

Reaction II

$$HSO_3^- + H_2O \rightleftharpoons H_3O^+ + SO_3^{2-} \quad K_a = 5.0 \times 10^{-6}$$

Reaction III

The concentration of H_2SO_3 in cleaning fluid was determined by titration with 0.10 M NaOH (strong base) as shown in Fig.1. Two equivalence points were determined using 30 ml and 60 ml of NaOH respectively:

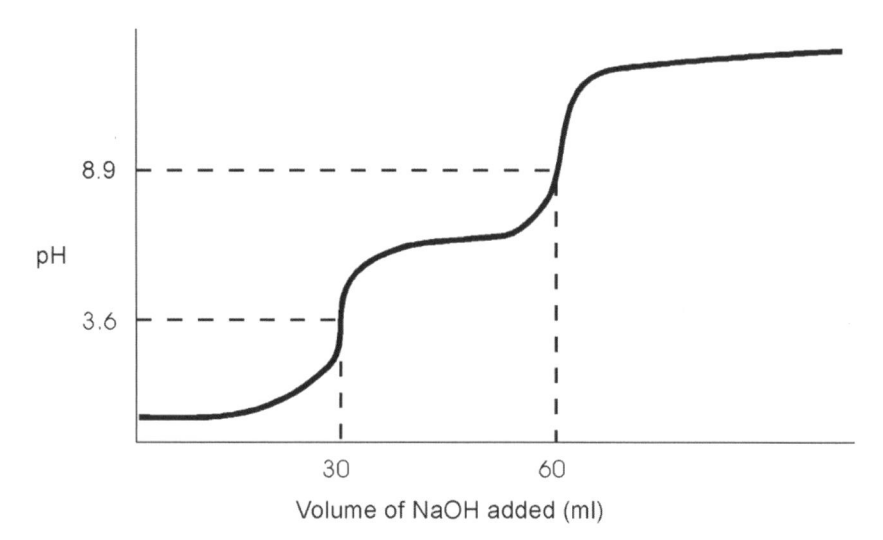

Figure 1

(Relative atomic mass: H = 1.0, N = 14.0, O = 16.0, S = 32, Cl = 35.5)

19. What is the oxidation number of sulfur in sulfurous acid?
    A +3
    B +4
    C +5
    D +6

20. What is the percent by mass of oxygen in sulfurous acid?
   - A 31.9%
   - B 19.7%
   - C 39.0%
   - D 58.5%

21. Which of the following acid-base indicators is most suitable for the determination of the first end point of the titration shown in Figure 1?
   - A Cresol red (color change between pH = 0.2 and pH = 1.8)
   - B p-Xylenol blue (color change between pH = 1.2 and pH = 2.8)
   - C Bromophenol blue (color change between pH = 3.0 and pH = 4.6)
   - D Bromocresol green (color change between pH = 3.8 and pH = 5.4)

22. The equilibrium constant K_a is also called the acid dissociation constant and K_b is the base dissociation constant. The value of K_a given in Reaction III is relatively low which would mean that, relatively, its:
   - A pK_a is low and the pK_b of its conjugate base is high.
   - B pK_a is high and the pK_b of its conjugate base is low.
   - C pK_a is low and the pK_b of its conjugate base is low.
   - D pK_a is high and the pK_b of its conjugate base is high.

23. If no catalyst was used in Reaction I, which of the following would experience a change in its partial pressure when the same system reaches equilibrium?
   - A There will be no change in the partial pressure of any of the reactants
   - B SO_3 (g)
   - C SO_2 (g)
   - D O_2 (g)

24. If the temperature was decreased in Reaction I, which of the following would experience an increase in its partial pressure when the same system reaches equilibrium?
   - A There will be no change in the partial pressure of any of the reactants
   - B SO_3 (g)
   - C SO_2 (g)
   - D O_2 (g) and SO_2 (g)

UNIT 7

Question 25

25. Apo-X is a drug which blocks prophase from occurring. When Apo-X is added to a tissue culture, in which phase of the cell cycle would most cells be arrested?
   - A Mitosis
   - B G_1
   - C G_2
   - D Synthesis

UNIT 8

Questions 26–31

Much of the study of evolution of *interspecific* interactions had focused on the results rather than the process of coevolution. In only a few cases has the genetic bases of interspecific interactions been explored. One of the most intriguing results has been the description of "gene-for-gene" systems governing the interaction between certain parasites and their hosts. In several crop plants, dominant alleles at a number of loci have been described that confer resistance to a pathogenic fungus; for each such gene, the fungus appears to have a recessive allele for "virulence" that enables the fungus to attack the otherwise resistant host. Cases of character displacement among competing species are among the best evidence that interspecific interactions can result in genetic change.

Assuming that parasites and their hosts coevolve in an "arms race," we might deduce that the parasite is "ahead" if local populations are more capable of attacking the host population with which they are associated than other populations. Whereas the host may be "ahead" if local populations are more resistant to the local parasite than to other populations of the parasite.

Several studies have been done to evaluate coevolutionary interactions between parasites and hosts, or predators and prey. In one, the fluctuations in populations of houseflies and of a wasp that parasitized them were recorded. The results of the experiment are shown in Fig. 1.

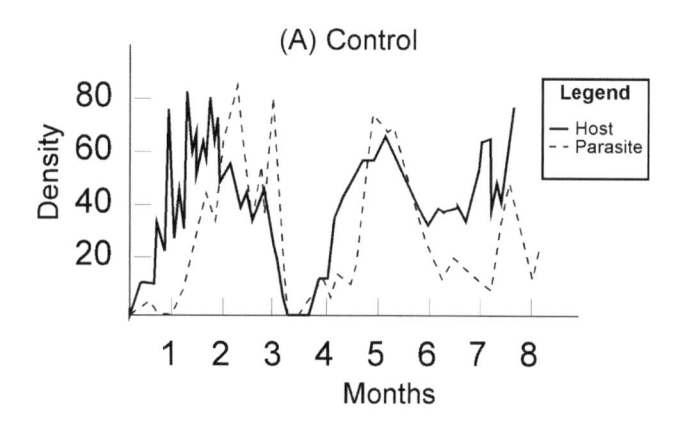

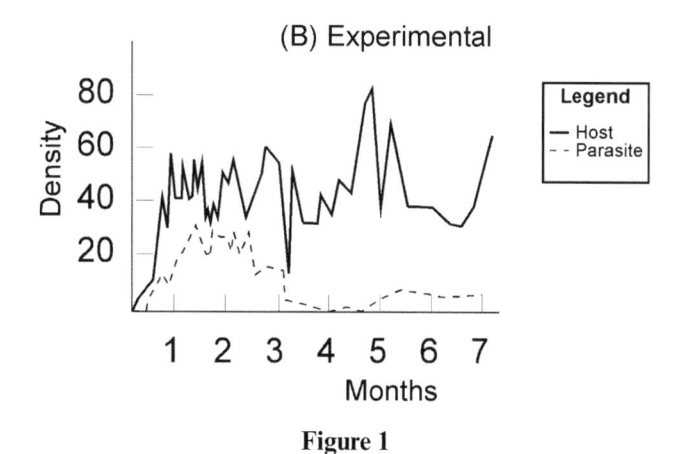

Figure 1

26. A pathogenic fungus is more capable of growth and reproduction on its native population of its sole host, the wild hog peanut, than on plants from other populations of the same species. It is reasonable to conclude that:
   A   the fungus, in this instance, was capable of more rapid adaptation to its host than vice versa.
   B   the fungus, in this instance, was capable of more rapid adaptation to all populations of the host species than vice versa.
   C   the host, in this instance, was capable of more rapid adaptation to the fungus than vice versa.
   D   all populations of the host species were capable of more rapid adaptation to the fungus than vice versa.

27. Allopatric refers to areas isolated geographically from one another whereas sympatric populations occupy the same or overlapping geographical areas. The passage suggests that one result of interspecific interactions might be:
   A   genetic drift within sympatric populations.
   B   genetic drift within allopatric populations.
   C   genetic mutations within sympatric populations.
   D   genetic mutations within allopatric populations.

28. According to Fig. 1, the experiment showed that over time:
   A   coevolution caused a decrease in both the host and parasite populations.
   B   coevolution caused both a decrease in fluctuation of the host and parasite populations, and a lowered density of the parasite population.
   C   coevolution caused a marked increase in the fluctuation of only the host population, and lowered the density of the parasite population.
   D   coevolution caused a decrease in the population density of the parasite population but caused a marked increase in the density of the host population.

29. The control in the experiment likely consisted of:
   A   members from different populations of the host and parasite species used in the experimental group, that had a short history of exposure to one another.
   B   members of the host and parasite species used in the experimental group, that had a long history of exposure to one another.
   C   members of the host and parasite species used in the experimental group that had no history of exposure to one another.
   D   members from different populations of the host and parasite species used in the experimental group, that had a long history of exposure to one another.

30. Which of the following is the least likely explanation of the results obtained for the control group in Fig. 1?
   A   A low parasite population results in a lowered host population by the sheer virulence of the parasite.
   B   A low host population can increase a parasite population by forcing the parasite to seek an alternate source for food.
   C   A high parasite population destroys the host population resulting in a lowered host population.
   D   A high host population creates a breeding ground for parasites thus increasing the parasite population.

31. Penicillin is an antibiotic which destroys bacteria by interfering with cell wall production. Could the development of bacterial resistance to Penicillin be considered similar to coevolution?
   A   Yes, a spontaneous mutation is likely to confer resistance to Penicillin.
   B   No, an organism can only evolve in response to another organism.
   C   Yes, as antibiotics continue to change there will be a selective pressure for bacterial genes which confer resistance.
   D   No, bacteria have plasma membranes and can survive without cell walls.

UNIT 9

Questions 32–37

The ninhydrin reaction is a useful analytical detection method for α-amino acids. The reagent ninhydrin produces a characteristic blue color with primary α-amino acids via the following series of reactions (see Fig. 1):

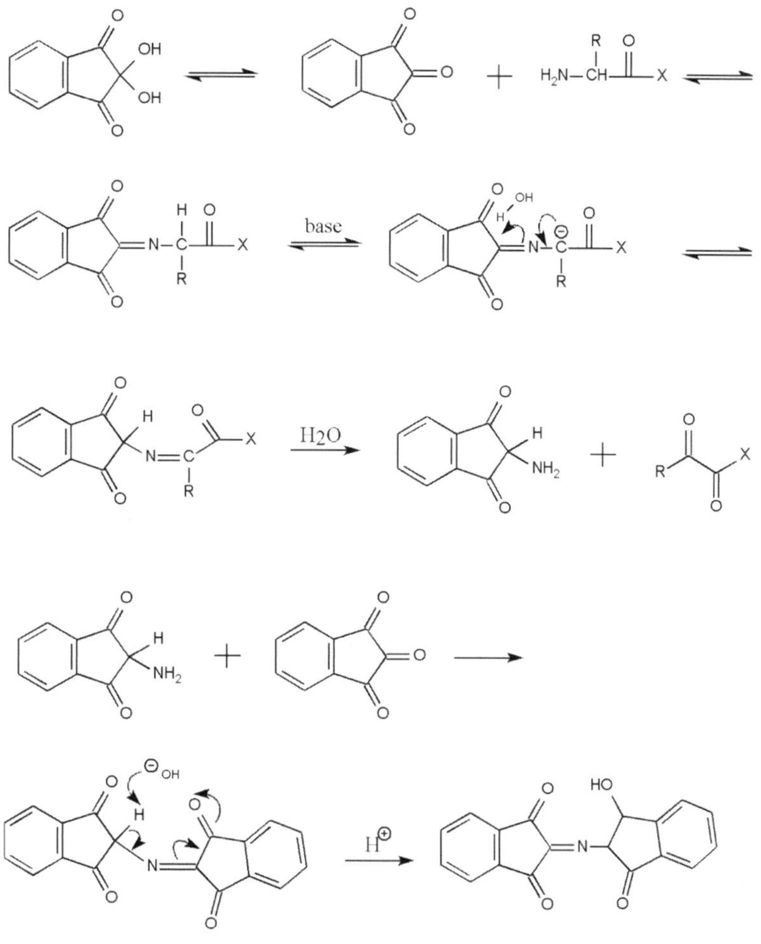

Figure 1

32. In the first reaction of Fig. 1, the inorganic product, which is not written, is:
   A CO_2
   B H_2O
   C HCl
   D H_2O_2

33. Which of the following compounds would be isotopically labeled if $H_2^{18}O$ were the only isotype source?

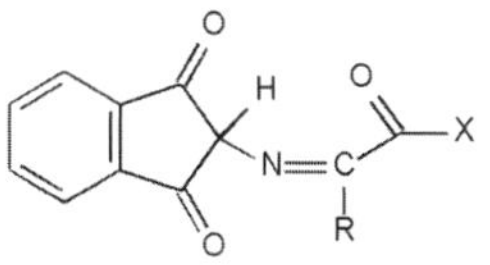

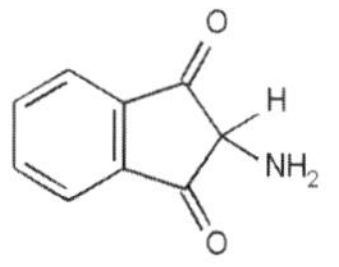

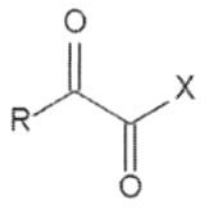

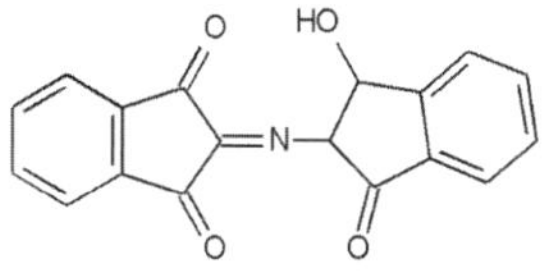

34. Base treatment of an amino acid usually results in the conversion of the acid to a derivative via the amino-carboxylate salt.

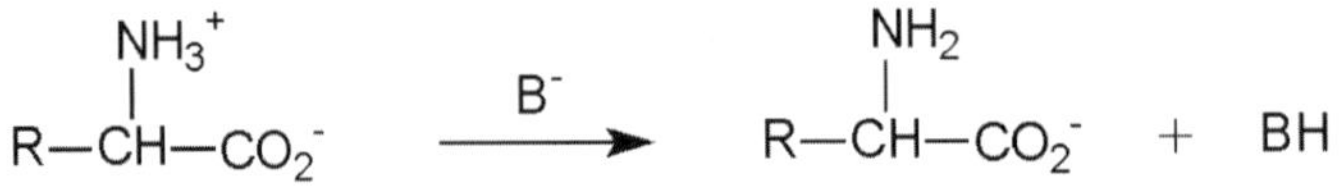

$$R-\underset{\underset{NH_3^+}{|}}{CH}-CO_2^- \xrightarrow{B^-} R-\underset{\underset{NH_2}{|}}{CH}-CO_2^- + BH$$

The above procedure:
A   decreases the rate of electrophilic reaction of the free amino group.
B   decreases the rate of nucleophilic reaction of the free amino group.
C   enhances the rate of nucleophilic reaction of the free amino group.
D   enhances the rate of electrophilic reaction of the free amino group.

35. A mixture of the amino acid alanine and the chemical benzoyl chloride is treated with dilute aqueous sodium hydroxide to yield compound X. What functional group would be present in compound X?
A   Ester
B   Aldehyde
C   Amide
D   Ether

36. Amino acids can be divided into the following four general categories based on their acid-base charge properties at intracellular pH (~6–7):

Positively charged
Negatively charged
Hydrophobic
Hydrophilic

Consider the following amino acids.

I. 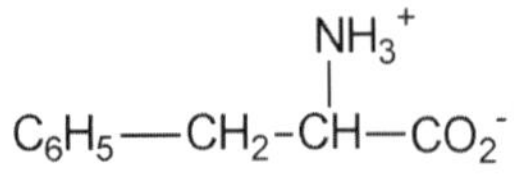 $C_6H_5-CH_2-\underset{\underset{NH_3^+}{|}}{CH}-CO_2^-$

II. 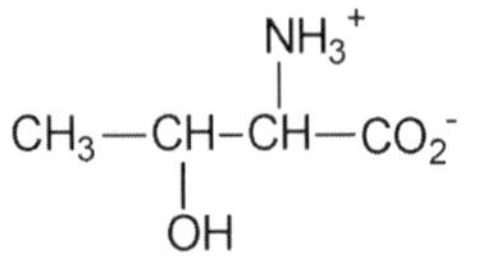 $CH_3-\underset{\underset{OH}{|}}{CH}-\underset{\underset{NH_3^+}{|}}{CH}-CO_2^-$

III. 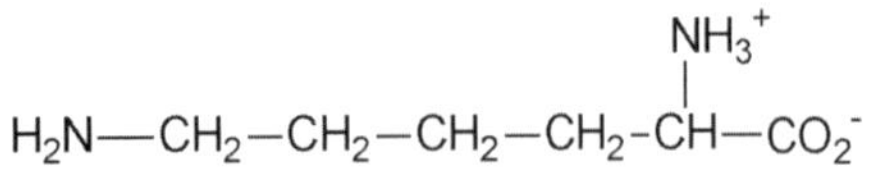 $H_2N-CH_2-CH_2-CH_2-CH_2-\underset{\underset{NH_3^+}{|}}{CH}-CO_2^-$

IV. 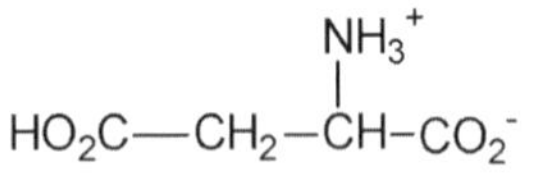 $HO_2C-CH_2-\underset{\underset{NH_3^+}{|}}{CH}-CO_2^-$

Which of the following classification series best represents amino acids I, II, III, and IV, respectively?
A   Hydrophobic, hydrophilic, positively charged, negatively charged
B   Hydrophobic, positively charged, hydrophilic, negatively charged
C   Hydrophilic, negatively charged, hydrophobic, positively charged
D   Positively charged, negatively charged, hydrophilic, hydrophobic

37. The structure of valine is shown below.

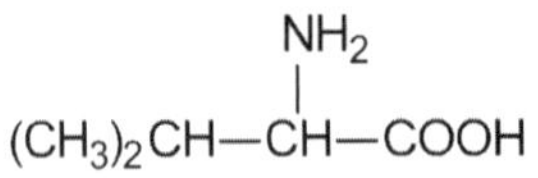

$$(CH_3)_2CH-\underset{\underset{NH_2}{|}}{CH}-COOH$$

In extremely basic solutions valine possesses 2 basic sites $-CO_2^-$ and $-NH_2$. Monoprotonation of such an alkaline solution would yield which of the following products?

A $(CH_3)_2CH-\underset{\underset{NH_2}{|}}{CH}-CH_2OH$

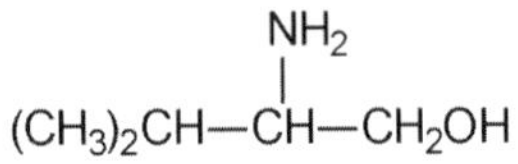

B $(CH_3)_2CH-\underset{\underset{NH_3^+}{|}}{CH}-COO^-$

C $(CH_3)_2CH-\underset{\underset{NH_3^+}{|}}{CH}-COOH$

D $(CH_3)_2CH-\underset{\underset{NH_2}{|}}{CH}-COOH$

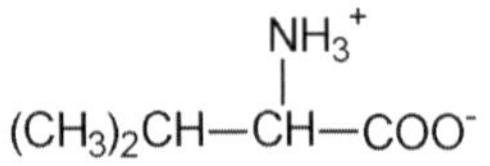

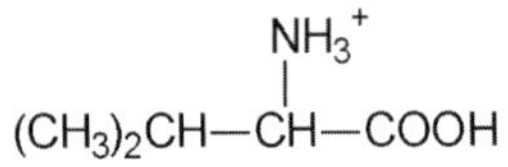

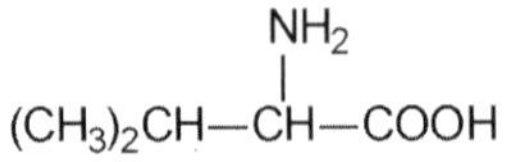

UNIT 10

Questions 38–43

The phenomenon of refraction has long intrigued scientists and was actually used to corroborate one of the major mysteries of early science: the determination of the speed of light.

The refractive index of a transparent material is related to a number of the physical properties of light. In terms of velocity, the refractive index represents the ratio of the velocity of light in a vacuum to its velocity in the material. From this ratio, it can be seen that light is retarded when it passes through most types of matter. It is worth noting that prisms break up white light into the seven "colors of the rainbow" because each color has a slightly different velocity in the medium.

Snell's law allows one to follow the behavior of light in terms of its path when moving from a material of one refractive index to another with the same, or different refractive index. It is given by: $n_1 \sin\theta_1 = n_2 \sin\theta_2$, where "1" refers to the first medium through which the ray passes, "2" refers to the second medium, and the angles refer to the angle of incidence in the first medium (θ_1) and the angle of refraction in the second (θ_2).

A ship went out on a search for a sunken treasure chest. In order to locate the chest, they shone a beam of light down into the water using a high intensity white light source as shown in Fig.1. The refractive index for sea water is 1.33 while that for air is 1.00.

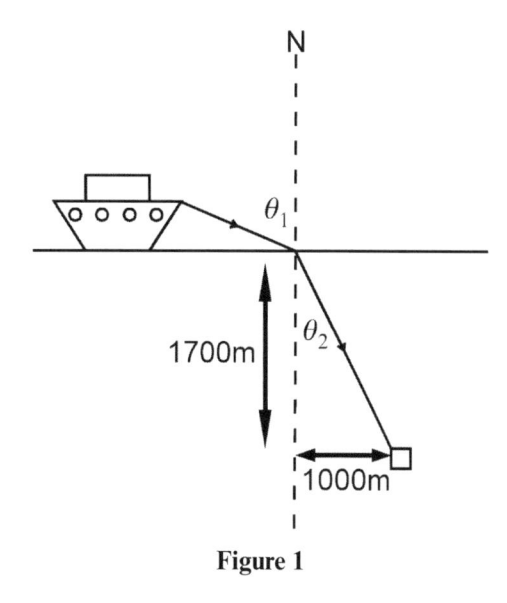

Figure 1

38. From the information in the passage, how would you expect the speed of light in air to compare with the speed of light in a vacuum (which is given by "c")?
    A   It would be approximately equal to c.
    B   It would be greater than c.
    C   It would be less than c.
    D   This cannot be determined from the information given.

39. Using the information in the passage, what must the approximate value of θ_2 be such that it hits the chest as shown in Figure 1?
    A   15°
    B   30°
    C   45°
    D   65°

40. How does the refractive index in water for violet light compare with that of red light given that violet light travels more slowly in water than red light?
   A $n_{violet} = n_{red}$
   B $n_{violet} < n_{red}$
   C $n_{violet} > n_{red}$
   D   This depends on the relative speeds of the different colors in a vacuum.

41. Total internal reflection first occurs when a beam of light travels from one medium to another medium which has a smaller refractive index at such an angle of incidence that the angle of refraction is 90°. This angle of incidence is called the critical angle. What is the value of the sine of this angle when the ray moves from water towards air?
   A 2π
   B   0.75
   C   0.50
   D   0

42. What would happen to the critical angle, in the previous question, if the beam of light was travelling from water to a substance with a greater refractive index than air, but a lower refractive index than water?
   A   It would increase.
   B   It would decrease.
   C   It would remain the same.
   D   Total internal reflection would not be possible.

43. Which of the following would you expect to remain constant when light travels from one medium to another and the media differ in their refractive indices?
   A   Velocity
   B   Frequency
   C   Wavelength
   D   Intensity

UNIT 11

Questions 44-49

Aside from diabetes, thyroid disease is the most common glandular disorder. Millions of people are treated for thyroid conditions, often an underactive or overactive gland. Overwhelmingly, women between the ages of 20 and 60 are much more likely than men to succumb to these conditions. The etiology lies in the failure of the immune system to recognize the thyroid gland as part of the body and thus antibodies are sent to attack the gland.

The plasma proteins that bind thyroid hormones are albumin, a prealbumin called thyroxine-binding prealbumin (TBPA), and a globulin with an electrophoretic mobility, thyroxine-binding globulin (TBG). The free thyroid hormones in plasma are in equilibrium with the protein-bound thyroid hormones in the tissues. Free thyroid hormones are added to the circulating pool by the thyroid. It is the free thyroid hormones in plasma that are physiologically active (increasing the metabolic rate) and imbalances in these hormones result in thyroid disease. In thyroid storm, a form of hyperthyroidism, the normal body temperature of 37.5 °C may rise to over 40 °C.

In addition, in humans there are four small parathyroid glands that produce the hormone, parathormone, which is a peptide composed of 84 amino acids. Parathormone and the thyroid hormone calcitonin work antagonistically to regulate the plasma calcium and phosphate levels. Overactive parathyroid glands, *hyperparathyroidism*, can lead to an increase in the level of calcium in plasma and tissues.

Table 1: Different plasma proteins and their binding capacity and affinity for thyroxine.

Protein	Plasma Level (mg/dl)	Thyroxine Binding Capacity (µg/dl)	Affinity for thyroxine	Amount of thyroxine bound in normal plasma (µg/dl)
Thyroxine binding globulin (TBG)	1.0	20	High	7
Thyroxine binding prealbumin (TBPA)	30.0	250	Moderate	1
Albumin	...	1000	Low	None
Total protein-bound thyroxine in plasma	...	...	...	8

44. Is it reasonable to conclude that thyroid disease is sex-linked?
    A   No, because thyroid disease appears to be caused by a defect of the immune system and not a defective DNA sequence.
    B   No, because if the disease was sex-linked, there would be a high incidence in the male, rather than the female, population.
    C   Yes, because the high incidence of the disease in women suggests that a gene found on the X chromosome codes for the disease.
    D   Yes, because the same factor increases the risk of women getting the disease, regardless of familial background.

45. According to Table 1, it would be expected that:
    A   TBG has the highest binding capacity for thyroxine while TBPA has the highest affinity.
    B   TBG has the highest binding capacity for thyroxine while albumin has the lowest affinity.
    C   albumin has the highest binding capacity for thyroxine while TBPA has the highest affinity.
    D   albumin has the highest binding capacity for thyroxine while TBG has the highest affinity.

Question 46 refers to Fig. 1.

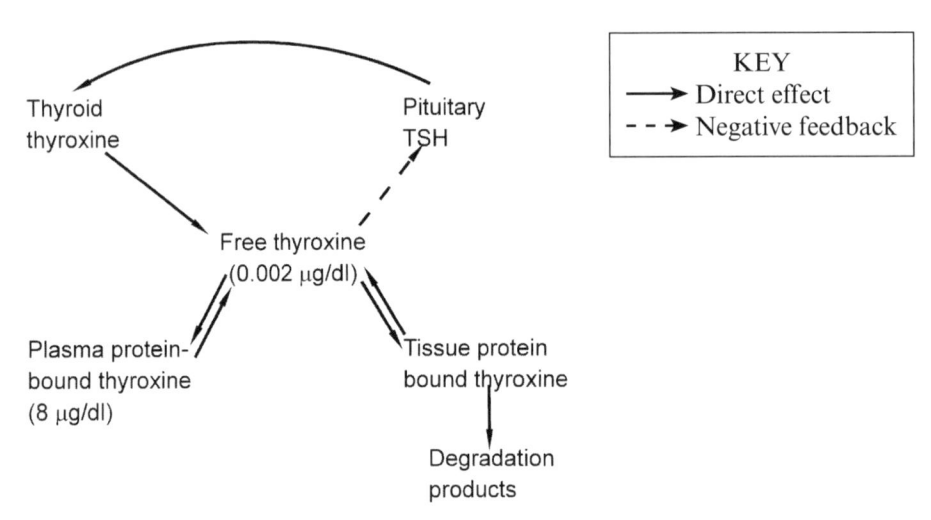

Figure 1

46. According to the equilibrium shown in Fig. 1, an elevation in the concentration of free thyroid hormone in the plasma is followed by:
    A an increase in tissue protein-bound thyroxine.
    B an increase in tissue protein-bound thyroxine and plasma protein-bound thyroxine.
    C an increase in the amount of TSH secreted from the pituitary gland.
    D an increase in both the amount of TSH secreted from the pituitary gland and the release of thyroxine from the thyroid gland.

47. Symptoms of hypothyroidism and hyperthyroidism, respectively, include:
    A a fine tremor and diminished concentration.
    B brittle nails and kidney stones.
    C rapid heart beat and increased irritability.
    D lethargy and nervous agitation.

48. Which of the following is an example of positive feedback?
    A A body temperature of 39 °C causes a further increase
    B Elevated TSH results in elevated thyroxine
    C Calcitonin and parathormone regulate calcium levels
    D Increased TBG leads to an increase in TSH

49. Parathormone influences calcium homeostasis by reducing tubular reabsorption of PO_4^{3-} in the kidneys. Which of the following, if true, would clarify the adaptive significance of this process?
    A PO_4^{3-} and Ca^{2+} feedback positively on each other.
    B Elevated levels of extracellular PO_4^{3-} result in calcification of bones and tissues.
    C Increased PO_4^{3-} levels cause an increase in parathormone secretion.
    D Decreased extracellular PO_4^{3-} levels cause a decrease in calcitonin production.

UNIT 12

Questions 50–54

The enthalpy of solution (ΔH_{soln}) of a salt depends on two other quantities: the energy released when free gaseous ions of the salt combine to give the solid salt (lattice energy: ΔH_{latt}) and the energy released when free gaseous ions of the salt dissolve in water via solute-solvent interactions to yield the solvated ions (enthalpy of hydration: ΔH_{solv}) where:

$$\Delta H_{soln} = \Delta H_{solv} - \Delta H_{latt} \qquad \text{Equation I}$$

From the formal definition of the quantities, it can be seen that both ΔH_{latt} and ΔH_{solv} are exothermic. Although these values seem to be in competition, the factors that affect ΔH_{latt} and ΔH_{solv} do so in the same way. Firstly, the smaller the ion, the closer the association of the ion with either other ions in the crystal lattice, or, with water molecules and thus the more negative ΔH_{latt} and ΔH_{solv} become. Also, the greater the charge on the ion, the greater the increase in electrostatic forces of attraction between itself and other ions or water molecules, and the more negative ΔH_{latt} and ΔH_{solv} become.

Although ΔH_{latt} and ΔH_{solv} undergo similar changes, the change in ΔH_{solv} up or down a group is much more profound than that of ΔH_{latt}. A good example of this is seen in the solubility changes of the Group II carbonates.

However, there is one exception to these general rules. If the cation of the salt is approximately the same size as the anion, the arrangement of ions in the crystal lattice is more uniform and hence the lattice is more stable and ΔH_{latt} is more negative.

Table 1: Note the order going down the periodic table is Mg, Ca, Sr, Ba.

Group II Carbonate	Solubility (mol L^{-1} H$_2$O)
MgCO$_3$	1.30×10^{-3}
CaCO$_3$	0.13×10^{-3}
SrCO$_3$	0.07×10^{-3}
BaCO$_3$	0.09×10^{-3}

50. It is often useful to determine the solubility product (K_{sp}) of compounds that are sparingly soluble like those in Table 1. In this context, K_{sp} can be defined as the mathematical product of ion concentrations raised to the power of their stoichiometric coefficients. The solubility product for MgCO$_3$ is:
    A 1.3×10^{-4}
    B 2.6×10^{-4}
    C 1.7×10^{-6}
    D 6.7×10^{-8}

51. Ca(OH)$_2$ has approximately the same K_{sp} as CaSO$_4$. Which of them has the greater solubility in terms of mol L^{-1}?
    A   They both have the same solubility.
    B   Ca(OH)$_2$
    C   CaSO$_4$
    D   It depends on the temperature at the time.

52. Given the information in the passage, the CO$_3^{2-}$ anion is approximately the same size as:
    A   Mg^{2+}.   B   Ca^{2+}.
    C   Sr^{2+}.   D   Ba^{2+}.

53. The ΔH$_{solv}$ for a doubly charged anion X^{2-} was found to be more negative than that for the carbonate anion. Given the information in the passage, which of the following is the most likely explanation?
    A   X^{2-} is the same size as the carbonate anion.
    B   X^{2-} is larger than the carbonate anion.
    C   X^{2-} is smaller than the carbonate anion.
    D   It depends on the H$_{latt}$ for the salt containing the anion.

54. A solution of SrCO$_3$ in water boils at a higher temperature than pure water. Why is this?
    A   SrCO$_3$ increases the density of water.
    B   SrCO$_3$ decreases the vapour pressure of the water.
    C   SrCO$_3$ has a low solubility in water.
    D   SrCO$_3$ decreases the surface tension of the water.

UNIT 13

Question 55

55. The following system includes a frictionless pulley and a cord of negligible mass. Since the system is at rest, what can be said about the force of friction between the platform and the large weight?

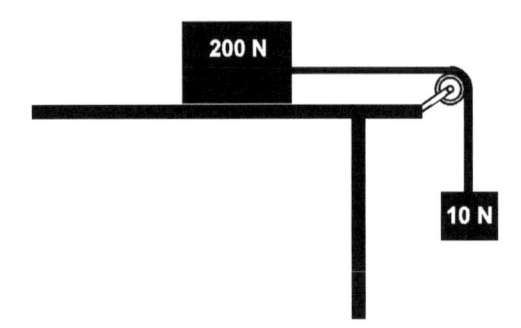

    A   It is 200 N.
    B   It is 10 N.
    C   It is 190 N.
    D   In this case, the force of friction is not necessarily present.

UNIT 14

Questions 56–61

In the simple model of a gas as described by the kinetic molecular theory, a gas is pictured as an assembly of particles travelling at high velocities in straight lines in all directions. The particles are constantly colliding, but they are supposed to be perfectly elastic so that no momentum is lost on impact. They are also supposed to be point masses, that is, they have mass but occupy no space. In addition, no attractive or repulsive forces are exerted between particles.

From this theory, and the work of other great scientists like Boyle and Charles, the ideal gas law was devised: PV = nRT where P = pressure of the gas, V = volume of the gas, n = number of moles of gas particles present, T = Kelvin temperature of the gas and R = universal gas constant.

However, no "real" gas conforms to this "ideal" gas theory, that is, no real gas obeys all of these laws at all temperatures and pressures. These deviations were investigated by the French physicist Amagat, who used pressures up to 320 atmospheres and a range of temperatures to investigate these deviations. The following diagram shows how the PV/nRT value varies with pressure for certain gases at 50 °C.

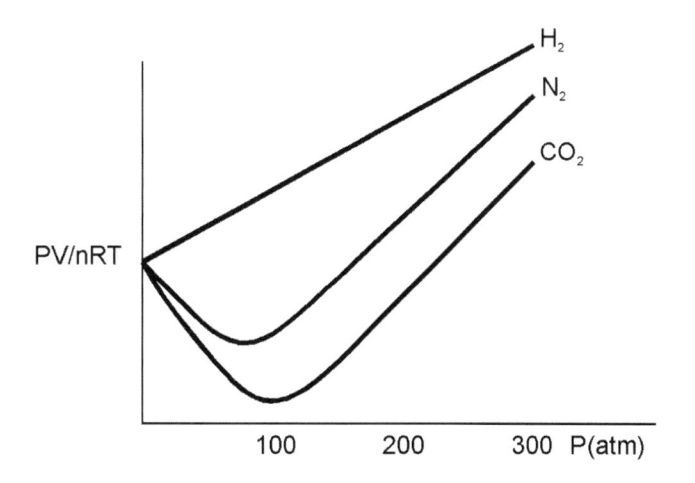

The deviations of real gases from ideality confers a number of properties on the gas which could not be explained by the kinetic molecular theory.

56. What would the PV/nRT versus P graph look like for an ideal gas?

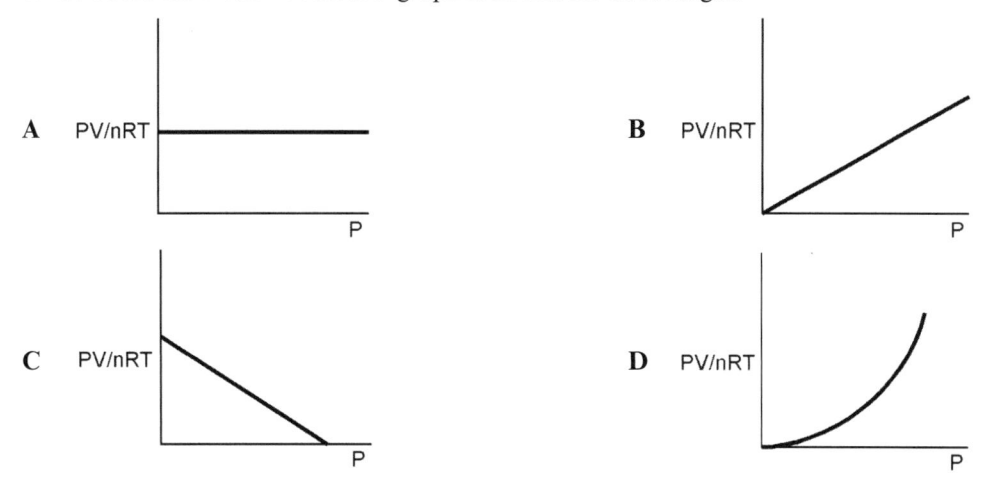

57. From the information in the passage, if 1 dm³ of H₂ gas initially at 50 atmospheres had its pressure increased to 100 atmospheres at a constant temperature, which of the following would be true?
- A   Volume = 500 cm³
- B   Volume > 500 cm³
- C   Volume < 500 cm³
- D   The change in volume will depend on the rate of increase of the external pressure.

58. Which of the following does not contribute to the explanation of the deviation of "real" gases from ideality?
- A   Gas particles occupy space.
- B   Gas particles have an attraction for each other.
- C   Gas particles possess mass.
- D   Gas particles do not undergo elastic collisions.

59. A sample of N_2, known to contain traces of water, occupied a volume of 200 dm³ at 25 °C and 1 atm. When passed over solid Na_2SO_4 (drying agent), the increase in mass of the salt was 35.0 grams. What was the partial pressure of the N_2 in the sample? (Assume ideality and molar volume at 25 °C = 24 dm³)
- A   0.1 atm
- B   0.2 atm
- C   0.4 atm
- D   0.8 atm

60. Which of the following would cause a gas to more closely resemble an ideal gas?
- A   Decreased pressure
- B   Decreased temperature
- C   Decreased volume
- D   None of the above

61. If a gas behaved ideally, which of the following would be expected on cooling the gas to 1 K?
- A   It would remain a gas.
- B   It would liquify.
- C   It would solidify.
- D   Cannot be determined from the information given.

UNIT 15

Question 62

62. Von Willebrand's disease is an autosomal dominant bleeding disorder. A man who does not have the disease has two children with a woman who is heterozygous for the condition. If the first child expresses the bleeding disorder, what is the probability that the second child will have the disease?
- A   0.25
- B   0.50
- C   0.75
- D   1.00

UNIT 16

Questions 63–68

Figure 1 illustrates chemical methods often used by organic chemists for qualitative analysis of water soluble unknowns. Table 1 lists characteristic chemical tests of organic compounds. For instance, Fehling's tests that are positive are indicative of an aldehyde.

```
                    Water
                   Soluble
                   Unknown
                      |
                 5% NaHCO₃
            No reaction │ Reaction
          ┌─────────────┘ └─────────────┐
       2,4-DNP                        KMnO₄
   Reaction │ No reaction       Reaction │ No immediate
   ┌────────┘ └──────┐          ┌────────┘    reaction
Fehling's         Lucas         ↓             ↓
  test            test          II            I
  No immediate
Reaction│reaction   No reaction│Reaction
┌───────┘ └──────┐      ┌──────┘ └──────┐
↓              Iodoform ↓              ↓
VII             test    IV             III
         No reaction│Reaction
         ┌──────────┘ └────────┐
         ↓                     ↓
         VI                    V
```

Figure 1

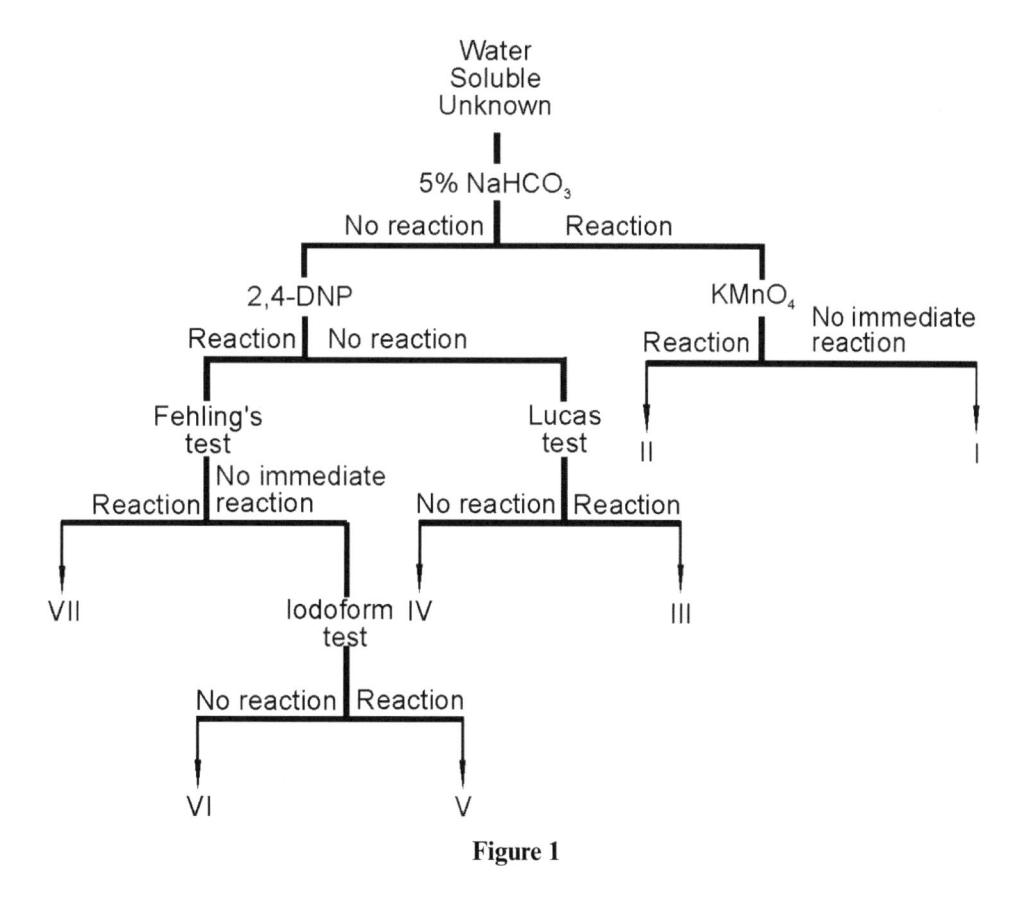

Table 1

Chemical Test	Compounds
Sodium hydroxide	Organic acids: carboxylic acids and phenols
Lucas	Alcohols with 5 or less carbon atoms
Sodium bicarbonate	Carboxylic acids
2,4-Dinitro- phenylhydrazine (DNP)	Aldehydes and ketones
Fehling's solution	Aldehydes
Iodine in sodium hydroxide (Iodoform)	Acetaldehydes and ketones with the CH_3-CO- group. Alcohols with the $CH_3CH(OH)$- as a structural feature
Sulfuric acid	Alcohols, ethers, alkenes Soluble Lewis bases
Potassium permanganate (Bayer)	Alkenes

63. Cyclohexanol should fall into which of the following groups?
   A   I
   B   II
   C   III
   D   IV

64. A water soluble unknown is unreactive in the presence of sodium bicarbonate, gives a positive 2,4-DNP test and negative Fehling's and Iodoform tests. In which of the following classes should this compound be classified?
   A   Aldehyde
   B   Ketone
   C   Carboxylic acid
   D   Alcohol

65. When an ether solution of an aldehyde is added to an ether solution of lithium aluminum hydride (LiAlH₄), the carbonyl group of the aldehyde will be:
   A   reduced to the corresponding primary alcohol.
   B   hydrated to the corresponding diol.
   C   reduced to the corresponding secondary alcohol.
   D   deoxygenated to the corresponding alkane.

66. Acetone should give positive test results for which of the following chemical tests?
   A   Lucas and sodium bicarbonate
   B   2,4-DNP and Fehling's
   C   Iodoform and 2,4-DNP
   D   Iodoform and potassium permanganate

67. 3-Pentanone falls into group VI, but acetone falls into group V. This is most likely due to the fact that acetone is:
   A   a cyclic ketone.
   B   an aldehyde.
   C   aromatic.
   D   a methyl ketone.

68. Sodium bicarbonate is a weak base and as such reacts readily with acetic acid. The evolution of bubbles which accompanies this acid-base neutralization reaction is due to the formation of which of the following gases?
   A $CO(g)$
   B $CO_2(g)$
   C $H_2(g)$
   D $O_2(g)$

UNIT 17

Question 69

69. The following equation is used to relate force and fluid viscosity η:

$$F = -2\pi r l \frac{v}{R} \eta$$

where F is force, r is radius, l is length, v is speed, R is distance and η is the viscosity. What are the dimensions of viscosity in the fundamental quantities of mass (M), length (L) and time (T)?

A $M \cdot L^3 \cdot T^{-3}$
B $M \cdot L^{-1} \cdot T^{-1}$
C $M \cdot L^2 \cdot T^{-1}$
D $M \cdot L^{-2} \cdot T^{-2}$

UNIT 18

Questions 70–74

Viral hepatitis type B (serum hepatitis) is an infection of humans that primarily damages the liver. The causative agent is a virus called HBV, which is transmitted in much the same way as the HIV virus.

If HBV could be cultivated in the laboratory in unlimited amounts, it could be injected into humans as a vaccine to stimulate immunity against hepatitis type B. Unfortunately, it is not yet possible to grow HBV in laboratory culture. However, the blood of chronically infected people contains numerous particles of a harmless protein component of the virus. This protein, called HBsAg, can be extracted from the blood, purified, and treated chemically to destroy any live virus that might also be present. When HBsAg particles are injected into humans, they stimulate immunity against the complete infectious virus.

Of late, a new source of HBsAg particles have become available. Thanks to genetic engineering, a technique for cloning the gene for HBsAg into cells of the common bread yeast *Saccharomyces cerevisiae* has been developed. The yeast expresses the gene and makes HBsAg particles that can be extracted after the cells are broken. Since yeast cells are easy to propagate, it is now possible to obtain unlimited amounts of HBsAg particles.

70. Before being injected into humans, the HBV virus would first have to:
   A be cloned in yeast cells to ensure that enough of the virus had been injected to elicit an immune response.
   B have its protein coat removed.
   C be purified.
   D be inactivated.

71. Which of the following physiological processes would be LEAST affected in someone who had viral hepatitis type B?
   A The production of the fat soluble vitamins A, D, E, and K
   B The production of fibrinogen and albumin
   C The breakdown of hemoglobin to amino acids
   D The conversion of amino acids into carbohydrates

72. HBsAg is likely a component of:
    A   the capsid of the virus.
    B   the nucleic acid core of the virus.
    C   the tail of the virus.
    D   the slimy mucoid-like capsule on the outer surface of the virus.

73. The following graph shows the immune response for an initial injection of HBsAg and a subsequent injection of the HBV virus. Which of the following best explains the differences in the two responses?

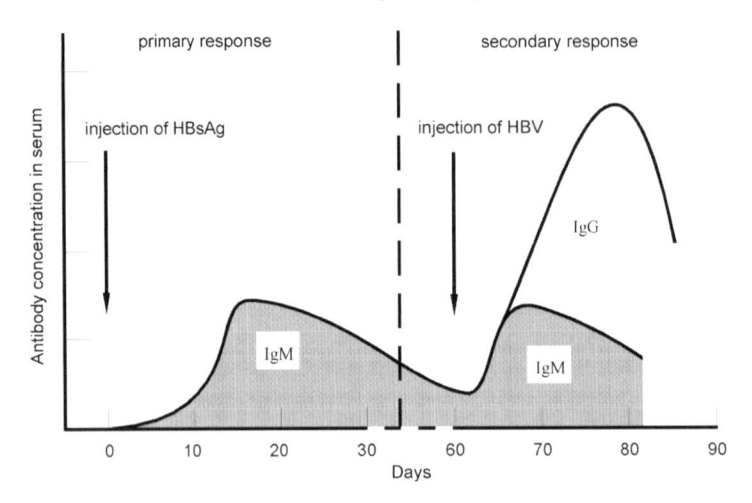

    A   During the initial response, the immune response was carried out primarily by macrophages and B-lymphocytes.
    B   During the secondary response, T-cells possessing membrane receptors, recognized and attacked the viral antigens.
    C   Memory cells produced by T- and B-cells during the first exposure made the second response faster and more intense.
    D   Memory cells produced by macrophages during the first infection recognized the viral antigens more quickly during the second infection, causing antibody production to be increased.

74. According to the preceding diagram, all of the following are correct EXCEPT:
    A   if the slope of the curve was taken at any time t, the units could be in mg/day.
    B   the time difference between the peak IgM and IgG secondary responses is less than the delay in the IgM primary response.
    C   the peak IgM primary response has a delay similar in duration to the peak IgG secondary response.
    D   the difference between peak IgG and peak IgM concentrations is greater than the peak IgM concentration.

UNIT 19

Question 75

75. A mass of 100 kg is placed on a uniform bar at a point 0.5 m to the left of a fulcrum. Where must a 75 kg mass be placed relative to the fulcrum in order to establish a state of equilibrium given that the bar was in equilibrium before any weights were applied?
    A   0.66 m to the right of the fulcrum
    B   0.66 m to the left of the fulcrum
    C   0.38 m to the right of the fulcrum
    D   0.38 m to the left of the fulcrum

UNIT 20

Questions 76–80

A 1200 kg car is travelling at 7.5 m s⁻¹ in a northerly direction on an icy road. It crashes into a 8000 kg truck moving in the same direction as the car with a velocity of 3.0 m s⁻¹ before the collision. The speed of the car after the collision is 3.0 m s⁻¹ in its original direction.

It may be helpful to keep in mind that momentum (p) is defined as the product of mass (m) times velocity (v):

$$p = mv.$$

The total momentum of an isolated system is constant. Frictional force (f) is given by the coefficient of friction (μ) times the force normal (N):

$$F = \mu N.$$

76. Which of the following is true regarding the relationship between energy and momentum in the passage?
 A The collision is not perfectly elastic, both momentum and energy are not conserved.
 B The collision is inelastic, kinetic energy is conserved but momentum is not.
 C The collision is not perfectly elastic, momentum is conserved but total energy is not.
 D The collision is not perfectly elastic, momentum is conserved but kinetic energy is not.

77. What is the velocity of the truck after the collision?
 A 7.5 m s⁻¹   B 3.7 m s⁻¹
 C 3.0 m s⁻¹   D 1.1 m s⁻¹

78. The car then proceeds to a garage. To get there, the driver turns off onto a smooth road with a coefficient of friction = 1/3. He then stops for a snack and then tries to drive off. What is the value of frictional force when the force the car exerts is 300 N?
 A 0 N   B 100 N
 C 300 N   D 4000 N

79. After leaving the garage, the driver of the car follows the same road and eventually has to go up a hill. How does the frictional force on the car now compare to the value when the car was driving on level ground?
 A No change
 B It increased.
 C It decreased.
 D The direction of change depends on the angle of elevation.

80. If the car is moving up the hill at 5 m s⁻¹ and the car is 40 m up the hill as shown in the diagram, how much potential energy does the car possess at that point?

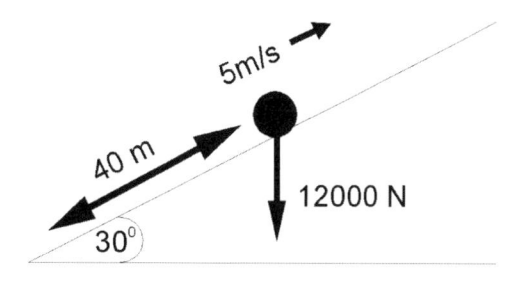

$g = 9.8$ m s⁻²

 A 2.40×10^5 J   B 2.40×10^4 J
 C 4.95×10^5 J   D 4.95×10^4 J

UNIT 21

Question 81

81. The free energy changes for the equilibria cis ⇌ trans of 1,2-, 1,3-, and 1,4- dimethylcyclohexane are shown below - though not necessarily for the following reaction directions:

I. 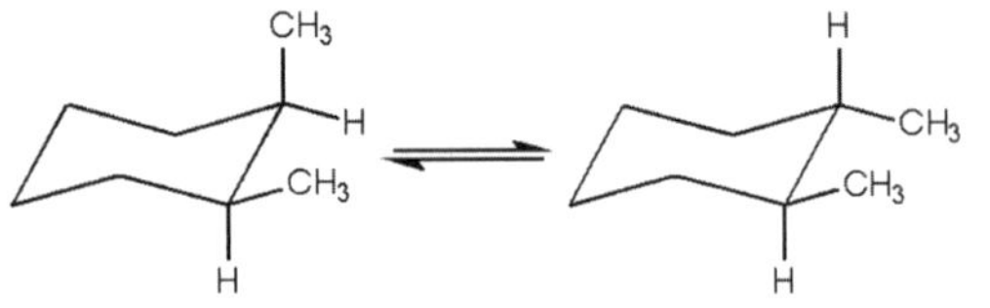 A ΔG = -1.87 Kcal/mol B

II. 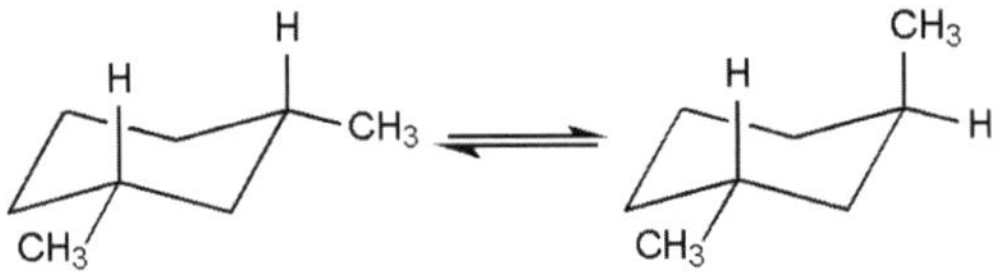 A ΔG = -1.96 Kcal/mol B

III. 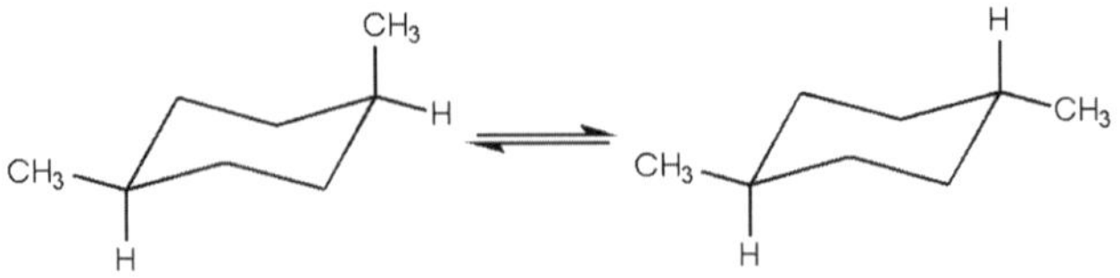 A ΔG = -1.90 Kcal/mol B

The most stable diastereomer in each case would be:
A   IA, IIB, IIIA
B   IB, IIA, IIIB
C   IA, IIA, IIIA
D   IA, IIB, IIIB

UNIT 22

Questions 82–87

Active transport is the energy-consuming transport of molecules against a concentration gradient. Energy is required because the substance must be moved in the opposite direction of its natural tendency to diffuse. Movement is usually unidirectional, unlike diffusion which is reversible.

When movement of ions is considered, two factors will influence the direction in which they diffuse: one is concentration, the other is electrical charge. An ion will usually diffuse from a region of its high concentration to a region of its low concentration. It will also generally be attracted towards a region of opposite charge, and move away from a region of similar charge. Thus ions are said to move down *electrochemical gradients*, which are the combined effects of both electrical and concentration gradients. Strictly speaking, active transport of ions is their movement against an electrochemical gradient powered by an energy source.

Research has shown that the cell surface membranes of most cells possess sodium pumps. Usually, though not always, the sodium pump is coupled with a potassium pump. The combined pump is called the sodium-potassium pump. This pump is an excellent example of active transport.

Table 1: Concentration of Na^+, K^+, and Cl^- inside and outside mammalian motor neurons. The sign of the potential (mV) is inside relative to the outside of the cell.

Ion	Concentration (mmol/L H₂O) Inside cell	Concentration (mmol/L H₂O) Outside cell	Equilibrium potential (mV)
Na^+	15.0	150.0	+60
K^+	150.0	5.5	–90
Cl^-	9.0	125.0	–75

Resting membrane potential (Vm) = –70 mV

The value of the equilibrium potential for any ion depends upon the concentration gradient for that ion across the membrane. The equilibrium potential for any ion can be calculated using the Nernst equation. The following is an approximation of the equation for the equilibrium potential for potassium (E_k in mV) at room temperature:

$$E_k = 60 \log_{10} \frac{[K^+]_o}{[K^+]_i}$$

$[K^+]_o$ = extracellular K^+ concentration in mM
$[K^+]_i$ = intracellular K^+ concentration in mM

82. All of the following explain the ionic concentrations in Table 1 EXCEPT:
 - **A** Na^+ and Cl^- ions passively diffuse more quickly into the extracellular fluid than K^+ ions.
 - **B** Na^+ ions are actively pumped out of the intracellular fluid.
 - **C** the negative charge of the cell contents repels Cl^- ions from the cell.
 - **D** the cell membrane is more freely permeable to K^+ ions than to Na^+ and Cl^- ions.

83. If the concentration of potassium outside a mammalian motor neuron were changed to 0.55 mol/L, what would be the predicted change in the equilibrium potential?
    A   12 mV
    B   120 mV
    C   60 mV
    D   600 mV

84. A graph of E_k vs $\log_{10}[K^+]_o$ would be:
    A   a straight line.
    B   a logarithmic curve.
    C   an exponential curve.
    D   a sigmoidal curve.

85. In the process of osmosis, the net flow of water molecules into or out of the cell depends primarily on the differences in the:
    A   concentration of protein on either side of the cell membrane.
    B   concentration of water molecules inside and outside the cell.
    C   rate of molecular transport on either side of the cell membrane.
    D   rate of movement of ions inside the cell.

86. Active transport assumes particular importance in all but which of the following structures?
    A   Cells of the large intestine
    B   Alveoli
    C   Nerve and muscle cells
    D   Loop of Henle

87. At inhibitory synapses, a hyperpolarization of the membrane known as an inhibitory postsynaptic potential is produced rendering V_m more negative. This occurs as a result of:
    A   an increase in the postsynaptic membrane's permeability to Na^+ and K^+ ions.
    B   an increase in the permeability of the presynaptic membrane to Ca^{2+} ions.
    C   the entry of Cl^- ions into the synaptic knob.
    D   an increase in the permeability of the postsynaptic membrane to Cl^- ions.

UNIT 23

Questions 88

Infrared (IR) spectroscopy is an instrumental technique used to identify substances by keying in on functional groups. By measuring the absorption of infrared radiation over a range of frequencies and then comparing such data to tables for known substances, it is possible to reveal the underlying identity of the chemical.

Table 1: IR Absorptions

Functional Group	Characteristic Absorption(s) (cm^{-1})	Notes
Alkyl C-H Stretch	2950–2850	Alkane C-H bonds are fairly ubiquitous and therefore usually less useful in determining structure.
Alkenyl C-H Stretch Alkenyl C=C Stretch	3100–3010 1680–1620	Absorption peaks above 3000 cm^{-1} are frequently diagnostic of unsaturation
Alcohol/Phenol O-H Stretch	3550–3200	Specifity of the absorption is in part dependent on surrounding functional groups.
Carboxylic Acid O-H Stretch	3000–2500	
Amine N-H Stretch	3500–3300	Primary amines produce two N-H stretch absorptions, secondary amides only one, and tetriary none.
Aldehyde C=O Stretch Ketone C=O Stretch Ester C=O Stretch Carboxylic Acid C=O Stretch Amide C=O Stretch	1740–1690 1750–1680 1750–1735 1780–1710 1690–1630	The carbonyl stretching absorption is one of the strongest IR absorptions, and is very useful in structure determination as one can determine both the number of carbonyl groups (assuming peaks do not overlap) but also an estimation of which types.
Amide N-H Stretch	3700–3500	As with amines, an amide produces zero to two N-H absorptions depending on its type.

All figures are for the typical case only – signal positions and intensities may vary depending on the particular bond environment.

88. Consider the following reaction.

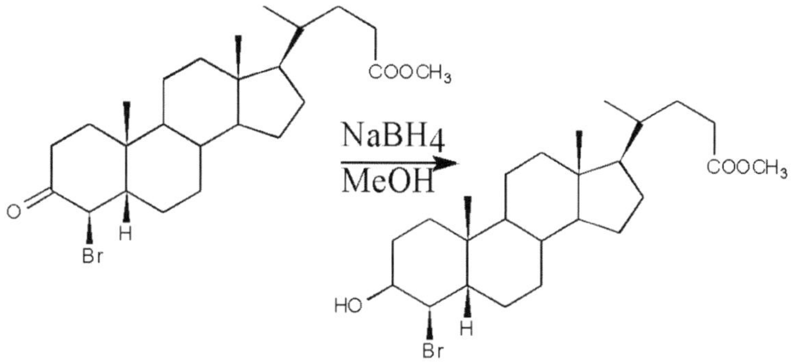

The infrared spectrum of the product can be distinguished from that of the starting material by the:
A   disappearance of IR absorption at 3360 cm^{-1}.
B   disappearance of IR absorption at 2820 cm^{-1}.
C   appearance of IR absorption at 3360 cm^{-1}.
D   appearance of IR absorption at 1740 cm^{-1}.

UNIT 24

Questions 89–94

It is well known that there are two major forms of carbon, that is, carbon has two main allotropes: graphite and diamond. These differ greatly from each other with respect to their physical properties as shown in Table 1. The physical properties of silicon are also shown in Table 1 for comparison as carbon and silicon belong to the same group in the periodic table.

Table 1

Physical properties	Graphite	Diamond	Silicon
Density (g cm^{-3})	2.26	3.51	2.33
Enthalpy of combustion to yield oxide (ΔHc) kJ mol^{-1}	−393.3	−395.1	−910
Melting point (°C)	2820	3730	1410
Boiling point (°C)		4830	2680
Conductivity (electrical)	Fairly good	Non-conductor	Good
Conductivity (thermal)	Fairly good	Non-conductivity	Good

Graphite possesses what is commonly known as a layer structure: carbon atoms form three covalent bonds with each other to yield layers of carbon assemblies parallel with each other. These layers are held together via weak Van der Waals' forces which permit some movement of the layers relative to one another.

A phase diagram is a graph that shows the relation between the solid, liquid and gaseous states. Any point in the graph is where 2 phases exist at equilibrium except the triple point where all 3 exist at equilibrium. Solid CO_2 is called "dry ice" because it can go directly from solid to vapour (sublimation) at room pressure (i.e. 101.3 kPa). The triple point of CO_2 occurs at 217 K and 515 kPa. A reduction in CO_2 pressure directly correlates with changes in its sublimation, melting and boiling points.

89. Which of the following is a correct representation of the phase diagram for carbon dioxide?

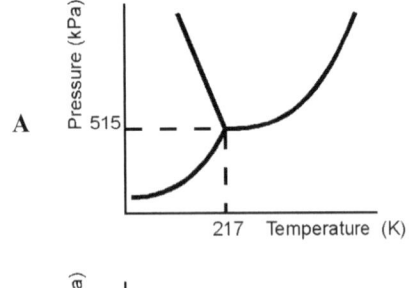

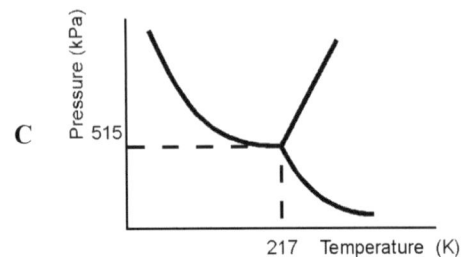

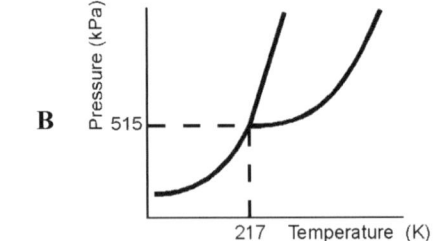

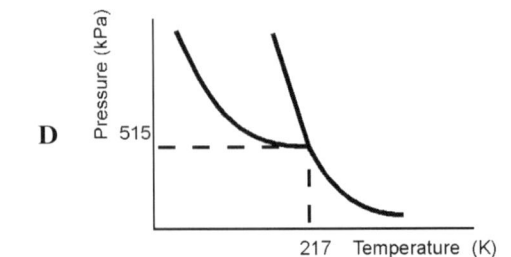

90. The properties of the layer-like structure of solid graphite stated in the passage would lend it to which of the following industrial uses?
    A   Insulator
    B   Structural
    C   Corrosive
    D   Lubricant

91. Using the information in the table, calculate the enthalpy change for the following process:

    $$C_{graphite} \rightarrow C_{diamond}$$

    A   +1.8 kJ mol^{-1}
    B   −1.8 kJ mol^{-1}
    C   +1.0 kJ mol^{-1}
    D   −1.0 kJ mol^{-1}

92. It is possible to convert graphite into diamond via various chemical processes. Based on the information in the passage, which of the following would facilitate increased amounts of diamond assuming that the system is in equilibrium?
    A   Higher pressures
    B   Lower temperatures
    C   A catalyst
    D   None of the above

Questions 93 and 94 refer to the following additional information:

At a given temperature T in kelvin, the relationship between the three thermodynamic quantities including the change in Gibbs free energy (ΔG), the change in enthalpy (ΔH) and the change in entropy (ΔS), can be expressed as follows:

$$\Delta G = \Delta H - T\Delta S$$

93. The sublimation of carbon dioxide occurs quickly at room temperature. What might be predicted for the three thermodynamic quantities for the reverse reaction?
    A   Only ΔS would be positive.
    B   Only ΔS would be negative.
    C   Only ΔH would be negative.
    D   Only ΔG would be positive.

94. Which of the following statements is consistent with the triple point of carbon dioxide?
    A   The absolute temperature dominates the effect on Gibbs free energy.
    B   The reaction is spontaneous, Gibbs free energy is negative.
    C   The enthalpy change is equal to the effect of the entropy change.
    D   The entropy change is negative because there is more disorder overall.

UNIT 25

Questions 95–97

A chemist studied the mechanisms of the reactions of isopropyl bromide with sodium t-butoxide and with sodium ethoxide.

In Reaction I, the treatment of isopropyl bromide with sodium t-butoxide at 40 °C gave almost exclusively one product. The reaction yielded Compound A which had a molecular formula of C_3H_6. The ^{1}HNMR spectrum of compound A revealed the presence of vinylic protons. The kinetic rate expression indicated second order kinetics for the reaction.

In Reaction II, the treatment of isopropyl bromide with sodium ethoxide (Na^+EtO^-) at 30 °C yielded an ether (Compound B) that had a molecular formula of $C_5H_{12}O$, and Compound A that had a molecular mass of 42 grams. Compound B accounted for only 20% of the total product. The remainder consisted of Compound A.

Compound B was found to be stable to base, dilute acid and most reducing agents. The infrared spectrum of Compound B revealed a strong band at 1100 cm^{-1} and the absence of stretching absorptions at 1730 cm^{-1} was noted.

Compound A was readily oxidized by a neutral solution of cold dilute potassium permanganate. During the oxidation process, the characteristic purple color of the permanganate ion (MnO_4^-) disappeared and was replaced by a brown precipitate indicating the formation of manganese dioxide (MnO_2).

95. Compound A belongs to which of the following classes of organic compounds?
   A   Alcohol
   B   Ketone
   C   Alkene
   D   Ester

96. Which of the following most accurately represents the activated complex formed in Reaction II and that subsequently led to Compound A?

   A   H—C(CH₃)(CH₃)···Br

   B   H—C⁺(CH₃)(CH₃)

   C   Et—O⁻ δ⁻ ···H···C(H)(H)···C(CH₃)(H)···Br δ⁻

   D   Et—O⁻ δ⁻ ···C(CH₃)(CH₃)···Br δ⁻ with H

97. Which of the following compounds is an accurate representation of Compound B?
   A CH_3OCH_3
   B $C_2H_5OC_2H_5$
   C $(CH_3)_2CHOCH_2CH_3$
   D $CH_3CH_2CH_2OCH_2CH_3$

UNIT 26

Question 98

98. 20 mL of 0.05 M Mg^{2+} in solution is desired. It is attempted to achieve this by adding 5 mL of 0.005 M $MgCl_2$ and 15 mL of $Mg_3(PO_4)_2$. What is the concentration of $Mg_3(PO_4)_2$?

- A   0.065 M
- B   0.022 M
- C   0.150 M
- D   0.100 M

UNIT 27

Question 99

99. The data in Table 1 were collected for Reaction I:

$$2X + Y \rightarrow Z \qquad \text{Reaction I}$$

Table 1

Exp.	[X] in M	[Y] in M	Initial rate of reaction
1	0.050	0.100	8.5×10^{-6}
2	0.050	0.200	3.4×10^{-5}
3	0.200	0.100	3.4×10^{-5}

What is the rate law for the reaction?

- A   Rate = $k[X]^2[Y]$
- B   Rate = $k[X]^2[Y]^2$
- C   Rate = $k[X][Y]^2$
- D   Rate = $k[X][Y]$

UNIT 28

Questions 100–102

The following represents a summary of nucleophilic acyl substitution followed by nucleophilic addition:

- Carboxylic esters, R'CO$_2$R", react with 2 equivalents of organolithium or Grignard reagents to give tertiary alcohols.
- The tertiary alcohol that results contains 2 identical alkyl groups (R in the mechanism shown).
- The reaction proceeds via a ketone intermediate [Step (1)] which then reacts with the second equivalent of the organometallic reagent or Grignard reagent [Step (2)].
- Et = ethyl

100. Which of the following represents the product of the reaction between propyl ethanoate and 1 equivalent of 2-butyl lithium (*sec*-butyllithium)?
    A. 2-hexanone
    B. 3-methyl-2-pentanone
    C. 4-methyl-3-hexanone
    D. 3-heptanone

101. Given the mechanism provided, in order to produce a secondary alcohol, which of the following must be true?
    A. R' must be a hydrogen
    B. One R must be a hydrogen
    C. R' and R" must be hydrogens
    D. Either one R or R' must be hydrogen

102. Using 2 equivalents of the first and 1 equivalent of the second, respectively, which of the following pairs of compounds can be used to form the following tertiary alcohol?

- A Propyl lithium and methyl butanoate
- B Butyl magnesium bromide and propyl butanoate
- C Butyl lithium and pentyl pentanoate
- D Propyl magnesium bromide and hexyl pentanoate

UNIT 29

Questions 103-106

The viscosity of a fluid, that is, a gas, a pure liquid or a solution is an index of its resistance to flow. The viscosity of a fluid in a cylindrical tube of radius R and length L is given by:

$$n = \pi \Delta P R^4 t / (8VL)$$ Equation I

where n = viscosity of fluid, ΔP = change in pressure, t = time, V = volume of fluid and V/t = rate of flow of fluid. This equation can be applied to the study of blood flow in our bodies. The heart pumps blood through the various vessels in our bodies to supply all of its tissues. At rest, the rate of blood flow is about 80 cm^3 s^{-1} and this is maintained in all blood vessels. However, the radii of the blood vessels decreases the further away blood moves from the heart. Therefore, in order to maintain the rate of blood flow, a pressure drop occurs as one moves from one blood vessel to another of smaller radius.

A great number of physiological conditions can be explained using Equation I, for example, hypertension.

103. What would be the pressure drop per cm of the blood in the first blood vessel leaving the heart if the blood vessel is of unit radius and the body is at rest?

$$n_{blood} = 0.04 \text{ dyn s cm}^{-3}$$

- A 25.6/π dyn cm^{-3}
- B 16000/π dyn cm^{-3}
- C π/25.6 dyn cm^{-3}
- D π/16000 dyn cm^{-3}

104. Which of the following has the greatest effect on the viscosity of a fluid per unit change in its value?
- A Volume of the fluid
- B Length of the tube
- C Pressure of the fluid
- D Radius of the tube

105. The equation for the rate of flow of a fluid (from Equation I) has often been compared to Ohm's law. Given that P can be likened to the voltage and flow rate can be likened to the current, which of the following can be likened to resistance?
   A πR⁴
   B πR⁴/(8Ln)
   C 8Ln/(πR⁴)
   D 8Ln

106. Hypertension involves the decrease in the radius of certain blood vessels. If the radius of a blood vessel is halved, by what factor must the pressure increase to maintain the normal rate of blood flow, all other factors being constant?
   A 2
   B 4
   C 8
   D 16

UNIT 30

Question 107

107. When a dilute solution of formaldehyde is dissolved in ¹⁸O-labeled water and allowed to equilibrate, ¹⁸O incorporation occurs thus indicating the existence of an intermediate product. Which of the following compounds best represents the intermediate product of this ¹⁸O exchange?

A [structure: CH₂=CH with O⁻]

B [structure: ketone with two methyl branches]

C [structure: CH₂(OH)₂ — methanediol]

D [structure: formaldehyde with OH⁺]

UNIT 31

Questions 108–109

Following blastula formation the developing embryo undergoes gastrulation, a tremendous reshaping with little or no additional cell growth. Since the blastulas vary in shape between different animals, the geometry of the reshaping also varies. Regardless of the type of animal, gastrulation results in the same fundamental cell layers: the ectoderm, the endoderm and the mesoderm. These three tissue types or *primordial layers* will form every organ in the developing embryo.

Research has recently shed light on the cells responsible for the continuation of the life cycle - the gametes. Early in the development of all animals, certain cells undergo determination producing primordial germ cells. Experiments have demonstrated an area in the egg cytoplasm of some animals which appears to be responsible for the determination of the primordial germ cell. This special region is the *germ plasm*.

To clarify the importance of the germ plasm, experiments have been carried out using microinjection of the developing fruit fly *Drosophila melanogaster*. Under normal conditions, pregametic cells arise from the posterior end of the syncytial blastoderm. Irradiation of this end of the egg produces a sterile fly. If cytoplasmic material from the posterior part of the developing egg is suctioned with a micropipette and injected into the anterior part of another developing egg, germ cells are formed at this abnormal site as well as the normal position. No nuclei are transferred in this experiment thus the evidence points to non-genetic material in the germ plasm of the egg being responsible for germ cell formation.

108. In the experiment described in the passage, which of the following materials in the germ plasm would likely be most functional in inducing germ cell function?
A   Nuclear DNA
B   Mitochondria
C   RNA and protein molecules
D   Microtubules

109. Which of the following experimental results would contradict the conclusion made from the experiment in the passage?
A   The only subunits detected after digesting the germ plasm were non-uracil containing nucleotides.
B   Microinjection of the midportion of a developing egg with germ plasm resulted in germ cell production at an abnormal site.
C   Microinjection of proteases into the posterior end of the syncytial blastoderm inhibited the production of germ cells.
D   The irradiated egg which produced a sterile fly demonstrated no post-radiation genetic abnormalities.

UNIT 32

Question 110

110. Consider the following conformations of tartaric acid.

A chiral carbon is one that is attached to 4 different atoms or groups. A diastereomer which has no enantiomer, thus is an achiral molecule, is called a *meso* compound. Thus meso compounds are superimposable on their mirror images. Given this information, which of the following statements is true regarding the 3 structures representing tartaric acid?
A   1 molecule is achiral and has no chiral carbons.
B   1 molecule is achiral but has more than 1 chiral carbon.
C   More than 1 molecule is achiral and each has more than 1 chiral carbon.
D   More than 1 molecule is achiral and they do not possess chiral carbons.

END OF REASONING IN BIOLOGICAL AND PHYSICAL SCIENCES. IF TIME REMAINS, YOU MAY GO BACK AND CHECK YOUR WORK IN THIS TEST BOOKLET.

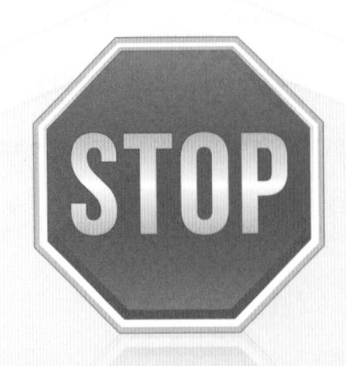

GAMSAT SCORE!

After you have completed test GS-1, you should spend the equivalent of a full day reviewing errors and guesses. Time must be taken to create "Gold Notes" which are high-density notes from your exam experience (preferably a maximum of 2 pages per exam section). By having a manageable number of pages, you can review all your exam experiences (ACER and GS tests) several times every week leading up to the real GAMSAT. This way you can always build on the progress you are making.

Worked solutions are available online for the original owner of this textbook by going to gamsat-prep.com, registering as an owner, clicking on Tests in the top Menu and scrolling down. Every question in the GS-1 exam also has a forum thread at gamsat-prep.com/forum so that if you do not understand the worked solution, we are happy to clarify any teaching points with you. There is no charge for this service.

The Gold Standard GAMSAT has put together a suite of home study materials, online courses, essay correction services and classroom lectures across Australia, Ireland and the UK. We recognize that everyone learns differently. Thus we created a multimedia integrated approach so you can choose the tools that help you study best. Good luck!

Answer Keys & Answer Documents

Answer Document

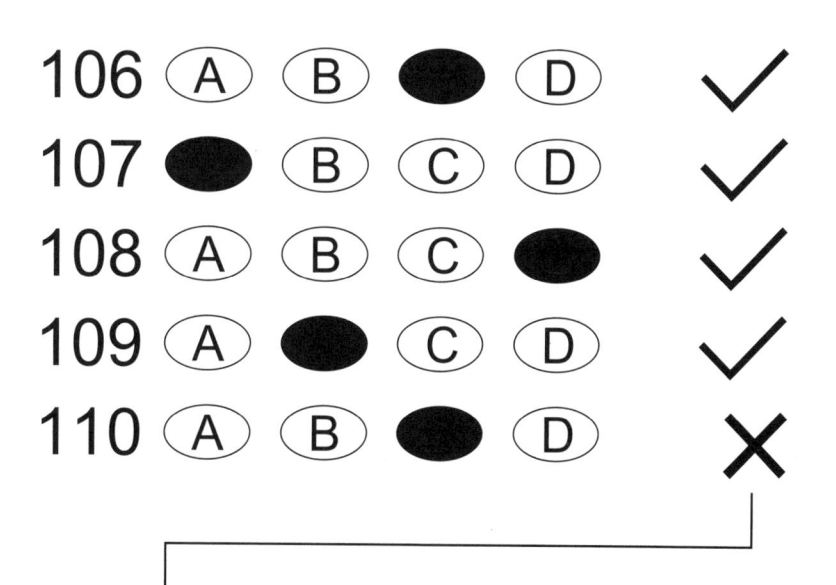

106 Ⓐ Ⓑ ● Ⓓ ✓
107 ● Ⓑ Ⓒ Ⓓ ✓
108 Ⓐ Ⓑ Ⓒ ● ✓
109 Ⓐ ● Ⓒ Ⓓ ✓
110 Ⓐ Ⓑ ● Ⓓ ✗

Answer Key

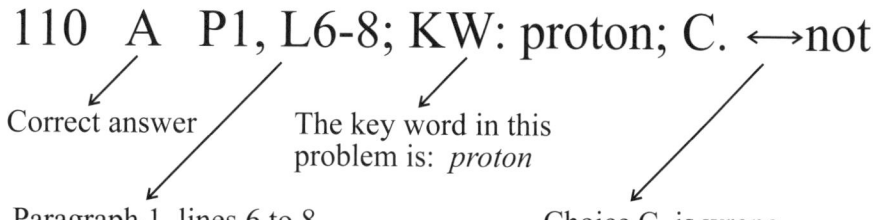

110   A   P1, L6-8; KW: proton; C. ⟷ not

- **A** — Correct answer
- **P1, L6-8** — Paragraph 1, lines 6 to 8, is where the answer can be found
- **KW: proton** — The key word in this problem is: *proton*
- **C. ⟷ not** — Choice C. is wrong because of the word "*not*"

The Gold Standard GAMSAT

GAMSAT is administered by ACER which is not associated with this product.

The Gold Standard GAMSAT

Answer Document 1

Test GS-1

CANDIDATE'S NAME ______________________ STUDENT ID ____________________

Mark one and only one answer to each question. Be sure to use a soft lead pencil and completely fill in the space for your intended answer. If you erase, do so completely. Make no stray marks.

Section I

1 (A) (B) (C) (D)
2 (A) (B) (C) (D)
3 (A) (B) (C) (D)
4 (A) (B) (C) (D)
5 (A) (B) (C) (D)
6 (A) (B) (C) (D)
7 (A) (B) (C) (D)
8 (A) (B) (C) (D)
9 (A) (B) (C) (D)
10 (A) (B) (C) (D)
11 (A) (B) (C) (D)
12 (A) (B) (C) (D)
13 (A) (B) (C) (D)
14 (A) (B) (C) (D)
15 (A) (B) (C) (D)
16 (A) (B) (C) (D)
17 (A) (B) (C) (D)
18 (A) (B) (C) (D)
19 (A) (B) (C) (D)
20 (A) (B) (C) (D)
21 (A) (B) (C) (D)
22 (A) (B) (C) (D)
23 (A) (B) (C) (D)
24 (A) (B) (C) (D)
25 (A) (B) (C) (D)
26 (A) (B) (C) (D)
27 (A) (B) (C) (D)
28 (A) (B) (C) (D)
29 (A) (B) (C) (D)
30 (A) (B) (C) (D)
31 (A) (B) (C) (D)
32 (A) (B) (C) (D)
33 (A) (B) (C) (D)
34 (A) (B) (C) (D)
35 (A) (B) (C) (D)
36 (A) (B) (C) (D)
37 (A) (B) (C) (D)
38 (A) (B) (C) (D)
39 (A) (B) (C) (D)
40 (A) (B) (C) (D)
41 (A) (B) (C) (D)
42 (A) (B) (C) (D)
43 (A) (B) (C) (D)
44 (A) (B) (C) (D)
45 (A) (B) (C) (D)
46 (A) (B) (C) (D)
47 (A) (B) (C) (D)
48 (A) (B) (C) (D)
49 (A) (B) (C) (D)
50 (A) (B) (C) (D)
51 (A) (B) (C) (D)
52 (A) (B) (C) (D)
53 (A) (B) (C) (D)
54 (A) (B) (C) (D)
55 (A) (B) (C) (D)
56 (A) (B) (C) (D)
57 (A) (B) (C) (D)
58 (A) (B) (C) (D)
59 (A) (B) (C) (D)
60 (A) (B) (C) (D)
61 (A) (B) (C) (D)
62 (A) (B) (C) (D)
63 (A) (B) (C) (D)
64 (A) (B) (C) (D)
65 (A) (B) (C) (D)
66 (A) (B) (C) (D)
67 (A) (B) (C) (D)
68 (A) (B) (C) (D)
69 (A) (B) (C) (D)
70 (A) (B) (C) (D)
71 (A) (B) (C) (D)
72 (A) (B) (C) (D)
73 (A) (B) (C) (D)
74 (A) (B) (C) (D)
75 (A) (B) (C) (D)

Section III

1 (A) (B) (C) (D)
2 (A) (B) (C) (D)
3 (A) (B) (C) (D)
4 (A) (B) (C) (D)
5 (A) (B) (C) (D)
6 (A) (B) (C) (D)
7 (A) (B) (C) (D)
8 (A) (B) (C) (D)
9 (A) (B) (C) (D)
10 (A) (B) (C) (D)
11 (A) (B) (C) (D)
12 (A) (B) (C) (D)
13 (A) (B) (C) (D)
14 (A) (B) (C) (D)
15 (A) (B) (C) (D)
16 (A) (B) (C) (D)
17 (A) (B) (C) (D)
18 (A) (B) (C) (D)
19 (A) (B) (C) (D)
20 (A) (B) (C) (D)
21 (A) (B) (C) (D)
22 (A) (B) (C) (D)
23 (A) (B) (C) (D)
24 (A) (B) (C) (D)
25 (A) (B) (C) (D)
26 (A) (B) (C) (D)
27 (A) (B) (C) (D)
28 (A) (B) (C) (D)
29 (A) (B) (C) (D)
30 (A) (B) (C) (D)
31 (A) (B) (C) (D)
32 (A) (B) (C) (D)
33 (A) (B) (C) (D)
34 (A) (B) (C) (D)
35 (A) (B) (C) (D)
36 (A) (B) (C) (D)
37 (A) (B) (C) (D)
38 (A) (B) (C) (D)
39 (A) (B) (C) (D)
40 (A) (B) (C) (D)
41 (A) (B) (C) (D)
42 (A) (B) (C) (D)
43 (A) (B) (C) (D)
44 (A) (B) (C) (D)
45 (A) (B) (C) (D)
46 (A) (B) (C) (D)
47 (A) (B) (C) (D)
48 (A) (B) (C) (D)
49 (A) (B) (C) (D)
50 (A) (B) (C) (D)
51 (A) (B) (C) (D)
52 (A) (B) (C) (D)
53 (A) (B) (C) (D)
54 (A) (B) (C) (D)
55 (A) (B) (C) (D)
56 (A) (B) (C) (D)
57 (A) (B) (C) (D)
58 (A) (B) (C) (D)
59 (A) (B) (C) (D)
60 (A) (B) (C) (D)
61 (A) (B) (C) (D)
62 (A) (B) (C) (D)
63 (A) (B) (C) (D)
64 (A) (B) (C) (D)
65 (A) (B) (C) (D)
66 (A) (B) (C) (D)
67 (A) (B) (C) (D)
68 (A) (B) (C) (D)
69 (A) (B) (C) (D)
70 (A) (B) (C) (D)
71 (A) (B) (C) (D)
72 (A) (B) (C) (D)
73 (A) (B) (C) (D)
74 (A) (B) (C) (D)
75 (A) (B) (C) (D)
76 (A) (B) (C) (D)
77 (A) (B) (C) (D)
78 (A) (B) (C) (D)
79 (A) (B) (C) (D)
80 (A) (B) (C) (D)
81 (A) (B) (C) (D)
82 (A) (B) (C) (D)
83 (A) (B) (C) (D)
84 (A) (B) (C) (D)
85 (A) (B) (C) (D)
86 (A) (B) (C) (D)
87 (A) (B) (C) (D)
88 (A) (B) (C) (D)
89 (A) (B) (C) (D)
90 (A) (B) (C) (D)
91 (A) (B) (C) (D)
92 (A) (B) (C) (D)
93 (A) (B) (C) (D)
94 (A) (B) (C) (D)
95 (A) (B) (C) (D)
96 (A) (B) (C) (D)
97 (A) (B) (C) (D)
98 (A) (B) (C) (D)
99 (A) (B) (C) (D)
100 (A) (B) (C) (D)
101 (A) (B) (C) (D)
102 (A) (B) (C) (D)
103 (A) (B) (C) (D)
104 (A) (B) (C) (D)
105 (A) (B) (C) (D)
106 (A) (B) (C) (D)
107 (A) (B) (C) (D)
108 (A) (B) (C) (D)
109 (A) (B) (C) (D)
110 (A) (B) (C) (D)

The Gold Standard GAMSAT

Answer Document 2

Test GS-1   Section II

CANDIDATE'S NAME _____   STUDENT ID _____

> When your timer is ready, you may turn the page and begin.

A A A A A

IF YOU NEED MORE SPACE, CONTINUE ON THE NEXT PAGE.

A A A A A

STOP HERE FOR WRITING TASK A.

B B B B B B

IF YOU NEED MORE SPACE, CONTINUE ON THE BACK OF THIS PAGE.

B   B   B   B   B

IF YOU NEED MORE SPACE, CONTINUE ON THE NEXT PAGE.

B   **B**   **B**   **B**   **B**

STOP HERE FOR WRITING TASK B.

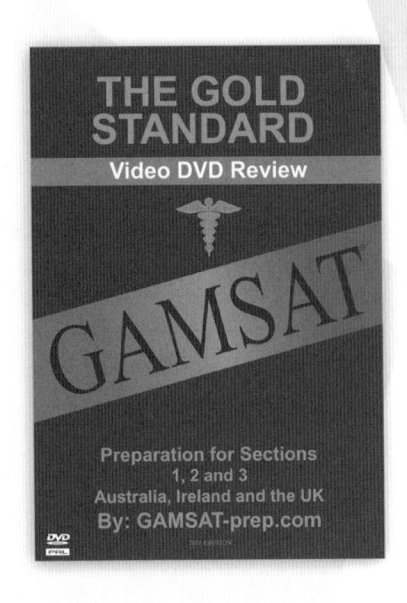

**Gold Standard
GAMSAT Preparation DVD
for Section 1, 2, 3
(Australia, Ireland, UK)
ISBN: 978-0986691546**

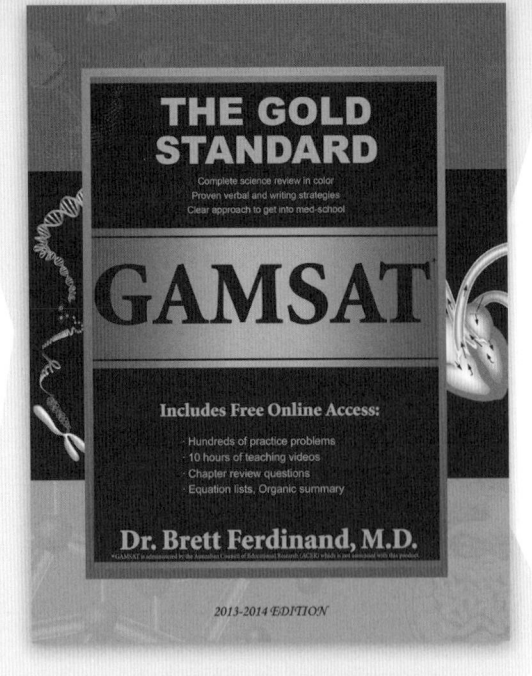

**Gold Standard
GAMSAT Textbook
(Australia, Ireland, UK)
ISBN: 978-1-927338-05-6**

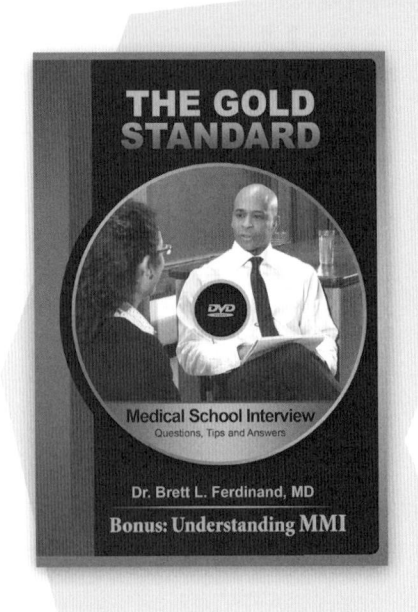

**The Medical School
Interview DVD:
Questions, Tips and Answers
(The Gold Standard)
ISBN: 978-0986691539**

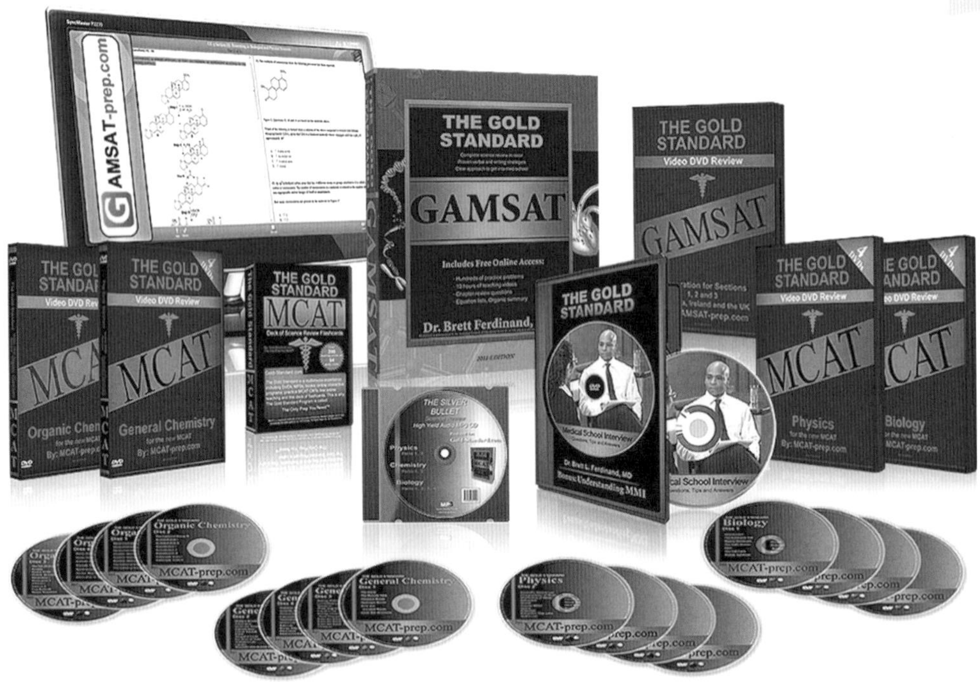

Complete GAMSAT Book Package for Home Study, 2013-2014 Edition
ASIN: B003PCQPA4

Also available at Amazon.co.uk, DrPrep.net, GAMSATtestpreparation.com and and participating bookstores.

Gold-Standard.com